THE WILLS EYE MANUAL

Office and Emergency Room
Diagnosis and Treatment of Eye Disease

SIXTH EDITION

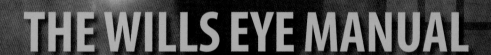

THE WILLS EYE MANUAL

Office and Emergency Room
Diagnosis and Treatment of Eye Disease

SIXTH EDITION

EDITORS

Adam T. Gerstenblith
Michael P. Rabinowitz

ASSOCIATE EDITORS

Behin I. Barahimi
Christopher M. Fecarotta

FOUNDING EDITORS

Mark A. Friedberg
Christopher J. Rapuano

Wolters Kluwer | Lippincott Williams & Wilkins
Health

Philadelphia · Baltimore · New York · London
Buenos Aires · Hong Kong · Sydney · Tokyo

Senior Executive Editor: Jonathan W. Pine, Jr.
Senior Product Manager: Emilie Moyer
Vendor Manager: Alicia Jackson
Senior Manufacturing Manager: Benjamin Rivera
Marketing Manager: Lisa Lawrence
Art Director: Doug Smock
Production Services: Aptara, Inc.

Fifth edition, © Lippincott Williams & Wilkins, 2008
Fourth edition, © Lippincott Williams & Wilkins, 2004
Third edition, © Lippincott Williams & Wilkins, 1999
Second edition, © Lippincott Williams & Wilkins, 1994
First edition, © Lippincott-Raven, 1990

Printed in China

Library of Congress Cataloging-in-Publication Data
available upon request

ISBN 13: 978-1-4511-0938-2
ISBN 10: 1-4511-0938-5

Care has been taken to confirm the accuracy of the information presented and to describe generally accepted practices. However, the authors, editors, and publisher are not responsible for errors or omissions or for any consequences from application of the information in this book and make no warranty, expressed or implied, with respect to the currency, completeness, or accuracy of the contents of the publication. Application of the information in a particular situation remains the professional responsibility of the practitioner.

The authors, editors, and publisher have exerted every effort to ensure that drug selection and dosage set forth in this text are in accordance with current recommendations and practice at the time of publication. However, in view of ongoing research, changes in government regulations, and the constant flow of information relating to drug therapy and drug reactions, the reader is urged to check the package insert for each drug for any change in indications and dosage and for added warnings and precautions. This is particularly important when the recommended agent is a new or infrequently employed drug.

Some drugs and medical devices presented in the publication have Food and Drug Administration (FDA) clearance for limited use in restricted research settings. It is the responsibility of the health care provider to ascertain the FDA status of each drug or device planned for use in their clinical practice.

To purchase additional copies of this book, call our customer service department at (800) 638-3030 or fax orders to (301) 223-2320. International customers should call (301) 223-2300.

Visit Lippincott Williams & Wilkins on the Internet at LWW.com. Lippincott Williams & Wilkins customer service representatives are available from 8:30 am to 6 pm, EST.

RRS1112

Contributors

CONTRIBUTORS TO THE SIXTH EDITION

Fatima K. Ahmad, M.D.
Christopher J. Brady, M.D.
Meg R. Gerstenblith, M.D.
Katherine G. Gold, M.D.
Sebastian B. Heersink, M.D.
Suzanne K. Jadico, M.D.
Brandon B. Johnson, M.D.
Jennifer H. Kim, M.D.
Amanda E. Matthews, M.D.
Melissa D. Neuwelt, M.D.
Anne M. Nguyen, M.D.
Linda H. Ohsie, M.D.
Kristina Yi-Hwa Pao, M.D.
Mindy R. Rabinowitz, M.D.
Vikram J. Setlur, M.D.
Gary Shienbaum, M.D.
Eileen Wang, M.D.
Douglas M. Wisner, M.D.

CONTRIBUTORS TO THE FIFTH EDITION

TEXT CONTRIBUTORS

Paul S. Baker, M.D.
Shaleen L. Belani, M.D.
Shawn Chhabra, M.D.
John M. Cropsey, M.D.
Emily A. DeCarlo, M.D.
Justis P. Ehlers, M.D.
Gregory L. Fenton, M.D.
David Fintak, M.D.
Robert E. Fintelmann, M.D.
Nicole R. Fram, M.D.
Susan M. Gordon, M.D.
Omesh P. Gupta, M.D., M.B.A.
Eliza N. Hoskins, M.D.
Dara Khalatbari, M.D.
Bhairavi V. Kharod, M.D.
Matthew R. Kirk, M.D.

Andrew Lam, M.D.
Katherine A. Lane, M.D.
Michael A. Malstrom, M.D.
Chrishonda C. McCoy, M.D.
Jesse B. McKey, M.D.
Maria P. McNeill, M.D.
Joselitio S. Navaleza, M.D.
Avni H. Patel, M.D.
Chirag P. Shah, M.D., M.P.H.
Heather N. Shelsta, M.D.
Bradley T. Smith, M.D.
Vikas Tewari, M.D.
Garth J. Willis, M.D.
Allison P. Young, M.D.

PHOTO CONTRIBUTORS

Elizabeth L. Affel, M.S., R.D.M.S.
Robert S. Bailey, Jr., M.D.
William E. Benson, M.D.
Jurij R. Bilyk, M.D.
Elisabeth J. Cohen, M.D.
Justis P. Ehlers, M.D.
Alan R. Forman, M.D.
Scott M. Goldstein, M.D.
Kammi B. Gunton, M.D.
Becky Killian
Donelson R. Manley, M.D.
Julia Monsonego
Christopher J. Rapuano, M.D.
Peter J. Savino, M.D.
Bruce M. Schnall, M.D.
Robert C. Sergott, M.D.
Chirag P. Shah, M.D., M.P.H.
Heather N. Shelsta, M.D.
Carol L. Shields, M.D.
Jerry A. Shields, M.D.
George L. Spaeth, M.D.
William Tasman, M.D.

MEDICAL ILLUSTRATOR
Paul Schiffmacher

CONTRIBUTORS TO THE FOURTH EDITION
Seema Aggarwal, M.D.
Edward H. Bedrossian, Jr., M.D.
Brian C. Bigler, M.D.
Vatinee Y. Bunya, M.D.
Christine Buono, M.D.
Jacqueline R. Carrasco, M.D.
Sandra Y. Cho, M.D.
Carolyn A. Cutney, M.D.
Brian D. Dudenhoefer, M.D.
John A. Epstein, M.D.
Colleen P. Halfpenny, M.D.
ThucAnh T. Ho, M.D.
Stephen S. Hwang, M.D.
Kunal D. Kantikar, M.D.
Derek Y. Kunimoto, M.D.
R. Gary Lane, M.D.
Henry C. Lee, M.D.
Mimi Liu, M.D.
Mary S. Makar, M.D.
Anson T. Miedel, M.D.
Parveen K. Nagra, M.D.
Michael A. Negrey, M.D.
Heather A. Nesti, M.D.
Vasudha A. Panday, M.D.
Nicholas A. Pefkaros, M.D.
Robert Sambursky, M.D.
Daniel E. Shapiro, M.D.
Derrick W. Shindler, M.D.

CONTRIBUTORS TO THE THIRD EDITION
Christine W. Chung, M.D.
Brian P. Connolly, M.D.
Vincent A. Deramo, M.D.
Kammi B. Gunton, M.D.
Mark R. Miller, M.D.
Ralph E. Oursler III, M.D.
Mark F. Pyfer, M.D.
Douglas J. Rhee, M.D.
Jay C. Rudd, M.D.
Brian M. Sucheski, M.D.

MEDICAL ILLUSTRATOR
Marlon Maus, M.D.

CONTRIBUTORS TO THE SECOND EDITION
Mark C. Austin, M.D.
Jerry R. Blair, M.D.
Benjamin Chang, M.D.
Mary Ellen Cullom, M.D.
R. Douglas Cullom, Jr., M.D.
Jack Dugan, M.D.
Forest J. Ellis, M.D.
C. Byron Faulkner, M.D.
Mary Elizabeth Gallivan, M.D.
J. William Harbour, M.D.
Paul M. Herring, M.D.
Allen C. Ho, M.D.
Carol J. Hoffman, M.D.
Thomas I. Margolis, M.D.
Mark L. Mayo, M.D.
Michele A. Miano, M.D.
Wynne A. Morley, M.D.
Timothy J. O'Brien, M.D.
Florentino E. Palmon, M.D.
William B. Phillips, M.D.
Tony Pruthi, M.D.
Carl D. Regillo, M.D.
Scott H. Smith, M.D.
Mark R. Stokes, M.D.
Janine G. Tabas, M.D.
John R. Trible, M.D.
Christopher Williams, M.D.

MEDICAL ILLUSTRATOR
Neal H. Atebara, M.D.

CONTRIBUTORS TO THE FIRST EDITION
Melissa M. Brown, M.D.
Catharine J. Crockett, M.D.
Bret L. Fisher, M.D.
Patrick M. Flaharty, M.D.
Mark A. Friedberg, M.D.
James T. Handa, M.D.
Victor A. Holmes, M.D.
Bruce J. Keyser, M.D.
Ronald L. McKey, M.D.
Christopher J. Rapuano, M.D.
Paul A. Raskauskas, M.D.
Eric P. Suan, M.D.

MEDICAL ILLUSTRATOR
Marlon Maus, M.D.

Consultants

CORNEA

MAJOR CONSULTANT
Christopher J. Rapuano, M.D.

CONSULTANTS
Brandon D. Ayers, M.D.
Elisabeth J. Cohen, M.D.
Brad H. Feldman, M.D.
Kristin M. Hammersmith, M.D.
Sadeer B. Hannush, M.D.
Irving M. Raber, M.D.

GLAUCOMA

MAJOR CONSULTANTS
L. Jay Katz, M.D.
George L. Spaeth, M.D.

CONSULTANTS
Mary J. Cox, M.D.
Scott J. Fudemberg, M.D.
Anand V. Mantravadi, M.D.
Marlene R. Moster, M.D.
Jonathan S. Myers, M.D.
Tara H. Uhler, M.D.

NEURO-OPHTHALMOLOGY

CONSULTANTS
Jennifer K. Hall, M.D.
Mark L. Moster, M.D
Peter J. Savino, M.D.
Robert C. Sergott, M.D.

OCULOPLASTICS

MAJOR CONSULTANTS
Jurij R. Bilyk, M.D.
Jacqueline R. Carrasco, M.D.
Robert B. Penne, M.D.
Mary A. Stefanyszyn, M.D.

CONSULTANTS
Edward H. Bedrossian, Jr., M.D.
Joseph C. Flanagan, M.D.
Scott M. Goldstein, M.D.
Ann P. Murchison, M.D., M.P.H.

ONCOLOGY

MAJOR CONSULTANTS
Carol L. Shields, M.D.
Jerry A. Shields, M.D.

CONSULTANTS
Sara A. Lally, M.D.
Arman Mashayekhi, M.D.

PEDIATRICS

MAJOR CONSULTANT
Alex V. Levin, M.D.

CONSULTANTS
Brian J. Forbes, M.D.
Kammi B. Gunton, M.D.
Sharon S. Lehman, M.D.
Leonard B. Nelson, M.D.
Jonathan H. Salvin, M.D.
Bruce M. Schnall, M.D.
Barry N. Wasserman, M.D.

RETINA

MAJOR CONSULTANTS
William E. Benson, M D
Sunir J. Garg, M.D.
Jason Hsu, M.D.
William Tasman, M.D.

CONSULTANTS
Mitchell S. Fineman, M.D.
Omesh P. Gupta, M.D., M.B.A.
Julia A. Haller, M.D.

Allen C. Ho, M.D.
Richard S. Kaiser, M.D.
Joseph I. Maguire, M.D.
Carl D. Regillo, M.D.
Marc J. Spirn, M.D.
James F. Vander, M.D.

INFECTIOUS DISEASE

CONSULTANT
Joseph A. DeSimone, Jr., M.D.

PATHOLOGY

CONSULTANT
Ralph C. Eagle, Jr., M.D.

GENERAL

CONSULTANTS
Michael A. DellaVecchia, M.D.
Alan R. Forman, M.D.
Edward A. Jaeger, M.D.
Bruce J. Markovitz, M.D.

RADIOLOGY

CONSULTANT
Adam E. Flanders, M.D.

VISUAL PHYSIOLOGY

CONSULTANTS
Elizabeth L. Affel, M.S., R.D.M.S.
Julia Monsonego, C.R.A.

FELLOW CONSULTANTS

F. Char DeCroos, M.D.
Darrell E. Baskin, M.D.
Allen Chiang, M.D.
Paul B. Johnson, M.D.
Nikolas J.S. London, M.D
Rajiv E. Shah, M.D.
Chirag P. Shah, M.D., M.P.H.
Andre J. Witkin, M.D.
Vladimir S. Yakopson, M.D.

MEDICAL ILLUSTRATOR

Paul Schiffmacher

Foreword

Wills Eye celebrated its 175th anniversary in 2009 and the Retina Service its 50th anniversary in 2010. Hard to believe. Now, in 2012, we are celebrating the sixth edition of *The Wills Eye Manual*. Conceived by Mark Friedberg and Christopher Rapuano when they were residents in 1990, the manual has had a great track record. To date, 150,000 copies have been sold, and it has been translated into ten languages. It is also now helping to disseminate educational information to physicians in developing countries, especially through the American Academy of Ophthalmology's Ophthalmic News & Education (ONE) network.

Adam Gerstenblith and Michael Rabinowitz, the editors of the sixth edition, have been extremely efficient in revising this latest volume. The previous edition, published in 2007, was the first to have illustrations enhancing the descriptions of various conditions, and the new edition includes additional and revised illustrations, where appropriate, as well as the latest information. In the past few years ophthalmology has taken giant steps forward, notably in the management of wet macular degeneration, use of computer chips for retinal function, the role of stem cells, and exponential progress in gene identification of disease entities.

Although tomorrow's future will soon be yesterday's history, we continue to learn more about the original Wills family. Thanks to the National Park Service, the deed to the original Wills house and grocery (which was located behind the house) between Second and Third on Chestnut has surfaced. The most interesting fact we learned was that James Sr. and Hannah Wills bought the property from Benjamin Rush, the renowned physician of the day. It was purchased for 700 pounds gold. Rush was a signer of the Declaration of Independence, and because of his fame, President Thomas Jefferson suggested that Meriwether Lewis pay him a visit before Lewis and William Clark left in 1804–1806 to explore the land acquired in the Louisiana Purchase.

So, Wills with its colorful history has grown up and continues to thrive. I am confident that it will continue to contribute new and exciting advances, some not yet even conceived.

William Tasman, M.D.

Preface

We are proud to present the Sixth Edition of *The Wills Eye Manual*. This edition builds upon the hard work of all previous contributors, and would not be possible without the collaborative effort of the Wills Eye Institute residents and faculty. Our goal is to continue to provide the most accurate and current information regarding the office and emergency room diagnosis, management, and treatment of ophthalmic disease.

The Sixth Edition includes the results of some of the most recent major clinical trials, including those relating to the care of patients with macular degeneration and retinal vein occlusion. Changing trends in the management of a variety of ophthalmic pathology, including orbital fractures, eyelid lacerations, strabismus, amblyopia, and ocular malignancies, are reflected in this newest edition. Many new high-definition photographs of external, anterior segment, and posterior segment disease processes have been added, including fundus photos of Sturge–Weber Syndrome, Wyburn-Mason Syndrome, and solar retinopathy. We have also updated the imaging modalities highlighted in the previous edition, with special attention to optical coherence tomography, magnetic resonance imaging, computed tomography, and ultrasound biomicroscopy. In addition, many updated chapters were expanded to include new, clinically relevant, topics.

With the addition of more illustrations and topics, it was necessary to streamline various sections. To that end, and with feedback from our readers, we have minimized redundancy throughout the manual and removed information more commonly found in other references.

We hope you continue to find the Sixth Edition of *The Wills Eye Manual* a fast, easy-to-use guide to managing ophthalmic disease.

Adam T. Gerstenblith, M.D.
Michael P. Rabinowitz, M.D.

Preface to the First Edition

Our goal has been to produce a concise book, providing essential diagnostic tips and specific therapeutic information pertaining to eye disease. We realized the need for this book while managing emergency room patients at one of the largest and busiest eye hospitals in the country. Until now, reliable information could only be obtained in unwieldy textbooks or inaccessible journals.

As residents at Wills Eye Hospital we have benefited from the input of some of the world-renowned ophthalmic experts in writing this book. More importantly, we are aware of the questions that the ophthalmology resident, the attending ophthalmologist, and the emergency room physician (not trained in ophthalmology) want answered immediately.

The book is written for the eye care provider who, in the midst of evaluating an eye problem, needs quick access to additional information. We try to be as specific as possible, describing the therapeutic modalities used at our institution. Many of these recommendations are, therefore, not the only manner in which to treat a particular disorder, but indicate personal preference. They are guidelines, not rules.

Because of the forever changing wealth of ophthalmic knowledge, omissions and errors are possible, particularly with regard to management. Drug dosages have been checked carefully, but the physician is urged to check the *Physicians' Desk Reference* or *Facts and Comparisons* when prescribing unfamiliar medications. Not all contraindications and side effects are described.

We feel this book will make a welcome companion to the many physicians involved with treating eye problems. It is everything you wanted to know and nothing more.

Christopher J. Rapuano, M.D.
Mark A. Friedberg, M.D.

Contents

Differential Diagnosis of Ocular Symptoms

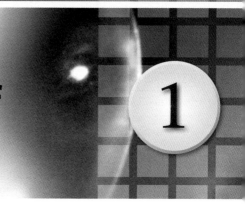

BURNING

More Common. Blepharitis, meibomitis, dry-eye syndrome, conjunctivitis (infectious, allergic, mechanical, chemical).

Less Common. Corneal defects (usually marked by fluorescein staining of the cornea), inflamed pterygium or pinguecula, episcleritis, superior limbic keratoconjunctivitis, ocular toxicity (medication, makeup, contact lens solutions), contact lens-related problems.

CROSSED EYES IN CHILDREN

See 8.4, *Esodeviations in Children* (eyes turned in), or 8.5, *Exodeviations in Children* (eyes turned out).

DECREASED VISION

1. **Transient visual loss** (vision returns to normal within 24 hours, usually within 1 hour).

More Common. Few seconds (usually bilateral): Papilledema. Few minutes: Amaurosis fugax (transient ischemic attack; unilateral), vertebrobasilar artery insufficiency (bilateral). Ten to 60 minutes: Migraine (with or without a subsequent headache).

Less Common. Impending central retinal vein occlusion, ischemic optic neuropathy, ocular ischemic syndrome (carotid occlusive disease), glaucoma, sudden change in blood pressure, central nervous system (CNS) lesion, optic disc drusen, giant cell arteritis, orbital lesion (vision loss may be associated with eye movement).

2. **Visual loss lasting >24 hours**

—**Sudden, painless loss**

More Common. Retinal artery or vein occlusion, ischemic optic neuropathy, vitreous hemorrhage, retinal detachment, optic neuritis (pain with eye movement in >50% of cases), sudden discovery of preexisting unilateral visual loss.

Less Common. Other retinal or CNS disease (e.g., stroke), methanol poisoning, ophthalmic artery occlusion (may also have extraocular motility deficits and ptosis).

—**Gradual, painless loss (over weeks, months, or years).**

More Common. Cataract, refractive error, open-angle glaucoma, chronic angle-closure glaucoma, chronic retinal disease [e.g., age-related macular degeneration (ARMD), diabetic retinopathy].

Less Common. Chronic corneal disease (e.g., corneal dystrophy), optic neuropathy/atrophy (e.g., CNS tumor).

—**Painful loss:** Acute angle-closure glaucoma, optic neuritis (may have pain with eye movements), uveitis, endophthalmitis, corneal hydrops (keratoconus).

3. **Posttraumatic visual loss:** Eyelid swelling, corneal irregularity, hyphema, ruptured globe, traumatic cataract, lens dislocation, commotio retinae, retinal detachment, retinal or vitreous hemorrhage, traumatic optic neuropathy, cranial neuropathies, CNS injury.

NOTE: Always remember nonphysiologic visual loss.

DISCHARGE

See "Red Eye" in this chapter.

1

DISTORTION OF VISION

More Common. Refractive error [including presbyopia, acquired myopia (e.g., from cataract, diabetes, ciliary spasm, medications, retinal detachment surgery), acquired astigmatism (e.g., from anterior segment surgery, chalazion, orbital fracture, and edema)], macular disease [e.g., central serous chorioretinopathy, macular edema, ARMD, and others associated with choroidal neovascular membranes (CNVMs)], corneal irregularity, intoxication (e.g., ethanol, methanol), pharmacologic (e.g., scopolamine patch).

Less Common. Keratoconus, topical eye drops (e.g., miotics, cycloplegics), retinal detachment, migraine (transient), hypotony, CNS abnormality (including papilledema), nonphysiologic.

DOUBLE VISION (DIPLOPIA)

1. **Monocular** (diplopia remains when the uninvolved eye is occluded)

More Common. Refractive error, incorrect spectacle alignment, corneal opacity or irregularity (including corneal or refractive surgery), cataract, iris defects (e.g., iridectomy).

Less Common. Dislocated natural lens or lens implant, macular disease, retinal detachment, CNS causes (rare), nonphysiologic.

2. **Binocular** (diplopia eliminated when either eye is occluded)

   —**Typically intermittent:** Myasthenia gravis, intermittent decompensation of an existing phoria.

   —**Constant:** Isolated sixth, third, or fourth nerve palsy; orbital disease [e.g., thyroid eye disease; idiopathic orbital inflammation (orbital pseudotumor), tumor]; cavernous sinus/superior orbital fissure syndrome; status-post ocular surgery (e.g., residual anesthesia, displaced muscle, undercorrection or overcorrection after muscle surgery, restriction from scleral buckle, severe aniseikonia after refractive surgery); status-post trauma (e.g., orbital wall fracture with extraocular muscle entrapment, orbital edema); internuclear ophthalmoplegia; vertebrobasilar artery insufficiency; other CNS lesions; spectacle problem.

DRY EYES

See 4.3, *Dry-Eye Syndrome.*

EYELASH LOSS

Trauma, burn, thyroid disease, Vogt–Koyanagi–Harada syndrome, eyelid infection or inflammation, radiation, chronic skin disease (e.g., alopecia areata), cutaneous neoplasm, trichotillomania.

EYELID CRUSTING

More Common. Blepharitis, meibomitis, conjunctivitis.

Less Common. Canaliculitis, nasolacrimal duct obstruction, dacryocystitis.

EYELIDS DROOPING (PTOSIS)

See 6.1, *Ptosis.*

EYELID SWELLING

1. **Associated with inflammation** (usually erythematous).

More Common. Hordeolum, blepharitis, conjunctivitis, preseptal or orbital cellulitis, trauma, contact dermatitis, herpes simplex or zoster dermatitis.

Less Common. Ectropion, corneal abnormality, urticaria or angioedema, blepharochalasis, insect bite, dacryoadenitis, erysipelas, eyelid or lacrimal gland mass, autoimmunities (e.g., discoid lupus, dermatomyositis).

2. **Noninflammatory:** Chalazion; dermatochalasis; prolapse of orbital fat (retropulsion of the globe increases the prolapse); laxity of the eyelid skin; cardiac, renal, or thyroid disease; superior vena cava syndrome; eyelid or lacrimal gland mass, foreign body.

EYELID TWITCH

Orbicularis myokymia (related to fatigue, excess caffeine, medication, or stress), corneal or conjunctival irritation (especially from an eyelash, cyst, or conjunctival foreign body), dry eye, blepharospasm (bilateral), hemifacial spasm, albinism (photosensitivity), serum electrolyte abnormality, tourettes, tic douloureux, anemia (rarely).

EYELIDS UNABLE TO CLOSE (LAGOPHTHALMOS)

Severe proptosis, severe chemosis, eyelid scarring, eyelid retractor muscle scarring, seventh cranial nerve palsy, status-post facial cosmetic or reconstructive surgery.

EYES "BULGING" (PROPTOSIS)

See 7.1, *Orbital Disease.*

EYES "JUMPING" (OSCILLOPSIA)

Acquired nystagmus, internuclear ophthalmoplegia, myasthenia gravis, vestibular function loss, opsoclonus/ocular flutter, superior oblique myokymia, various CNS disorders.

FLASHES OF LIGHT

More Common. Retinal break or detachment, posterior vitreous detachment, migraine, rapid eye movements (particularly in darkness), oculodigital stimulation.

Less Common. CNS (particularly occipital lobe) disorders, vestibulobasilar artery insufficiency, optic neuropathies, retinitis, entoptic phenomena, hallucinations.

FLOATERS

See "Spots in Front of the Eyes" in this chapter.

FOREIGN BODY SENSATION

Dry-eye syndrome, blepharitis, conjunctivitis, trichiasis, corneal abnormality (e.g., corneal abrasion or foreign body, recurrent erosion, superficial punctate keratopathy), contact lens-related problem, episcleritis, pterygium, pinguecula.

GLARE

Cataract, pseudophakia, posterior capsular opacity, corneal irregularity or opacity, altered pupillary structure or response, status-post refractive surgery, posterior vitreous detachment, pharmacologic (e.g., atropine).

HALLUCINATIONS (FORMED IMAGES)

Posterior vitreous detachments (white lightning streaks of Moore), retinal detachment, optic neuropathies, blind eyes, bilateral eye patching, Charles Bonnet syndrome, psychosis, parietotemporal area lesions, other CNS causes, medications.

HALOS AROUND LIGHTS

Cataract, pseudophakia, posterior capsular opacity, acute angle-closure glaucoma or corneal edema from another cause (e.g., aphakic or pseudophakic bullous keratopathy, contact lens overwear), corneal dystrophies, status-post refractive surgery, corneal haziness, discharge, pigment dispersion syndrome, vitreous opacities, drugs (e.g., digitalis, chloroquine).

HEADACHE

See 10.26, *Headache.*

ITCHY EYES

Conjunctivitis (especially allergic, vernal, and viral), blepharitis, dry-eye syndrome, topical drug allergy or contact dermatitis, giant papillary conjunctivitis, or another contact lens-related problem.

LIGHT SENSITIVITY (PHOTOPHOBIA)

1. **Abnormal eye examination**

More Common. Corneal abnormality (e.g., abrasion or edema), anterior uveitis.

Less Common. Conjunctivitis (mild photophobia), posterior uveitis, scleritis, albinism, total color blindness, aniridia, mydriasis of any etiology (e.g., pharmacologic, traumatic), congenital glaucoma.

2. **Normal eye examination:** Migraine, meningitis, retrobulbar optic neuritis, subarachnoid hemorrhage, trigeminal neuralgia, or a lightly pigmented eye.

NIGHT BLINDNESS

More Common. Refractive error (especially undercorrected myopia), advanced glaucoma or optic atrophy, small pupil (especially from miotic drops), retinitis pigmentosa, congenital stationary night blindness, status-post panretinal photocoagulation drugs (e.g., phenothiazines, chloroquine, quinine).

Less Common. Vitamin A deficiency, gyrate atrophy, choroideremia.

PAIN

1. **Ocular**

   —**Typically mild to moderate:** Dry-eye syndrome, blepharitis, infectious conjunctivitis, episcleritis, inflamed pinguecula or pterygium, foreign body (corneal or conjunctival), corneal disorder (e.g., superficial punctate keratopathy), superior limbic keratoconjunctivitis, ocular medication toxicity, contact lens-related problems, postoperative, ocular ischemic syndrome, eye strain from uncorrected refractive error.

   —**Typically moderate to severe:** Corneal disorder (e.g., abrasion, erosion, infiltrate/ulcer/keratitis, chemical injury, ultraviolet burn), trauma, anterior uveitis, scleritis, endophthalmitis, acute angle-closure glaucoma.

2. **Periorbital:** Trauma, hordeolum, preseptal cellulitis, dacryocystitis, dermatitis (e.g., contact, chemical, varicella zoster, or herpes simplex), referred pain (e.g., dental, sinus), tic douloureux.

3. **Orbital:** Sinusitis, trauma, orbital cellulitis, idiopathic orbital inflammatory syndrome orbital tumor or mass, optic neuritis, acute dacryoadenitis, migraine or cluster headache, diabetic cranial nerve palsy.

4. **Asthenopia:** Uncorrected refractive error, phoria or tropia, convergence insufficiency, accommodative spasm, pharmacologic (miotics).

RED EYE

1. **Adnexal causes:** Trichiasis, distichiasis, floppy eyelid syndrome, entropion or ectropion, lagophthalmos (incomplete eyelid closure), blepharitis, meibomitis, acne rosacea, dacryocystitis, canaliculitis.

2. **Conjunctival causes:** Ophthalmia neonatorum in infants, conjunctivitis (bacterial, viral, chemical, allergic, atopic, vernal, medication toxicity), subconjunctival hemorrhage, inflamed pinguecula, superior limbic keratoconjunctivitis, giant papillary conjunctivitis, conjunctival foreign body, symblepharon and associated etiologies (e.g., ocular cicatricial pemphigoid, Stevens–Johnson syndrome, toxic epidermal necrolysis), conjunctival neoplasia.

3. **Corneal causes:** Infectious or inflammatory keratitis, contact lens-related problems (see 4.21, *Contact Lens-Related Problems*), corneal foreign body, recurrent corneal erosion, pterygium, neurotrophic keratopathy, medicamentosa, ultraviolet or chemical burn.

4. **Other:** Trauma, postoperative, dry-eye syndrome, endophthalmitis, anterior uveitis, episcleritis, scleritis, pharmacologic (e.g., prostaglandin analogs), angle-closure glaucoma, carotid–cavernous fistula (corkscrew conjunctival vessels), cluster headache.

"SPOTS" IN FRONT OF THE EYES

1. **Transient:** Migraine.

2. **Permanent or long-standing**

More Common. Posterior vitreous detachment, intermediate or posterior uveitis, vitreous hemorrhage, vitreous condensations/debris.

Less Common. Microhyphema, hyphema, retinal break or detachment, corneal opacity or foreign body.

NOTE: Some patients are referring to a blind spot in their visual field caused by a retinal, optic nerve, or CNS disorder.

TEARING

1. **Adults**

   —**Pain present:** Corneal abnormality (e.g., abrasion, foreign body or rust ring, recurrent erosion, edema), anterior uveitis, eyelash or eyelid disorder (e.g., trichiasis, entropion), conjunctival foreign body, dacryocystitis, dacryoadenitis, canaliculitis, trauma.

   —**Minimal/no pain:** Dry-eye syndrome, blepharitis, nasolacrimal duct obstruction, punctal occlusion, lacrimal sac mass, ectropion, conjunctivitis (especially allergic and toxic), emotional states, crocodile tears (congenital or seventh nerve palsy).

2. **Children:** Nasolacrimal duct obstruction, congenital glaucoma, corneal or conjunctival foreign body, or other irritative disorder.

Differential Diagnosis of Ocular Signs

ANTERIOR CHAMBER/ANTERIOR CHAMBER ANGLE

Hyphema

Traumatic, iatrogenic (e.g., intraocular surgery or laser), iris neovascularization, herpes simplex or zoster iridocyclitis, blood dyscrasia or clotting disorder (e.g., hemophilia), anticoagulation, Fuchs heterochromic iridocyclitis, intraocular tumor (e.g., juvenile xanthogranuloma, retinoblastoma, angioma).

Hypopyon

Infectious corneal ulcer, endophthalmitis, severe iridocyclitis (e.g., HLA-B27 associated, Behcet disease), reaction to an intraocular lens (sterile hypopyon), retained lens particle, device contaminant after cataract surgery (toxic anterior segment syndrome), intraocular tumor necrosis (e.g., pseudohypopyon from retinoblastoma), retained intraocular foreign body, tight contact lens, chronic corneal edema with ruptured bullae, severe inflammatory reaction from a recurrent corneal erosion, drugs (e.g., rifampin).

Blood in Schlemm Canal on Gonioscopy

Compression of episcleral vessels by a gonioprism (iatrogenic), Sturge–Weber syndrome, arteriovenous fistula [e.g., carotid–cavernous sinus fistula (c-c fistula)], superior vena cava obstruction, hypotony.

CORNEA/CONJUNCTIVAL FINDINGS

Conjunctival Swelling (Chemosis)

Allergy, any ocular or periocular inflammation, postoperative, drugs, venous congestion (e.g., c-c fistula), angioneurotic edema, myxedema.

Conjunctival Dryness (Xerosis)

Vitamin A deficiency, postcicatricial conjunctivitis, Stevens–Johnson syndrome, ocular cicatricial pemphigoid, exposure (e.g., lagophthalmos, absent blink reflex, proptosis), radiation, chronic dacryoadenitis, Sjogren syndrome.

Corneal Crystals

See 4.14, *Crystalline Keratopathy.*

Corneal Edema

1. **Congenital:** Congenital glaucoma, congenital hereditary endothelial dystrophy (autosomal recessive form is present at birth, autosomal dominant form has later onset), posterior polymorphous dystrophy (PPMD), birth trauma (forceps injury).

2. **Acquired:** Postoperative edema, aphakic or pseudophakic bullous keratopathy, Fuchs endothelial dystrophy, contact lens overwear, traumatic, exposure, chemical injuries, acute increase in intraocular pressure (e.g. angle-closure glaucoma), corneal hydrops (decompensated keratoconus), herpes simplex or zoster keratitis, iritis, failed corneal graft, iridocorneal endothelial (ICE) syndrome, PPMD.

Dilated Episcleral Vessels (Without Ocular Irritation or Pain)

Underlying uveal neoplasm, arteriovenous fistula (e.g., c-c fistula), polycythemia vera, leukemia, ophthalmic vein or cavernous sinus thrombosis, extravascular blockage of ophthalmic/orbital venous outflow.

Enlarged Corneal Nerves

Most Important. Multiple endocrine neoplasia type IIb (medullary carcinoma of the thyroid gland, pheochromocytoma, mucosal neuromas; may have marfanoid habitus).

Others. Acanthamoeba keratitis, chronic keratitis, keratoconus, neurofibromatosis, Fuchs endothelial dystrophy, Refsum syndrome, trauma, congenital glaucoma, failed corneal graft, leprosy, ichthyosis, idiopathic, normal variant.

Follicles on the Conjunctiva

See 5.1, *Acute Conjunctivitis,* and 5.2, *Chronic Conjunctivitis.*

Membranous Conjunctivitis

(Removal of the membrane is difficult and causes bleeding). Streptococci, pneumococci, chemical burn, ligneous conjunctivitis, *Corynebacterium diphtheriae,* adenovirus, herpes simplex virus, ocular vaccinia. (Compare with "Pseudomembranous Conjunctivitis".)

Pseudomembranous Conjunctivitis

(Removal of the pseudomembrane is easy without bleeding). See earlier for causes of membranous conjunctivitis, as well as ocular cicatricial pemphigoid, Stevens–Johnson syndrome, superior limbic keratoconjunctivitis, gonococci, staphylococci, chlamydia in newborns, and others.

Opacification of the Cornea in Infancy

Congenital glaucoma, birth trauma (forceps injury), congenital hereditary endothelial or stromal dystrophy (bilateral), PPMD, developmental abnormality of the anterior segment (e.g., Peters anomaly), metabolic abnormalities (bilateral; e.g., mucopolysaccharidoses, mucolipidoses), interstitial keratitis, herpes simplex virus, corneal ulcer, corneal dermoid, sclerocornea.

Pannus (Superficial Vascular Invasion of the Cornea)

Ocular rosacea, tight contact lens or contact lens overwear, phlyctenule, chlamydia (trachoma and inclusion conjunctivitis), superior limbic keratoconjunctivitis (micropannus only), staphylococcal hypersensitivity, vernal keratoconjunctivitis, herpes simplex or zoster virus, chemical burn, ocular cicatricial pemphigoid, aniridia, molluscum contagiosum, leprosy.

Papillae on the Conjunctiva

See 5.1, *Acute Conjunctivitis,* and 5.2, *Chronic Conjunctivitis.*

Pigmentation/Discoloration of the Conjunctiva

Racial melanosis (perilimbal), nevus, primary acquired melanosis, melanoma, ocular and oculodermal melanocytosis (congenital, blue-gray, not conjunctival but episcleral), Addison disease, pregnancy, radiation, jaundice, resolving subconjunctival hemorrhage, mascara, conjunctival or subconjunctival foreign body, pharmacologic (e.g., chlorpromazine, topical epinephrine).

Symblepharon (Fusion of the Palpebral Conjunctiva with the Bulbar Conjunctiva)

Ocular cicatricial pemphigoid, Stevens–Johnson syndrome, chemical burn, trauma, drugs, long-standing conjunctival or episcleral inflammation, epidemic keratoconjunctivitis, atopic conjunctivitis, radiation, congenital, iatrogenic (postsurgical).

Whorl-Like Opacity in the Corneal Epithelium (Verticillata)

Amiodarone, chloroquine, Fabry disease and carrier state, phenothiazines, indomethacin.

EYELID ABNORMALITIES

Eyelid Edema

See "Eyelid Swelling" in Chapter 1, *Differential Diagnosis of Ocular Symptoms.*

Eyelid Lesion

See 6.11, *Malignant Tumors of the Eyelid.*

Ptosis and Pseudoptosis

See 6.1, *Ptosis.*

FUNDUS FINDINGS

Bone Spicules (Widespread Pigment Clumping)

See 11.28, *Retinitis Pigmentosa and Inherited Chorioretinal Dystrophies.*

Bull's-Eye Macular Lesion

Age-related macular degeneration (ARMD), Stargardt disease or fundus flavimaculatus, albinism, cone dystrophy, chloroquine or hydroxychloroquine retinopathy, Spielmeyer–Vogt syndrome, central areolar choroidal dystrophy. See 11.32, *Chloroquine/Hydroxychloroquine Toxicity.*

Choroidal Folds

Orbital or choroidal tumor, idiopathic orbital inflammatory syndrome, thyroid eye disease, posterior scleritis, hypotony, retinal detachment, marked hyperopia, scleral laceration, papilledema, postoperative.

Choroidal Neovascularization (Gray-Green Membrane or Blood Seen Deep to the Retina)

More Common. ARMD, ocular histoplasmosis syndrome, high myopia, idiopathic polypoidal choroidal vasculopathy, angioid streaks, choroidal rupture (trauma).

Less Common. Drusen of the optic nerve head, tumors, retinal scarring after laser photocoagulation, idiopathic.

Cotton–Wool Spots

See 11.5, *Cotton–Wool Spot.*

Embolus

See 10.22, *Transient Visual Loss/Amaurosis Fugax;* 11.6, *Central Retinal Artery Occlusion;* 11.7, *Branch Retinal Artery Occlusion;* 11.33, *Crystalline Retinopathy.*

- Platelet–fibrin (dull gray and elongated): Carotid disease, less common cardiac.

- Cholesterol (sparkling yellow, usually at an arterial bifurcation): Carotid disease.

- Calcium (dull white, typically around or on the disc): Cardiac disease.

- Cardiac myxoma (common in young patients, particularly in the left eye; often occludes the ophthalmic or central retinal artery behind the globe and is not seen).

- Talc and cornstarch (small yellow-white glistening particles in macular arterioles; may produce peripheral retinal neovascularization): Intravenous (i.v.) drug abuse.

- Lipid or air (cotton–wool spots, not emboli, are often seen): Results from chest trauma (Purtscher retinopathy) and fracture of long bones.

- Others (tumors, parasites, other foreign bodies).

Macular Exudates

More Common. Diabetes, choroidal (subretinal) neovascular membrane, hypertension.

Less Common. Macroaneurysm, Coats disease (children), peripheral retinal capillary hemangioma, retinal vein occlusion, papilledema, radiation retinopathy.

Normal Fundus in the Presence of Decreased Vision

Retrobulbar optic neuritis, cone degeneration, Stargardt disease or fundus flavimaculatus, other optic neuropathy (e.g., Leber hereditary optic neuropathy, tumor, alcohol or tobacco), rod monochromatism, amblyopia, nonphysiologic visual loss.

Optociliary Shunt Vessels on the Disc

Orbital or intracranial tumor (especially meningioma), previous central retinal vein occlusion, chronic papilledema (e.g., pseudotumor cerebri), chronic open-angle glaucoma, optic nerve glioma.

Retinal Neovascularization

1. **Posterior pole:** Diabetes, after central retinal vein occlusion.

2. **Peripheral:** Sickle cell retinopathy, after branch retinal vein occlusion, diabetes, sarcoidosis, syphilis, ocular ischemic syndrome (carotid occlusive disease), pars planitis, Coats disease, retinopathy of prematurity, embolization from i.v. drug abuse (talc retinopathy), chronic uveitis, others (e.g., leukemia, anemia, Eales disease, familial exudative vitreoretinopathy).

Roth Spots (Retinal Hemorrhages with White Centers)

More Common. Diabetes, leukemia, septic chorioretinitis (e.g., secondary to bacterial endocarditis).

Less Common. Pernicious anemia (and rarely other forms of anemia), sickle cell disease, scurvy, systemic lupus erythematosus, other connective tissue diseases.

Sheathing of Retinal Veins (Periphlebitis)

More Common. Syphilis, sarcoidosis, pars planitis, sickle cell disease.

Less Common. Tuberculosis, multiple sclerosis, Eales disease, viral retinitis (e.g., human immunodeficiency virus, herpes), Behçet disease, fungal retinitis, bacteremia.

Tumor

See 11.36, *Choroidal Nevus and Malignant Melanoma of the Choroid.*

INTRAOCULAR PRESSURE

Acute Increase in Intraocular Pressure

Acute angle-closure glaucoma, glaucomatocyclitic crisis (Posner–Schlossman syndrome), inflammatory open-angle glaucoma, malignant glaucoma, postoperative (see "Postoperative Problems," this chapter), suprachoroidal hemorrhage, hyphema, c-c fistula, retrobulbar hemorrhage, or other orbital disease.

Chronic Increase in Intraocular Pressure

See 9.1, *Primary Open-Angle Glaucoma.*

Decreased Intraocular Pressure (Hypotony)

Ruptured globe, phthisis bulbi, retinal/choroidal detachment, iridocyclitis, severe dehydration, cyclodialysis cleft, ocular ischemia, drugs (e.g., glaucoma medications), postoperative (see "Postoperative Problems," this chapter), traumatic ciliary body shutdown.

IRIS

Iris Heterochromia (Irides of Different Colors)

1. **Involved iris is lighter than normal:** Congenital Horner syndrome, most cases of Fuchs heterochromic iridocyclitis, chronic uveitis, juvenile xanthogranuloma, metastatic carcinoma, Waardenburg syndrome.

2. **Involved iris is darker than normal:** Ocular melanocytosis or oculodermal melanocytosis, hemosiderosis, siderosis, retained intraocular foreign body, ocular malignant melanoma, diffuse iris nevus, retinoblastoma, leukemia, lymphoma, ICE syndrome, some cases of Fuchs heterochromic iridocyclitis.

Iris Lesion

1. **Melanotic (brown):** Nevus, melanoma, adenoma, or adenocarcinoma of the iris pigment epithelium.

NOTE: Cysts, foreign bodies, neurofibromas, and other lesions may appear pigmented in heavily pigmented irides.

---

2. **Amelanotic (white, yellow, or orange):** Amelanotic melanoma, inflammatory nodule or granuloma (e.g., sarcoidosis, tuberculosis, leprosy, other granulomatous disease), neurofibroma, patchy hyperemia of syphilis, juvenile xanthogranuloma, foreign body, cyst, leiomyoma, seeding from a posterior segment tumor.

Neovascularization of the Iris

Diabetic retinopathy, ocular ischemic syndrome, after central or branch retinal vein or artery occlusion, chronic uveitis, chronic retinal detachment, intraocular tumor (e.g., retinoblastoma, melanoma), other retinal vascular disease.

LENS (SEE ALSO 13.1, *ACQUIRED CATARACT*)

Dislocated Lens (Ectopia Lentis)

See 13.10, *Subluxed or Dislocated Crystalline Lens.*

Iridescent Lens Particles

Drugs, hypocalcemia, myotonic dystrophy, hypothyroidism, familial, idiopathic.

Lenticonus

1. **Anterior (marked convexity of the anterior lens):** Alport syndrome (hereditary nephritis).

2. **Posterior (marked concavity of the posterior lens surface):** Usually idiopathic, may be associated with persistent fetal vasculature.

NEUROOPHTHALMIC ABNORMALITIES

Afferent Pupillary Defect

1. **Severe (2+ to 3+):** Optic nerve disease (e.g., ischemic optic neuropathy, optic neuritis,

2

tumor, glaucoma); central retinal artery or vein occlusion; less commonly, a lesion of the optic chiasm or tract.

2. **Mild (1+):** Any of the preceding, amblyopia, dense vitreous hemorrhage, advanced macular degeneration, branch retinal vein or artery occlusion, retinal detachment, or other retinal disease.

Anisocoria (Pupils of Different Sizes)

See 10.1, *Anisocoria.*

Limitation of Ocular Motility

1. **With exophthalmos and resistance to retropulsion:** See 7.1, *Orbital Disease.*

2. **Without exophthalmos and resistance to retropulsion:** Isolated third, fourth, or sixth cranial nerve palsy; multiple ocular motor nerve palsies [see 10.10, *Cavernous Sinus and Associated Syndromes (Multiple Ocular Motor Nerve Palsies)*], myasthenia gravis, chronic progressive external ophthalmoplegia and associated syndromes, orbital blow-out fracture with muscle entrapment, ophthalmoplegic migraine, Duane syndrome, other central nervous system (CNS) disorders.

Optic Disc Atrophy

More Common. Glaucoma; after central retinal vein or artery occlusion; previous ischemic optic neuropathy; chronic optic neuritis; chronic papilledema; compression of the optic nerve, chiasm, or tract by a tumor or aneurysm; previous traumatic optic neuropathy.

Less Common. Syphilis, retinal degeneration (e.g., retinitis pigmentosa), toxic or metabolic optic neuropathy, Leber hereditary optic atrophy, Leber congenital amaurosis, lysosomal storage disease (e.g., Tay–Sachs), radiation neuropathy, other forms of congenital or hereditary optic atrophy (nystagmus almost always present in congenital forms).

Optic Disc Swelling (Edema)

See 10.15, *Papilledema.*

Optociliary Shunt Vessels

See "Fundus Findings" in this chapter.

Pardoxical Pupillary Reaction (Pupil Dilates in Light and Constricts in Darkness)

Congenital stationary night blindness, congenital achromatopsia, optic nerve hypoplasia, Leber congenital amaurosis, Best disease, optic neuritis, dominant optic atrophy, albinism, retinitis pigmentosa. Rarely amblyopia.

ORBIT

Extraocular Muscle Thickening on Imaging

More Common. Thyroid orbitopathy (often spares tendon), idiopathic orbital inflammatory syndrome.

Less Common. Tumor (e.g., lymphoma, metastasis, or spread of lacrimal gland tumor to muscle), c-c fistula, superior ophthalmic vein thrombosis, cavernous hemangioma (usually appears in the muscle cone without muscle thickening), rhabdomyosarcoma (children).

Lacrimal Gland Lesions

See 7.6, *Lacrimal Gland Mass/Chronic Dacryoadenitis.*

Optic Nerve Lesion (Isolated)

More Common. Optic nerve glioma (especially children), optic nerve meningioma (especially adults).

Less Common. Metastasis, leukemia, idiopathic orbital inflammatory syndrome, sarcoidosis, increased intracranial pressure with secondary optic nerve swelling.

Orbital Lesions/Proptosis

See 7.1, *Orbital Disease.*

PEDIATRICS

Leukocoria (White Pupillary Reflex)

See 8.1, *Leukocoria.*

Nystagmus In Infancy (See Also 10.21, *Nystagmus*)

Congenital nystagmus, albinism, Leber congenital amaurosis, CNS (thalamic) injury, spasmus nutans, optic nerve or chiasmal glioma, optic nerve hypoplasia, congenital cataracts, aniridia, congenital corneal opacities.

POSTOPERATIVE COMPLICATIONS

Shallow Anterior Chamber

1. **Accompanied by increased intraocular pressure:** Pupillary block glaucoma, suprachoroidal hemorrhage, malignant glaucoma.

2. **Accompanied by decreased intraocular pressure:** Wound leak, choroidal detachment, over filtration after glaucoma filtering procedure.

Hypotony

Wound leak, choroidal detachment, cyclodialysis cleft, retinal detachment, ciliary body shutdown, pharmacologic aqueous suppression.

REFRACTIVE PROBLEMS

Progressive Hyperopia

Orbital tumor pressing on the posterior surface of the eye, serous elevation of the retina (e.g., central serous chorioretinopathy), posterior scleritis, presbyopia, hypoglycemia, cataracts, after radial keratotomy, or other refractive surgery.

Progressive Myopia

High (pathologic) myopia, diabetes, cataract, staphyloma and elongation of the globe, corneal ectasia (keratoconus or after corneal refractive surgery), medications (e.g., miotic drops, sulfa drugs, tetracycline), childhood (physiologic).

VISUAL FIELD ABNORMALITIES

Altitudinal Field Defect

More Common. Ischemic optic neuropathy, hemi or branch retinal artery or vein occlusion, optic neuritis.

Less Common. Glaucoma, optic nerve or chiasmal lesion, optic nerve coloboma.

Arcuate Scotoma

More Common. Glaucoma.

Less Common. Ischemic optic neuropathy (especially nonarteritic), optic disc drusen, high myopia, optic neuritis.

Binasal Field Defect

More Common. Glaucoma, bitemporal retinal disease (e.g., retinitis pigmentosa).

Rare. Bilateral occipital disease, tumor or aneurysm compressing both optic nerves or chiasm, chiasmatic arachnoiditis, nonphysiologic.

Bitemporal Hemianopsia

More Common. Chiasmal lesion (e.g., pituitary adenoma, meningioma, craniopharyngioma, aneurysm, glioma).

Less Common. Tilted optic discs.

Rare. Nasal retinitis pigmentosa.

Blind Spot Enlargement

Papilledema, glaucoma, optic nerve drusen, optic nerve coloboma, myelinated (medullated) nerve fibers off the disc, drugs, myopic disc with a crescent, multiple evanescent white dot syndrome (MEWDS), acute idiopathic blind spot enlargement syndrome [(AIBSE) may be on spectrum with MEWDS].

Central Scotoma

Macular disease; optic neuritis; ischemic optic neuropathy (more typically produces an altitudinal field defect); optic atrophy (e.g., from tumor compressing the nerve, toxic or metabolic disease); rarely, an occipital cortex lesion.

Constriction of the Peripheral Fields Leaving a Small Residual Central Field (Tunnel Vision)

Glaucoma; retinitis pigmentosa, or other peripheral retinal disorders (e.g., gyrate atrophy); chronic papilledema; status-post panretinal photocoagulation or cryotherapy, central retinal artery occlusion with cilioretinal artery sparing; bilateral occipital lobe infarction with macular sparing; nonphysiologic visual loss; carcinoma, melanoma, and autoimmune-associated retinopathy;

rarely, medications (e.g., phenothiazines); vitamin A deficiency.

Homonymous Hemianopsia

Optic tract or lateral geniculate body lesion; temporal, parietal, or occipital lobe lesion of the brain (stroke and tumor more common; aneurysm and trauma less common). Migraine may cause a transient homonymous hemianopsia.

VITREOUS

Vitreous Opacities

Asteroid hyalosis; synchysis scintillans; vitreous hemorrhage; inflammatory cells from vitritis or posterior uveitis; snowball opacities of pars planitis or sarcoidosis; normal vitreous strands from age-related vitreous degeneration; tumor cells; foreign body; hyaloid remnants; rarely, amyloidosis or Whipple disease.

Trauma

3

3.1 CHEMICAL BURN

Treatment should be instituted IMMEDIATELY, even before testing vision, unless an open globe is suspected.

NOTE: This includes alkali (e.g., lye, cements, plasters, airbag powder, bleach, ammonia), acids (e.g., battery acid, pool cleaner, vinegar), solvents, detergents, and irritants (e.g., mace).

Emergency Treatment

1. Copious but gentle irrigation using saline or Ringer lactate solution for at least 30 minutes. Tap water can be used in the absence of these solutions and may be more efficacious in inhibiting elevated intracameral pH than normal saline for alkali burns. NEVER use acidic solutions to neutralize alkalis or vice versa as acid–base reactions themselves can generate harmful substrates. An eyelid speculum and topical anesthetic (e.g., proparacaine) can be placed prior to irrigation. Upper and lower fornices must be everted and irrigated. After exclusion of open globe, particulate matter should be flushed or manually removed. Manual use of intravenous tubing connected to an irrigation solution facilitates the irrigation process.

2. Wait 5 to 10 minutes after irrigation is stopped to allow the dilutant to be absorbed, then check the pH in the fornices using litmus paper. Irrigation is continued until neutral pH is achieved (i.e., 7 to 7.4).

NOTE: The volume of irrigation fluid required to reach neutral pH varies with the chemical and with the duration of the chemical exposure. The volume required may range from a few liters to many liters (more than 8 to 10 L).

3. Conjunctival fornices should be swept with a moistened cotton-tipped applicator or glass rod to remove any sequestered particles of caustic material and necrotic conjunctiva, especially in the case of a persistently abnormal pH. Double eversion of the eyelids with Desmarres eyelid retractors is especially important in identifying and removing particles in the deep fornix. Calcium hydroxide particles may be more easily removed with a cotton-tipped applicator soaked in disodium ethylenediaminetetraacetic acid.

4. Acidic or basic foreign bodies embedded in the conjunctiva, cornea, sclera, or surrounding tissues may require surgical debridement or removal.

MILD-TO-MODERATE BURNS

Signs

(See Figure 3.1.1.)

Critical. Corneal epithelial defects range from scattered superficial punctate keratopathy (SPK), to focal epithelial loss, to sloughing of the entire epithelium. No significant

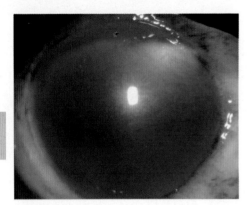

FIGURE 3.1.1. Alkali burn.

areas of peri limbal ischemia are seen (i.e., no blanching of the conjunctival or episcleral vessels).

Other. Focal areas of conjunctival epithelial defect, chemosis, hyperemia, hemorrhages, or a combination of these; mild eyelid edema; mild anterior chamber (AC) reaction; first- and second-degree burns of the periocular skin with or without lash loss.

NOTE: If you suspect an epithelial defect but do not see one with fluorescein staining, repeat the fluorescein application to the eye. Sometimes the defect is slow to take up the dye. If the entire epithelium sloughs off, only Bowman membrane remains, which may take up fluorescein poorly.

Work-Up

1. History: Time of injury? Specific type of chemical? Time between exposure until irrigation was started? Duration of and type of irrigation? Eye protection? Sample of agent, package or label, or material safety data sheets are helpful in identifying and treating the exposing agent.

2. Slit-lamp examination with fluorescein staining. Eyelid eversion to search for foreign bodies. Evaluate for conjunctival or corneal ulcerations or defects. Check the intraocular pressure (IOP). In the presence of a distorted cornea, IOP may be most accurately measured with a Tono-Pen or pneumotonometer. Gentle palpation may be used if necessary.

Treatment

1. See *Emergency Treatment* above.

2. Cycloplegic (e.g., scopolamine 0.25%). If limbal ischemia is suspected, avoid phenylephrine because of its vasoconstrictive properties.

3. Topical antibiotic ointment (e.g., erythromycin) q1–2h while awake or pressure patch for 24 hours.

4. Oral pain medication (e.g., acetaminophen with or without codeine) as needed.

5. If IOP is elevated, acetazolamide 250 mg p.o. q.i.d., acetazolamide 500 mg sequel p.o. b.i.d. or methazolamide 25 to 50 mg p.o. b.i.d. or t.i.d. may be given. Electrolytes, especially potassium, should be monitored in patients on these medications. Add a topical beta-blocker (e.g., timolol 0.5% b.i.d.) if additional IOP control is required. Alpha-agonists may be avoided because of their vasoconstrictive properties.

6. Frequent (e.g., q1h while awake) use of preservative-free artificial tears or gel if not pressure patched.

Follow-Up

Daily initially and then every few days until the corneal epithelial defect is healed. Topical steroids may then be used to reduce significant inflammation. Monitor for corneal epithelial breakdown, stromal thinning, and infection.

SEVERE BURNS

Signs (in addition to the above)

Critical. Pronounced chemosis and conjunctival blanching, corneal edema and opacification, a moderate-to-severe AC reaction (may not be appreciated if the cornea is opaque).

Other. Increased IOP, second- and third-degree burns of the surrounding skin, and local necrotic retinopathy as a result of direct penetration of alkali through the sclera.

Work-Up

Same as for mild-to-moderate burns.

Treatment

1. See *Emergency Treatment* above.

2. Hospital admission rarely needed for close monitoring of IOP and corneal healing.

3. Debride necrotic tissue containing foreign matter.

4. Cycloplegic (e.g., scopolamine 0.25% or atropine 1%, b.i.d. to t.i.d.). Avoid phenylephrine because it is a vasoconstrictor.

5. Topical antibiotic (e.g., trimethoprim/polymyxin B or fluoroquinolone drops q.i.d.; erythromycin or bacitracin ointment four to nine times per day).

6. Topical steroid (e.g., prednisolone acetate 1% or dexamethasone 0.1% four to nine times per day) if significant AC or corneal inflammation is present. May use a combination antibiotic—steroids such as tobramycin/dexamethasone drops or ointment q1–2h.

7. Consider a pressure patch between drops or ointment.

8. Antiglaucoma medications as above if the IOP is increased or cannot be determined.

9. Frequent (e.g., q1h while awake) use of preservative-free artificial tears or gel if not using frequent ointments.

10. Oral tetracyclines may also reduce collagenolysis and stromal melting (e.g., doxycycline 100 mg p.o. b.i.d.).

11. Lysis of conjunctival adhesions b.i.d. by using a glass rod or a moistened cotton-tipped applicator covered with an antibiotic ointment to sweep the fornices may be helpful. If symblepharon begins to form despite attempted lysis, consider using a scleral shell or ring to maintain the fornices.

12. Other considerations:

    —Therapeutic soft contact lens, collagen shield, amniotic membrane graft (e.g., Pro-Kera or sutured/glued), or tarsorrhaphy (usually used if healing is delayed beyond 2 weeks).

    —Ascorbate and citrate for alkali burns has been reported to speed healing time and allow better visual outcome. Administration has been studied intravenously (i.v.), orally (ascorbate 500 to 2,000 mg q.d.), and topically (ascorbate 10% q1h). Caution in patients with renal compromise secondary to potential renal toxicity.

    —If any melting of the cornea occurs, other collagenase inhibitors may be used. (e.g., acetylcysteine 10% to 20% drops q4h).

    —If the melting progresses (or the cornea perforates), consider cyanoacrylate tissue adhesive. An emergency patch graft or corneal transplantation may be necessary; however, the prognosis is better if this procedure is performed at least 12 to 18 months after the injury.

Follow-Up

These patients need to be monitored closely, either in the hospital or daily as outpatients. Topical steroids should be tapered after 7 to 10 days because they can promote corneal melting. Long-term use of preservative-free artificial tears q1–6h and lubricating ointments q.h.s to q.i.d may be required. A severely dry eye may require a tarsorrhaphy or a conjunctival flap. Conjunctival or limbal stem cell transplantation from the fellow eye may be performed in unilateral injuries that fail to heal within several weeks to several months.

SUPER GLUE (CYANOACRYLATE) INJURY TO THE EYE

NOTE: Rapid-setting super glues harden quickly on contact with moisture.

Treatment

1. If the eyelids are glued together, they can be separated with gentle traction. Lashes may need to be cut to separate the eyelids. Misdirected lashes, hardened glue mechanically rubbing the cornea, and glue adherent to the cornea should be carefully removed

with fine forceps. Copious irrigation with warm normal saline or warm compresses may be used to loosen hardened glue on the lids, lashes, cornea, or conjunctiva.

2. Epithelial defects are treated as corneal abrasions (see 3.2, *Corneal Abrasion*).

3. Warm compresses q.i.d. may help remove any remaining glue stuck in the lashes that did not require urgent removal.

Follow-Up

Daily until corneal epithelial defects are healed.

3.2 CORNEAL ABRASION

Symptoms

Sharp pain, photophobia, foreign body sensation, tearing, discomfort with blinking, history of scratching, or hitting the eye.

Signs

(See Figure 3.2.1.)

Critical. Epithelial defect that stains with fluorescein, absence of underlying corneal opacification (presence of which indicates infection or inflammation).

Other. Conjunctival injection, swollen eyelid, mild AC reaction.

Differential Diagnosis

- Recurrent erosion (see 4.2, *Recurrent Corneal Erosion*).

- Herpes simplex keratitis (see 4.15, *Herpes Simplex Virus*).

- Confluent SPK (see 4.1, *Superficial Punctate Keratopathy*).

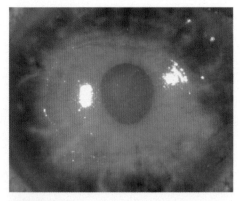

FIGURE 3.2.1. Corneal abrasion with fluorescein staining.

Work-Up

1. Slit-lamp examination: Use fluorescein dye, measure the size (e.g., height and width) of the abrasion, and diagram its location. Evaluate for an AC reaction, infiltrate (underlying corneal opacification), corneal laceration, and penetrating trauma.

2. Evert the eyelids to ensure that no foreign body is present, especially in the presence of vertical or linear abrasions.

Treatment

1. Antibiotic

   —Noncontact lens wearer: Antibiotic ointment (e.g., erythromycin, bacitracin, or bacitracin/polymyxin B q2–4h) or antibiotic drops (e.g., polymyxin B/trimethoprim or a fluoroquinolone q.i.d.). Abrasions secondary to fingernails or vegetable matter should be covered with a fluoroquinolone drop (e.g., ciprofloxacin, moxifloxacin) or ointment (e.g., ciprofloxacin) at least q.i.d.

   —Contact lens wearer: Must have antipseudomonal coverage. May use antibiotic ointment or antibiotic drops at least q.i.d.

   NOTE: The decision to use drops versus ointment depends on the needs of the patient. Ointments offer better barrier and lubricating function between eyelid and abrasion but tend to blur vision temporarily. They may be used to augment drops at bedtime. We prefer frequent ointments.
   ---

2. Cycloplegic agent (e.g., cyclopentolate 1% to 2% b.i.d or t.i.d.) for traumatic iritis which may develop 24 to 72 hours after trauma.

Avoid steroid use for iritis with epithelial defects because it may retard epithelial healing and increase the risk of infection. Avoid use of long-acting cycloplegics for small abrasions to allow for faster visual recovery.

3. Patching is rarely necessary. Patching may be helpful for comfort, but DO NOT patch if the mechanism of injury involves vegetable matter, fingernails, or if the patient wears contact lenses. Be careful that the patch is properly placed so that the upper lid is totally prevented from opening as this can cause a serious abrasion.

4. Consider topical nonsteroidal anti-inflammatory drug (NSAID) drops (e.g., ketorolac 0.4% to 0.5% q.i.d. for 3 days) for pain control. Avoid in patients with other ocular surface disease and in postoperative patients. Oral acetaminophen, NSAIDs, or narcotics (in severe cases) can also be used for pain control.

5. Debride loose or hanging epithelium because it may inhibit healing. A cotton-tipped applicator soaked in topical anesthetic (e.g., proparacaine) or a sterile jewelers forceps (used with caution) may be utilized.

6. No contact lens wear. Some clinicians use bandage contact lenses for therapy. We rarely do unless the size of the abrasion and discomfort warrants it and there is poor healing in the absence of infection. If a bandage contact lens is used, patients should use prophylactic topical antibiotics (e.g., polymyxin B/trimethoprim or a fluoroquinolone q.i.d.) and should be followed-up daily for evaluation and contact lens replacement.

Follow-Up

Noncontact Lens Wearer

1. If patched or given bandage contact lens, the patient should return in 24 hours (or sooner if the symptoms worsen) for re-evaluation.

2. Central or large corneal abrasion: Return the next day to determine if the epithelial defect is improving. If the abrasion is healing, may see 2 to 3 days later. Instruct the patient to return sooner if symptoms worsen. Revisit every 3 to 5 days until healed.

3. Peripheral or small abrasion: Return 2 to 5 days later. Instruct the patient to return sooner if symptoms worsen. Revisit every 3 to 5 days until healed.

Contact Lens Wearer

Close follow-up until the epithelial defect resolves, and then treat with topical fluoroquinolone or tobramycin drops for an additional 1 or 2 days. The patient may resume contact lens wear after the eye feels normal for a week after the cessation of a proper course of medication. A new contact lens should be instituted at that time.

3.3 CORNEAL AND CONJUNCTIVAL FOREIGN BODIES

Symptoms

Foreign body sensation, tearing, history of trauma.

Signs

(See Figure 3.3.1.)

Critical. Conjunctival or corneal foreign body with or without a rust ring.

Other. Conjunctival injection, eyelid edema, mild AC reaction, and SPK. A small infiltrate may surround a corneal foreign body; it is usually reactive and sterile. Vertically oriented linear corneal abrasions or SPK may indicate a foreign body under the upper eyelid.

Work-Up

1. History: Determine the mechanism of injury [e.g., metal striking metal, power tools or weed-whackers may suggest an intraocular foreign body (IOFB), direct pathway with no safety glasses, distance of the patient from the site, etc.]. Attempt to determine

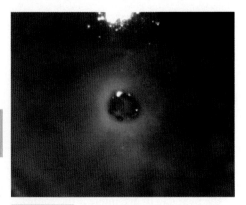

FIGURE 3.3.1. Corneal metallic foreign body with rust ring.

the size, weight, velocity, force, shape, and composition of the object.

2. Document visual acuity before any procedure is performed. One or two drops of topical anesthetic may be necessary to control blepharospasm and pain.

3. Slit-lamp examination: Locate and assess the depth of the foreign body. Examine closely for possible entry sites (rule out self-sealing lacerations) pupil irregularities, iris tears and trans-illumination defects (TIDs), capsular perforations, lens opacities, hyphema, AC shallowing (or deepening in scleral perforations), and asymmetrically low IOP in the involved eye.

NOTE: There may be multiple IOFBs with power equipment or explosive debris.

If there is no evidence of perforation, evert the eyelids and inspect the fornices for additional foreign bodies. Double everting the upper eyelid with a Desmarres eyelid retractor may be necessary. Carefully inspect a conjunctival laceration to rule out a scleral laceration or perforation. Measure the dimensions of any infiltrate and the degree of any AC reaction for monitoring therapy response and progression of possible infection.

NOTE: An infiltrate accompanied by a significant AC reaction, purulent discharge, or extreme conjunctival injection and pain should be cultured to rule out an infection, treated aggressively with antibiotics, and followed intensively (see 4.11, *Bacterial Keratitis*).

4. Dilate the eye and examine the posterior segment for a possible IOFB (see 3.15, *Intraocular Foreign Body*).

5. Consider a B-scan ultrasonography, a computed tomography (CT) scan of the orbit (axial and coronal views, 1-mm sections), or ultrasonographic biomicroscopy (UBM) to exclude an intraocular or intraorbital foreign body. Avoid magnetic resonance imaging (MRI) if there is a history of possible metallic foreign body.

Treatment

Corneal Foreign Body (Superficial or Partial Thickness)

1. Apply topical anesthetic (e.g., proparacaine). Remove the corneal foreign body with a foreign body spud, fine forceps, or small-gauge needle at a slit lamp. Multiple superficial foreign bodies may be more easily removed by irrigation.

NOTE: If there is concern for full-thickness corneal foreign body, exploration and removal should be performed in the operating room.

2. Remove the rust ring as completely as possible on the first attempt. This may require an ophthalmic burr (see Figure 3.3.2). It is sometimes safer to leave a deep, central rust ring to allow time for the rust to migrate to the corneal surface, at which point it can be removed more easily.

3. Measure the size of the resultant corneal epithelial defect.

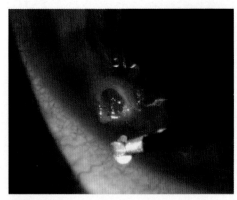

FIGURE 3.3.2. Burr removal of metallic rust ring.

4. Treat as for corneal abrasion (see 3.2, *Corneal Abrasion*).

NOTE: Erythromycin ointment should not be used for residual epithelial defects from corneal foreign bodies as it does not provide strong enough antibiotic coverage.

---

5. Alert the patient to return as soon as possible if there is any worsening of symptoms.

Conjunctival Foreign Body

1. Remove foreign body under topical anesthesia.

—Multiple or loose superficial foreign bodies can often be removed with saline irrigation.

—A foreign body can be removed with a cotton-tipped applicator soaked in topical anesthetic or with fine forceps. For deeply embedded foreign bodies, consider pre-treatment with a cotton-tipped applicator soaked in phenylephrine 2.5% to reduce conjunctival bleeding.

—Small, relatively inaccessible, buried subconjunctival foreign bodies may sometimes be left in the eye without harm unless they are infectious or proinflammatory. Occasionally they will surface with time, at which point they may be removed more easily. Conjunctival excision is sometimes indicated.

—Check the pH if an associated chemical injury is suspected (e.g., alkali from fireworks). See 3.1, *Chemical Burn*.

2. Sweep the conjunctival fornices with a glass rod or cotton-tipped applicator soaked with a topical anesthetic to remove any remaining pieces.

3. See 3.4, *Conjunctival Laceration* if there is a significant conjunctival laceration.

4. A topical antibiotic (e.g., bacitracin ointment, trimethoprim/polymyxin B drops, or fluoroquinolone drops q.i.d.) may be used.

5. Preservative-free artificial tears may be given as needed for irritation.

Follow-Up

1. **Corneal foreign body:** Follow-up as with corneal abrasion (see 3.2, *Corneal Abrasion*). If residual rust ring remains, re-evaluate in 24 hours.

2. **Conjunctival foreign body:** Follow-up as needed, or in 1 week if residual foreign bodies were left in the conjunctiva.

3.4 CONJUNCTIVAL LACERATION

Symptoms

Mild pain, red eye, foreign body sensation; usually, a history of ocular trauma.

Signs

Fluorescein staining of the conjunctiva. The conjunctiva may be torn and rolled up on itself. Exposed white sclera may be noted. Conjunctival and subconjunctival hemorrhages are often present.

Work-Up

1. History: Determine the nature of the trauma and whether a ruptured globe or intraocular or intraorbital foreign body may be present. Evaluate the mechanism for possible foreign body involvement, including size, shape, weight, and velocity of object.

2. Complete ocular examination, including careful exploration of the sclera (after topical anesthesia, e.g., proparacaine or viscous lidocaine) in the region of the conjunctival laceration to rule out a scleral laceration or a subconjunctival foreign body. The entire area of sclera under the conjunctival laceration must be inspected. Since the conjunctiva is mobile, inspect a wide area of the sclera under the laceration. Use a proparacaine-soaked, sterile cotton-tipped applicator to manipulate the conjunctiva. Irrigation with saline may be helpful in removing scattered debris. A Seidel test may be helpful (see Appendix 5, *Seidel Test to Detect a Wound Leak*). Dilated fundus examination, especially

3

evaluating the area underlying the conjunctival injury, must be carefully performed with indirect ophthalmoscopy.

3. Consider a CT scan of the orbit (axial and coronal views, 1-mm sections) to exclude an intraocular or intraorbital foreign body. B-scan ultrasound may be helpful.

4. Exploration of the site in the operating room under general anesthesia may be necessary when a ruptured globe is suspected, especially in children.

5. Children often do not give an accurate history of trauma. They and nearby observers must be questioned and ophthalmic examination must be especially detailed.

Treatment

In case of a ruptured globe or penetrating ocular injury, see 3.14, *Ruptured Globe and Penetrating Ocular Injury.* Otherwise:

1. Antibiotic ointment (e.g., erythromycin, bacitracin or bacitracin/polymyxin B q.i.d.). A pressure patch may rarely be used for the first 24 hours for comfort.

2. Most lacerations will heal without surgical repair. Some large lacerations (≥1 to 1.5 cm) may be sutured with 8-0 polyglactin 910 (e.g., Vicryl). When suturing, take care not to bury folds of conjunctiva or incorporate Tenon capsule into the wound. Avoid suturing the plica semilunaris or caruncle to the conjunctiva.

Follow-Up

If there is no concomitant ocular damage, patients with large conjunctival lacerations are re-examined within 1 week. Patients with small injuries are seen as needed and told to return immediately if there is a worsening of symptoms.

3.5 TRAUMATIC IRITIS

Symptoms

Dull, aching or throbbing pain, photophobia, tearing, onset of symptoms usually within 3 days of trauma.

Signs

Critical. White blood cells (WBCs) and flare in the AC (seen under high-power magnification by focusing into the AC with a small, bright, tangential beam from the slit lamp).

Other. Pain in the traumatized eye when light enters either eye; lower (due to ciliary body shock) or higher (due to inflammatory debris and/or trabeculitis) IOP; smaller, poorly dilating pupil or larger pupil (due to iris sphincter tears) in the traumatized eye; perilimbal conjunctival injection; decreased vision; occasionally floaters.

Differential Diagnosis

■ Nongranulomatous anterior uveitis: No history of trauma, or the degree of trauma

is not consistent with the level of inflammation. See 12.1, *Anterior Uveitis (Iritis/ Iridocyclitis).*

■ Traumatic microhyphema or hyphema: Red blood cells (RBCs) suspended in the AC. See 3.6, *Hyphema and Microhyphema.*

■ Traumatic corneal abrasion: May have an accompanying AC reaction. See 3.2, *Corneal Abrasion.*

■ Traumatic retinal detachment: May produce an AC reaction or may see pigment in the anterior vitreous. See 11.3, *Retinal Detachment.*

Work-Up

Complete ophthalmic examination, including IOP measurement and dilated fundus examination.

Treatment

Cycloplegic agent (e.g., cyclopentolate 2% t.i.d. or scopolamine 0.25% b.i.d.). May use a steroid drop (e.g., prednisolone acetate

0.125% to 1% q.i.d.). Avoid topical steroids if an epithelial defect is present.

Follow-Up

1. Recheck in 5 to 7 days.

2. If resolved, the cycloplegic agent is discontinued and the steroid is tapered.

3. One month after trauma, perform gonioscopy to look for angle recession and indirect ophthalmoscopy with scleral depression to detect retinal breaks or detachment.

3.6 HYPHEMA AND MICROHYPHEMA

TRAUMATIC HYPHEMA

Symptoms

Pain, blurred vision, history of blunt trauma.

Signs

(See Figure 3.6.1.)
Blood or clot or both in the AC, usually visible without a slit lamp. A total (100%) hyphema may be black or red. When black, it is called an "8-ball" or "black ball" hyphema, indicating deoxygenated blood; when red, the circulating blood cells may settle with time to become less than a 100% hyphema.

Work-Up

1. History: Mechanism (including force, velocity, type, and direction) of injury? Protective eyewear? Time of injury? Time and extent of visual loss? Usually the visual compromise occurs at the time of injury; decreasing vision over time suggests a rebleed or continued bleed (which may cause an IOP rise). Use of medications with anticoagulant properties (aspirin, NSAIDs, warfarin, or clopidogrel)? Personal or family history of sickle cell disease or trait? Symptoms of coagulopathy (e.g., bloody nose blowing, bleeding gums with tooth brushing, easy bruising, bloody stool)?

2. Ocular examination, first ruling out a ruptured globe (see 3.14, *Ruptured Globe and Penetrating Ocular Injury*). Evaluate for other traumatic injuries. Document the extent (e.g., measure the hyphema height) and location of any clot and blood. Measure the IOP. Perform a dilated retinal evaluation without scleral depression. Consider a gentle B-scan ultrasound if the view of the fundus is poor. Avoid gonioscopy unless intractable increased IOP develops. If gonioscopy is necessary, perform gently. Consider UBM to evaluate the anterior segment if the view is poor and lens capsule rupture, IOFB, or other anterior-segment abnormalities are suspected.

3. Consider a CT scan of the orbits and brain (axial and coronal views, with 1-mm sections through the orbits) when indicated (e.g., suspected orbital fracture or IOFB, loss of consciousness).

4. Patients should be screened for sickle cell trait or disease (order Sickledex screen; if necessary, may check hemoglobin electrophoresis) as clinically appropriate.

Treatment

Many aspects remain controversial, including whether hospitalization and absolute bed rest

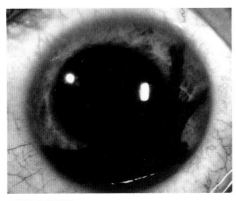

FIGURE 3.6.1. Hyphema.

are necessary, but an atraumatic upright environment is essential. Consider hospitalization for noncompliant patients, patients with bleeding diathesis or blood dyscrasia, patients with other severe ocular or orbital injuries, and patients with concomitant significant IOP elevation and sickle cell. In addition, consider hospitalization and aggressive treatment for children, especially those at risk for amblyopia (e.g., those under age 7 to 10), when a thorough clinical exam is difficult, or when child abuse is suspected.

1. Confine either to bed rest with bathroom privileges or to limited activity. Elevate the head of bed to allow blood to settle. Discourage bending or heavy lifting.

2. Place a shield (metal or clear plastic) over the involved eye at all times. Do not patch because this prevents recognition of sudden visual change in the event of a rebleed.

3. Atropine 1% solution b.i.d. to t.i.d. or scopolamine 0.25% b.i.d. to t.i.d.

4. Avoid aspirin-containing products or NSAIDs unless otherwise medically necessary. Consult with prescribing physicians regarding the need for anticoagulant therapy.

5. Mild analgesics only (e.g., acetaminophen). Avoid sedatives.

6. Use topical steroids (e.g., prednisolone acetate 1% q.i.d. to q1h) if any suggestion of iritis (e.g., photophobia, deep ache, ciliary flush), evidence of lens capsule rupture, any protein (e.g., fibrin), or definitive WBCs in AC. Taper the frequency of steroids quickly as soon as signs and symptoms resolve to reduce the likelihood of steroid-induced glaucoma.

NOTE: No definitive evidence exists regarding the use of steroids in improving outcomes for hyphemas. Use must be balanced with the risks of topical steroids (increased infection potential, increased IOP, cataract). In children, particular caution must be used regarding topical steroids. Children often get rapid rises in IOP and with prolonged use there is a significant risk for cataract. As outlined above, in certain cases steroids may be beneficial, but steroids should be prescribed in an individualized manner. Children

must be monitored closely for increased IOP and should be tapered off the steroids as soon as possible.

7. For increased IOP:

NOTE: Increased IOP, especially soon after trauma, may be transient, secondary to acute mechanical plugging of the trabecular meshwork. Elevating the patient's head may decrease the IOP by causing RBCs to settle inferiorly and clot.

—Non—sickle-cell disease or trait (≥30 mm Hg):

• Start with a beta-blocker (e.g., timolol or levobunolol 0.5% b.i.d.).

• If IOP is still high, add topical alpha-agonist (e.g., apraclonidine 0.5% or brimonidine 0.15% t.i.d.) or topical carbonic anhydrase inhibitor (e.g., dorzolamide 2% or brinzolamide 1% t.i.d.). Avoid prostaglandin analogs and miotics (may increase inflammation). In children under 5, topical alpha-agonists are contraindicated.

• If topical therapy fails, add acetazolamide (500 mg p.o. q12h for adults, 20 mg/kg/day divided three times per day for children) or mannitol [1 to 2 g/kg i.v. over 45 minutes q24h]. If mannitol is necessary to control the IOP, surgical evacuation may be imminent.

—Sickle-cell disease or trait (≥24 mm Hg):

• Start with a beta-blocker (e.g., timolol or levobunolol 0.5% b.i.d.).

• All other agents must be used with extreme caution: Topical dorzolamide and brinzolamide may reduce aqueous pH and induce increased sickling; topical alpha-agonists (e.g., brimonidine or apraclonidine) may affect iris vasculature; miotics and prostaglandins may promote inflammation.

• If possible, avoid systemic diuretics because they promote sickling by inducing systemic acidosis and volume contraction. If a carbonic anhydrase inhibitor is necessary, use methazolamide 50 mg p.o. q8h instead of acetazolamide (controversial). If mannitol is necessary to control the IOP, surgical evacuation may be imminent.

- AC paracentesis may be considered if IOP cannot be safely lowered medically (see Appendix 13, *Anterior Chamber Paracentesis*). This procedure is often only a temporizing measure when the need for surgical evacuation is anticipated.

8. If hospitalized, use antiemetics p.r.n. for severe nausea or vomiting [e.g., prochlorperazine 10 mg intramuscularly (i.m.) q8h or 25 mg q12h p.r.n.; ≤12 years of age, trimethobenzamide suppositories, 100 mg PR q6h p.r.n.].

9. Indications for surgical evacuation of hyphema:

—Corneal stromal blood staining.

—Significant visual deterioration.

—Hyphema that does not decrease to ≤50% by 8 days (to prevent peripheral anterior synechiae).

—IOP ≥60 mm Hg for ≥48 hours, despite maximal medical therapy (to prevent optic atrophy).

—IOP ≥25 mm Hg with total hyphema for ≥5 days (to prevent corneal stromal blood staining).

—IOP 24 mm Hg for ≥24 hours (or any transient increase in IOP ≥30 mm Hg) in sickle trait or disease patients.

—Consider early surgical intervention for children at risk for amblyopia.

NOTE: Previously, systemic aminocaproic acid was used in hospitalized patients to stabilize the clot and to prevent rebleeding. This therapy is rarely used now. Topical aminocaproic acid is currently under research and development. Preliminary studies suggest that it may be useful in reducing the risk of rebleeding. Further research is needed before the role for topical aminocaproic acid in the management of hyphemas can be determined.

Follow-Up

1. The patient should be seen daily after initial trauma to check visual acuity, IOP, and for a slit-lamp examination. Look for new bleeding (most commonly occurs within the first 5 to 10 days), increased IOP, corneal blood staining, and other intraocular injuries as the blood clears (e.g., iridodialysis; subluxated or dislocated lens, or cataract). Hemolysis, which may appear as bright red fluid, should be distinguished from a rebleed, which forms a new, bright red clot. If the IOP is increased, treat as described earlier. Time between visits may be increased once consistent improvement in clinical exam is documented.

2. The patient should be instructed to return immediately if a sudden increase in pain or decrease in vision is noted (which may be symptoms of a rebleed or increased IOP).

3. If a significant rebleed or an intractable IOP increase occurs, hospitalization or surgical evacuation should be considered.

4. After the initial close follow-up period, the patient may be maintained on a long-acting cycloplegic (e.g., atropine 1% solution q.d. to b.i.d., scopolamine 0.25% q.d. to b.i.d.), depending on the severity of the condition. Topical steroids may be tapered as the blood, fibrin, and WBCs resolve.

5. Glasses or eye shield during the day and eye shield at night. As with any patient, protective eyewear (polycarbonate shatterproof lenses) should be worn any time significant potential for an eye injury exists.

6. The patient must refrain from strenuous physical activities (including bearing down or Valsalva maneuvers) for 1 week after the initial injury or rebleed. Normal activities may be resumed once the hyphema has resolved and patient is out of rebleed time frame.

7. Future outpatient follow-up:

—If the patient was hospitalized, see 2 to 3 days after discharge. If not hospitalized, see several days to 1 week after initial daily follow-up period, depending on the severity of condition (amount of blood, potential for IOP increase, other ocular or orbital pathologic processes).

—Four weeks after trauma for gonioscopy and dilated fundus examination with scleral depression for all patients.

—Some experts suggest annual follow-up because of the potential for development of angle-recession glaucoma.

—If any complications arise, more frequent follow-up is required.

—If filtering surgery was performed, follow-up and activity restrictions are based on the surgeon's specific recommendations.

TRAUMATIC MICROHYPHEMA

Symptoms

See *Hyphema* above.

Signs

Suspended RBCs only in the AC, visible only with a slit lamp. Sometimes there may be enough suspended RBCs to see a haziness of the AC (e.g., poor visualization of iris details) without a slit lamp; in these cases, the RBCs may settle out as a frank hyphema.

Work-Up

See *Hyphema* above.

Treatment

1. Most microhyphemas can be treated on an outpatient basis.

2. Scopolamine 0.25% b.i.d. or atropine 1% q.d. In children, scopolamine is usually preferred.

3. Otherwise, see treatment for *Hyphema* above.

Follow-Up

1. The patient should return on the third day after the initial trauma and again at 1 week. If the IOP is >25 mm Hg at presentation, the patient should be followed for 3 consecutive days for pressure monitoring, and again at 1 week. Sickle-cell–positive patients with initial IOP of ≥24 mm Hg should also be followed for 3 consecutive days.

2. Otherwise, see follow-up for hyphema above.

NONTRAUMATIC (SPONTANEOUS) AND POSTSURGICAL HYPHEMA OR MICROHYPHEMA

Symptoms

May present with decreased vision or with transient visual loss (intermittent bleeding may cloud vision temporarily).

Etiology of Spontaneous Hyphema or Microhyphema

- Occult trauma: must be excluded, evaluate for child or elder abuse.

- Neovascularization of the iris or angle (e.g., from diabetes, old central retinal vein occlusion, ocular ischemic syndrome, chronic uveitis).

- Blood dyscrasias and coagulopathies.

- Iris–intraocular lens chafing.

- Herpetic keratouveitis.

- Use of anticoagulants (e.g., ethanol, aspirin, warfarin).

- Other (e.g., iris microaneurysm, leukemia, iris or ciliary body melanoma, retinoblastoma, juvenile xanthogranuloma, Fuchs heterochromic iridocyclitis).

Work-Up

As for traumatic hyphemas, plus:

1. Gentle gonioscopy initially to evaluate neovascularization or masses in the angle.

2. Consider the following studies:

—Prothrombin time/INR, partial thromboplastin time, complete blood count with platelet count, bleeding time, proteins C and S.

—Fluorescein angiogram of iris.

—UBM to evaluate position of intraocular lens haptics, ciliary body masses or other anterior-segment pathology.

Treatment

Cycloplegia with atropine 1% solution q.d. to t.i.d., or scopolamine 0.25% q.d. to t.i.d., limited activity, elevation of head of bed, and avoidance of medically unnecessary anticoagulants (e.g., aspirin and NSAIDs). Recommend protective plastic or metal shield if etiology unclear. Monitor IOP. Post-surgical hyphemas and microhyphemas are usually self-limited and often require observation only, with close attention to IOP.

3.7 IRIDODIALYSIS/CYCLODIALYSIS

3

Definitions

Iridodialysis: Disinsertion of the iris from the scleral spur. Elevated IOP can result from damage to the trabecular meshwork or from the formation of peripheral anterior synechiae.

Cyclodialysis: Disinsertion of the ciliary body from the scleral spur. Increased uveoscleral outflow occurs initially resulting in hypotony. IOP elevation can later result from closure of a cyclodialysis cleft, leading to glaucoma.

Symptoms

Usually asymptomatic unless glaucoma or hypotony/hypotony maculopathy develop. Large iridodialyses may be associated with monocular diplopia, glare, and photophobia. Both are associated with blunt trauma or penetrating globe injuries. Typically unilateral.

Signs

(See Figure 3.7.1.)

Critical. Characteristic gonioscopic findings as described above.

Other. Decreased or elevated IOP, glaucomatous optic nerve changes (see 9.1, *Primary Open-Angle Glaucoma*), angle recession, and hypotony syndrome (see 13.11, *Hypotony Syndrome*). Other signs of trauma include hyphema, cataract and pupillary irregularities.

Differential Diagnosis

In setting of glaucoma, see 9.1, *Primary Open-Angle Glaucoma.*

Work-Up

See 9.6, *Angle-Recession Glaucoma.*

Treatment

1. Sunglasses, contact lenses with an artificial pupil, or surgical correction if large iridodialysis and patient symptomatic.

2. If glaucoma develops, treatment is similar to that for primary open-angle glaucoma (see 9.1, *Primary Open-Angle Glaucoma*). Aqueous suppressants are usually first-line therapy. Miotics are generally avoided because they may reopen cyclodialysis clefts, causing hypotony. Strong mydriatics may close clefts, resulting in pressure spikes. Often these spikes are transient, as the meshwork resumes aqueous filtration.

3. If hypotony syndrome develops due to cyclodialysis clefts, first-line treatment is usually atropine b.i.d to approximate the ciliary body to the sclera and steroids to decrease inflammation. Further surgical treatment as described in section 13.11, *Hypotony Syndrome.*

Follow-Up

1. See section 9.1, *Primary Open-Angle Glaucoma.*

2. Carefully monitor both eyes due to the high incidence of delayed open-angle and steroid-response glaucoma in the uninvolved as well as the traumatized eye.

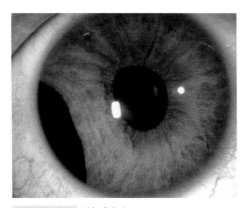

FIGURE 3.7.1. Iridodialysis.

| 3.8 | EYELID LACERATION |

Symptoms

Periorbital pain, tearing.

Signs

(See Figure 3.8.1.)
Partial or full-thickness defect in the eyelid involving the skin and subcutaneous tissues. Superficial laceration/abrasion may mask a deep laceration or injury to the lacrimal drainage system (e.g., puncta, canaliculi, common canaliculus, lacrimal sac), the orbit, globe, or cranial vault.

Work-Up

1. History: Determine the mechanism of injury: bite, foreign body potential, etc.

2. Complete ocular examination, including bilateral dilated fundus evaluation. Make sure there is no injury to the globes and optic nerves before attempting eyelid repair.

NOTE: In cases of deep eyelid lacerations, extensive examination of the underlying cornea and sclera should be undertaken to ensure no lacerations and/or corneal, scleral, or IOFBs.

---

3. Determine the depth of the laceration (can look deceptively superficial). Flip lids, and use toothed forceps or cotton-tipped applicators to gently pull open one edge of the wound to determine the depth of penetration.

4. CT scan of brain and orbits (axial and coronal views, 1- to 2-mm sections) should be obtained with any history suggestive of penetrating injury or severe blunt trauma to rule out fracture, retained foreign body, ruptured globe, or intracranial injury. Loss of consciousness usually mandates a CT scan of the brain. Depending on the mechanism of injury, the cervical spine may need to be cleared.

5. If laceration is nasal to either the upper or lower eyelid punctum, even if not obviously through the canalicular system, perform punctal dilation and irrigation of the canalicular system to exclude canalicular involvement (see Figures 3.8.2 and 3.8.3, and Appendix 7, *Technique for Diagnostic Probing and Irrigation of the Lacrimal System*).

6. Be suspicious in glancing blunt trauma to the cheek or zygoma. This type of blow puts tremendous stress on the medial canthal anatomy and may result in avulsion of the medial canthus with concomitant canalicular laceration. This type of laceration may be missed because of the blunt mechanism and because the medial canthal tissues often reapose into a reasonable position, camouflaging the extent of the injury.

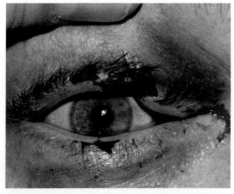

FIGURE 3.8.1. Marginal eyelid laceration.

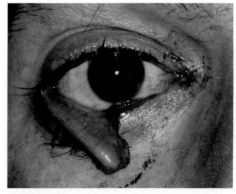

FIGURE 3.8.2. Canalicular laceration.

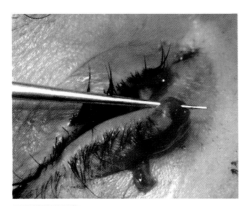

FIGURE 3.8.3. Canalicular laceration showing exposed tip after probing the punctum.

NOTE: Dog bites are notorious for causing canalicular lacerations. Probing should be performed in all such cases, even with lacerations that appear to be superficial. With uncooperative children, conscious sedation or an examination under anesthesia may be necessary to thoroughly examine the eyelids and globes.

Treatment

1. Consider tetanus prophylaxis (see Appendix 2, *Tetanus Prophylaxis,* for indications).

2. Give systemic antibiotics if contamination or foreign body is suspected [e.g., dicloxacillin or cephalexin, 250 to 500 mg p.o. q.i.d. (adults); 25 to 50 mg/kg/day divided into four doses (children); for human or animal bites, consider penicillin V (same dose as dicloxacillin)]. Continue for 5 to 7 days. For animal bites, if indicated, consider rabies prophylaxis.

NOTE: In most states, animal bites are required to be reported to the local department of health.

---

3. Assess eyelid laceration.

The following laceration characteristics are an indication for repair in the operating room and are beyond the scope of this book:

—Associated with ocular trauma requiring surgery (e.g., ruptured globe or intraorbital foreign body).

—Involving the lacrimal drainage apparatus (i.e., punctum, canaliculus, common duct, or lacrimal sac), except when uncomplicated and near the punctum in a cooperative patient. Note that repair of canalicular lacerations is not an ophthalmic emergency. Repair can be delayed for 3 to 7 days with no negative effects.

—Involving the levator aponeurosis of the upper eyelid (producing ptosis) or the superior rectus muscle.

—Visible orbital fat in an eyelid laceration, indicating penetration of the orbital septum. All such patients require CT imaging and careful documentation of levator and extraocular muscle function. Exploration of deeper tissue planes may be necessary.

—Medial canthal tendon avulsion (exhibits displacement, excessive rounding, or abnormal laxity of the medial canthus).

—Extensive tissue loss (especially more than one-third of the eyelid) or severe distortion of anatomy.

Procedure for eyelid lacerations repairable in the minor surgical environment:

4. Clean the area of injury and the surrounding skin (e.g., copious irrigation and ophthalmic povidone–iodine).

5. Administer local subcutaneous anesthetic (e.g., 2% lidocaine with epinephrine). Since direct injection of local anesthetic causes tissue distortion and bleeding, use the minimal amount of anesthetic needed or perform field blocks (e.g., supraorbital and/or infraorbital nerves).

6. Irrigate the wound aggressively with saline in a syringe and angiocath.

NOTE: Goggles or splash shields are mandatory.

---

7. Explore the wound carefully for foreign bodies. If foreign bodies are suspected, obtain CT imaging prior to initial

exploration to evaluate the depth and extent of penetration. Do NOT remove any foreign body prior to surgery if there is a possibility of globe penetration, or extension into the orbit. If there is any possibility of deeper penetration into the orbit, cavernous sinus, or brain, the patient requires an extensive preoperative evaluation and a multidisciplinary approach, sometimes necessitating angiography and ENT or neurosurgical consultation.

NOTE: Lacerations resulting from human or animal bites or those with significant risk of contamination may require minimal debridement of necrotic tissue. Contaminated wounds may be left open for delayed repair, although some believe that the excellent blood supply of the eyelid allows for primary repair. If electing primary repair, proceed to the subsequent steps.

---

8. Isolate the surgical field with a sterile eye drape.

9. Place a drop of topical anesthetic (e.g., proparacaine) into the eye. Place a protective eye shell over the eye before suturing.

10a. Marginal Eyelid Laceration Repair. Lacerations involving the eyelid margin may be repaired by using one of many methods. Two methods are described below.

10b. Nonmarginal Eyelid Laceration Repair.

—See steps 1 to 9 above. Then close the skin with interrupted 6-0 absorbable (e.g., plain gut) sutures. Avoid deep sutures. Never suture the orbital septum.

Final Steps:

11. Remove the protective eye shell.

12. Apply antibiotic ointment (e.g., bacitracin ophthalmic) to the wound t.i.d.

13. Dress the wound if appropriate and consider oral antibiotics.

Key Points:

—The most important step is to reapproximate the tarsus along its vertical axis with several sutures to allow for proper eyelid alignment and healing. Marginal repair alone will not provide structural integrity to the eyelid; the injured tarsus will splay apart, resulting in eyelid notching (see Figure 3.8.4c).

—If unsure about patient reliability or in patients who will not cooperate for suture removal (e.g., young children, patients with advanced dementia, etc.), use absorbable 6-0 polyglactin suture (e.g., Vicryl) in the margin, instead of nonabsorbable silk.

—Be careful to avoid deeper, buried subcutaneous sutures that can incorporate the orbital septum, resulting in eyelid tethering. In general, deep sutures should be avoided outside of the tarsal zone (upper eyelid = 10 mm from eyelid margin, lower eyelid = 5 mm from eyelid margin).

—Deep tarsal sutures placed anteriorly should be lamellar (half thickness), especially in the upper eyelid, to avoid penetration through the underlying conjunctiva and a subsequent corneal abrasion.

Procedure Steps—Traditional Method

(See Figure 3.8.4.)

A. Place a 6-0 silk suture from gray line to gray line, entering and exiting the gray line 2 to 3 mm from the laceration edge. (As already noted, in difficult or unreliable patients, use absorbable suture material only.) Put the suture on traction with a hemostat to ensure good reapproximation of the splayed tarsus and gray line. Leave suture untied.

NOTE: This marginal suture provides no structural integrity to the eyelid; its main function is to align the eyelid margin anatomy to ensure a good cosmetic repair.

B. Realign the tarsal edges with multiple interrupted sutures placed through an anterior approach (5-0 or 6-0 polyglactin on a spatulated needle). This is the most important step in marginal laceration closure. In the upper eyelid, 3 to 4 sutures can usually

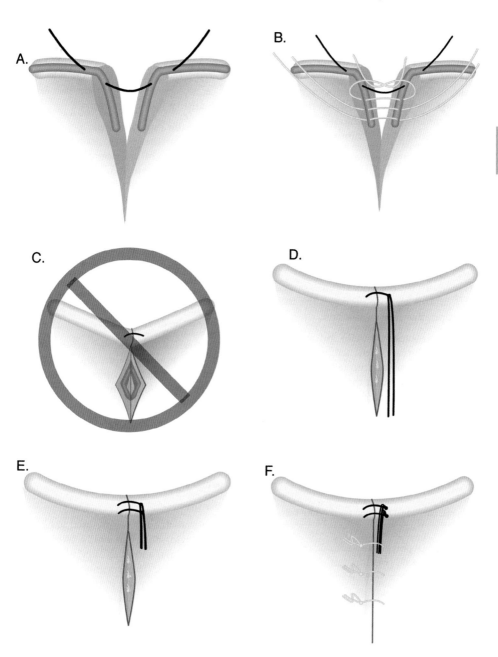

FIGURE 3.8.4. Marginal eyelid laceration repair, traditional method: **A:** Reapproximate the gray line with a 6-0 silk suture. **B:** The most important step is to realign the tarsal edges with multiple interrupted 5-0 or 6-0 absorbable (e.g., Vicryl) sutures. Take partial-thickness bites. **C:** Failure to realign the tarsus will compromise the integrity of the eyelid, resulting in splaying and notching. **D:** Tie the tarsal and gray line sutures. **E:** Place another marginal 6-0 silk suture. **F:** Suture the skin with interrupted 6-0 plain gut, securing the tails of the marginal sutures.

NOTE: If patient reliability is questionable, use absorbable (e.g., 6-0 Vicryl) sutures for every step.

3

be placed. In the lower eyelid, 2 to 3 sutures are typically the maximum. A single tarsal suture is inadequate for appropriate tarsal realignment. It is important to take only lamellar (half-thickness) bites through the tarsus and to avoid the underlying conjunctiva to minimize the risk of postoperative corneal injury.

C. Failure to reapproximate the tarsus will result in eyelid splaying and notching.

D. Tie down and trim the tarsal sutures. Tie down the marginal silk suture leaving long tails.

E. Place and tie another 6-0 silk marginal suture either anterior or posterior to the gray-line suture, again leaving long tails. Frequently, the posterior suture is unnecessary and its absence decreases the risk of postoperative corneal abrasion.

F. Use interrupted 6-0 plain gut sutures to close the skin along the length of the laceration. Incorporate the tails of both silk marginal sutures into the skin suture closest to the eyelid margin to keep tails away from corneal surface.

Procedure Steps—Alternative Method

(See Figure 3.8.5)

NOTE: In this method, the only knots are at the nonmarginal edge of the wound, eliminating the risk of corneal abrasion from suture tails.

A. Pass a 5-0 polyglactin suture, preferably on a P2 needle (small radius of curvature, spatulated), in a vertical mattress fashion through the tarsal plate to realign the eyelid margin. Ensure good reapproximation of the tarsus and gray line, then tie the suture.

B. Close the skin using a 6-0 nylon suture in running fashion beginning at the nonmar-

ginal extent of the laceration and extending towards the eyelid margin. Approaching the eyelid margin, pass the needle anterior to the lash line on one side of the laceration and come out in the lash line on the other side of the laceration.

C. Realign the anterior lamella by passing the needle into the parallel lash line on the opposite side of the laceration, and come out through the meibomian gland orifices on the original side of the laceration. Care must be taken to ensure even placement of the suture to avoid lid margin override.

D. To realign the posterior lamella, pass the next bite into the parallel meibomian gland orifices and come out through the gray line on the original side of the laceration. Then pass the needle into the parallel gray line, and come out anterior to the lash line on the original side.

E. A pattern of three parallel passes through the lash line, gray line, and meibomian gland line is thereby achieved to reapproximate the eyelid margin without any loose marginal sutures.

F. Run the suture back toward the nonmarginal extent of the laceration, crisscrossing the previously placed sutures. Tie the suture securely, its tails distant from the ocular surface.

Follow-Up

If nonabsorbable sutures are used (e.g., silk), eyelid margin sutures should be left in place for 5 to 10 days, and other superficial sutures for 4 to 7 days. The integrity of an eyelid margin repair is in the longer lasting tarsal sutures. Therefore, the eyelid margin sutures can be removed as soon as 5 days postoperatively. If a small notch is present, it can be followed over the ensuing 3 to 6 months to allow for scar maturation. A small eyelid notch will often soften and disappear on its own.

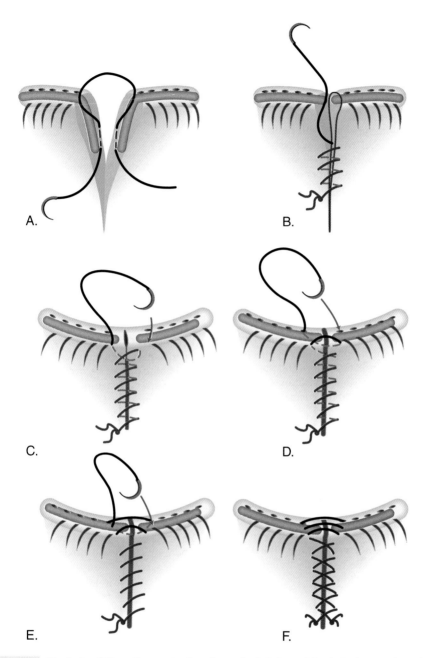

FIGURE 3.8.5. Marginal eyelid laceration repair, alternative method: **A:** Pass a 5-0 polyglactin suture in vertical mattress fashion through the tarsal plate to realign the eyelid margin. **B:** Close the skin with a 6-0 nylon suture in a running fashion beginning at the nonmarginal extent of the laceration. **C:** Pass the needle anterior to the lash line and emerge in the lash line on the other side of the laceration. Then pass the needle into the parallel lash line on the opposite side of the laceration, and emerge in the meibomian gland line on the original side. **D:** Pass the needle through the parallel meibomian gland orifices, and emerge through the gray line on the original side. **E:** Place the next bite into the parallel gray line, and emerge anterior to the lash line on the original side of the laceration. **F:** Run the suture back toward the nonmarginal extent of the laceration, crisscrossing the previously placed sutures. Tie the suture securely.

3

3.9   ORBITAL BLOW-OUT FRACTURE

Symptoms

Pain on attempted eye movement (orbital floor fracture: pain with vertical eye movement; medial wall fracture: pain with horizontal eye movement), local tenderness, eyelid edema, binocular diplopia, crepitus (particularly after nose blowing), recent history of trauma. Tearing may be a symptom of nasolacrimal duct obstruction or injury seen with medial buttress, Leforte II, or nasoethmoidal complex fractures, but this is typically a late complaint. Acute tearing is usually due to ocular irritation (e.g., chemosis, corneal abrasion, iritis).

Signs

Critical. Restricted eye movement (especially in upward gaze, lateral gaze, or both), subcutaneous or conjunctival emphysema, hypesthesia in the distribution of the infraorbital nerve (ipsilateral cheek and upper lip), point tenderness, enophthalmos (may initially be masked by orbital edema).

Other. Nosebleed, eyelid edema, and ecchymosis. Superior rim and orbital roof fractures may show hypesthesia in the distribution of the supratrochlear or supraorbital nerve (ipsilateral forehead) and ptosis. Trismus, malar flattening, and a palpable step-off deformity of the inferior orbital rim are characteristic of tripod (zygomatic complex) fractures. Optic neuropathy may be present secondary to traumatic optic neuropathy (TON) or orbital compartment syndrome secondary to retrobulbar hemorrhage (see below).

Differential Diagnosis of Muscle Entrapment in Orbital Fracture

- Orbital edema and hemorrhage without a blow-out fracture: May have limitation of ocular movement, periorbital swelling, and ecchymosis due to soft-tissue edema and hemorrhage, but these resolve over 7 to 10 days.

- Cranial nerve palsy: Limitation of ocular movement, but no restriction on forced-duction testing. Will have abnormal results on force generation testing. In cases of suspected traumatic cranial neuropathy, skull base and intracranial processes should be ruled out with CT imaging.

Work-Up

1. Complete ophthalmologic examination, including measurement of extraocular movements and globe displacement. Compare the sensation of the affected cheek with that on the contralateral side; palpate the eyelids for crepitus (subcutaneous emphysema); palpate the orbital rim for step-off deformities; evaluate the globe carefully for a rupture, hyphema or microhyphema, traumatic iritis, and retinal or choroidal damage. Measure IOP. Check pupils and color vision to rule out a TON (see 3.11, *Traumatic Optic Neuropathy*). If eyelid and periocular edema limit the view, special techniques may be necessary [e.g., use of Desmarres retractors or clean paperclips (see Figure 3.9.1), lateral cantholysis, examination under general anesthesia].

NOTE: It is of paramount importance to rule out intraocular and optic nerve injury as quickly as possible in ALL patients presenting with suspected orbital fracture.

NOTE: Pediatric patients are particularly at risk for "trapdoor" fractures, as their bones tend to be cartilaginous and bendable. Children may have a benign external periocular appearance with a remarkable paucity of eyelid signs but with significant extraocular muscle restriction (usually vertical) on examination ("white-eyed blow-out fracture" or WEBOF). Younger children often do not complain of binocular diplopia, and may simply close one eye. Further, pediatric patients may present with a severe oculocardiac reflex (nausea or vomiting, bradycardia, syncope, dehydration from an inability to eat or drink) and a vague history and may therefore be misdiagnosed as having an intracranial injury (e.g., concussion). CT evidence of an orbital fracture may be minimal, or may be missed if only a CT of the head is obtained. Alternatively, CT may

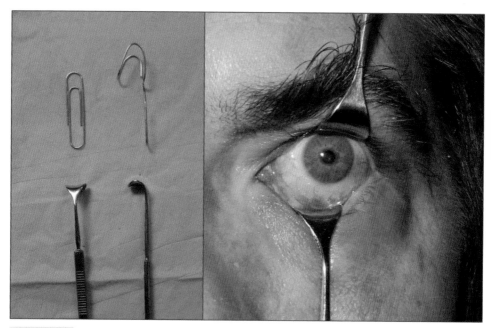

FIGURE 3.9.1. Lid retraction with Desmarres retractors or clean paperclips.

show a trapdoor fracture with rectus muscle incarceration or a "missing" inferior rectus. The narrow configuration of the typical WEBOF is often missed on CT imaging, particularly when fine cuts through the orbits are not obtained. Careful examination of coronal views is critical in such cases.

2. Forced-duction testing may be performed if limitation of eye movement persists beyond 1 week and restriction is suspected. Although in the early phase it is often difficult to distinguish soft-tissue edema or contusion from soft-tissue entrapment in the fracture. See Appendix 6, *Forced-Duction Test and Active Force Generation Test.*

3. CT of the orbit and midface (axial and coronal views, 1- to 1.5-mm sections, without contrast) is obtained in all cases of suspected orbital fractures. Bone windows are especially helpful in the evaluation of fractures (see Figures 3.9.2 and 3.9.3), including the narrow, oft-missed WEBOF. Inclusion of the

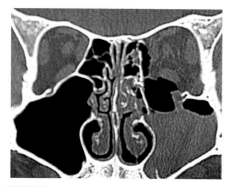

FIGURE 3.9.2. CT of orbital blow-out fracture.

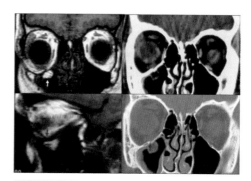

FIGURE 3.9.3. Coronal and sagittal cuts of a WEBOF in a patient with an entrapped inferior rectus.

midfacial skeleton is also recommended in such cases to rule out zygomatic complex or LeForte fractures. If there is any history of loss of consciousness, brain imaging is recommended.

NOTE: In the absence of visual symptoms (subjective change in vision, diplopia, periocular pain, photophobia, floaters or flashes), patients with orbital fractures are unlikely to have an ophthalmic condition requiring intervention within 24 hours. However, all patients with orbital fractures should undergo a complete ophthalmologic examination within 48 hours of injury. Any patient complaining of blurred vision, severe pain, or any other significant visual symptoms should undergo more urgent ophthalmic evaluation.

Treatment

1. Consider broad-spectrum oral antibiotics (e.g., cephalexin 250 to 500 mg p.o. q.i.d.; or erythromycin 250 to 500 mg p.o. q.i.d; or doxycycline 100 mg po b.i.d.) for 7 days. Antibiotics may be considered if the patient has a history of chronic sinusitis, diabetes, or is otherwise immunocompromised. This is based on limited, anecdotal evidence. In all other patients, the decision about antibiotic use is left to the treating physician. Prophylactic antibiotics should not be considered mandatory in patients with orbital fractures.

2. Instruct the patient not to blow his or her nose.

3. Nasal decongestants (e.g., oxymetazoline nasal spray b.i.d.) for 3 days. Use is limited to 3 days to minimize the chance of rebound nasal congestion.

4. Apply q1–2h ice packs for 20 minutes each hour to the eyelids for the first 24 to 48 hours and 30-degree incline when at rest.

5. Consider oral corticosteroids (e.g., Medrol dose pack) if extensive swelling limits examination of ocular motility and globe position. Some experts advise the use of oral antibiotics if corticosteroid therapy is considered, but there are no data to support the effectiveness of such a regimen.

6. Neurosurgical consultation is recommended for all fractures involving the orbital roof, frontal sinus, or cribriform plate, and for all fractures associated with intracranial hemorrhage. Otolaryngology or oral maxillofacial surgery consultation may be useful for frontal sinus, midfacial, and mandibular fractures.

7. Surgical repair should be considered based on the following criteria:

Immediate Repair (Within 24 to 72 hours)

If there is clinical evidence of muscle entrapment and nonresolving bradycardia, heart block, nausea, vomiting, or syncope. These may be present despite "negative" CT findings (see above, WEBOF).

NOTE: Patients with WEBOF require urgent orbital exploration to release any incarcerated muscle in the hope of decreasing the chance of permanent restrictive strabismus from muscle ischemia and fibrosis, as well as to alleviate the systemic symptoms from the oculocardiac reflex.

Repair in 1 to 2 Weeks

—Persistent, symptomatic diplopia in primary or downgaze that has not improved over 1 week. CT may show muscle distortion or herniation around fractures. Forced ductions may be useful in identifying bony restriction.

—Large orbital floor fractures (>50%) or large combined medial wall and orbital floor fractures that are likely to cause cosmetically unacceptable enophthalmos over time. Enophthalmos and/or hypoglobus at initial presentation is indicative of a large fracture. It is also reasonable to wait several months to see if enophthalmos develops before offering repair. There is no clear evidence that early repair is more effective in preventing or reversing globe malposition compared to delayed repair. However, many surgeons prefer early repair simply because dissection planes and abnormal (fractured) bony anatomy is more easily discernable before post-traumatic fibrosis sets in.

—Complex trauma involving the orbital rim, or displacement of the lateral wall and/or the zygomatic arch. Complex fractures of the midface (zygomatic complex,

Leforte II) or skull base (Leforte III). Naso-ethmoidal complex fractures. Superior or superomedial orbital rim fractures involving the frontal sinuses.

Delayed Repair

—Old fractures that have resulted in enophthalmos or hypoglobus can be repaired at any later date.

NOTE: The role of anticoagulation in postoperative or post-trauma patients is debatable. Anecdotal reports have described orbital hemorrhage in patients with orbital and midfacial fractures who were anticoagulated for prophylaxis against deep vein thrombosis (DVT). On the other hand, multiple large studies have also demonstrated an increased risk of DVT and pulmonary embolism (PE) in postoperative patients who are obtunded or cannot ambulate. At the very least, all in-patients with orbital fractures awaiting surgery and all postoperative orbital fracture patients should be placed on intermittent pneumatic compression (IPC) therapy and encouraged to ambulate. In patients at high risk for DVT, including those who are obtunded from concomitant intracranial injury, a detailed discussion with the primary team regarding anticoagulation should be documented, and the risks for and against such therapy should be discussed in detail with the patient and family.

Follow-Up

Patients should be seen at 1 and 2 weeks after trauma to be evaluated for persistent diplopia and/or enophthalmos after the acute orbital edema has resolved. If sinusitis symptoms develop or were present prior to the injury, the patient should be seen within a few days of the injury. If only a limited fundus examination was performed initially, it should be repeated to assure there is no peripheral retinal damage. Depending on the level of associated ocular injury, patients should also be monitored for the development of associated ocular injuries (e.g., orbital cellulitis, angle-recession glaucoma, and retinal detachment). Gonioscopy of the AC angle and dilated retinal examination with scleral depression is performed 3 to 4 weeks after trauma if a hyphema or microhyphema was present. Warning symptoms of retinal detachment and orbital cellulitis are explained to the patient.

3.10 TRAUMATIC RETROBULBAR HEMORRHAGE

Symptoms

Pain, decreased vision, inability to open the eyelids due to severe swelling, recent history of trauma or surgery to the eye or orbit.

NOTE: Most orbital hemorrhages following eyelid surgery occur within the first 3 hours postoperatively. The risk decreases dramatically after the first 24 hours, but bleeding may occur days later.

Signs

(See Figure 3.10.1.)

Critical. Proptosis with resistance to retropulsion, tense eyelids ("rock hard") that are very difficult to open, diffuse subconjunctival hemorrhage, variable degree of vision loss, increased IOP, afferent pupillary defect, dyschromatopsia, evidence of retinal vascular occlusion (boxcarring of the retinal arterioles, or signs of retinal vein or artery occlusion).

Other. Eyelid ecchymosis, chemosis, congested conjunctival vessels; often, limited extraocular

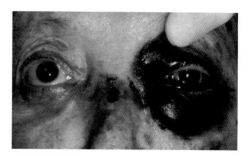

FIGURE 3.10.1. Retrobulbar hemorrhage.

motility in any or all fields of gaze. Funduscopy may show disc swelling from compressive optic neuropathy.

Differential Diagnosis

■ Orbital cellulitis: Fever, proptosis, chemosis, limitation or pain with eye movement; also may follow trauma, but usually not as acutely. See 7.3.1, *Orbital Cellulitis.*

■ Severe orbital emphysema ("tension pneumo-orbit"): Tight orbit, tight lids, crepitus, decreased extraocular motility; may follow orbital fracture with or without nose blowing.

■ Orbital fracture: Limited extraocular motility, enophthalmos or proptosis may be present. See 3.9, *Orbital Blow-Out Fracture.*

■ Ruptured globe: Subconjunctival edema and hemorrhage may mask a ruptured globe. See 3.14, *Ruptured Globe and Penetrating Ocular Injury.*

■ Carotid–cavernous fistula: May follow trauma. Pulsating exophthalmos, ocular bruit, corkscrew-arterialized conjunctival vessels, chemosis, and increased IOP may be seen. Usually unilateral, although bilateral signs from a unilateral fistula may be seen occasionally. See 10.10, *Cavernous Sinus and Associated Syndromes (Multiple Ocular Motor Nerve Palsies).*

■ Varix: Increased proptosis with Valsalva maneuver. Is not usually seen acutely, and there is usually no history of trauma or surgery.

■ Lymphangioma: Usually in younger patients. May have acute proptosis, ecchymosis, and external ophthalmoplegia after minimal trauma or upper respiratory tract infection. MRI is usually diagnostic.

■ Spontaneous retrobulbar hemorrhage: Signs and symptoms are identical to those of traumatic or postoperative hemorrhage. May occur in patients who are chronically anticoagulated or with an underlying coagulopathy from other systemic disease (e.g., hemophilia). Occasionally reported in pregnant women.

Work-Up

1. Complete ophthalmic examination; check specifically for an afferent pupillary defect, loss of color vision (color plates or red desaturation), increased IOP, pulsations of the central retinal artery (often precede artery occlusion), and choroidal folds (sign of globe distortion from severe optic nerve stretching). Assess the degree of tightness of the eyelids and any resistance to retropulsion.

2. CT orbit (axial and coronal views). When vision and/or optic nerve function is threatened, CT can be delayed until after definitive treatment has been instituted. CT rarely shows a discreet hematoma. Typically, retrobulbar hemorrhage manifests as a diffuse, increased reticular pattern of the intraconal orbital fat. The so-called "teardrop" or "tenting" sign may be seen: the optic nerve is at maximum stretch and distorts (tents) the back of the globe into a teardrop shape. This is an ominous radiologic sign, especially if the posterior scleral angle is <130°.

NOTE: Retrobulbar hemorrhage is a clinical diagnosis and does not require imaging. A delay while CT is being obtained may result in further visual compromise. Imaging can be obtained once the orbital compartment syndrome has been reversed and visual function has been stabilized.

Treatment

The key to effective management of retrobulbar hemorrhage is timely and aggressive decompression. Retrobulbar hemorrhage results in an orbital compartment syndrome, and the initial goal is to decrease the compression on critical soft tissue, mainly the optic nerve. All patients should be treated utilizing the same guidelines, even if the hemorrhage is thought to have occurred hours or days ago (unless intraoperative, there is no way to know when the orbital hemorrhage reached a critical threshold causing optic neuropathy and/or retinal ischemia).

1. If optic neuropathy is present, immediately release orbital pressure with lateral canthotomy and inferior cantholysis (see below and Figure 3.10.2). The procedure can be performed in an office or ER setting with

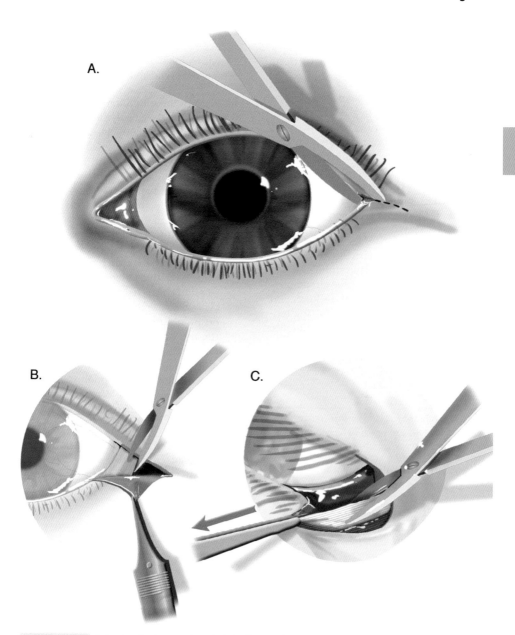

FIGURE 3.10.2. Lateral canthotomy and cantholysis: **A:** Lateral canthotomy. **B:** Grasp the lateral lower eyelid with toothed forceps. **C:** Pull the eyelid anteriorly. Point the scissors toward the patient's nose, strum the lateral canthal tendon, and cut.

basic instrumentation and local anesthetic injection. Conscious sedation can be used in the ER setting if this does not delay treatment, but is usually unnecessary.

2. If there are no orbital signs and no evidence of ocular ischemia or compressive optic neuropathy but the IOP is increased (e.g., ≥30 mm Hg in a patient with a normal optic nerve, or ≥20 mm Hg in a patient with glaucoma who normally has a lower IOP), the patient is treated in a more stepwise fashion in an effort to reduce the IOP (see below and 9.1, *Primary Open-Angle Glaucoma*).

Canthotomy and Cantholysis (See Figure 3.10.2)

The goal of canthotomy and cantholysis is to perform an adequate soft-tissue decompression of the orbit by disinserting the lower eyelid from its periosteal attachments. The retina's infarct time is approximately 90 minutes, and so decreased perfusion of longer duration as a result of an orbital compartment syndrome may lead to retinal nerve fiber death and permanent vision loss.

NOTE: A canthotomy alone is inadequate treatment. A cantholysis also needs to be performed.

---

a. Subdermal injection of lidocaine 2% with epinephrine (inject away from the eye).

b. Consider placing a hemostat horizontally at the lateral canthus and clamp for 1 minute to compress the tissue and reduce bleeding (optional step). Because of the eyelid edema and acidotic local environment, local anesthesia may not be effective. A field block may be used. The patient should be warned that the procedure may be painful, but fortunately in most cases cantholysis can be performed quickly.

c. Only two instruments are needed for canthotomy and cantholysis: A pair of blunt-tipped scissors (e.g., Wescott or Stevens) and forceps with heavy teeth (e.g., Bishop Harmon or Addson). Avoid sharp-tipped scissors to minimize the chance of globe injury. Delicate forceps (e.g., 0.12-mm Castroviejo) will not provide enough traction to effectively disinsert the eyelid and should not be used.

d. Perform the canthotomy. Place the scissors across the lateral canthus and incise the canthus full thickness (from conjunctiva to skin). Forceps are not needed for this step. This step simply gains access to the inferior crux of the lateral canthal tendon. It provides very little soft-tissue decompression.

e. Perform inferior cantholysis. With the toothed forceps, grasp the lower eyelid at the inner edge of the incised canthus. With the patient supine, traction should be directed upward, toward the ceiling. Place the scissors in an open position just beneath the skin, with the tips pointing toward the tip of the nose, and strum the lateral canthal tendon to determine its location. Begin to cut. As the canthal tendon is released, the eyelid should come completely away from the globe.

NOTE: The canthotomy/cantholysis is critical to decompress the orbit, and is done exclusively by feel. Do not search for a specific tendon or anatomic landmark.

---

f. There are several clues to a successful cantholysis. The eyelid should release completely away from the globe. Once the forceps are released, the lateral portion of the eyelid margin should move medially, usually to the lateral aspect of the limbus of the globe. If any eyelid margin still remains in its normal position lateral to the temporal limbus, the cantholysis is incomplete: keep cutting!

g. Because of the eyelid edema, the incision will bleed. Cautery is usually unnecessary. Pressure over the bone of the lateral orbital rim (but not on the globe and orbit) for several minutes will usually result in good control.

h. The results of a successful cantholysis are usually evident within the first 15 minutes. IOP should decrease and the retina should re-perfuse. Cadaver studies have shown a reliable correlation between IOP and intraorbital pressure. A significant decrease in IOP after cantholysis is indicative of a successful orbital decompression. Depending on the timing of the cantholysis in relation to the hemorrhage, vision may dramatically improve. Superior cantholysis is usually unnecessary: Cadaver studies have not shown a dramatic decrease in intraorbital pressure with superior cantholysis. In addition, superior cantholysis may result in lacrimal gland incision, which can bleed profusely. A limited orbital floor (bony) decompression using a curved hemostat placed blindly through the lateral canthotomy is also discouraged, because this maneuver may lacerate the infraorbital artery. By far the most common reason for persistent signs of orbital compartment syndrome following cantholysis is inadequate cantholysis. Make sure the cantholysis is performed effectively.

3. Close observation is indicated in all cases of orbital hemorrhage affecting visual function and in cases of acute retrobulbar hemorrhage (<6 hours), even if visual function is normal. Most cases of postoperative hemorrhages evolve over the first 6 to 8 hours. It is therefore dangerous to assume that a patient with recent injury, retrobulbar hemorrhage, and normal optic nerve function is stable enough for discharge. In such cases, it is best to follow the patient over 8 to 12 hours with frequent serial examinations in the ER or hospital.

4. Anticoagulants (e.g., warfarin) and antiplatelet agents (e.g., aspirin) are often discontinued, if possible, to prevent rebleed. This decision should be made in conjunction with an internist or cardiologist. Intravenous corticosteroids may be indicated to further decrease soft-tissue edema when no traumatic head injury is present. Antibiotics may be indicated, depending on the etiology of the hemorrhage (e.g., fracture). Frequent ice compresses (20 minutes on, 20 minutes off) are important and their compliant use should be emphasized to the patient and the nursing staff.

5. Medical IOP control as needed:

—Oral carbonic anhydrase inhibitor (e.g., acetazolamide, two 250-mg pills, not extended release).

—Topical beta-blocker (e.g., timolol 0.5% or levobunolol 0.5%), alpha-agonist (e.g., brimonidine 0.15%), or topical carbonic anhydrase inhibitor (e.g., dorzolamide 2% or brinzolamide 1%). May repeat each drop after 30 minutes.

—Hyperosmotic agent (e.g., mannitol, 1 to 2 g/kg i.v. over 45 minutes).

NOTE: A 500-mL bag of mannitol 20% contains 100 g of mannitol.

Follow-Up

In cases where vision is threatened, monitor patient closely until stable, with frequent vision and IOP checks.

Any patient with a post-traumatic orbital hemorrhage older than 6 to 8 hours with normal visual function should be instructed in detail on how to serially measure visual function, especially over the first 24 hours, and to return immediately if vision deteriorates. Wounds may be left for spontaneous healing, or be closed with a secondary canthoplasty within 1 to 2 weeks. If reconstruction of the lateral canthus is indicated, it may be performed as an outpatient procedure under local anesthesia. The inferior canthal tendon is sutured back to the inner aspect of the lateral orbital rim. Interestingly, a significant portion of eyelids will heal adequately without any surgery. If a residual optic neuropathy is present, the patient should be followed with serial examinations and visual fields. It is not uncommon for visual function to continue to improve over the first 6 months.

3

3.11 TRAUMATIC OPTIC NEUROPATHY

Symptoms

Decreased visual acuity or visual field after a traumatic injury to the eye or periocular area; other trauma symptoms (e.g., pain).

Signs

Critical. A new afferent pupillary defect in a traumatized eye that cannot be accounted for by previously existing ocular pathology.

Other. Decreased color vision in the affected eye, a visual field defect, and other signs of trauma. The optic disc acutely appears normal in most cases of posterior indirect TON. In cases of anterior TON, optic disc avulsion may be obvious on funduscopic examination unless obscured by vitreous hemorrhage. Extraocular motility may be compromised in these cases because of associated extraocular muscle avulsion or contusion. TON is often associated with intracranial injury.

NOTE: Optic disc pallor usually does not appear for weeks after a traumatic optic nerve injury. If pallor is present immediately after trauma, a preexisting optic neuropathy should be suspected.

Differential Diagnosis of a Traumatic Afferent Pupillary Defect

- Severe retinal trauma: Lesion evident on examination.

- Traumatic vitreous hemorrhage: Obscured view of retina, relative afferent papillary defect (RAPD) is rare and mild if present.

- Intracranial trauma with asymmetric damage to the optic chiasm.

- Bilateral, asymmetric TON.

Etiology

TON is typically categorized based on location of injury (anterior or posterior) and mechanism of injury (direct or indirect). Anterior TON is arbitrarily defined as occurring anterior to the entrance of the central retinal artery into the optic nerve. Direct TON is usually due to compression, contusion, and/or laceration of the optic nerve. Indirect TON is typically due to deceleration injury with shearing of the nerve and vascular supply in the optic canal and less commonly due to rapid rotation of the globe leading to avulsion.

- Compressive optic neuropathy from orbital hemorrhage: Most common TON. See 3.10, *Traumatic Retrobulbar Hemorrhage.*

- Compressive optic neuropathy from orbital foreign body: A subcategory of direct TON. See 3.12, *Intraorbital Foreign Body.*

- Bony impingement: A posterior direct TON that results from impingement of the apical optic nerve from a fracture at the orbital apex. Mechanisms vary widely. Direct bony impingement on the optic canal may result from a skull base fracture of any structure, including the cavernous sinus, with resultant cranial neuropathy (see Figure 3.11.1).

- Optic nerve sheath hematoma: Extremely rare and difficult to diagnose direct or indirect TON. Imaging may show perineural blood in the optic nerve sheath. Often a presumptive diagnosis requiring an abnormal fundus appearance, typically a combination of retinal venous and arterial occlusions (e.g., central retinal artery occlusion, central retinal vein occlusion). Progressive visual loss may occur as the hematoma expands. In most cases, optic nerve sheath hematoma is seen in conjunction with retinal hemorrhages and a subarachnoid intracranial bleed (Terson syndrome).

- Deceleration injury: The second most common form of TON, specifically known as posterior indirect TON, but often simply referred to as TON. The head hits a static object (steering wheel, handlebars, pavement) while the soft tissue within the orbit continues to move forward. Since the optic nerve is tethered at the optic canal, shearing of the nutrient pial vessels may occur with subsequent optic nerve edema within the confined space of the optic canal. Visual

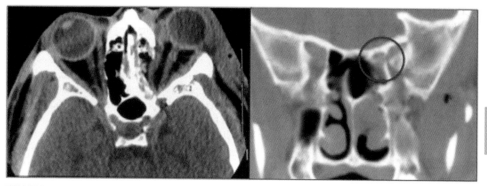

FIGURE 3.11.1. CT of bony impingement of the optic nerve.

loss from posterior indirect TON is typically immediate and does not progress.

- Others (e.g., optic nerve laceration, optic nerve avulsion).

Work-Up

1. History: Mechanism of injury (e.g., deceleration)? Loss of consciousness, nausea and/or vomiting, headache, clear nasal discharge (suggestive of cerebrospinal fluid leakage)? Past ocular history including history of amblyopia, strabismus surgery, previous optic neuropathy, retinal detachment, glaucoma, etc.?

2. Complete ocular examination including an assessment of visual acuity and pupils. This may be difficult depending on the patient's mental status, use of sedatives, narcotics, etc.

NOTE: If a bilateral, symmetric TON is present, a RAPD may be absent. In addition, if an RAPD is present, the patient may have either a unilateral TON or a bilateral asymmetric TON. Do not assume that vision is not compromised in the fellow eye, especially in comatose or sedated patients.

---

3. Color vision testing in each eye. Checking red desaturation is a useful alternative if color plates are not available.

4. Visual fields by confrontation. Formal visual field testing is helpful if available.

5. CT scan of the head and orbit (coronal and axial views) with thin (i.e., 1 mm) sections through the optic canal and skull base to rule out an intraorbital foreign body or bony impingement on the optic nerve. There may be fractures along the cribriform plate, the sphenoid sinus, and the medial wall of the cavernous sinus. A normal CT in no way rules out posterior indirect TON.

6. B-scan ultrasound if optic nerve head avulsion is suspected but is obscured clinically by a hyphema, vitreous hemorrhage, or other media opacity.

Treatment

Depends on the type of TON:

1. Compressive optic neuropathy from orbital hemorrhage: See 3.10, *Traumatic Retrobulbar Hemorrhage.*

2. Compressive optic neuropathy from orbital foreign body: See 3.12, *Intraorbital Foreign Body.*

3. Optic nerve sheath hematoma: Optic nerve sheath fenestration may be helpful in the acute stage if optic neuropathy is progressing and no other cause is evident.

4. Optic nerve laceration: No effective treatment.

5. Optic nerve head avulsion· No effective treatment.

6. Deceleration injury· Effective treatment of posterior indirect TON is, at best, extremely limited. Given the results of the CRASH study, high-dose corticosteroids should never be offered by ophthalmologists to patients with concomitant traumatic brain injury (TBI) or if the TON is older than

8 hours. In the vast majority of cases, we recommend observation alone. If steroids are considered (no evidence of TBI, injury within 8-hour window, no medical comorbidities), the lack of definitive therapeutic evidence and significant side effects must be discussed with the patient and/or family and the primary team. Dosing of methylprednisolone includes a loading dose of 30 mg/kg and then 5.4 mg/kg q6h for 48 hours. Histamine type 2 receptor antagonists should be given concomitantly.

7. Bone impingement of the optic canal: Endoscopic optic canal and orbital apex decompression may be offered in select cases, especially if the optic neuropathy is progressive. However, this option should be approached with extreme caution because of the proximity to the cavernous sinus and carotid siphon and possible bony instability of the skull base. The procedure should only be performed by an otolaryngologist experienced in stereotactic endoscopic sinus and skull base surgery. The patient and/or family should also be informed that there is no definitive data that proves efficacy of this procedure in TON and that optic canal decompression may result in additional damage to the intracanalicular optic nerve.

Follow-Up

For cases of indirect TON, vision, pupillary reactions, and color vision must be evaluated daily for 1 to 2 days, especially in cases where progression is suspected. If a secondary etiology is causing a TON, follow-up may be closer and longer, and depend on the intervention offered. If facial and orbital fracture repair is indicated, it is crucial to document the preoperative visual acuity and visual fields, and to explain to the patient and family that TON is present in order to avoid later claims of iatrogenic optic nerve injury. In comatose patients with suspected TON who require facial or orbital fracture repair, the family should be informed that only limited assessment of visual function is possible preoperatively, but significant traumatic visual compromise may have occurred. Anecdotally, mild-to-moderate posterior indirect TON may show significant spontaneous improvement over 3 to 6 months, while severe initial visual loss seems to carry a worse prognosis.

Reference

Edwards P, Arango M, Balica L, et al. Final results of MRC CRASH, a randomised placebo-controlled trial of intravenous corticosteroid in adults with head injury-outcomes at 6 months. *Lancet.* 2005;365:1957–1959.

3.12   INTRAORBITAL FOREIGN BODY

Symptoms

Decreased vision, pain, double vision, or may be asymptomatic. History of trauma, may be remote.

Signs

(See Figures 3.12.1 and 3.12.2.)

Critical. Orbital foreign body identified by clinical examination, radiograph, CT scan, orbital ultrasonography, or a combination of these.

Other. A palpable orbital mass, limitation of ocular motility, proptosis, eyelid or conjunctival laceration, erythema, edema, or ecchymosis of eyelids. The presence of an afferent pupillary defect may indicate TON.

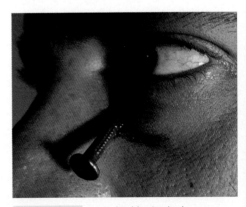

FIGURE 3.12.1. Intraorbital foreign body.

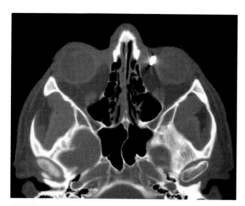

FIGURE 3.12.2. CT of intraorbital foreign body.

Types of Foreign Bodies

1. Poorly tolerated (often lead to inflammation or infection): Organic (e.g., wood or vegetable matter), chemical [e.g., diesel fuel (see Figure 3.12.3)], and certain retinotoxic metallic foreign bodies (especially copper).

2. Fairly well tolerated (typically produce a chronic low-grade inflammatory reaction): Alloys that are <85% copper (e.g., brass, bronze).

3. Well tolerated (inert materials): Stone, glass, plastic, iron, lead, steel, aluminum, and most other metals and alloys, assuming that they were relatively clean on entry and have a low potential for microbe inoculation.

Work-Up

1. History: Determine the nature of the injury and the foreign body. Must have a high index of suspicion in all trauma. Remember that children are notoriously poor historians.

2. Complete ocular and periorbital examination with special attention to pupillary reaction, IOP, and retinal evaluation. Carefully examine for an entry wound. Rule out occult globe rupture. Gentle gonioscopy may be needed.

3. CT scan of the orbit and brain (axial and coronal views, with no larger than 1-mm sections of the orbit) is always the initial study of choice regardless of foreign body material to rule out a possible metallic foreign body. CT may miss certain materials (e.g., wood may look like air). If wood or vegetative matter is suspected, it is helpful to let the radiologist know in advance. Any lucency within the orbit can then be measured in Hounsfield units to differentiate wood from air. MRI is never the initial study and is contraindicated if a metal foreign body is suspected or cannot be excluded, but may be a helpful adjunct to CT once metallic foreign bodies are ruled out.

4. Based on imaging studies, determine the location of the intraorbital foreign body, and rule out optic nerve or central nervous system involvement (frontal lobe, cavernous sinus, carotid artery).

5. Conduct orbital B-scan if a foreign body is suspected, but not detected, by CT scan. B-scan is only helpful in the anterior orbit.

6. Culture any drainage sites or foreign material as appropriate.

Treatment

1. NEVER remove an intraorbital foreign body at the slit lamp without first obtaining imaging to evaluate the depth and direction of penetration. Premature removal may result in intracranial bleeding, cerebrospinal fluid leakage, etc.

2. Surgical exploration, irrigation, and extraction, based on the following indications:

   —Signs of infection or inflammation (e.g., fever, proptosis, restricted motility, severe chemosis, a palpable orbital mass, abscess on CT scan).

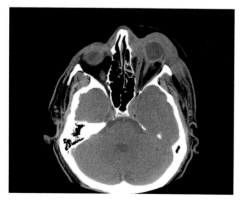

FIGURE 3.12.3. CT of intraorbital diesel fuel causing severe retrobulbar inflammation.

3

—Any organic or wooden foreign body (because of the high risk for infection and sight-threatening complications). Many copper foreign bodies need to be removed because of a marked inflammatory reaction.

—Infectious fistula formation.

—Signs of optic nerve compression or gaze-evoked amaurosis (decreased vision in a specific gaze).

—A large or sharp-edged foreign body (independent of composition) that can be easily extracted.

—Removal of an orbital foreign body should never be attempted in the setting of a ruptured globe. The globe must be repaired first. The orbital foreign body may be removed as necessary thereafter.

NOTE: Posteriorly located foreign bodies are often simply observed if inert and not causing optic nerve compression due to the risk of iatrogenic optic neuropathy or diplopia if surgical removal is attempted. Alternatively, even an inert and otherwise asymptomatic metallic foreign body that is anterior and easily accessed may be removed with relatively low morbidity.

---

3. Tetanus toxoid as indicated (see Appendix 2, *Tetanus Prophylaxis*).

4. Consider hospitalization.

—Administer systemic antibiotics promptly (e.g., cefazolin, 1 g i.v. q8h, for clean, inert objects). If the object is contaminated or organic, treat as orbital cellulitis (see 7.3.1, *Orbital Cellulitis*).

—Follow vision, degree (if any) of afferent pupillary defect, extraocular motility, proptosis, and eye discomfort daily.

—Surgical exploration and removal of the foreign body when indicated (as above). Warn the patient and the family preoperatively that it may be impossible to find and remove the foreign body. Wood is notorious for splintering on entry, and multiple procedures may be necessary to entirely remove it. Organic foreign bodies frequently cause recurrent or smoldering infection within the orbit, which may require months of antibiotic therapy and additional surgical exploration. This may result in progressive orbital soft-tissue fibrosis and restrictive strabismus.

—If the decision is made to leave the orbital foreign body in place, discharge when stable with oral antibiotics (e.g., amoxicillin–clavulanate 250 to 500 mg p.o. q8h) to complete a 10- to 14-day course.

5. Patients with small inorganic foreign bodies not requiring surgical intervention may be discharged without hospitalization with oral antibiotics for a 10- to 14-day course.

Follow-Up

The patient is told to return within 1 week of discharge (or immediately if the condition worsens). Close follow-up is indicated for several weeks after the antibiotic is stopped to assure that there is no clinical evidence of infection or migration of the orbital foreign body toward a critical orbital structure (e.g., the optic nerve, extraocular muscle, globe). Re-image patient as clinically necessary. See 3.14, *Ruptured Globe and Penetrating Ocular Injury*; 3.11, *Traumatic Optic Neuropathy*; and 7.3.1, *Orbital Cellulitis*.

3.13   CORNEAL LACERATION

PARTIAL-THICKNESS LACERATION

Signs

(See Figure 3.13.1.)
The AC is not entered and, therefore, the cornea is not perforated.

Work-Up

1. Careful slit-lamp examination should be performed to exclude ocular penetration. Carefully evaluate the conjunctiva, sclera, and cornea, checking for extension beyond the limbus in cases involving the corneal

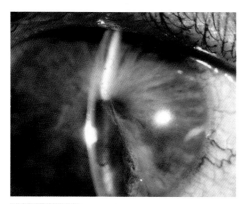

FIGURE 3.13.1. Corneal laceration.

periphery. Evaluate the depth of the AC and compare with the fellow eye. A shallow AC indicates an actively leaking wound or a self-sealed leak (see *Full-Thickness Corneal Laceration* below). A deeper AC in the involved eye can be an indication of a posterior rupture. Check the iris for TIDs and evaluate the lens for a cataract or a foreign body tract (must have a high level of suspicion with projectile objects). The presence of TIDs and lens abnormalities indicate a ruptured globe. IOP should be measured only after a ruptured globe is ruled out. Use applanation only if the laceration site can be avoided. Otherwise, use a Tono-Pen to check the IOP.

2. Seidel test (see Appendix 5, *Seidel Test to Detect a Wound Leak*). If the Seidel test is positive, a full-thickness laceration is present (see *Full-Thickness Corneal Laceration* below). A negative Seidel test indicates either a partial-thickness laceration or a self-sealed full-thickness laceration.

Treatment

1. A cycloplegic (e.g., scopolamine 0.25%) and an antibiotic (e.g., frequent polymyxin B/bacitracin ointment or fluoroquinolone drops, depending on the nature of the wound).

2. When a moderate to deep corneal laceration is accompanied by wound gape, it is often best to suture the wound closed in the operating room to avoid excessive

scarring and corneal irregularity, especially in the visual axis.

3. If corneal foreign bodies are present and superficial, treat per section 3.3, *Corneal and Conjunctival Foreign Bodies.* If foreign bodies are in the deeper cornea, there are no signs of infection or inflammation, and are well tolerated (see 3.15, *Intraocular Foreign Body,* for inert foreign bodies), they may be left and watched closely. If the patient is symptomatic or signs of infection or inflammation occur, deeper corneal foreign bodies should be removed in the operating room.

4. Tetanus toxoid for dirty wounds (see Appendix 2, *Tetanus Prophylaxis*).

Follow-Up

Re-evaluate daily until the epithelium heals.

FULL-THICKNESS CORNEAL LACERATION

(See Figure 3.13.2.)
See 3.14, *Ruptured Globe and Penetrating Ocular Injury.* Note that small, self-sealing, or slow-leaking lacerations may be treated with aqueous suppressants, bandage soft contact lenses, fluoroquinolone drops q.i.d., and precautions as listed in 3.14. Alternatively, a pressure patch and twice-daily antibiotics may be used. Avoid topical steroids. If an IOFB is present, see 3.15, *Intraocular Foreign Body.*

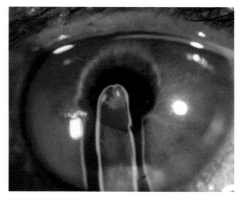

FIGURE 3.13.2. Full-thickness corneal laceration with positive Seidel test.

3.14   RUPTURED GLOBE AND PENETRATING OCULAR INJURY

Symptoms

Pain, decreased vision, loss of fluid from eye. History of trauma, fall, or sharp object entering globe.

Signs

(See Figure 3.14.1.)

Critical. Full-thickness scleral or corneal laceration, severe subconjunctival hemorrhage (especially involving 360 degrees of bulbar conjunctiva, often bullous), a deep or shallow AC compared to the fellow eye, peaked or irregular pupil, iris TIDs, lens material or vitreous in the AC, foreign body tract or new cataract in the lens, or limitation of extraocular motility (greatest in the direction of rupture). Intraocular contents may be outside of the globe.

Other. Low IOP (although it may be normal or rarely increased), iridodialysis, cyclodialysis, hyphema, periorbital ecchymosis, vitreous hemorrhage, dislocated or subluxed lens, and TON. Commotio retinae, choroidal rupture, and retinal breaks may be seen but are often obscured by vitreous hemorrhage.

Work-Up/Treatment

Once the diagnosis of a ruptured globe is made, further examination should be deferred until the time of surgical repair in the operating room. This is to avoid placing any pressure on the globe and risking extrusion of the intraocular contents. Diagnosis should be made by penlight, indirect ophthalmoscope, or, if possible, by slit-lamp examination (with very gentle manipulation). Once the diagnosis is made, the following measures should be taken:

1. Protect the eye with a shield at all times. Do not patch the eye.

2. CT scan of the brain and orbits (axial and coronal views, 1-mm sections) to rule out IOFB in most cases.

3. Gentle B-scan ultrasound may be needed to localize posterior rupture site(s) or to rule out IOFBs not visible on CT scan (nonmetallic, wood, etc.). However, B-scan should not be done in patients with an obvious anterior rupture for the risk of extrusion of intraocular contents. A trained ophthalmologist should evaluate the patient before B-scan or other manipulation is performed on a ruptured globe suspect.

4. Admit patient to the hospital with no food or drink (NPO).

5. Place patient on bed rest with bathroom privileges. Avoid bending over and Valsalva maneuvers.

6. Systemic antibiotics should be administered within 6 hours of injury. For adults, give cefazolin 1 g i.v. q8h or vancomycin 1 g i.v. q12h. Also give ciprofloxacin 400 mg p.o. or i.v. b.i.d. (fourth-generation fluoroquinolones, such as gatifloxacin 400 mg q.d. or moxifloxacin 400 mg q.d. may have better vitreous penetration). For children ≤12 years, give cefazolin 25 to 50 mg/kg/ day i.v. in three divided doses, and gentamicin 2 mg/kg i.v. q8h.

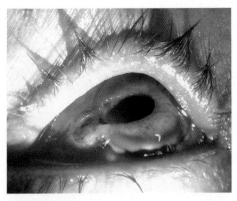

FIGURE 3.14.1. Ruptured globe showing flat AC, iris prolapse, and peaked pupil.

NOTE: Antibiotic doses may need to be reduced if renal function is impaired. Gentamicin peak and trough levels are obtained one-half hour before and after the fifth dose, and blood urea nitrogen and creatinine levels are evaluated every other day.

7. Administer tetanus toxoid p.r.n. (see Appendix 2, *Tetanus Prophylaxis*).

8. Administer antiemetic (e.g., prochlorperazine 10 mg i.m. q8h) p.r.n. for nausea and vomiting to prevent Valsalva and possible expulsion of intraocular contents.

9. Pain medicine before and after surgery p.r.n.

10. Determine the time of the patient's most recent meal. The timing of surgical repair is often influenced by this information.

11. Arrange for surgical repair to be done as soon as possible.

NOTE: In any severely traumatized eye in which there is no chance of restoring vision, enucleation should be considered initially or within 7 to 14 days after the trauma to prevent the rare occurrence of sympathetic ophthalmia.

Infection is more likely to occur in eyes with dirty injuries, retained IOFBs, rupture of lens capsule, and in patients with a long delay until primary surgical repair. In patients at high risk of infection, some groups recommend intravitreal antibiotics (see 12.15, *Traumatic Endophthalmitis*).

TABLE 3.14.1	Calculating the OTS	
Variable		**Raw Points**
Initial Vision		
NLP		60
LP/HM		70
1/200–19/200		80
20/200–20/50		90
>20/40		100
Rupture		−23
Endophthalmitis		−17
Perforating injury		−14
Retinal detachment		−11
Afferent pupillary defect		−10

NOTE: *Several studies have examined prognostic factors for ocular trauma and open globe injuries. One commonly used and validated system is the Ocular Trauma Score (OTS). See Tables 3.14.1 and 3.14.2.*

Reference

This article was published in *Ophthalmol Clin N Am*, Volume 15, Kuhn F, Maisiak R, Mann L, Mester V, Morris R, Witherspoon CD. *The Ocular Trauma Score (OTS)*, 163-165, Elsevier Limited, 2002.

TABLE 3.14.2	Visual Prognosis per OTS					
Sum of Raw Points	**OTS**	**No Light Perception**	**Light Perception/ Hand Motion**	**1/200– 19/200**	**20/200– 20/50**	**>20/40**
0–44	1	74%	15%	7%	3%	1%
45–65	2	27%	26%	18%	15%	15%
66–80	3	2%	11%	15%	31%	41%
81–91	4	1%	2%	3%	22%	73%
92–100	5	0%	1%	1%	5%	94%

3.15   INTRAOCULAR FOREIGN BODY

Symptoms

Eye pain, decreased vision, or may be asymptomatic; often suggestive history (e.g., hammering metal).

Signs

(See Figure 3.15.1.)

Critical. May have a clinically detectable corneal or scleral perforation site, hole in the iris, or an IOFB. IOFBs are often seen on CT scan, UBM, and/or B-scan.

Other. See 3.14, *Ruptured Globe and Penetrating Ocular Injury.* Also, microcystic (epithelial) edema of the peripheral cornea (a clue that a foreign body may be hidden in the AC angle in the same sector of the eye). Longstanding iron-containing IOFBs may cause siderosis, manifesting as anisocoria, heterochromia, corneal endothelial and epithelial deposits, anterior subcapsular cataracts, lens dislocation, and optic atrophy.

Types of Foreign Bodies

1. Frequently produce severe inflammatory reactions and may encapsulate within 24 hours if on the retina.

    a. Magnetic: Iron, steel, and tin.

    b. Nonmagnetic: Copper and vegetable matter (may be severe or mild).

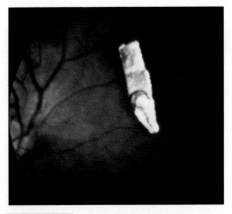

FIGURE 3.15.1.   Intraocular foreign body.

2. Typically produce mild inflammatory reactions.

    a. Magnetic: Nickel.

    b. Nonmagnetic: Aluminum, mercury, zinc, vegetable matter (may be severe or mild).

3. Inert foreign bodies: Carbon, gold, coal, glass, lead, plaster, platinum, porcelain, rubber, silver, and stone. Brass, an alloy of copper and zinc, is also relatively nontoxic. However, even inert foreign bodies can be toxic to the eye because of a coating or chemical additive. Most BBs and gunshot pellets are made of 80% to 90% lead and 10% to 20% iron.

Work-Up

1. History: Composition of the foreign body and the time of last meal.

2. Perform ocular examination, including visual acuity assessment and careful evaluation of whether the globe is intact. If there is an obvious perforation site, the remainder of the examination may be deferred until surgery. If there does not appear to be a risk of extrusion of the intraocular contents, the globe is inspected gently to localize the site of perforation and to detect the foreign body.

    a. Slit-lamp examination; search the AC and iris for a foreign body and look for an iris TID. Examine the lens for disruption, cataract, or embedded foreign body. Check the IOP.

    b. Consider gonioscopy of the AC angle if no wound leak can be detected and the globe appears intact.

    c. Dilated retinal examination using indirect ophthalmoscopy.

3. Obtain a CT scan of the orbits and brain (coronal and axial views with no larger than 1-mm sections through the orbits). MRI is contraindicated in the presence of a metallic foreign body. It may be difficult to visualize wood, glass, or plastic on a CT scan, especially acutely.

4. Gentle B-scan of the globe and orbit. Intraocular air can mimic a foreign body. UBM to inspect the AC if IOFB not visible on clinical exam (e.g., foreign body in the AC angle or sulcus) if needed. These steps should be deferred in patients with an anterior rupture or suspicion thereof given risk for extrusion of intraocular contents.

5. Culture the wound site, if it appears infected.

6. Determine whether the foreign body is magnetic (e.g., examine material from which the foreign body came).

Treatment

1. Hospitalization with no food or drink (NPO) until repair.

2. Place a protective shield over the involved eye. Do not patch the eye.

3. Tetanus prophylaxis as needed (see Appendix 2, *Tetanus Prophylaxis*).

4. Antibiotics (e.g., vancomycin 1 g i.v. q12h; and ceftazidime 1 g i.v. q12h or ciprofloxacin 400 mg i.v. q12 hr or moxifloxacin 400 mg i.v. q.d. or gatifloxacin 400 mg i.v. q.d.).

NOTE: Fluoroquinolones are contraindicated in children and pregnant women.

---

5. Cycloplegic (e.g., atropine 1% t.i.d.) for posterior-segment foreign bodies.

6. Urgent surgical removal of any acute IOFB is advisable to reduce the risk of infection. For some metallic foreign bodies, a magnet may be useful during surgical extraction. Copper or contaminated foreign bodies require especially urgent removal. A chronic IOFB may require removal if associated with severe recurrent inflammation, if in the visual axis, or if causing siderosis.

7. If endophthalmitis is present, treat as per 12.15, *Traumatic Endophthalmitis*.

Follow-Up

Observe the patient closely in the hospital for signs of inflammation or infection. If the surgeon is uncertain as to whether the foreign body was entirely removed, postoperative imaging should be considered with B-scan or UBM as above. Periodic follow-up for years is required; watch for a delayed inflammatory reaction. When an IOFB is left in place, an electroretinogram (ERG) should be obtained as soon as it can be done safely. Serial ERGs should be followed to look for a toxic retinopathy, which will often reverse if the foreign body is removed.

3.16 COMMOTIO RETINAE

Symptoms

Decreased vision or asymptomatic; history of recent ocular trauma.

Signs

(See Figure 3.16.1.)
Confluent area of retinal whitening. When occurring in the posterior pole is called Berlin's edema. The retinal blood vessels are undisturbed in the area of retinal whitening. However, other signs of ocular trauma may be noted including retinal hemorrhages.

NOTE: Visual acuity does not always correlate with the degree of retinal whitening.

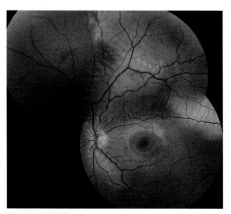

FIGURE 3.16.1. Commotio retinae.

Etiology

Contrecoup injury. Blunt trauma to the globe causes shock waves which travel posteriorly and lead to disruption of the photoreceptors. The whitening is the result of fragmentation of the photoreceptor outer segments and intracellular edema of the retinal pigment epithelium (RPE). There is little to no intercellular edema.

Differential Diagnosis

- Retinal detachment: Retina elevated associated with retinal break or dialysis. See 11.3, *Retinal Detachment.*

- Branch retinal artery occlusion: Rarely follows trauma. Whitening of the retina along the distribution of an artery. See 11.7, *Branch Retinal Artery Occlusion.*

- White without pressure: Common benign peripheral retinal finding. May be associated with a prominent vitreous base.

- Myelinated nerve fiber layer: Develops postnatally (see Figure 11.5.2).

Work-Up

Complete ophthalmic evaluation, including dilated fundus examination. Scleral depression is performed except when a ruptured globe, hyphema, microhyphema, or iritis is present.

Treatment

No treatment is required because this condition usually clears without therapy. Rarely, some patients with foveal involvement may be left with chronic visual impairment secondary to photoreceptor damage.

Follow-Up

Dilated fundus examination is repeated in 1 to 2 weeks. Patients are instructed to return sooner if retinal detachment symptoms are experienced (see 11.3, *Retinal Detachment*).

3.17   TRAUMATIC CHOROIDAL RUPTURE

Symptoms

Decreased vision or asymptomatic; history of ocular trauma.

Signs

(See Figure 3.17.1.)

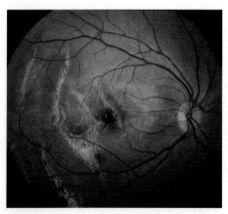

FIGURE 3.17.1. Choroidal rupture.

Critical. A yellow or white crescent-shaped subretinal streak, usually concentric to the optic disc. It may be single or multiple. Often the rupture cannot be seen until several days or weeks after trauma because it may be obscured by overlying blood.

Other. Rarely, the rupture may be radially oriented. Choroidal neovascularization (CNV) may develop later. TON may be present.

Differential Diagnosis

- Lacquer cracks of high myopia: Often bilateral. A tilted disc, a scleral crescent adjacent to the disc, and a posterior staphyloma may also be seen. CNV also may develop in this condition. See 11.22, *High Myopia.*

- Angioid streaks: Bilateral subretinal streaks that radiate from the optic disc, sometimes associated with CNV. See 11.23, *Angioid Streaks.*

Work-Up

1. Complete ocular examination, including dilated fundus evaluation to rule out retinal breaks and to detect CNV which is best seen using slit-lamp biomicroscopy with either a fundus contact or 60- or 90-diopter lens.

2. Consider fluorescein angiography to confirm the presence and location of CNV.

Treatment

Intravitreal anti-vascular endothelial growth factor (VEGF) drugs are the treatment of choice for all types of CNV. Surgical removal of the CNV, laser photocoagulation, or photodynamic therapy may be considered depending on location of CNV. See 11.17, *Neovascular or Exudative (Wet) Age-Related Macular Degeneration,* for more information on CNV treatment.

Follow-Up

After ocular trauma, patients with hemorrhage obscuring the underlying choroid are re-evaluated every 1 to 2 weeks until the choroid can be well visualized. If a choroidal rupture is present, patients are instructed in the use of an Amsler grid and told to return if a change in the appearance of the grid is noted (see Appendix 4, *Amsler Grid*). Although CNV is rare overall, ruptures that are particularly long or closer to the fovea are at greater risk for development of CNV. Fundus examinations may be performed every 6 to 12 months depending on the severity and risk of progression to CNV. Patients treated for CNV must be followed closely after treatment to watch for persistent or new CNV (see 11.17, *Neovascular or Exudative (Wet) Age-Related Macular Degeneration,* for further follow-up guidelines).

3

3.18 CHORIORETINITIS SCLOPETARIA

Symptoms

Visual loss, severity depends on region of involvement, history of high-velocity missile injury to orbit (e.g., a BB, bullet, or shrapnel).

Signs

(See Figure 3.18.1.)

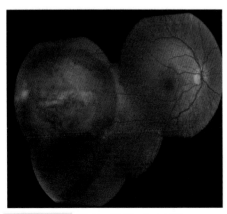

FIGURE 3.18.1. Chorioretinitis sclopetaria.

Critical. Areas of choroidal and retinal rupture and necrosis leaving bare sclera on fundus examination; subretinal, intraretinal, preretinal, and vitreous hemorrhage often involving the macula. Eventually blood is resorbed and the resultant defects are replaced by fibrous tissue.

Other. Intraorbital foreign body, "claw-like" break in the Bruch membrane and choriocapillaris. Can have associated avulsion of vitreous base which can cause peripheral retinal dialysis.

Etiology

Caused by a high-velocity missile passing through the orbit without directly contacting the globe. Shock waves produced by the missile's passage through the orbit lead to the chorioretinal injury.

Differential Diagnosis

- Ruptured globe: Severe subconjunctival hemorrhage and chemosis, often with deep or shallow AC, low IOP, and peaked, irregular pupil. See 3.14, *Ruptured Globe and Penetrating Ocular Injury.*

- Choroidal rupture: White or yellow crescent-shaped subretinal streak usually concentric to the optic nerve. No retinal break is present. Initially retinal hemorrhage in the posterior pole may obscure a choroidal rupture which then becomes apparent only over the following several weeks as the blood clears. See 3.17, *Traumatic Choroidal Rupture.*

- Optic nerve avulsion: Decreased vision with RAPD on examination and hemorrhagic depression or excavation of the optic disc if partial or retraction of entire nerve if complete. Often associated with vitreous hemorrhage. No treatment is available and visual prognosis depends on extent of injury. See 3.11, *Traumatic Optic Neuropathy.*

Work-Up

1. History: Known injury with a projectile?

2. Complete ocular evaluation including dilated retinal examination. Look for areas of retinal and choroidal rupture with underlying bare sclera. Carefully examine the conjunctiva and anterior sclera ruling out ruptured globe. Rule out IOFB. Carefully examine the retinal periphery for retinal tears or dialysis especially if the vitreous base has avulsed.

3. Protect the eye with a shield.

4. CT of the orbits (axial and coronal) to check for intrascleral, intraocular, or intraorbital foreign bodies. B-scan or UBM may be helpful to rule out intraocular or intraorbital foreign bodies.

Treatment

There is no effective treatment, and typically patients are observed. Complications, including retinal dialysis and retinal detachment, are treated appropriately. Surgery can also be considered for nonclearing vitreous hemorrhage (VH).

Follow-Up

Sequential examinations are required every 2 to 4 weeks looking for signs of retinal detachment as blood clears. Patients should be followed until an atrophic scar replaces areas of hemorrhage.

3.19 PURTSCHER RETINOPATHY

Symptoms

Decreased vision, often sudden, can be severe. There may be a history of compression injury to the chest, head, or lower extremities, but not a direct ocular injury.

Signs

(See Figure 3.19.1.)

Critical. Multiple cotton wool spots and/or superficial hemorrhages in a configuration around the optic nerve; can also have larger areas of superficial retinal whitening. Changes are typically bilateral but may be asymmetric or unilateral.

Other. Serous macular detachment; dilated tortuous vessels; hard exudates; optic disc edema, though the disc usually appears normal; RAPD; optic atrophy when chronic.

Differential Diagnosis

- Pseudo-Purtscher retinopathy: Several entities with the same or similar presentation that

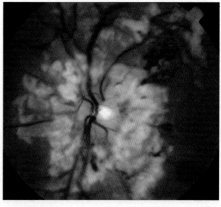

FIGURE 3.19.1. Purtscher retinopathy.

are not associated with trauma (Purtscher retinopathy by definition occurs with trauma). Causes include acute pancreatitis, malignant hypertension, collagen vascular diseases (e.g., systemic lupus erythematosis, scleroderma, dermatomyositis, Sjögren syndrome), thrombotic thrombocytopenic purpura (TTP), chronic renal failure, amniotic fluid embolism, retrobulbar anesthesia, orbital steroid injection, alcohol use, and long bone fractures.

▪ Central retinal vein occlusion: Unilateral, multiple hemorrhages and cotton wool spots diffusely throughout the retina. See 11.8, *Central Retinal Vein Occlusion*.

▪ Central retinal artery occlusion: Unilateral retinal whitening with a cherry-red spot, see 11.6, *Central Retinal Artery Occlusion*.

Etiology

Not well understood. It is felt that the findings are due to occlusion of small arterioles in the peripapillary retina by different particles depending on the associated systemic condition: complement activation, fibrin clots, platelet–leukocyte aggregates, or fat emboli.

Work-Up

1. History: Determine if there is a history of compression injury to the head or chest. If not, then inquire as to symptoms associated with causes of pseudo-Purtscher (see above e.g., renal failure, rheumatologic disease).

2. Complete ocular examination including dilated retinal evaluation. Rule out direct globe injury.

3. If the characteristic findings occur in association with severe head or chest trauma, then the diagnosis is established and no further work-up is required. However, if not, then the patient needs a systemic work-up to investigate other causes (e.g., basic metabolic panel, amylase, lipase, complete blood count, blood pressure measurement, rheumatologic evaluation).

4. CT of the head, chest, or long bones as indicated.

5. Fluorescein angiography: Shows patchy capillary nonperfusion in regions of retinal whitening.

Treatment

No ocular treatment available. Must treat the underlying condition if possible to prevent further damage.

Follow-Up

Repeat dilated fundus examination in 2 to 4 weeks. Retinal lesions resolve over a few weeks to months. Visual acuity may remain reduced, but may return to baseline in 50% of cases.

3.20 SHAKEN BABY SYNDROME/INFLICTED CHILDHOOD NEUROTRAUMA

Definition

Syndrome of intracranial hemorrhage, skeletal fractures and/or multilayered retinal hemorrhages thought due to the acceleration–deceleration forces of violent shaking. May be associated with other injuries (e.g., long bone or rib fractures). External signs of trauma are frequently absent.

Symptoms

Change in mental status, new onset seizures, poor feeding, irritability, inability to track or follow with eyes. Child is usually <1 year old and rarely >3 years of age. Symptoms and signs often inconsistent with history.

Signs

Critical. Multilayered (pre-, intra-, and subretinal) retinal hemorrhages are present in ~80%. Markedly asymmetric hemorrhages in up to 20% of cases, unilateral in approximately 2% of cases. Hemorrhages can be few in number, exclusively intraretinal, and confined to the posterior pole. In approximately two-thirds of the cases, the hemorrhages are too numerous to count and extend to the ora serrata. Macular retinoschisis (hemorrhagic macular cysts) may be seen. Most commonly associated brain lesions are subarachnoid and subdural hemorrhages.

Other. Subretinal and vitreous hemorrhage less common. Retinal detachment, papilledema, late optic atrophy, optic nerve avulsion, optic nerve sheath hemorrhage, avulsion fractures, periosteal reactions in long bones as well as many signs of acute and old trauma can be seen.

Differential Diagnosis

- Severe accidental injury: Accompanied by other external injuries consistent with the history. Even in the most severe accidental injuries, retinal hemorrhages are rare. If present, they are typically mild and do not extend to the ora serrata.

- Birth trauma: Retinal hemorrhages can be extensive but typically resolve within 4 to 6 weeks. Clinical history must be consistent. Most common cause of mild retinal hemorrhage in neonates.

- Coagulopathies, leukemia, and other blood dyscrasias. Rare, but should be ruled out. May be source of extensive retinal hemorrhages.

- Terson syndrome: Intraocular hemorrhage due to intracranial hemorrhage and elevated intracranial pressure. Subhyaloid hemorrhage is classic, but can be in any level (i.e., sub-, intra-, or preretinal, or vitreous hemorrhage). Most often after subarachnoid hemorrhage due to ruptured cerebral aneurysms. Rarely, if ever, occurs in children.

- Severe hypertension: Peripapillary retinal hemorrhages are most common. See 11.10, *Hypertensive Retinopathy.*

Work-Up

1. Obtain a thorough history from caregiver(s), separately if possible. Be alert for history incompatible with injuries or changing versions of history.

2. Check vitals and obtain systemic evaluation by a pediatrician.

3. Complete ophthalmic examination, including pupils and dilated fundus examination.

4. Laboratory: Complete blood count, platelet count, PT/INR, and PTT. Consider additional evaluation including fibrinogen, D-dimer, factor levels, von Willebrand factor, as well as other tests based on initial screening results.

5. Obtain appropriate imaging: CT or MRI, as well as a bone scan.

6. Admit patient to the hospital if shaken baby syndrome is suspected. Requires coordinated care by neurosurgery, pediatrics, psychiatry, and social services.

NOTE: Careful documentation is an integral part of the evaluation as the medical record may be used as a legal document. Ocular photography is perhaps the gold standard for documenting retinal hemorrhages, although fundus photography can be difficult to obtain and is not universally available.

Treatment

Predominantly supportive. Focus is on systemic complications. Ocular manifestations are usually observed. In cases of dense vitreous hemorrhage, vitrectomy may be considered due to the risk of amblyopia and high myopia.

NOTE: All physicians are legally mandated to report suspected child abuse. There is legal precedence for prosecution of non-reporters.

Follow-Up

Prognosis is variable and unpredictable. Approximately a 30% mortality rate. Survivors can suffer from significant cognitive disabilities, and severe visual loss occurs in 20% of children, usually from optic atrophy or brain injury.

Cornea

4

4.1   SUPERFICIAL PUNCTATE KERATOPATHY

Symptoms

Pain, photophobia, red eye, foreign body sensation, mildly decreased vision.

Signs

(See Figure 4.1.1.)

Critical. Pinpoint corneal epithelial defects that stain with fluorescein. May be confluent if severe. Staining pattern may allude to etiology. Pain is relieved by the instillation of anesthetic drops.

NOTE: Relief of pain with the instillation of anesthetic drops (e.g., proparacaine) strongly suggests corneal epithelial disease as the etiology of pain. Although anesthetic drop instillation is an essential part of the ocular examination, patients should NEVER be prescribed topical anesthetic drops and the clinician should ensure the patient does not take anesthetic drops from the office. When used chronically, these drops inhibit epithelial healing and may cause ring corneal ulcers.

Other. Conjunctival injection, watery discharge.

Etiology

Superficial punctate keratopathy (SPK) is non-specific but is most commonly seen in the following disorders, which may be associated with a specific staining pattern:

- Superior staining

  —Contact lens-related disorder: e.g., chemical toxicity, tight lens syndrome, contact lens overwear syndrome, giant papillary conjunctivitis. See 4.21, *Contact Lens-Related Problems.*

  —Foreign body under the upper eyelid: Typically linear SPK, fine epithelial defects arranged vertically.

  —Floppy eyelid syndrome: Extremely loose upper eyelids that evert easily. See 6.6, *Floppy Eyelid Syndrome.*

  —Superior limbic keratoconjunctivitis (SLK): Superior bulbar conjunctival inflammation. See 5.4, *Superior Limbic Keratoconjunctivitis.*

  —Vernal conjunctivitis: Atopy, large conjunctival papillae under the upper eyelid and/or limbus. See 5.1, *Acute Conjunctivitis.*

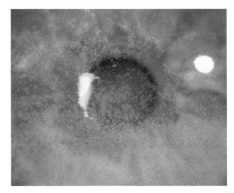

FIGURE 4.1.1. Superficial punctate keratopathy with fluorescein.

■ Interpalpebral staining

—Dry-eye syndrome: Poor tear lake, decreased tear break-up time, decreased Schirmer test. See 4.3, *Dry-Eye Syndrome*.

—Neurotrophic keratopathy: May progress to corneal ulceration. See 4.6, *Neurotrophic Keratopathy*.

—Ultraviolet burn/photokeratopathy: Often in welders or from sun lamps. See 4.7, *Thermal/Ultraviolet Keratopathy*.

■ Inferior staining

—Blepharitis: Erythema, telangiectasias, or crusting of the eyelid margins, meibomian gland dysfunction. See 5.8, *Blepharitis/Meibomitis*.

—Exposure keratopathy: Poor eyelid closure with failure of eyelids to cover the entire globe. See 4.5, *Exposure Keratopathy*.

—Topical drug toxicity: e.g., neomycin, gentamicin, trifluridine, atropine, any drops with preservatives, including artificial tears, or any frequently used drop.

—Conjunctivitis: Discharge, conjunctival injection, eyelids stuck together on awakening. See 5.1, *Acute Conjunctivitis*, and 5.2, *Chronic Conjunctivitis*.

—Trichiasis/distichiasis: One or more eyelashes rubbing against the cornea (superior SPK if misdirected lashes from upper eyelid). See 6.5, *Trichiasis*.

—Entropion or ectropion: Eyelid margin turned in or out (superior SPK if upper eyelid abnormality). See 6.3, *Ectropion*, and 6.4, *Entropion*.

■ Other

—Trauma: Can occur from relatively mild trauma, such as chronic eye rubbing.

—Mild chemical injury: See 3.1, *Chemical Burn*.

—Thygeson SPK: Bilateral, recurrent epithelial keratitis (raised epithelial staining lesions, not SPK) without conjunctival injection. See 4.8, *Thygeson Superficial Punctate Keratopathy*.

NOTE: Presence of underlying inflammation and infiltrates indicates punctate epithelial keratitis, which appears as granular opalescent devitalized epithelial cells that stain relatively poorly with fluorescein. May stain with rose bengal. May indicate a viral etiology.

Work-Up

1. History: Trauma? Contact lens wear? Eye drops? Discharge or eyelid matting? Chemical or ultraviolet light exposure? Time of day when worse? Snoring or sleep apnea?

2. Evaluate the cornea, eyelid margin, and tear film with fluorescein. Evert the upper and lower eyelids. Check eyelid closure, position, and laxity. Look for inward-growing lashes.

3. Inspect contact lenses for fit (if still in the eye) and for the presence of deposits, sharp edges, and cracks.

NOTE: A soft contact lens should be removed before placing fluorescein in the eye.

Treatment

See the appropriate section to treat the underlying disorder. SPK is often treated nonspecifically as follows:

1. Noncontact lens wearer with a small amount of SPK

   —Artificial tears q.i.d., preferably preservative free.

   —Can add a lubricating ointment q.h.s.

2. Noncontact lens wearer with a large amount of SPK

   —Preservative-free artificial tears q2h.

   —Antibiotic (e.g., bacitracin/polymyxin B or erythromycin ointment q.i.d. for 3 to 5 days).

   —Consider a cycloplegic drop (e.g., cyclopentolate 1% to 2% t.i.d., or scopolamine 0.25% b.i.d.) for relief of pain and photophobia.

3. Contact lens wearer with a small amount of SPK

—Discontinue contact lens wear.

—Artificial tears four to six times per day, preferably preservative free.

—Can add a lubricating ointment q.h.s.

4. Contact lens wearer with a large amount of SPK

—Discontinue contact lens wear.

—Antibiotic: Fluoroquinolone (e.g., gatifloxacin, moxifloxacin, or besifloxacin) or tobramycin drops four to six times per day, and tobramycin, ciprofloxacin, or bacitracin/polymyxin B ointment q.h.s. If confluent SPK, consider bacitracin/polymyxin B, ciprofloxacin, or tobramycin ointment four to six times per day.

—Consider a cycloplegic drop (e.g., cyclopentolate 1% to 2% t.i.d.) for relief of pain and photophobia.

NOTE: DO NOT patch contact lens-related SPK or epithelial defects because they can quickly develop into severe infectious ulcers.

Follow-Up

1. Non-contact lens wearers with SPK are not seen again solely for the SPK unless the patient is a child or is unreliable. Reliable patients are told to return if their symptoms worsen or do not improve within 2 to 3 days. When underlying ocular disease is responsible for the SPK, follow-up is in accordance with the guidelines for the underlying problem.

2. Contact lens wearers with a large amount of SPK are seen daily until significant improvement is demonstrated. Contact lenses are not to be worn until the condition clears. Antibiotics may be discontinued when the SPK resolves. The patient's contact lens regimen (e.g., wearing time, cleaning routine) must be corrected or the contact lenses changed if either is thought to be responsible (see 4.21, *Contact Lens-Related Problems*). Contact lens wearers with a small amount of SPK are rechecked in several days to 1 week, depending on their symptoms and degree of SPK.

NOTE: Contact lens wearers should be told not to wear their lenses when their eyes feel irritated.

4.2 RECURRENT CORNEAL EROSION

Symptoms

Recurrent attacks of acute ocular pain, photophobia, foreign body sensation, and tearing. Typically occur at the time of awakening, when the eyelids are rubbed or opened. There is often a history of prior corneal abrasion in the involved eye. The unpredictability of recurrent erosions may cause patients intense anxiety.

Signs

Critical. Localized roughening of the corneal epithelium (fluorescein dye may lightly outline the area) or a corneal abrasion. Epithelial changes may resolve within hours of the onset of symptoms so that an abnormality is difficult to detect or absent when the patient is examined.

Other. Corneal epithelial dots or small cysts (microcysts), a fingerprint pattern, or maplike lines may be seen in both eyes if epithelial basement membrane (map–dot–fingerprint) dystrophy is present.

Etiology

Damage to the corneal epithelium or epithelial basement membrane from one of the following:

- Anterior corneal dystrophy: e.g., epithelial basement membrane (most common), Reis–Bücklers, and Meesmann dystrophies.

- Previous traumatic corneal abrasion: Injury may have been years before the current presentation.

- Stromal corneal dystrophy: Lattice, granular, and macular dystrophies.

- Corneal degeneration: Band keratopathy, Salzmann nodular degeneration.

- Keratorefractive, corneal transplant, or cataract surgery.

Work-Up

1. History: History of a corneal abrasion? Ocular surgery? Family history (corneal dystrophy)?

2. Slit-lamp examination with fluorescein staining (visualization of abnormal basement membrane lines may be enhanced by staining the tear film thickly with fluorescein and looking for areas of rapid tear break-up, referred to as "negative staining").

Treatment

1. Acute episode: Cycloplegic drop (e.g., cyclopentolate 1%) and antibiotic ointment (e.g., erythromycin, bacitracin) four to six times daily. Can use 5% sodium chloride ointment q.i.d. in addition to antibiotic ointment. If the defect is large, a pressure patch or bandage contact lens and topical antibiotic drops q.i.d. may be placed (NEVER patch contact lens wearers). Oral analgesics as needed.

2. Never prescribe topical anesthetic drops for home use.

3. After epithelial healing is complete, artificial tears four to eight times per day and artificial tear ointment q.h.s. for at least 3 to 6 months, or 5% sodium chloride drops four times per day and 5% sodium chloride ointment q.h.s. for at least 3 to 6 months.

4. If the corneal epithelium is loose or heaped and is not healing, consider epithelial debridement. Apply a topical anesthetic (e.g., proparacaine) and use a sterile cotton-tipped applicator or cellulose sponge to gently remove the loose epithelium.

5. For erosions not responsive to the preceding treatment, consider the following:

—Prophylactic medical treatment with 5% sodium chloride ointment q.h.s. or oral doxycycline (matrix metalloproteinase inhibitor) 50 mg b.i.d. with or without a short course of topical corticosteroid drops (e.g., fluorometholone 0.1% b.i.d. to q.i.d. for 2 to 4 weeks).

—Extended-wear bandage soft contact lens for several months with a topical antibiotic until epithelial adhesion is obtained.

—Anterior stromal puncture can be applied to localized erosions, often after trauma, outside the visual axis in cooperative patients. It can be performed with or without an intact epithelium. Stromal puncture may be applied manually at the slit lamp or more recently with a Nd:YAG laser. This treatment may cause small permanent corneal scars that are usually of no visual significance.

—Epithelial debridement with diamond burr polishing of Bowman membrane. Effective for large areas of epithelial irregularity and lesions in the visual axis.

—Phototherapeutic keratectomy (PTK): Excimer laser ablation of the superficial stroma is successful in up to 90% of patients with recurrent erosions. Diamond burr polishing is at least as effective.

—Other treatment options may include alcohol delamination of the corneal epithelium and autologous serum drops.

Follow-Up

Every 1 to 2 days until the epithelium has healed, and then every 1 to 3 months, depending on the severity and frequency of the episodes.

4.3 DRY-EYE SYNDROME

Symptoms

Burning, dryness, foreign body sensation, mildly to moderately decreased vision, excess tearing. Often exacerbated by smoke, wind, heat, low humidity, or prolonged use of the eye (commonly when working on a computer). May worsen later in the day. Usually bilateral and chronic (although patients sometimes are seen with recent onset in one eye). Discomfort often out of proportion to clinical signs.

Signs

Critical.

- Scanty or irregular tear meniscus seen at the inferior eyelid margin: The normal meniscus should be at least 1 mm in height and have a convex shape.

- Decreased tear break-up time (measured from a blink to the appearance of a tear film defect, by using fluorescein stain): Less than 10 seconds indicates tear film instability.

NOTE: Tear film defects must be randomly located, as isolated areas of repeated early tear break-up may indicate a focal corneal surface irregularity.

Other. Punctate corneal or conjunctival fluorescein, rose bengal, or lissamine green staining; usually inferiorly or in the interpalpebral area. Excess mucus or debris in the tear film and filaments on the cornea may be found in severe cases.

Differential Diagnosis

See 4.1, *Superficial Punctate Keratopathy.*

Etiology

- Idiopathic: Commonly found in menopausal and postmenopausal women.

  —Evaporative: Outer lipid layer tear deficiency; often associated with blepharitis or meibomian gland dystrophy.

  —Hyposecretory: Middle aqueous layer tear deficiency; production decrease with age.

  —Combination: Often an inner mucin layer tear deficiency.

- Lifestyle related: Arid climate, allergen exposure, smoking, extended periods of reading/computer work/television viewing.

- Connective tissue diseases: e.g., Sjögren syndrome, rheumatoid arthritis, Wegener granulomatosis, systemic lupus erythematosus.

- Conjunctival scarring: e.g., ocular cicatricial pemphigoid, Stevens–Johnson syndrome, trachoma, chemical burn.

- Drugs: e.g., oral contraceptives, anticholinergics, antihistamines, antiarrhythmics, antipsychotics, antispasmotics, tricyclic antidepressants, beta blockers, diuretics, retinoids, selective serotonin reuptake inhibitors, chemotherapy.

- Infiltration of the lacrimal glands: e.g., sarcoidosis, tumor.

- Post-radiation fibrosis of the lacrimal glands.

- Vitamin A deficiency: Usually from malnutrition, intestinal malabsorption, or bariatric surgery. See 13.7, *Vitamin A Deficiency.*

- After laser in situ keratomileusis (LASIK): Likely secondary to disruption of corneal nerves and interference with normal reflex tearing.

Work-Up

1. History and external examination to detect underlying etiology.

2. Slit-lamp examination with fluorescein stain to examine the tear meniscus and tear break-up time. May also use rose bengal or lissamine green stain to examine the cornea and conjunctiva.

3. Schirmer test. Technique: After drying the eye of excess tears, Schirmer filter paper is placed at the junction of the middle and lateral one-third of the lower eyelid in each eye for 5 minutes. Eyes are to remain open with normal blinking.

—Unanesthetized: Measures basal and reflex tearing. Normal is wetting of at least 15 mm in 5 minutes.

—Anesthetized: Topical anesthetic (e.g., proparacaine) is applied before drying the eye and placing the filter paper. Measures basal tearing only. Abnormal is wetting of 5 mm or less in 5 minutes. Less than 10 mm may be considered borderline. We prefer the less irritating anesthetized method.

Treatment

Mild Dry Eye

Artificial tears q.i.d.

Moderate Dry Eye

1. Increase the frequency of artificial tear application up to q1–2h; use unit dose preservative-free artificial tears.

2. Add a lubricating ointment or gel q.h.s.

3. Lifestyle modification (e.g., humidifiers and smoking cessation).

4. Cyclosporine 0.05% b.i.d. is effective for patients with chronic dry eye and decreased tears secondary to ocular inflammation. Cyclosporine often burns with application for the first several weeks and takes 1 to 3 months for significant clinical improvement. To hasten improvement and lessen side effects, consider treating patients concomitantly with a mild topical corticosteroid drop (e.g., loteprednol 0.5%) b.i.d. to q.i.d. for 1 month while beginning cyclosporine therapy.

5. If these measures are inadequate or impractical, consider punctal occlusion. Use collagen inserts (temporary) or silicone or acrylic plugs (reversible). Be sure any inflammatory component including blepharitis is treated prior to punctal occlusion.

Severe Dry Eye

1. Cyclosporine 0.05%, as described earlier.

2. Punctal occlusion, as described earlier (both lower and upper puncta if necessary), and preservative-free artificial tears up to q1–2h as needed. Consider permanent occlusion by thermal cautery if plugs fall out.

3. Add lubricating ointment or gel b.i.d. to q.i.d., p.r.n.

4. Moisture chamber (plastic film sealed at orbital rim) or goggles with lubrication at night.

5. If mucus strands or filaments are present, remove with forceps and consider 10% acetylcysteine q.i.d.

6. Other therapies may include oral flaxseed oil, oral omega-3 fatty acids, autologous serum tears, topical vitamin A, bandage contact lens, or a scleral lens.

7. Consider a permanent lateral tarsorrhaphy if all of the previous measures fail. A temporary adhesive tape tarsorrhaphy (to tape the lateral one-third of the eyelid closed) can also be used, pending a surgical tarsorrhaphy.

NOTE:

1. In addition to treating the dry eye, treatment for contributing disorders (e.g., blepharitis, exposure keratopathy) should be instituted if these conditions are present.

2. Always use preservative-free artificial tears if dosing is more frequent than q.i.d. to prevent preservative toxicity.

3. If the history suggests the presence of a connective tissue disease (e.g., history of arthritic pain, dry mouth), referral should be made to an internist or rheumatologist for further evaluation.

Follow-Up

In days to months, depending on the severity of the drying changes and the symptoms. Anyone with severe dry eyes caused by an underlying chronic systemic disease (e.g., rheumatoid arthritis, sarcoidosis, ocular pemphigoid) may need to be monitored more closely.

NOTE: Patients with significant dry eye should be discouraged from contact lens wear and LASIK surgery. However, daily disposable contact lenses can be successful if fit loosely and combined with cyclosporine 0.05% and plugs, if needed.

Patients with Sjögren syndrome have an increased incidence of lymphoma and mucous membrane problems and may require internal medicine, rheumatologic, dental, and gynecologic follow-up.

FILAMENTARY KERATOPATHY

Symptoms

Moderate-to-severe pain, red eye, foreign body sensation, photophobia.

Signs

Critical. Short fluorescein-staining strands of epithelial cells and mucus attached to the anterior surface of the cornea at one end of the strand.

Other. Conjunctival injection, poor tear film, punctate epithelial defects.

Etiology

- Dry-eye syndrome: Most common cause. See 4.3, *Dry-Eye Syndrome.*

- Superior limbic keratoconjunctivitis: Filaments are located in the superior cornea, in association with superior conjunctival injection and fluorescein staining, and with superior corneal pannus. See 5.4, *Superior Limbic Keratoconjunctivitis.*

- Recurrent corneal erosions: Recurrent spontaneous corneal abrasions often occurring upon awakening. See 4.2, *Recurrent Corneal Erosion.*

- Adjacent to irregular corneal surface (e.g., postoperative, near a surgical wound).

- Patching: e.g., postoperative, after corneal abrasions.

- Neurotrophic keratopathy: See 4.6, *Neurotrophic Keratopathy.*

- Chronic bullous keratopathy: See 4.28, *Aphakic Bullous Keratopathy/Pseudophakic Bullous Keratopathy.*

Work-Up

1. History, especially for the previously mentioned conditions.

2. Slit-lamp examination with fluorescein staining.

Treatment

1. Treat the underlying condition.

2. Consider debridement of the filaments. After applying topical anesthesia (e.g., proparacaine), gently remove filaments at their base with fine forceps or a cotton-tipped applicator. This gives temporary relief, but the filaments will recur if the underlying etiology is not treated.

3. Lubrication with one of the following regimens:

   —Preservative-free artificial tears six to eight times per day and lubricating ointment q.h.s.

   —Punctal occlusion.

   —Acetylcysteine 10% q.i.d.

   _____

   NOTE: Acetylcysteine is not commercially available as a drop but can be made by a compounding pharmacy.

   _____

4. If the symptoms are severe or treatment fails, then consider a bandage soft contact lens (unless the patient has severe dry eyes). Extended-wear bandage soft contact lenses may need to be worn for weeks to months. Consider concomitant topical antibiotic use.

Follow-Up

In 1 to 4 weeks, if the condition is not improved, consider repeating the filament removal or applying a bandage soft contact lens. Long-term lubrication must be maintained if the underlying condition cannot be eliminated.

4.5   EXPOSURE KERATOPATHY

Symptoms

Ocular irritation, burning, foreign body sensation, and redness of one or both eyes. Usually worse in the morning.

Signs

Critical. Inadequate blinking or closure of the eyelids, leading to corneal drying. Punctate epithelial defects are found in the lower one-third of the cornea or as a horizontal band in the region of the palpebral fissure (see Figure 4.5.1).

Other. Conjunctival injection and chemosis, corneal erosion, infiltrate or ulcer, eyelid deformity, or abnormal eyelid closure.

Etiology

- Seventh nerve palsy: Orbicularis oculi weakness (e.g., Bell palsy). See 10.9, *Isolated Seventh Nerve Palsy.*

- Sedation or altered mental status.

- Eyelid deformity: e.g., ectropion or eyelid scarring from trauma, chemical burn, or herpes zoster ophthalmicus (HZO).

- Nocturnal lagophthalmos: Failure to close the eyes during sleep.

- Proptosis: e.g., due to an orbital process, such as thyroid eye disease. See 7.1, *Orbital Disease.*

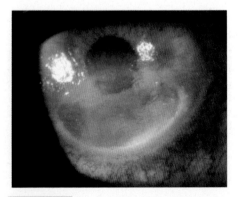

FIGURE 4.5.1. Exposure keratopathy with fluorescein.

- After ptosis repair or blepharoplasty procedures.

- Floppy eyelid syndrome: See 6.6, *Floppy Eyelid Syndrome.*

- Poor blink from Parkinson disease.

Work-Up

1. History: Previous Bell palsy or eyelid surgery? Thyroid disease?

2. Evaluate eyelid closure and corneal exposure. Ask the patient to close his or her eyes gently (as if sleeping). Assess Bell phenomenon (the patient is asked to close the eyelids forcefully against resistance; abnormal when the eyes do not rotate upward). Check for eyelid laxity.

3. Check corneal sensation before instillation of anesthetic drops. If sensation is decreased, there is greater risk for corneal complications.

4. Slit-lamp examination: Evaluate the tear film and corneal integrity with fluorescein dye. Look for signs of secondary infection (e.g., corneal infiltrate, anterior chamber reaction, severe conjunctival injection).

5. Investigate any underlying disorder (e.g., etiology of seventh nerve palsy).

Treatment

Prevention is critical. All patients who are sedated or obtunded are at risk for exposure keratopathy and should receive lubrication as recommended in the following.

In the presence of secondary corneal infection, see 4.11, *Bacterial Keratitis.*

1. Correct any underlying disorder.

2. Preservative-free artificial tears q2–6h. Punctal occlusion with plugs may also be considered.

3. Lubricating ointment q.h.s. or q.i.d.

4. Consider eyelid taping or patching q.h.s. to maintain the eyelids in the closed position. If severe, consider taping the lateral

one-third of the eyelids closed (leaving the visual axis open) during the day. Taping is rarely definitive but may be tried when the underlying disorder is thought to be temporary.

5. When maximal medical therapy fails to prevent progressive corneal deterioration, one of the following surgical procedures may be beneficial:

—Partial tarsorrhaphy (eyelids sewn together).

—Eyelid reconstruction (e.g., for ectropion).

—Eyelid gold weight implant (e.g., for seventh nerve palsy).

—Orbital decompression (e.g., for proptosis).

—Conjunctival flap or amniotic membrane graft (for severe corneal decompensation if the preceding fail).

Follow-Up

Reevaluate every 1 to 2 days in the presence of corneal ulceration. Less frequent examinations (e.g., in weeks to months) are required for less severe corneal disease.

4.6 NEUROTROPHIC KERATOPATHY

Symptoms

Red eye, foreign body sensation, swollen eyelid.

Signs

Critical. Loss of corneal sensation, epithelial defects with fluorescein staining.

Other.

- Early: Perilimbal injection progressing to corneal punctate epithelial defects or a frank nonhealing epithelial defect with rolled edges, stromal edema, and Descemet folds.

- Late: Corneal ulcer with associated iritis. The ulcer often has a gray, heaped-up epithelial border, tends to be in the lower one-half of the cornea, and is horizontally oval. A descemetocele (corneal stromal loss down to Descemet membrane) or perforation may occur.

Differential Diagnosis

See 4.1, *Superficial Punctate Keratopathy.*

Etiology

- Postinfection with varicella zoster virus (VZV) or herpes simplex virus (HSV).
- Post-LASIK (or other refractive) eye surgery.
- Chronic contact lens wear.

- Stroke, multiple sclerosis, Riley–Day syndrome.
- Diabetic neuropathy.
- Extensive panretinal photocoagulation: may damage the long ciliary nerves.
- Complication of trigeminal nerve or dental surgery.
- Complication of irradiation to the eye or an adnexal structure.
- Tumor (especially an acoustic neuroma).
- Topical anesthetic abuse.
- Chronic topical medications (e.g., timolol, diclofenac, sulfacetamide).
- Crack keratopathy: Often bilateral. Take careful history for crack cocaine smoking or potential exposure. Often helpful to admit patient and remove them from their environment.

Work-Up

1. History: Previous episodes of a red and painful eye (herpes)? Previous ocular shingles rash? Diabetes? Previous irradiation, stroke, or hearing problem? Previous refractive procedure or other eye surgery?

4

2. Prior to anesthesia instillation, test corneal sensation bilaterally with a sterile cotton wisp.

3. Slit-lamp examination with fluorescein staining of cornea and conjunctiva.

4. Check the skin for herpetic lesions or scars from a previous herpes zoster infection.

5. Look for signs of a corneal exposure problem (e.g., inability to close an eyelid, seventh nerve palsy, absent Bell phenomenon).

6. If suspicious of a central nervous system lesion, obtain a computed tomography (CT) or magnetic resonance imaging (MRI) of the brain.

Treatment

1. Mild-to-moderate punctate epithelial staining: Preservative-free artificial tears q2–4h and artificial tear ointment q.h.s. Consider punctal plugs.

2. Small corneal epithelial defect: Antibiotic ointment (e.g., erythromycin or bacitracin) four to eight times per day for 3 to 5 days or until resolved. Usually requires prolonged artificial tear treatment, as described previously.

3. Corneal ulcer: See 4.11, *Bacterial Keratitis,* for the work-up and treatment of an infected ulcer. Antibiotic ointment q2h without patching may be used. Alterna-

tively, if the ulcer is sterile, apply antibiotic ointment, cycloplegic drop, and a pressure patch and re-evaluate in 24 hours. Repeat procedure daily until healed. Collagenase inhibitors (e.g., topical acetylcysteine, oral tetracyclines) may promote re-epithelization. A tarsorrhaphy (eyelids sewn together), bandage soft contact lens, conjunctival flap, amniotic membrane graft, or keratoprosthesis may be required. Autologous serum, albumin, or umbilical cord serum eye drops may also be beneficial.

NOTE: Patients with neurotrophic keratopathy and corneal exposure often do not respond to treatment unless a tarsorrhaphy is performed. A temporary adhesive tape tarsorrhaphy (the lateral one-third of the eyelid is taped closed) may be beneficial, pending more definitive treatment.

Follow-Up

1. Mild-to-moderate epithelial staining: In 3 to 14 days.

2. Corneal epithelial defect: Every 1 to 3 days until improvement demonstrated, and then every 5 to 7 days until resolved.

3. Corneal ulcer: Daily until significant improvement is demonstrated. Hospitalization may be required for severe ulcers (see 4.11, *Bacterial Keratitis*).

4.7 THERMAL/ULTRAVIOLET KERATOPATHY

Symptoms

Moderate-to-severe ocular pain, foreign body sensation, red eye, tearing, photophobia, blurred vision; often a history of welding or using a sunlamp without adequate protective eyewear. Symptoms typically worse 6 to 12 hours after the exposure. Usually bilateral.

Signs

Critical. Confluent punctate epithelial defects in an interpalpebral distribution, seen with fluorescein staining.

Other. Conjunctival injection, mild-to-moderate eyelid edema, mild-to-no corneal edema, relatively miotic pupils that react sluggishly, and mild anterior chamber reaction.

Differential Diagnosis

■ Toxic epithelial keratopathy from exposure to a chemical (e.g., solvents, alcohol) or drug (e.g., neomycin, gentamicin, antiviral agents).

■ Exposure keratopathy: Poor eyelid closure. See 4.5, *Exposure Keratopathy.*

- Floppy eyelid syndrome: Loose upper eyelids that evert easily during sleep. See 6.6, *Floppy Eyelid Syndrome.*

Work-Up

1. History: Welding? Sunlamp use? Topical medications? Chemical exposure? Prior episodes?

2. Slit-lamp examination: Use fluorescein stain. Evert the eyelids to search for a foreign body.

3. If chemical exposure suspected, check pH of tear lake in lower conjunctival fornix. If not neutral (6.8 to 7.5), treat as chemical burn. See 3.1, *Chemical Burn.*

Treatment

1. Cycloplegic drop (e.g., cyclopentolate 1%).

2. Antibiotic ointment (e.g., erythromycin or bacitracin) four to eight times per day.

3. Consider a pressure patch for the more affected eye for 24 hours in reliable patients.

4. Oral analgesics as needed.

Follow-Up

1. Reliable patients are asked to assess their own symptoms after 24 hours (if a patch was placed, it is removed at this time).

2. If much improved, the patient continues with topical antibiotics (e.g., erythromycin or bacitracin ointment q.i.d.).

3. If still significantly symptomatic, the patient should return for re-evaluation. If significant punctate staining is still present, the patient is retreated with a cycloplegic, antibiotic, and possible pressure patch, as discussed previously.

4. Unreliable patients or those with an unclear etiology should not be patched and should be re-examined in 24 to 48 hours.

4.8 THYGESON SUPERFICIAL PUNCTATE KERATOPATHY

Symptoms

Mild-to-moderate foreign body sensation, photophobia, and tearing. No history of red eye. Usually bilateral with a chronic course of exacerbations and remissions.

Signs

Critical. Coarse stellate gray-white corneal epithelial opacities that are often central, slightly elevated, stain lightly with fluorescein, with or without underlying subepithelial infiltrates (see Figure 4.8.1).

Other. No conjunctival injection, corneal edema, anterior chamber reaction, or eyelid abnormalities.

Differential Diagnosis

See 4.1, *Superficial Punctate Keratopathy.*

Treatment

Mild

1. Artificial tears four to eight times per day.

2. Artificial tear ointment q.h.s.

3. Consider therapeutic soft contact lens.

4. Treatment based more on patient symptoms than corneal appearance.

Moderate to Severe

1. Mild topical steroid (e.g., fluorometholone 0.1% or loteprednol 0.2% to 0.5% q.i.d.) for

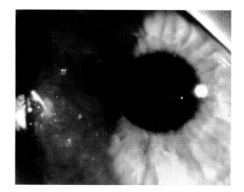

FIGURE 4.8.1. Thygeson superficial punctate keratopathy.

1 to 4 weeks. Then taper very slowly. May need prolonged low-dose topical steroid therapy.

2. If no improvement with topical steroids, a therapeutic soft contact lens can be tried.

3. Cyclosporine 0.05% drops q.d. to q.i.d. may be an alternative or adjunctive treatment, especially in patients with side effects from steroids.

Follow-Up

Weekly during an exacerbation, then every 3 to 6 months. Patients receiving topical steroids require intraocular pressure (IOP) checks every 4 to 12 weeks.

4.9 PTERYGIUM/PINGUECULA

Symptoms

Irritation, redness, decreased vision; may be asymptomatic.

Signs

Critical. One of the following, almost always located at the 3- or 9-o'clock position at the limbus.

- Pterygium: Wing-shaped fold of fibrovascular tissue arising from the interpalpebral conjunctiva and extending onto the cornea. Usually nasal in location (see Figure 4.9.1).

- Pinguecula: Yellow-white, flat or slightly raised conjunctival lesion, usually in the interpalpebral fissure adjacent to the limbus, but not involving the cornea.

Other. Either lesion may be highly vascularized and injected or may be associated with SPK or delle (thinning of the adjacent cornea secondary to drying). An iron line (Stocker line) may be seen in the cornea just beyond the leading edge of a pterygium.

Differential Diagnosis

- Conjunctival intraepithelial neoplasia (CIN): Unilateral papillomatous jelly-like, velvety, or leukoplakic (white) mass, often elevated, vascularized, not in a wing-shaped configuration, not in the typical 3- or 9-o'clock location of a pterygium or pinguecula. See 5.12, *Conjunctival Tumors.*

NOTE: Atypical pterygia require biopsy to rule out CIN or melanoma.

- Limbal dermoid: Congenital rounded white lesion, usually at the inferotemporal limbus. May be a manifestation of Goldenhar syndrome if accompanied by preauricular skin tags or vertebral skeletal defects. See 5.12, *Conjunctival Tumors.*

- Other conjunctival tumors: e.g., papilloma, nevus, melanoma; see 5.12, *Conjunctival Tumors.*

- Pseudopterygium: Conjunctival tissue adherent to the peripheral cornea. May appear in location of previous trauma, corneal ulceration, or cicatrizing conjunctivitis.

- Pannus: Blood vessels growing into the cornea, often secondary to chronic contact lens wear, blepharitis, ocular rosacea, herpes keratitis, phlyctenular keratitis, atopic disease,

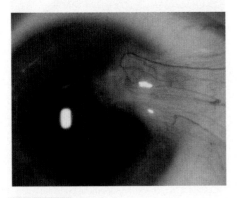

FIGURE 4.9.1. Pterygium.

trachoma, trauma, and others. Usually at the level of Bowman membrane with minimal to no elevation.

- Sclerokeratitis: See 5.7, *Scleritis*.

Etiology

Elastotic degeneration of deep conjunctival layers, related to sunlight exposure and chronic irritation. More common in individuals from equatorial regions.

Work-Up

Slit-lamp examination to identify the lesion and evaluate the adjacent corneal integrity and thickness. Check for corneal astigmatism in the axis of the pterygium.

Treatment

1. Protect eyes from sun, dust, and wind (e.g., sunglasses or goggles if appropriate).

2. Lubrication with artificial tears four to eight times per day to reduce ocular irritation.

3. For an inflamed pterygium or pinguecula:

—Mild: Artificial tears q.i.d.

—Moderate to severe: A mild topical steroid (e.g., fluorometholone 0.1% q.i.d., or loteprednol 0.2% to 0.5% q.i.d.). A nonsteroidal anti-inflammatory drop (e.g., ketorolac 0.4% to 0.5%) may be used two to four times per day to decrease symptoms.

4. If a delle is present, then apply artificial tear ointment q2h. See 4.24, *Dellen*.

5. Surgical removal is indicated when:

—The pterygium progresses toward the visual axis.

—The patient is experiencing excessive irritation not relieved by the aforementioned treatment.

—The lesion is interfering with contact lens wear.

NOTE: Pterygia can recur after surgical excision. Bare sclera dissection with a conjunctival autograft or amniotic membrane graft reduces the recurrence rate. Intraoperative application of an antimetabolite (5-fluorouracil or mitomycin-C) also reduces recurrence. Complications are reduced if no bare sclera remains.

Follow-Up

1. Asymptomatic patients may be checked every 1 to 2 years.

2. Pterygia should be measured periodically (every 3 to 12 months, initially) to determine the rate at which they are growing toward the visual axis.

3. If treating with a topical steroid, check after a few weeks to monitor inflammation and IOP. Taper and discontinue the steroid drop over several weeks once the inflammation has abated. A nonsteroidal drop may be used periodically for short times for recurrent inflammation.

4.10 BAND KERATOPATHY

Symptoms

Decreased vision, foreign body sensation, corneal whitening; may be asymptomatic.

Signs

(See Figure 4.10.1.)

Critical. Anterior corneal plaque of calcium at the level of Bowman membrane, typically within the interpalpebral fissure, and separated from the limbus by clear cornea. Lucid spaces are often present in the plaque, giving it a Swiss cheese appearance. The plaque usually begins at the 3- and 9-o'clock positions, adjacent to the limbus, and can extend across the cornea.

Other. May have other signs of chronic eye disease.

Etiology

More Common. Chronic uveitis (e.g., juvenile idiopathic arthritis), interstitial keratitis (IK), corneal edema, repeated trauma, phthisis bulbi,

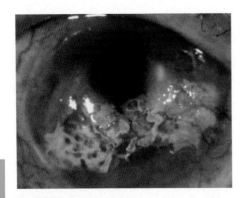

FIGURE 4.10.1. Band keratopathy.

long-standing glaucoma, dry eye, ocular surgery (especially retinal detachment repair with silicone oil), idiopathic.

Less Common. Hypercalcemia (may result from hyperparathyroidism, renal failure, sarcoidosis, multiple myeloma, Paget disease of bone, vitamin D excess, etc.), hyperphosphatemia, gout, corneal dystrophy, myotonic dystrophy, long-term exposure to irritants (e.g., mercury fumes), and other causes.

Work-Up

1. History: Chronic eye disease? Previous ocular surgery? Chronic exposure to environmental irritants? Systemic disease?

2. Slit-lamp examination.

3. If no signs of chronic anterior segment disease or long-standing glaucoma are present and the band keratopathy cannot be accounted for, then consider the following work-up:

   —Serum calcium, albumin, magnesium, and phosphate levels. Blood urea nitrogen and creatinine. Uric acid level if gout is suspected.

Treatment

Mild (e.g., Foreign Body Sensation)

Artificial tears four to six times per day and artificial tear ointment q.h.s. or q.i.d., p.r.n. Consider bandage contact lens for comfort.

Severe (e.g., Obstruction of Vision, Irritation not Relieved by Lubricants, Cosmetic Problem)

Removal of the calcium may be performed at the slit lamp or under the operating microscope by chelation using disodium ethylenediamine tetraacetic acid (EDTA):

1. Dilute a solution of 15% EDTA to create a 3% mixture by mixing in a 1.0-mL tuberculin syringe, 0.2 mL of 15% EDTA with 0.8 mL of 0.9% normal saline.

2. Anesthetize the eye with a topical anesthetic (e.g., proparacaine) and place an eyelid speculum.

3. Debride the corneal epithelium with a sterile scalpel or a sterile cotton-tipped applicator dipped in topical anesthetic or EDTA solution.

4. Wipe a cellulose sponge or cotton swab saturated with the 3% disodium EDTA solution over the band keratopathy until the calcium clears (which may take 10 to 30 minutes).

5. Irrigate with normal saline, place an antibiotic ointment (e.g., erythromycin), a cycloplegic drop (e.g., cyclopentolate 1% to 2%), and a pressure patch on the eye for 24 hours. (A bandage soft contact lens or an amniotic membrane may be used to cover the epithelial defect.)

6. Consider giving the patient an analgesic (e.g., acetaminophen with codeine).

Follow-Up

1. If surgical removal has been performed, the patient should be examined every 1 to 2 days with repatching (optional), frequent antibiotic ointment, and a cycloplegic until the epithelial defect heals.

2. Residual anterior stromal scarring may be amenable to excimer laser PTK to improve vision. PTK may also be used to try to improve the ocular surface and prevent recurrent erosions.

3. The patient should be checked every 3 to 12 months, depending on the severity of symptoms. Surgical removal can be repeated if the band keratopathy recurs.

4.11 BACTERIAL KERATITIS

Symptoms

Red eye, moderate-to-severe ocular pain, photophobia, decreased vision, discharge, acute contact lens intolerance.

Signs

(See Figure 4.11.1.)

Critical. Focal white opacity (infiltrate) in the corneal stroma. An ulcer exists if there is also stromal loss with an overlying epithelial defect that stains with fluorescein.

NOTE: An examiner using a slit beam cannot see through an infiltrate or ulcer to the iris, whereas stromal edema or mild anterior stromal scars are more transparent.

Other. Epithelial defect, mucopurulent discharge, stromal edema, anterior chamber reaction with or without hypopyon formation (which, in the absence of globe perforation, usually represents sterile inflammation), conjunctival injection, corneal thinning, folds in Descemet membrane, upper eyelid edema. Posterior synechiae, hyphema, and increased IOP may occur in severe cases.

Differential Diagnosis

- Fungal: Must be considered after any traumatic corneal injury, particularly from vegetable matter (e.g., a tree branch), which

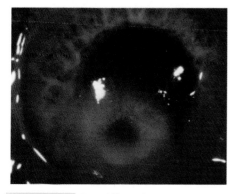

FIGURE 4.11.1. Bacterial keratitis.

may lead to filamentous fungal keratitis. Contact lens wear is another risk factor. Infiltrates commonly have feathery borders and may be surrounded by satellite lesions. Candida infections generally occur in eyes with pre-existing ocular surface disease and look like bacterial ulcers. See 4.12, *Fungal Keratitis.*

- *Acanthamoeba:* This protozoan causes an extremely painful epithelial keratitis and/or stromal infiltrate. It usually occurs in daily-wear soft contact lens wearers who may or may not practice poor lens hygiene, have a history of swimming while wearing contact lenses, or a history of trauma. In the early stages, the slit-lamp appearance typically looks more like HSV keratitis than a bacterial ulcer. In the late stages (3 to 8 weeks), the infiltrate often becomes ring shaped. See 4.13, *Acanthamoeba Keratitis.*

- HSV: May have eyelid vesicles or corneal epithelial dendrites. A history of recurrent unilateral eye disease or known ocular herpes is common. Bacterial superinfections may develop in patients with chronic herpes simplex keratitis. It is unusual for HSV to have a staining infiltrate; if present, one needs to rule out a superinfection. See 4.15, *Herpes Simplex Virus.*

- Atypical mycobacteria: Usually follows ocular injuries with vegetable matter or ocular surgery, such as cataract extraction, corneal grafts, and refractive surgery (especially LASIK). It has a more indolent course. Culture plates (on Lowenstein Jensen media) must be kept for 8 weeks. An acid-fast bacillus smear is very helpful

- Sterile corneal thinning and ulcers: Usually less painful, minimal or no discharge, iritis, or corneal edema, no infiltrates, and negative cultures. The melting is caused by the associated disease. See 4.23, *Peripheral Corneal Thinning/Ulceration.*

- Staphylococcal hypersensitivity: Peripheral corneal infiltrates, sometimes with an

4

overlying epithelial defect, usually multiple, often bilateral, with a clear space between the infiltrate and the limbus. Conjunctival injection is localized rather than diffuse, and there is less pain. There is minimal-to-no anterior chamber reaction. Often with coexisting blepharitis. See 4.19, *Staphylococcal Hypersensitivity.*

- Sterile corneal infiltrates: Typically from an immune reaction to contact lens solutions or hypoxia. Usually multiple small, often peripheral, subepithelial infiltrates with an intact overlying epithelium and minimal or no anterior chamber reaction. Usually a diagnosis of exclusion after ruling out an infectious process. Similar lesions can occur after adenoviral conjunctivitis, but these are often more central and more gray. See 5.1, *Acute Conjunctivitis.*

- Residual corneal foreign body or rust ring: History of foreign body injury. May be accompanied by corneal stromal inflammation, edema, and sometimes, a sterile infiltrate. There may be a mild anterior chamber reaction. The infiltrate and inflammation usually clear after the foreign body and rust ring are removed, but a superinfection may occur.

- Topical anesthetic abuse: A type of neurotrophic ulcer that should be suspected when there is poor response to appropriate therapy. In the late stages of anesthetic abuse, the corneal appearance may mimic an infectious process despite negative cultures. A large ring opacity, edema, and anterior chamber reaction are characteristic. Crack cocaine keratopathy has a similar appearance. Healing, with or without scarring, typically occurs when the exposure to anesthetic is stopped.

Etiology

Bacterial organisms are the most common cause of infectious keratitis. In general, corneal infections are assumed to be bacterial until proven otherwise by laboratory studies or until a therapeutic trial of topical antibiotics is unsuccessful. At the Wills Eye Institute, the most common causes of bacterial keratitis are *Staphylococcus,* *Pseudomonas, Streptococcus, Moraxella,* and Serratia species. Clinical findings vary widely depending on the severity of disease and on the organism involved. The following clinical characteristics may be helpful in predicting the organism involved. However, clinical impression should never take the place of broad-spectrum initial treatment and appropriate laboratory evaluation. See Appendix 8, *Corneal Culture Procedure.*

- Staphylococcal ulcers typically have a well-defined, gray-white stromal infiltrate that may enlarge to form a dense stromal abscess.

- Streptococcal infiltrates may be either very purulent or crystalline (see 4.14, *Crystalline Keratopathy*). Severe anterior chamber reaction and hypopyon formation are common in the former, and the latter tends to occur in patients on chronic topical steroids.

- Pseudomonas typically presents as a rapidly progressive, suppurative, necrotic infiltrate associated with a hypopyon and mucopurulent discharge in the setting of soft contact lens use (see Figure 4.11.2).

- Moraxella may cause infectious keratitis in patients with preexisting ocular surface disease and in patients who are immunocompromised. Infiltrates are typically indolent, located in the inferior portion of the cornea, and have a tendency to be full-thickness and may perforate.

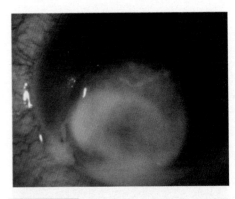

FIGURE 4.11.2. Pseudomonal keratitis.

Work-Up

1. History: Contact lens wear and care regimen should always be discussed. Sleeping in contact lenses (this greatly increases the risk of bacterial keratitis and should be strongly discouraged)? Daily or extended-wear lenses? Conventional, frequent replacement, or single use? Disinfecting solutions used? Recent changes in routine? Swimming or hot tub use with lenses? Trauma or corneal foreign body? Corneal surgery? History of refractive surgery? Eye care before visit (e.g., antibiotics or topical steroids)? Previous corneal disease? Systemic illness?

2. Slit-lamp examination: Stain with fluorescein to determine if there is epithelial loss overlying the infiltrate; document the size, depth, and location of the corneal infiltrate and epithelial defect; assess the anterior chamber reaction and look for a hypopyon; and measure the IOP by Tono-Pen.

3. Corneal scrapings for smears and cultures if appropriate. We routinely culture infiltrates larger than 1 to 2 mm, in the visual axis, unresponsive to initial treatment, or if we suspect an unusual organism based on history or examination. See Appendix 8, *Corneal Culture Procedure*.

4. In contact lens wearers suspected of having an infectious ulcer, the contact lenses and case are cultured, if possible. Explain to the patient that the cultured contact lenses will be discarded.

Treatment

Ulcers and infiltrates are initially treated as bacterial unless there is a high index of suspicion of another form of infection. Initial therapy needs to be broad spectrum.

1. Cycloplegic drops for comfort and to prevent synechiae formation (e.g., scopolamine 0.25% t.i.d.). Use atropine 1% t.i.d. when a hypopyon is present.

2. Topical antibiotics according to the following algorithm:

Low Risk of Visual Loss

Small, nonstaining peripheral infiltrate with at most minimal anterior chamber reaction and no discharge:

—Noncontact lens wearer: Broad-spectrum topical antibiotics [e.g., fluoroquinolone (moxifloxacin, gatifloxacin, besifloxacin, levofloxacin) drops q1–2h].

—Contact lens wearer: Fluoroquinolone (e.g., gatifloxacin, moxifloxacin, ciprofloxacin, besifloxacin, levofloxacin) drops q1–2h; can add tobramycin or ciprofloxacin ointment q.h.s. If using ointment more than q.i.d., use ciprofloxacin ointment.

Borderline Risk of Visual Loss

Medium size (1- to 1.5-mm diameter) peripheral infiltrate, or any smaller infiltrate with an associated epithelial defect, mild anterior chamber reaction, or moderate discharge:

—Fluoroquinolone (e.g., moxifloxacin, gatifloxacin, besifloxacin, levofloxacin) q1h around the clock. Consider starting with a loading dose of q5 min for five doses and then q30 min until midnight then q1h. Moxifloxacin has better Gram-positive coverage. Gatifloxacin and ciprofloxacin have better Pseudomonas and Serratia coverage.

Vision Threatening

Our current practice at Wills Eye is to start fortified antibiotics for most ulcers larger than 1 to 2 mm, in the visual axis, or unresponsive to initial treatment. See Appendix 9, *Fortified Topical Antibiotics/Antifungals*, for directions on making fortified antibiotics.

—Fortified tobramycin or gentamicin (15 mg/mL) q1h, alternating with fortified cefazolin (50 mg/mL) or vancomycin (25 mg/mL) q1h. This means that the patient will be placing a drop in the eye every one-half hour around the clock. Vancomycin drops should be reserved for resistant organisms, patients at risk for

4

resistant organisms (e.g., due to hospital or antibiotic exposure, unresponsive to initial treatment), and for patients who are allergic to penicillin or cephalosporins. An increasing number of methicillin-resistant *Staphylococcus aureus* (MRSA) infections are now community acquired. If the ulcer is severe and pseudomonas is suspected, start fortified tobramycin every 30 minutes and fortified cefazolin q1h; in addition, consider fortified ceftazidime q1h.

NOTE: All patients with borderline risk of visual loss or severe vision-threatening ulcers are initially treated with loading doses of antibiotics using the following regimen: One drop every 5 minutes for five doses, then every 30 to 60 minutes around the clock.

---

3. In some cases, topical corticosteroids are added after the bacterial organism and sensitivities are known, the infection is under control, and severe inflammation persists. Infectious keratitis may worsen significantly with topical corticosteroids, especially when caused by fungus, atypical mycobacteria, or Pseudomonas.

4. Eyes with corneal thinning should be protected by a shield without a patch (a patch is never placed over an eye thought to have an infection). The use of an anti-metalloproteinase (e.g., doxycycline 100 mg b.i.d.) may help to suppress connective tissue breakdown and prevent the perforation of the cornea.

5. No contact lens wear.

6. Oral pain medication as needed.

7. Oral fluoroquinolones (e.g., ciprofloxacin 500 mg p.o. b.i.d.; moxifloxacin 400 mg p.o. q.d.) penetrate the cornea well. These may have added benefit for patients with scleral extension or for those with frank or impending perforation. Ciprofloxacin is preferred for Pseudomonas and Serratia.

8. Systemic antibiotics are also necessary for Neisseria and Haemophilus infections [e.g., ceftriaxone 1 g intravenously (i.v.) if corneal involvement, or intramuscularly (i.m.) q12–24h if there is only conjunctival involvement]. Oral fluoroquinolones have been used for *Neisseria gonorrhea,* but there is increasing resistance in some locations and in men who have sex with men.

9. Admission to the hospital may be necessary if:

   —Infection is sight threatening.

   —Patient has difficulty administering the antibiotics at the prescribed frequency.

   —High likelihood of noncompliance with drops or daily follow-up.

   —Suspected topical anesthetic abuse.

   —Intravenous antibiotics are needed (e.g., corneal perforation, scleral extension of the infection, gonococcal conjunctivitis with corneal involvement).

10. For atypical mycobacteria, consider prolonged treatment (q1h for 1 week, then gradually tapering) with one of the following topical agents: fluoroquinolones [e.g., moxifloxacin or gatifloxacin), amikacin (15 mg/mL), clarithromycin (1% to 4%), or tobramycin (15 mg/mL)]. Consider oral treatment with clarithromycin 500 mg b.i.d. Previous LASIK has been implicated as a risk factor for atypical mycobacteria infections (although recently, Staphylococcal infections have been more common post-LASIK).

11. Bacterial coinfection may occasionally complicate fungal (especially candidal) and *Acanthamoeba* keratitis. Mixed bacterial infections can also occur.

Follow-Up

1. Daily evaluation at first, including repeated measurements of the size of the infiltrate and epithelial defect. The most important criteria in evaluating treatment response are the amount of pain, the epithelial defect size, the size and depth of the infiltrate, and the anterior chamber reaction. The IOP must be checked and treated if elevated (see 9.7, *Inflammatory Open-Angle Glaucoma*). Reduced pain is often the first sign of a positive response to treatment.

2. If improving, the antibiotic regimen is gradually tapered but is never tapered past the minimum dose to inhibit the emergence of resistance (usually t.i.d. to q.i.d. depending on the agent). Otherwise, the antibiotic regimen is adjusted according to the culture and sensitivity results.

3. If cultures were not taken or the cultures were negative and the infiltrate or ulcer does not respond or subsequently worsens, then new cultures (without stopping treatment), stains, and treatment with fortified antibiotics are needed. Treatment is modified based on the culture results. Hospitalization may be recommended. See Appendix 8, *Corneal Culture Procedure.*

4. A corneal biopsy may be required if the condition is worsening and infection is still suspected despite negative cultures.

5. For an impending or a complete corneal perforation, a corneal transplant or patch graft is considered. Cyanoacrylate tissue glue may also work in a treated corneal ulcer that has perforated despite infection control. Due to concern about drug penetration, antibiotics are often given for 1 to 2 days prior to glue application over an active area of infection.

NOTE: Outpatients are told to return immediately if the pain increases, vision decreases, or they notice an increase in the size of the ulcer when they look in the mirror.

4

4.12   FUNGAL KERATITIS

Symptoms

Pain, photophobia, red eye, tearing, discharge, foreign body sensation. Often history of minor trauma particularly with vegetable matter (e.g., a tree branch), contact lens wear, chronic eye disease, and/or a history of poor response to conventional antibacterial therapy. Usually more indolent than bacterial keratitis.

Signs

Critical.
Filamentous fungi: Corneal stromal gray-white opacity (infiltrate) with a feathery border. The epithelium over the infiltrate may be elevated above the remainder of the corneal surface, or there may be an epithelial defect with stromal thinning (ulcer).

Nonfilamentous fungi: A yellow-white stromal infiltrate similar to a bacterial ulcer.

Other. Satellite lesions surrounding the primary infiltrate, conjunctival injection, mucopurulent discharge, anterior chamber reaction, hypopyon. The infiltrate is more likely to extend beyond the epithelial defect than in bacterial ulcers.

Differential Diagnosis

See 4.11, *Bacterial Keratitis.*

Etiology

■ Filamentous fungi (e.g., Fusarium or Aspergillus species most commonly): Usually from trauma with vegetable matter in previously healthy eyes. There was a Fusarium keratitis epidemic in contact lens wearers associated with Bausch & Lomb's ReNu with MoistureLoc solution (recalled May 2006).

■ Nonfilamentous fungi (e.g., Candida species): Usually in previously diseased eyes, e.g., dry eyes, herpes simplex or zoster keratitis, exposure keratopathy, and chronic use of corticosteroid drops (see Figure 4.12.1).

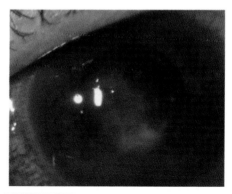

FIGURE 4.12.1. Candida fungal keratitis.

Work-Up

See 4.11, *Bacterial Keratitis* for complete work-up and culture procedure.

NOTE:

1. Whenever smears and cultures are done, include a Gram, Giemsa, calcofluor white, or KOH stain for organisms (periodic acid–Schiff, Gomori methenamine silver, and H&E stains also can be used) and scrape deep into the edge of the ulcer for material. See Appendix 8, *Corneal Culture Procedure*.

2. If an infectious etiology is still suspected despite negative cultures, consider a corneal biopsy to obtain further diagnostic information.

3. Consider cultures and smears of contact lens case and solution.

4. Sometimes all tests are negative and therapeutic penetrating keratoplasty is necessary for diagnosis and treatment.

Treatment

Corneal infiltrates and ulcers of unknown etiology are treated as bacterial until proven otherwise (see 4.11, *Bacterial Keratitis*). If the stains or cultures indicate a fungal keratitis, institute the following measures:

1. Admission to the hospital may be necessary, unless the patient is reliable. It may take weeks to achieve complete healing.

2. Natamycin 5% drops (especially for filamentous fungi) or amphotericin B 0.15% drops (especially for Candida), initially q1–2h around the clock, then taper over 4 to 6 weeks. Alternatively, use topical fortified voriconazole 1% q1h around the clock (see Appendix 9, *Fortified Topical Antibiotics/Antifungals*).

NOTE: Natamycin is the only commercially available topical antifungal agent; all others must be compounded from intravenous solutions with sterile techniques.

3. Cycloplegic (e.g., scopolamine 0.25% t.i.d.). Use atropine 1% t.i.d. if hypopyon is present.

4. No topical steroids. If the patient is currently taking steroids, they should be tapered rapidly and discontinued.

5. Consider adding oral antifungal agents (e.g., fluconazole 200 to 400 mg p.o. loading dose, then 100 to 200 mg p.o. q.d., or voriconazole 200 mg p.o. b.i.d.). Oral fluconazole and voriconazole are often used for deep corneal ulcers or suspected fungal endophthalmitis.

6. Consider epithelial debridement to facilitate the penetration of antifungal medications. Topical antifungals do not penetrate the cornea well, especially through an intact epithelium.

7. Measure IOP with Tono-Pen. Treat elevated IOP if present (see 9.7, *Inflammatory Open-Angle Glaucoma*).

8. Eye shield, without patch, in the presence of corneal thinning.

Follow-Up

Patients are re-examined daily. However, the initial clinical response to treatment in fungal keratitis is much slower compared to bacterial keratitis. Stability of infection after initiation of treatment is often a favorable sign. Unlike bacterial ulcers, epithelial healing in fungal keratitis is not always a sign of positive response. Fungal infections in deep corneal stroma are frequently recalcitrant to therapy. These ulcers may require weeks to months of treatment, and corneal transplantation may be necessary for infections that progress despite maximal medical therapy or corneal perforation.

4.13 ACANTHAMOEBA KERATITIS

Acanthamoeba keratitis should be considered in any patient with a history of soft contact lens wear, poor contact lens hygiene (e.g., using tap water to clean lenses, infrequent disinfection), or swimming, fishing, hot-tub use, or trauma while wearing contact lenses. Heat disinfection and hydrogen peroxide systems with at least 8 hours of contact time are effective in killing *Acanthamoeba* cysts and trophozoites, but are not commercially available in the United States. Sorbic acid, EDTA, and quaternary ammonium compounds are mostly ineffective against *Acanthamoeba* cysts. The best approach to prevention is to use daily disposable (single-use) lenses. The best available solutions involve hydrogen peroxide exposure before neutralization, such as Oxysept UltraCare or Clear Care. Boston rigid gas-permeable (RGP) solutions are effective, but contact with tap water must be avoided. A multipurpose RGP solution (e.g., Boston Simplus) and patient education against rinsing RGP lenses in tap water is the best approach. Although most patients with *Acanthamoeba* have a history of contact lens use, some patients do not and often have a delayed diagnosis.

Symptoms

Severe ocular pain (often out of proportion to the early clinical findings), redness, and photophobia over a period of several weeks.

Signs

(See Figure 4.13.1.)

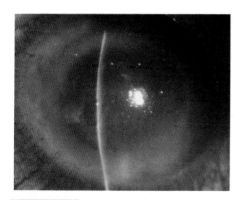

FIGURE 4.13.1. *Acanthamoeba* keratitis.

Critical.
Early: Pseudodendrites on the epithelium. Less corneal and anterior segment inflammation than expected for the degree of pain the patient is experiencing, subepithelial infiltrates (sometimes along corneal nerves, producing a radial keratoneuritis).

Late (3 to 8 weeks): Ring-shaped corneal stromal infiltrate.

NOTE: Cultures for bacteria are negative. The condition usually does not improve with antibiotic or antiviral medications and commonly follows a chronic, progressive, downhill course. Patients are often initially misdiagnosed as having herpes simplex keratitis. *Acanthamoeba* is important to consider in patients with unresponsive HSV keratitis, as HSV keratitis usually responds well to appropriate treatment.

Other. Eyelid swelling, conjunctival injection (especially circumcorneal), cells, and flare in the anterior chamber. Minimal discharge or corneal vascularization. Corneal ulceration and bacterial superinfection may occur later in the course.

Differential Diagnosis

HSV keratitis is first in the differential. See 4.11, *Bacterial Keratitis,* and 4.15, *Herpes Simplex Virus.*

Work-Up

See 4.11, *Bacterial Keratitis* for a general work-up. One or more of the following are obtained when *Acanthamoeba* is suspected:

1. Corneal scrapings for Gram, Giemsa, and calcofluor white stains (Giemsa and periodic acid-Schiff stains may show typical cysts). See Appendix 8, *Corneal Culture Procedure.*

2. Consider a culture on non-nutrient agar with *E. coli* overlay.

3. Consider a corneal biopsy if the stains and cultures are negative and the condition is not improving on the current regimen.

4. Consider cultures and smears of contact lens and case.

5. Confocal biomicroscopy may be helpful if available.

Treatment

One or more of the following are usually used in combination, sometimes in the hospital initially:

1. Polyhexamethylene biguanide 0.02% (PHMB) drops q1h. Chlorhexidine 0.02% can be used as an alternative to PHMB.

2. Propamidine isethionate 0.1% drops q1h. Dibromopropamidine isethionate 0.15% ointment is also available.

3. Consider polymyxin B/neomycin/gramicidin drops q1h. No longer used by most doctors.

4. Itraconazole 400 mg p.o. for one loading dose, then 100 to 200 mg p.o. q.d., ketoconazole 200 mg p.o. q.d., or voriconazole 200 mg p.o. q.d. to b.i.d.

NOTE: Alternative therapy includes hexamidine, clotrimazole 1% drops, miconazole 1% drops, or paromomycin drops q2h. Low-dose corticosteroid drops may be helpful in reducing inflammation after the infection is controlled, but steroid use is controversial.

All patients:

5. Discontinue contact lens wear in both eyes.

6. Cycloplegic (e.g., scopolamine 0.25% t.i.d.)

7. Oral nonsteroidal anti-inflammatory agent (e.g., naproxen 250 to 500 mg p.o. b.i.d.) for inflammation, for pain, and for scleritis, if present. Additional narcotic oral analgesics are often needed.

NOTE: Corneal transplantation may be indicated for medical failures, but this procedure can be complicated by recurrent infection. It is best delayed for 3 to 12 months after medical treatment is completed.

Follow-Up

Every 1 to 4 days until the condition is consistently improving, and then every 1 to 3 weeks. Medication may then be tapered judiciously. Treatment is usually continued for 3 months after resolution of inflammation, which may take up to 6 to 12 months.

NOTE:

1. Propamidine isethionate 0.1% drops is available in the United Kingdom and other countries; it may be compounded in the United States (e.g., Leiter pharmacy, www.leiterrx.com).

2. PHMB is available in the United Kingdom as Cosmocil; it can be prepared by a compounding pharmacy in the United States from Baquacil, a swimming pool disinfectant.

4.14   CRYSTALLINE KERATOPATHY

Signs

Crystals seen in subepithelial and/or stromal regions of the cornea.

Symptoms

Decreased vision, photophobia, decreased corneal sensation may occur, may be asymptomatic.

Etiology

■ Infectious crystalline keratopathy: Seen in corneal grafts and chronically inflamed corneas. *Streptococcus viridans* is the most common organism; other organisms include *Staphylococcus epidermidis*, Corynebacterium species, *Pseudomonas aeruginosa*, and fungi. Patients with refractive surgery are at a higher risk for atypical mycobacteria and alternaria.

■ Schnyder corneal dystrophy: Slowly progressive, autosomal dominant. Subepithelial corneal crystals in 50% of patients (cholesterol and phospholipids), central and midperipheral corneal opacification, dense arcus, decreased corneal sensation. Local disorder of corneal lipid metabolism but can be associated with hyperlipidemia and hypercholesterolemia. Higher prevalence in patients with Swede–Finn descent. See 4.26, *Corneal Dystrophies*.

- Bietti crystalline corneoretinal dystrophy: Rare, autosomal recessive. Retinal crystals (decrease with time). Sparkling, yellow-white spots at the corneal limbus in the superficial stroma and subepithelial layers of the cornea.

- Cystinosis: Rare, autosomal recessive, systemic metabolic defect. Infantile form (nephropathic): dwarfism, progressive renal dysfunction, polychromatic cystine crystals in conjunctiva, corneal stroma (densest in peripheral cornea but present throughout anterior stroma), trabecular meshwork. Intermediate/adolescent form: less severe renal involvement. Adult form: normal life expectancy.

- Lymphoproliferative disorders, including monoclonal gammopathy of undetermined significance, essential cryoglobulinemia, or multiple myeloma.

Work-Up

1. Fasting lipid profile in patients with Schnyder corneal dystrophy.

2. Electroretinogram may be decreased in later stages of Bietti crystalline dystrophy.

3. Cystinosis: Very high level of suspicion required, especially for infantile form, which can be fatal in the first decade of life without a renal transplant. Conjunctival biopsy, blood or bone marrow smear.

4. Infectious crystalline keratopathy: Culture as outlined in Appendix 8, *Corneal Culture Procedure*. Obtain mycobacterial cultures/acid-fast bacillus stain (especially in patients after refractive surgery).

5. If a lymphoproliferative disorder is suspected, consult Hematology and consider complete blood count with differential, serum chemistries (including calcium), creatinine, albumin, lactate dehydrogenase, beta-2 microglobulin, c-reactive protein (CRP), serum protein electrophoresis (SPEP), urine protein electrophoresis (UPEP), and peripheral/bone marrow smear.

Treatment

1. Schnyder corneal dystrophy: PTK may be effective for subepithelial crystals. Corneal transplantation for severe cases. Diet and/or medications for elevated cholesterol.

2. No specific treatment for Bietti crystalline dystrophy.

3. Cystinosis: Topical cysteamine drops reduce the density of crystalline deposits and corneal pain. Penetrating keratoplasty for severe cases (although corneal deposits may recur). Patients must get systemic evaluation by primary care physician and/or geneticist.

4. Infectious keratopathy: Treat as outlined in 4.11, *Bacterial Keratitis,* and 4.30, *Corneal Refractive Surgery Complications*.

5. Lymphoproliferative disorder: Consult a hematologist and/or oncologist.

4.15 HERPES SIMPLEX VIRUS

Symptoms

Red eye, pain, photophobia, tearing, decreased vision, skin (e.g., eyelid) vesicular rash, history of previous episodes, fever blisters; usually unilateral.

Signs

Primary HSV infection is usually not apparent clinically. However, neonatal primary herpes infection is a rare, potentially devastating disease associated with localized skin, eye, or oral infection and severe central nervous system and multiorgan system infection [see 8.9, *Opthalmia Neonatorum (Newborn Conjunctivitis)*]. In older children, primary HSV infection may be associated with extensive eyelid involvement with or without oral facial HSV, follicular conjunctivitis, and often multiple conjunctival and corneal dendrites. Triggers for recurrence are commonly thought to include fever, stress, trauma, and ultraviolet light exposure [although this clinical suspicion was not confirmed by the Herpetic Eye Disease Study (HEDS)]. Infection may be characterized by any or all of the following:

Eyelid/Skin Involvement

Clear vesicles on an erythematous base that progress to crusting, heal without scarring and cross dermatomes.

Conjunctivitis

Conjunctival injection with acute unilateral follicular conjunctivitis, with or without conjunctival dendrites, geographic ulcers.

Corneal Epithelial Disease

(See Figure 4.15.1.)
May be seen as macropunctate, dendritic keratitis (a thin, linear, branching epithelial ulceration with club-shaped terminal bulbs at the end of each branch), or a geographic ulcer (a large, amoeba-shaped corneal ulcer with a dendritic edge). The edges of herpetic lesions are heaped up with swollen epithelial cells that stain well with rose bengal or lissamine green; the central ulceration stains well with fluorescein. Corneal sensitivity may be decreased. Scars (ghost dendrites) may develop underneath the epithelial lesions.

Neurotrophic Ulcer

A sterile ulcer with smooth epithelial margins over an area of interpalpebral stromal disease that persists or worsens despite antiviral therapy. May be associated with stromal melting and perforation.

Corneal Stromal Disease

- Disciform keratitis (non-necrotizing keratitis): Disc-shaped stromal edema with an intact epithelium. A mild iritis with localized granulomatous keratic precipitates is typical, and increased IOP may be present. No necrosis or corneal neovascularization is present.

- Necrotizing interstitial keratitis (IK) (uncommon): Appearance of multiple or diffuse, whitish corneal stromal infiltrates with or without an epithelial defect, often accompanied by stromal inflammation, thinning, and neovascularization. Concomitant iritis, hypopyon, or glaucoma may be present. Microbial (bacterial and fungal) superinfection should be ruled out.

Uveitis

An anterior chamber reaction may develop as a result of corneal stromal involvement. Less commonly, anterior chamber reaction and granulomatous keratic precipitates can develop without active corneal disease and may be associated with very high IOP.

Retinitis

Rare. In neonates, it is usually associated with a severe systemic HSV infection and is often bilateral.

Differential Diagnosis of Corneal Dendrites

- Varicella zoster virus (VZV): Typically painful skin vesicles are found along a dermatomal distribution of the face, not crossing the midline. Moderate-to-severe pain may be present before vesicles appear. Skin involvement is very helpful in distinguishing VZV from HSV. Early VZV dendrites can mimic HSV dendrites. Late pseudodendrites in VZV are raised mucous plaques. They do not have true terminal bulbs and do not stain well with fluorescein. See 4.16, *Herpes Zoster Ophthalmicus/Varicella Zoster Virus.*

- Recurrent corneal erosion: A healing erosion often has a dendritiform appearance. Recurrent erosions in patients with lattice

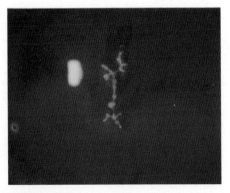

FIGURE 4.15.1. Herpes simplex dendritic keratitis.

dystrophy can have a geographic shape. See 4.2, *Recurrent Corneal Erosion.*

■ *Acanthamoeba* keratitis pseudodendrites: History of soft contact lens wear, pain out of proportion to inflammation, chronic course. These are raised epithelial lesions, not epithelial ulcerations. See 4.13, *Acanthamoeba Keratitis.*

■ Vaccinia keratitis: Recent history of smallpox vaccination or vaccine exposure. See 4.17, *Ocular Vaccinia.*

Work-Up

1. History: Previous episodes? History of corneal abrasion; contact lens wear; or previous nasal or oral sores? Recent topical or systemic steroids? Immune deficiency state? Recent fever or sun/UV exposure?

2. External examination: Note the distribution of skin vesicles if present. The lesions are more suggestive of HSV than VZV if concentrated around the eye without extension onto forehead, scalp, and tip of nose. HSV often involves both eyelids.

3. Slit-lamp examination with IOP measurement.

4. Check corneal sensation (before instillation of topical anesthetic), which may be decreased in HSV and VZV.

5. Herpes simplex is usually diagnosed clinically and requires no confirmatory laboratory tests. If the diagnosis is in doubt, any of the following tests may be helpful:

—Scrapings of a corneal or skin lesion (scrape the edge of a corneal ulcer or the base of a skin lesion) for Giemsa stain, which shows multinucleated giant cells. Enzymelinked immunosorbent assay testing also is available.

—Viral culture: A sterile, cotton-tipped applicator is used to swab the cornea, conjunctiva, or skin (after unroofing vesicles with a sterile needle) and is placed in the viral transport medium.

—HSV antibody titers are frequently present in patients. They rise after primary but not recurrent infection. The absence of HSV1 antibodies helps rule out HSV as a cause of stromal keratitis. Positive titer is nonspecific.

Treatment

The treatment of HSV eye disease has been refined by the findings of the HEDS. Treatment modalities supported by evidence from HEDS are indicated by an asterisk (*).

Eyelid/Skin Involvement

1. Topical acyclovir ointment, five times per day, is an option, although it has not been proven effective. This is not an ocular preparation and should be used on the skin only. It may be better to use antiviral ointment rather than antibacterial ointment, though erythromycin or bacitracin ophthalmic ointment is often used b.i.d. Ganciclovir 0.15% ophthalmic gel (now available in the United States) five times per day may also be effective.

2. Warm or cool soaks to skin lesions t.i.d. or p.r.n.

3. Eyelid margin involvement: Add ganciclovir 0.15% ophthalmic gel or trifluridine 1% drops, five times per day, to the eye. Vidarabine 3% ointment five times per day is useful for small children; it is currently available in Canada, Europe, and in the USA from Leiter pharmacy (www.leiterrx.com). These medications are continued for 7 to 14 days until resolution of the symptoms.

NOTE: Many physicians give oral acyclovir 400 mg five times per day, for 7 to 14 days, to adults suspected of having primary herpetic disease.

Conjunctivitis

Ganciclovir 0.15% ophthalmic gel, trifluridine 1% drops, or vidarabine 3% ointment five times per day. Discontinue the antiviral agent when the conjunctivitis has resolved after 7 to 14 days.

Corneal Epithelial Disease

1. Ganciclovir 0.15% ophthalmic gel five times per day, trifluridine 1% drops nine times per day, or vidarabine 3% ointment five times per day. Oral antiviral agents (e.g., acyclovir 400 mg p.o. five times per day, for 7 to 10 days) may be used to avoid

4

the toxicity of topical antiviral drops or when drops cannot be given due to compliance problems, especially in children.

2. Consider cycloplegic agent (e.g., scopolamine 0.25% b.i.d.) if an anterior chamber reaction or photophobia is present.

3. Patients taking topical steroids should have them tapered rapidly.

4. Consider gentle debridement of the infected epithelium as an adjunct to the antiviral agents.

   —Technique: After topical anesthesia, a sterile, moistened cotton-tipped applicator or semisharp instrument is used carefully to peel off the lesions at the slit lamp. After debridement, antiviral treatment should be instituted as described earlier.

5. For epithelial defects that do not resolve after 1 to 2 weeks, noncompliance, topical antiviral toxicity, neurotrophic ulcer or *Acanthamoeba* keratitis should be suspected. At that point, the topical antiviral agent should be discontinued, and a nonpreserved artificial tear ointment or an antibiotic ointment (e.g., erythromycin) should be used four to eight times per day for several days with careful follow-up. Smears for *Acanthamoeba* should be performed whenever the diagnosis is suspected.

NOTE: Oral acyclovir does not prevent the development of stromal keratitis or uveitis in patients with HSV epithelial keratitis.*

However, a short course of systemic acyclovir may be used when frequent topical antivirals cannot be given.

Neurotrophic Ulcer

See 4.6, *Neurotrophic Keratopathy*.

Corneal Stromal Disease

1. Disciform keratitis

   Mild. Consider treatment with cycloplegic (e.g., scopolamine 0.25% b.i.d.) alone.

   Severe or central (i.e., vision is reduced).

   —Cycloplegic, as above.

   —Topical steroid (e.g., prednisolone acetate 1% q.i.d.).*

—Antiviral prophylaxis: Ganciclovir 0.15% ophthalmic gel three to five times a day, trifluridine 1% t.i.d. to q.i.d., or acyclovir 400 mg p.o. b.i.d.* Oral acyclovir alone is not effective treatment of stromal keratitis.* Acyclovir 400 mg p.o. b.i.d. is also recommended for prophylaxis of subsequent episodes of HSV stromal keratitis.

—Adjunctive medications which may be used include:

- Antibiotic (e.g., erythromycin ointment q.h.s.) in the presence of epithelial defects.

- Aqueous suppressants for increased IOP. Avoid prostaglandin analogues due to association with recurrent HSV infections.

2. Necrotizing IK: Treated as severe disciform keratitis. The first priority is to diagnose and treat any associated overlying epithelial defect and bacterial superinfection with antibiotic drops or ointment (see 4.11, *Bacterial Keratitis*). Tissue adhesive or corneal transplantation may be required if the cornea perforates (this is more common with neurotrophic keratitis). Oral acyclovir treatment may be beneficial, but necrotizing IK was too rare in the HED study to know definitively.

NOTE:

1. Topical steroids are contraindicated in those with infectious epithelial disease.

2. Rarely, a systemic steroid (e.g., prednisone 40 to 60 mg p.o. q.d., tapered rapidly) is given to patients with severe stromal disease accompanied by an epithelial defect and hypopyon. Cultures should be done to rule out a superinfection.

3. Valacyclovir has greater bioavailability than acyclovir but is more expensive. Little has been published on famciclovir for HSV, but it may be better tolerated in patients who have side effects to acyclovir such as headache, fatigue, or gastrointestinal upset.

4. Acyclovir needs to be adjusted in patients with renal insufficiency. Checking BUN and creatinine is recommended in patients at risk for renal disease before starting high-dose acyclovir.

5. Oral antivirals (e.g., acyclovir, famciclovir, and valacyclovir) have not been shown to be

beneficial in the treatment of stromal disease but may be beneficial in the treatment of herpetic uveitis* [see 12.1, *Anterior Uveitis (Iritis/Iridocyclitis)*].

6. The persistence of an ulcer with stromal keratitis is commonly due to the underlying inflammation (requiring cautious steroid therapy); however, it may be due to antiviral toxicity or active HSV epithelial infection. When an ulcer deepens, a new infiltrate develops, or the anterior chamber reaction increases, and smears and cultures should be taken for bacteria and fungi. See Appendix 8, *Corneal Culture Procedure.*

Follow-Up

1. Patients are reexamined in 2 to 7 days to evaluate the response to treatment and then every 1 to 2 weeks, depending on the clinical findings. The following clinical parameters are evaluated: the size of the epithelial defect and ulcer, the corneal thickness and the depth of corneal involvement, the anterior chamber reaction, and the IOP (see 9.7, *Inflammatory Open-Angle Glaucoma,* for glaucoma management).

2. Antiviral medications for corneal dendrites and geographic ulcers should be continued five to nine times per day for 7 to 14 days until healed, then four times per day for 4 to 7 days, then stopped.

3. Topical steroids used for corneal stromal disease are tapered slowly (often over months to years). The initial concentration of the steroid (e.g., prednisolone acetate 1%) is eventually reduced (e.g., loteprednol 0.5% or prednisolone acetate 0.125%). Extended taper includes dosing q.o.d., twice weekly, once weekly, etc., especially with a history of flare-ups when steroids are stopped. Prophylactic topical antiviral agents (e.g., ganciclovir 0.15% or trifluridine 1% t.i.d.) or systemic agents (e.g., acyclovir 400 mg b.i.d.) are used until steroids are used once daily or less.

4. Corneal transplantation may eventually be necessary if inactive postherpetic scars significantly affect vision, though an RGP lens should be tried first.

5. Recommend long-term oral antiviral prophylaxis (e.g., acyclovir 400 mg b.i.d.) if a patient has had multiple episodes of herpetic stromal disease.*

NOTE: Topical antivirals can cause a local toxic or allergic reaction (usually a papillary or follicular conjunctivitis) typically after 3 weeks of therapy. In this setting, the patient can be switched to an oral antiviral agent.

4.16 HERPES ZOSTER OPHTHALMICUS/ VARICELLA ZOSTER VIRUS

Symptoms

Dermatomal pain, paresthesias, and skin rash or discomfort. May be preceded by headache, fever, malaise, blurred vision, eye pain, and red eye.

Signs

Critical. Acute vesicular dermatomal skin rash along the first division of the fifth cranial nerve. Characteristically, the rash is unilateral, respects the midline, and does not involve the lower eyelid. Hutchinson sign (tip of the nose involved in the distribution of the nasociliary branch of V1) predicts higher risk of ocular involvement.

Other. Less commonly, the lower eyelid and cheek on one side (V2), and, rarely, one side of the jaw (V3) are involved. Conjunctivitis, corneal involvement [e.g., multiple small epithelial dendritiform lesions early, followed by larger pseudodendrites (raised mucous plaques which may be present on cornea or conjunctiva, see Figure 4.16.1), SPK, immune stromal keratitis, neurotrophic keratitis], uveitis, sectoral iris atrophy, scleritis, retinitis, choroiditis, optic neuritis, cranial nerve palsies, and elevated IOP can occur. Late postherpetic neuralgia also may occur.

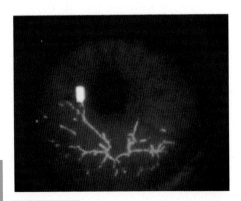

FIGURE 4.16.1. Herpes zoster keratitis with pseudo-dendrites.

NOTE: Corneal disease may follow the acute skin rash by several days to weeks or months and last for years. Occasionally, it can precede the skin rash or there is no rash, making the diagnosis more difficult. There is a rise in VZV titers after zoster.

HZO may be the initial manifestation of HIV, particularly in patients <40 years without known immunocompromisation.

Differential Diagnosis

■ HSV: Patients are often young; rash is not dermatomal and crosses the midline. See 4.15, *Herpes Simplex Virus*.

Work-Up

1. History: Duration of rash and pain? Immunocompromised or risk factors for HIV/AIDS?

Hearing changes, facial pain or weakness, vertigo [cranial nerve VII involvement (Ramsay–Hunt syndrome)]? Rashes elsewhere?

2. Complete ocular examination, including a slit-lamp evaluation with fluorescein or rose bengal staining, IOP check, and dilated fundus examination with careful exam for progressive outer retinal necrosis (PORN), an immunodeficiency-related manifestation of VZV. See 12.8, *Acute Retinal Necrosis (ARN)*.

3. Systemic evaluation:

—Patients <40 years: Consider medical evaluation for immunocompromised status, particularly HIV.

—Patients aged 40 to 60 years: None, unless immunodeficiency is suspected from the history.

—Patients >60 years: If systemic steroid therapy is to be instituted, obtain a steroid work-up as required.

—If any other organ systems or non-ophthalmic sites are involved, consider evaluation by internal medicine or other subspecialists as needed.

NOTE: Immunocompromised patients should not receive systemic steroids.

Treatment

See Table 4.16.1 for the treatment of VZV in immunocompromised patients.

TABLE 4.16.1	Herpes Zoster Ophthalmicus in Immunosuppressed Patients		
Drug	**Dosing Information**	**Toxicities**	**Contraindications**
Acyclovir	10 mg/kg i.v. q8h (q12h if creatinine >2.0) for 7–10 d. Consider maintenance with 800 mg p.o. five times per day to prevent reactivation.	Intravenous: reversible renal and neurologic toxicity.	Use with caution in patients with a history of renal impairment.
Famciclovir	500 mg p.o. q8h. Adjust dosage for creatinine clearance <60 mL/min.	Headache, nausea, diarrhea, dizziness, fatigue	Use with caution in patients with a history of renal impairment.
Valacyclovir HCl	1 g p.o. q8h. Adjust dosage for creatinine clearance <60 mL/min.	Headache, nausea, vomiting, diarrhea	TTP/HUS has been reported in patients with advanced HIV/AIDS.

Skin Involvement

1. In adults with a moderate-to-severe skin rash for <4 days in which active skin lesions are present and (consider) if the patient presents later in the first week with active lesions:

    —Oral antiviral agent (e.g., acyclovir 800 mg p.o. five times per day; famciclovir 500 mg p.o. t.i.d.; or valacyclovir 1,000 mg p.o. t.i.d.) for 7 to 10 days; if the condition is severe, as manifested by orbital, optic nerve, or cranial nerve involvement, or the patient is systemically ill, hospitalize and prescribe acyclovir 5 to 10 mg/kg i.v. q8h for 5 to 10 days.

    —Bacitracin or erythromycin ointment to the skin lesions b.i.d.

    —Warm compresses to periocular skin t.i.d.

2. Adults with a skin rash of more than 1 week duration or without active skin lesions.

    —Warm compresses to periocular skin t.i.d.

    —Bacitracin or erythromycin ointment to skin lesions b.i.d.

3. Children: Discuss with a pediatrician and consider adjusted-dose acyclovir. Otherwise, treat as in (2) unless evidence of systemic spread. For systemic spread, hospitalize and prescribe acyclovir (if >12 years of age, 30 mg/kg/day in three divided doses; if <12 years of age, 60 mg/kg/day in three divided doses) for 7 days. Consult Pediatrics and Infectious Disease to manage the systemic disease.

Ocular Involvement

1. Conjunctival involvement: Cool compresses and erythromycin ointment to the eye b.i.d.

2. SPK: Lubrication with preservative-free artificial tears q1–2h and ointment q.h.s.

3. Corneal or conjunctival pseudodendrites. Lubrication with preservative-free artificial tears q1–2h and ointment q.h.s. Topical antivirals (e.g., ganciclovir 0.15% or vidarabine 3% ointment) t.i.d. to q.i.d. may also be helpful. Consider antibiotic ointment to prevent bacterial superinfection.

4. Immune stromal keratitis: Topical steroid (e.g., prednisolone acetate 1%, start q.i.d.,

adjust according to the response), tapering over months to years using weaker steroids and less than daily dosing.

5. Uveitis (with or without immune stromal keratitis): Topical steroid (e.g., prednisolone acetate 1%) q.i.d. and cycloplegic (e.g., scopolamine 0.25% b.i.d.). See 12.1, *Anterior Uveitis (Iritis/Iridocyclitis).* Treat increased IOP with aggressive aqueous suppression; avoid prostaglandin analogues.

6. Neurotrophic keratitis: Treat mild epithelial defects with erythromycin ointment four to eight times per day. If corneal ulceration occurs, obtain appropriate smears and cultures to rule out infection (see 4.11, *Bacterial Keratitis*). If the ulcer is sterile, and there is no response to ointment, consider a bandage contact lens, tarsorrhaphy, amniotic membrane graft, or conjunctival flap (see 4.6, *Neurotrophic Keratopathy*).

7. Scleritis: See 5.7, *Scleritis.*

8. Retinitis, choroiditis, optic neuritis, or cranial nerve palsy: Acyclovir 5 to 10 mg/kg i.v. q8h for 1 week and prednisone 60 mg p.o. for 3 days, then taper over 1 week. Management of acute retinal necrosis or PORN may require intraocular antivirals [see 12.8, *Acute Retinal Necrosis (ARN)*]. Consult Infectious Disease. Recommend neurologic consultation to rule out central nervous system involvement. Patients with severe disease can develop a large vessel cranial arteritis resulting in a massive CVA.

9. Increased IOP: May be steroid response or secondary to inflammation. If uveitis is present, increase the frequency of the steroid administration for a few days and use topical aqueous suppressants (e.g., timolol 0.5% b.i.d., brimonidine 0.2% t.i.d., or dorzolamide 2% t.i.d.) (see 9.7, *Inflammatory Open-Angle Glaucoma,* and 9.9, *Steroid-Response Glaucoma*). Oral carbonic anhydrase inhibitors may be necessary if the IOP is >30 mm Hg. If IOP remains increased and the inflammation is controlled, substitute fluorometholone 0.25%, rimexolone 1%, or loteprednol 0.5% drops for prednisolone acetate and attempt to taper the dose.

4

NOTE: Pain may be severe during the first 2 weeks, and narcotic analgesics may be required. An antidepressant (e.g., amitriptyline 25 mg p.o. t.i.d.) may be beneficial for both postherpetic neuralgia and depression that can develop in VZV. Capsaicin 0.025% or doxepin ointment may be applied to the skin t.i.d. to q.i.d. after the rash heals (not around the eyes) for postherpetic neuralgia. Oral gabapentin or pregabalin can be helpful for acute pain and for postherpetic neuralgia. Management of postherpetic neuralgia should involve the patient's primary medical doctor.

Follow-Up

If ocular involvement is present, examine the patient every 1 to 7 days, depending on the severity. Patients without ocular involvement can be followed every 1 to 4 weeks. After the acute episode resolves, check the patient every 3 to 6 months (3 if on steroids) because relapses may occur months to years later, particularly as steroids are tapered. Systemic steroid use is controversial and requires collaboration with the patient's internist.

NOTE: VZV is contagious for children and adults who have not had chickenpox or the chickenpox vaccine and is spread by inhalation. Varicella-naïve pregnant women must be especially careful to avoid contact with an VZV-infected patient. A vaccine for VZV is recommended by the FDA for people aged 60 years or older; it was demonstrated to decrease the frequency and severity of HZO versus placebo.

VARICELLA ZOSTER VIRUS (CHICKEN POX)

Symptoms

Facial rash, red eye, foreign body sensation.

Signs

Acute conjunctivitis with vesicles or papules at the limbus, on the eyelid, or on the conjunctiva. Pseudodendritic corneal epithelial lesions, stromal keratitis, anterior uveitis, optic neuritis, retinitis, and ophthalmoplegia occur rarely.

Late (weeks to months after the outbreak). Immune stromal or neurotrophic keratitis.

Treatment

1. Conjunctival involvement and/or corneal epithelial lesions: Cool compresses and erythromycin ointment t.i.d. to the eye and periorbital lesions.

2. Stromal keratitis with uveitis: Topical steroid (e.g., prednisolone acetate 1% q.i.d.), cycloplegic (e.g., scopolamine 0.25% b.i.d.), and erythromycin ointment q.h.s.

3. Neurotrophic keratitis: Uncommon; see 4.6, *Neurotrophic Keratopathy.*

4. Canalicular obstruction: Uncommon. Managed by intubation of puncta.

NOTE:

1. Aspirin is contraindicated because of the risk of Reye syndrome in children.

2. Immunocompromised children with chicken pox may require i.v. acyclovir.

3. Varicella zoster virus vaccination is available and will likely prevent ophthalmic complications of chicken pox in immunocompetent patients if given at least 8 to 12 weeks before exposure.

Follow-Up

1. Follow-up in 1 to 7 days, depending on the severity of ocular disease. Taper the topical steroids slowly.

2. Watch for stromal or neurotrophic keratitis approximately 4 to 6 weeks after the chicken pox resolves. Stromal keratitis can have a chronic course requiring long-term topical steroids with a very gradual taper.

4.17 OCULAR VACCINIA

Symptoms

Red eye, pain, photophobia, tearing, itching, decreased vision, eyelid swelling, vesicular or pustular skin rash; malaise, fever, history of recent smallpox vaccination or exposure to vaccine directly or indirectly.

Signs

Eyelid/Skin Involvement

Acute blepharitis: Nondermatomal distribution of vesicles that progress into pustules, which umbilicate and indurate. Severe eyelid edema and erythema; periorbital cellulitis. Lymphadenopathy may be present.

Conjunctivitis

Acute papillary conjunctivitis, often with mucopurulent discharge and an inflammatory membrane. Ulcers of the conjunctiva are common. Symblepharon may follow. Limbal pustules have also been noted.

Keratitis (Uncommon)

Similar to HSV: SPK, corneal dendrites, or a geographic epithelial ulcer. Focal or diffuse stromal edema; stromal infiltrate or ulceration, sometimes with necrosis and rarely perforation; late corneal scarring or clouding may develop; secondary uveitis and elevated IOP may occur.

Differential Diagnosis

- HSV: Vesicles do not become pustules. Dendrites of HSV have true terminal bulbs and stain well with fluorescein. See 4.15, *Herpes Simplex Virus.*

- HZO: Vesicles obey the midline, are dermatomal in distribution, and do not become pustules. See 4.16, *Herpes Zoster Ophthalmicus/Varicella Zoster Virus.*

- Chicken pox (Varicella zoster): Systemic illness, common during childhood. See 4.16, *Herpes Zoster Ophthalmicus/Varicella Zoster Virus.*

- Molluscum contagiosum: Skin lesions are umbilicated, but not vesicular or pustular. See 5.2, *Chronic Conjunctivitis.*

Etiology

Vaccinia virus may be shed from the inoculation site for 3 weeks after vaccination. The virus is spread by contact and replicates at a new site. The most common sites for inadvertent vaccinia inoculation are the eye and ocular adnexae. Patients with past or current inflammatory skin diseases (e.g., atopic dermatitis, seborrheic dermatitis) are at higher risk. The incubation period is 5 to 19 days. Approximately one per 30,000 to 40,000 vaccinations results in ocular vaccinia.

Work-Up

1. History: Recent smallpox vaccination? Exposure to someone recently vaccinated? History of work with vaccinia (laboratory)? History of previous nasal or oral sores? History of exposure to chicken pox? Recent topical or systemic steroids? Immune deficiency state? History of atopic dermatitis?

2. External examination: Note the distribution of skin vesicles, if present.

3. Slit-lamp examination with IOP measurement.

4. Check corneal sensation (before instillation of anesthetic), which may be decreased in HSV and HZO.

5. Most cases of ocular vaccinia are diagnosed clinically and require no confirmatory laboratory tests. If the diagnosis is in doubt, viral studies may be obtained (including culture, polymerase chain reaction, and restriction endonuclease analysis).

NOTE: Smears and cultures for bacteria should be taken to rule out superinfection if a corneal ulceration suddenly worsens. See Appendix 8, *Corneal Culture Procedure.*

Treatment

Ocular vaccinia is usually self-limiting. The goal of treatment is to decrease the severity of the disease. Counsel patients on contact precautions to prevent disease spread.

Eyelid/Skin Involvement (Without Keratitis)

1. Ganciclovir 0.15% ophthalmic gel or trifluridine 1% drops five times per day for 2 weeks (may substitute vidarabine 3% ointment five times per day for children, if available).

2. Topical antibiotic ointment (e.g., bacitracin) to skin lesions b.i.d.

3. If severe (e.g., cellulitis and fever), add vaccinia immune globulin (VIG) 100 mg/kg i.m. Repeat in 48 hours if not improved.

Conjunctivitis (Without Keratitis)

1. Ganciclovir 0.15% ophthalmic gel five times a day or trifluridine 1% drops eight times per day for 2 weeks (may substitute vidarabine 3% ointment five times per day for children, if available).

2. Topical antibiotic ointment (e.g., bacitracin) b.i.d.

3. VIG 100 mg/kg i.m. or 6,000 units/kg i.v.

4. If severe (e.g., with ulceration, membrane, fever) and no improvement in 48 hours, VIG administration may be repeated.

Keratitis

1. Ganciclovir 0.15% ophthalmic gel five times a day or trifluridine 1% drops eight times per day for 1 to 2 weeks, then taper, and discontinue over a week (may substitute vidarabine 3% ointment five times per day for children, if available).

2. Topical antibiotic ointment (e.g., bacitracin) b.i.d. to q.i.d. (if epithelial defect).

3. If severe (e.g., with infiltrate or ulcer), add

   a. Cycloplegic agent (e.g., scopolamine 0.25% b.i.d.).

   b. After the epithelium heals, cautiously add topical steroid (dose depends on severity) and slowly taper (while using prophylactic topical antivirals).

4. VIG is relatively contraindicated for patients with isolated vaccinia keratitis. However, it should not be withheld from patients when keratitis accompanies a serious nonocular condition (e.g., progressive vaccinia, eczema vaccinatum), or the ocular involvement is progressing on topical antivirals.

NOTE: VIG is currently available only through the US Centers for Disease Control and Prevention (CDC).

Follow-Up

1. Vaccinia dermatitis and conjunctivitis usually resolve in 7 days. Patients are reexamined in 2 to 7 days to evaluate the response to treatment and then every 7 to 14 days, depending on the clinical findings.

2. The following clinical parameters are evaluated: epithelial defect and ulcer size, corneal thinning and the depth to which the cornea is involved, the anterior chamber reaction, and the IOP (see 9.7, *Inflammatory Open-Angle Glaucoma,* for glaucoma management).

3. Topical antiviral medications should be continued for 2 weeks.

4. Topical steroids used for corneal stromal disease are tapered slowly. Prophylactic topical antiviral agents are used while on steroids.

4.18   INTERSTITIAL KERATITIS

Acute symptomatic IK most commonly occurs within the first or second decade of life. Signs of old IK often persist through life.

Signs

Acute Phase

Critical. Marked corneal stromal blood vessels and edema.

Other. Anterior chamber cells and flare, fine keratic precipitates on the corneal endothelium, conjunctival injection.

Chronic Phase

(See Figure 4.18.1.)
Deep corneal haze or scarring, corneal stromal blood vessels containing minimal or no blood (ghost vessels), stromal thinning.

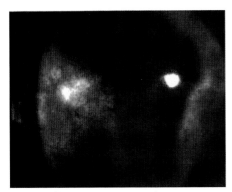

FIGURE 4.18.1. Interstitial keratitis.

Etiology

More Common. Congenital syphilis (usu-ally bilateral, often occurs in the first or sec-ond decade of life, affects both eyes within 1 year of each other, common for late inac-tive, uncommon for acute).

Common. Acquired syphilis (unilateral, often sectoral); tuberculosis (TB) (unilateral, often sectoral); Cogan syndrome [bilateral involvement, vertigo, tinnitus, hearing loss, negative syphilis serologies, often associated with systemic vasculitis (typically polyarteritis nodosa), can occur at any age]; leprosy; HSV; VZV; EBV; Lyme disease.

Work-Up

For active IK and old, previously untreated IK:

1. History: Venereal disease in the mother during pregnancy or in the patient? Diffi-culty hearing or tinnitus?

2. External examination: Look for saddle-nose deformity, Hutchinson teeth, frontal bossing, or other signs of congenital syphilis. Look for hypopigmented or anesthetic skin lesions and thickened skin folds, loss of the temporal eyebrow, and loss of eyelashes, as in leprosy.

3. Slit-lamp examination: Examine corneal nerves for segmental thickening, like beads on a string (leprosy). Examine the iris for nodules (leprosy) and hyperemia with fleshy, pink nodules (syphilis). Check IOP.

4. Dilated fundus examination: Classic salt-and-pepper chorioretinitis or optic atrophy of syphilis.

5. Venereal Disease Research Laboratory test (VDRL, correlates with disease activity) or rapid plasma reagin (RPR); fluorescent trepo-nemal antibody absorption (FTA-ABS, stays positive after treatment) or microhemagglu-tination-*Treponema pallidum* (MHA-TP). See 12.12, *Syphilis.*

6. Purified protein derivative (PPD).

7. Chest radiograph if negative FTA-ABS (or MHA-TP) or positive PPD.

8. Consider erythrocyte sedimentation rate, antinuclear antibody, rheumatoid factor, complete blood count, Lyme, and EBV titers.

Treatment

1. Acute disease

   —Topical cycloplegic.

   —Topical steroid (e.g., prednisolone acetate 1% q2h depending on the degree of inflam-mation).

   —Treat any underlying disease.

2. Old inactive disease with central scarring

   —Corneal transplantation may improve vision if minimal amblyopia is present.

   —Late decrease in vision often due to cata-racts.

3. Acute or old inactive disease

   —If FTA-ABS is positive and the patient has not been treated for syphilis in the past (or is unsure about treatment), there are signs of active syphilitic disease (e.g., active chorioret-initis or papillitis), or if the VDRL or RPR titer is positive and has not declined the expected amount after treatment, then treatment for syphilis is indicated. See 12.12, *Syphilis.*

   —If PPD is positive and the patient is <35 years and has not been treated for TB in the past, or there is evidence of active systemic TB (e.g., positive finding on chest radio-graph), then refer the patient to an inter-nist for TB treatment.

   —If Cogan syndrome is present, refer the patient to an otolaryngologist and rheuma-tologist.

   —If Lyme titers are positive, treat per 13.3, *Lyme Disease.*

Follow-Up

1. Acute disease: Every 3 to 7 days initially, and then every 2 to 4 weeks. The frequency of steroid administration is slowly reduced as the inflammation subsides over the course of months (may take up to 2 years). IOP is monitored closely and reduced with medications based on the degree of elevation and health of the optic nerve (see 9.7, *Inflammatory Open-Angle Glaucoma*).

2. Old inactive disease: Yearly follow-up, unless treatment is required for underlying etiology.

4.19   STAPHYLOCOCCAL HYPERSENSITIVITY

Symptoms

Mild photophobia, mild pain, localized red eye, chronic eyelid crusting, foreign body sensation or dryness. History of recurrent acute episodes, chalazia, or styes.

Signs

(See Figure 4.19.1.)

Critical. Singular or multiple, unilateral or bilateral, peripheral corneal stromal infiltrates with a clear space between the infiltrates and the limbus, and variable staining with fluorescein. Minimal anterior chamber inflammation. Sectoral conjunctival injection, typically.

Other. Blepharitis, inferior SPK, phlyctenule (a wedge-shaped, raised, vascularized sterile infiltrate near the limbus, usually in children), peripheral scarring and corneal neovascularization in the contralateral eye or elsewhere in the same eye.

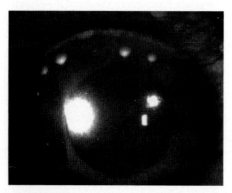

FIGURE 4.19.1. Staphylococcal hypersensitivity.

Differential Diagnosis

■ Infectious corneal infiltrates: Often round, painful, and associated with an anterior chamber reaction. Not usually multiple and recurrent. See 4.11, *Bacterial Keratitis*.

■ Other causes of marginal thinning/infiltrates: See 4.23, *Peripheral Corneal Thinning/Ulceration*.

Etiology

Infiltrates are believed to be a noninfectious reaction of the host's antibodies to bacterial antigens in the setting of staphylococcal blepharitis.

NOTE: Patients with ocular rosacea (e.g., meibomian gland inflammation and telangiectasias of the eyelids) are also susceptible to this condition.

Work-Up

1. History: Recurrent episodes? Contact lens wearer (a risk factor for infection)?

2. Slit-lamp examination with fluorescein staining and IOP check.

3. If an infectious infiltrate is suspected, then corneal scrapings for cultures and smears should be obtained. See Appendix 8, *Corneal Culture Procedure*.

Treatment

Mild

Warm compresses, eyelid hygiene, and a fluoroquinolone antibiotic q.i.d. and bacitracin ophthalmic ointment q.h.s. (see 5.8, *Blepharitis/Meibomitis*).

Moderate to Severe

—Treat as described earlier, but add a low-dose topical steroid (e.g., loteprednol 0.2% to 0.5% or prednisolone 0.25% q.i.d.) with an antibiotic (e.g., trimethoprim/polymyxin B or a fluoroquinolone q.i.d.). A combination antibiotic/steroid can also be used q.i.d. (e.g., loteprednol 0.5%/tobramycin or dexamethasone/tobramycin). Never use steroids without antibiotic coverage. Maintain until the symptoms improve and then slowly taper.

—If episodes recur despite eyelid hygiene, add systemic tetracycline (250 mg p.o. q.i.d. for 1 to 2 weeks, then b.i.d. for 1 month, and then q.d.) or doxycycline (100 mg p.o. b.i.d., for 2 weeks, and then q.d. for 1 month, and then 50 to 100 mg q.d., titrated as necessary) until the ocular disease is controlled for several months. These medications have an anti-inflammatory effect on the sebaceous glands in addition to their antimicrobial action. Topical azithromycin q.h.s. or cyclosporine b.i.d. may be helpful in controlling eyelid inflammation.

—Low-dose antibiotics (e.g., bacitracin ointment q.h.s.) may have to be maintained indefinitely.

NOTE: Tetracycline and doxycycline are contraindicated in children <8 years, pregnant women, and breast-feeding mothers. Erythromycin 200 mg p.o. one to two times per day can be used in children to decrease recurrent disease.

4

Follow-Up

In 2 to 7 days, depending on the clinical picture. IOP is monitored while patients are taking topical steroids.

4.20 PHLYCTENULOSIS

Symptoms

Tearing, irritation, pain, mild-to-severe photophobia. History of similar episodes, styes, or chalazia. Corneal phlyctenules more symptomatic than conjunctival phlyctenules.

Signs

Critical.

- Conjunctival phlyctenule: A small, white nodule on the bulbar conjunctiva, often at limbus, in the center of a hyperemic area.

- Corneal phlyctenule: A small, white nodule, initially at the limbus, with dilated conjunctival blood vessels approaching it. Often associated with epithelial ulceration and central corneal migration, producing wedge-shaped corneal neovascularization and scarring behind the leading edge of the lesion. Can be bilateral (see Figure 4.20.1).

Other. Conjunctival injection, blepharitis, corneal scarring.

Differential Diagnosis

- Inflamed pinguecula: Uncommon in children. Located in the palpebral fissure. Connective tissue often seen from lesion to the limbus. Usually bilateral. See 4.9, *Pterygium/Pinguecula*.

- Infectious corneal ulcer: With migration, corneal phlyctenules produce a sterile ulcer surrounded by a white infiltrate. When an

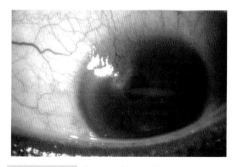

FIGURE 4.20.1. Corneal phlyctenule.

infectious ulcer is suspected (e.g., increased pain, anterior chamber reaction), appropriate antibiotic treatment and diagnostic smears and cultures are necessary. See Appendix 8, *Corneal Culture Procedure.*

■ Staphylococcal hypersensitivity: Peripheral corneal infiltrates, sometimes with an overlying epithelial defect, usually multiple, often bilateral, with a clear space between the infiltrate and the limbus. Minimal anterior chamber reaction. See 4.19, *Staphylococcal Hypersensitivity.*

■ Ocular rosacea: Corneal neovascularization with thinning and subepithelial infiltration may develop in an eye with rosacea. See 5.9, *Ocular Rosacea.*

■ Herpes simplex keratitis: May produce corneal neovascularization associated with a stromal infiltrate. Usually unilateral. See 4.15, *Herpes Simplex Virus.*

Etiology

Delayed hypersensitivity reaction usually as a result of one of the following:

■ *Staphylococcus:* Often related to blepharitis. See 4.19, *Staphylococcal Hypersensitivity.*

■ TB, rarely, or another infectious agent (e.g., Coccidiomycosis, Candidiasis, Lymphogranuloma venereum).

Work-Up

1. History: TB or recent infection?

2. Slit-lamp examination: Inspect the eyelid margin for signs of Staphylococcal anterior blepharitis and rosacea.

3. PPD in patients without blepharitis and those at high risk for TB.

4. Chest radiograph if the PPD is positive or TB is suspected.

Treatment

Indicated for symptomatic patients.

1. Topical steroid (e.g., loteprednol 0.5% or prednisolone acetate 1% q.i.d., depending on the severity of symptoms). A combination antibiotic/steroid can also be used q.i.d. (e.g., loteprednol 0.5%/tobramycin 0.3% or dexamethasone 0.1%/tobramycin 0.3%). If there is significant tearing, a steroid/antibiotic ointment (e.g., dexamethasone/tobramycin) may be more effective.

2. Topical antibiotic in the presence of corneal ulcer. See 4.11, *Bacterial Keratitis.*

3. Eyelid hygiene b.i.d. to t.i.d. for blepharitis. See 5.8, *Blepharitis/Meibomitis.*

4. Artificial tears four to six times per day.

5. Bacitracin ophthalmic ointment q.h.s.

6. In severe cases of blepharitis or acne rosacea, use doxycycline 100 mg p.o. q.d. to b.i.d., or erythromycin 200 mg p.o. q.d. to b.i.d. See 5.8, *Blepharitis/Meibomitis.*

7. If the PPD or chest radiograph is positive for TB, refer the patient to an internist or infectious disease specialist for management.

Follow-Up

Recheck in several days. Healing usually occurs over a 10- to 14-day period, with a residual stromal scar. When the symptoms have significantly improved, slowly taper the steroid. Maintain the antibiotic ointment and eyelid hygiene indefinitely. Continue oral antibiotics for 3 to 6 months. Topical azithromycin or cyclosporine may be beneficial steroid-sparing agents in patients with recurrent inflammation.

4.21 CONTACT LENS-RELATED PROBLEMS

Symptoms

Pain, photophobia, foreign body sensation, decreased vision, red eye, itching, discharge, burning, contact lens intolerance.

NOTE: Any contact lens wearer with pain or redness should remove the lens immediately and have a thorough ophthalmic examination as soon as possible if symptoms persist or worsen.

Signs

See the distinguishing characteristics of each etiology.

Etiology

- Infectious corneal infiltrate/ulcer (bacterial, fungal, *Acanthamoeba*): White corneal lesion that may stain with fluorescein. Must always be ruled out in contact lens patients with eye pain. See 4.11, *Bacterial Keratitis,* 4.12, *Fungal Keratitis,* and 4.13, *Acanthamoeba Keratitis.*

- Giant papillary conjunctivitis: Itching, mucous discharge and lens intolerance in a patient with large superior tarsal conjunctival papillae. See 4.22, *Contact Lens-Induced Giant Papillary Conjunctivitis.*

- Hypersensitivity/toxicity reactions to preservatives in solutions: Conjunctival injection and ocular irritation typically develop shortly after lens cleaning and insertion, but can be present chronically. A recent change from one type or brand of solution is common. Occurred more often in patients using older preserved solutions (e.g., thimerosal or chlorhexidine as a component), but also is seen with newer "all-purpose" solutions. May be due to inadequate rinsing of lenses after enzyme use. Signs include SPK, conjunctival injection, bulbar conjunctival follicles, subepithelial or stromal corneal infiltrates, superior epithelial irregularities, and superficial scarring.

- Contact lens deposits: Multiple small deposits on the contact lens, leading to corneal and conjunctival irritation. The contact lens is often old and may not have been cleaned or enzyme-treated properly in the past.

- Tight lens syndrome: Symptoms may be severe and often develop within 1 or 2 days of contact lens fitting (usually a soft lens), especially if patient sleeps overnight with daily-wear lenses. No lens movement with blinking and lens appears "sucked-on" to the cornea (this can occur after rewearing a soft lens that has dried out and then been rehydrated). An imprint in the conjunctiva is often observed after the lens is removed. Central corneal edema, SPK, anterior chamber reaction, and sometimes a sterile hypopyon may develop.

- Corneal warpage: Seen predominantly in long-term polymethylmethacrylate hard contact lens wearers. Initially, the vision becomes blurred with glasses ("spectacle blur") but remains good with contact lenses. Keratometry reveals distorted mires and corneal topography shows irregular astigmatism that eventually resolves after lens discontinuation.

- Corneal neovascularization: Patients are often asymptomatic until the visual axis is involved. Superficial corneal neovascularization for 1 mm is common and usually not a concern in aphakic contact lens wearers. With any sign of chronic hypoxia, the goal is to increase oxygen permeability, increase movement, and discontinue extended-wear lenses.

- Dry eyes/inadequate/incomplete blinking/thick RGP lenses: Can lead to chronic inflammation, staining, and in some cases scarring, at the 3- and 9-o'clock positions.

- Contact lens keratopathy (pseudosuperior limbic keratoconjunctivitis): Hyperemia and fluorescein staining of the superior bulbar conjunctiva, particularly at the limbus. SPK, subepithelial infiltrates, haze, and irregularity may be found on the superior cornea. This may represent a hypersensitivity or toxicity reaction to preservatives in contact lens solutions (classically thimerosal, but newer preservatives as well). No corneal filaments, papillary reaction, or association with thyroid disease.

- Displaced contact lens: Most commonly the lens has actually fallen out of the eye and been lost. If retained, lens usually found in the superior fornix and may require double-eversion of the upper eyelid to remove. Fluorescein will stain a soft lens to aid in finding it.

- Others: Contact lens inside out, corneal abrasion (see 3.2, *Corneal Abrasion*), poor lens fit, damaged contact lens, change in refractive error.

Work-Up

1. History: Main complaint (mild-to-severe pain, discomfort, itching)? Type of contact

lens (soft, hard, gas permeable, daily wear, extended wear, or frequent replacement, or single-use daily disposable)? Age of the lenses? Continuous time lenses are worn? Sleeping in lenses? How are the lenses cleaned and disinfected? Are enzyme tablets used? Preservative-free products? Recent changes in contact lens habits or solutions? How is the pain related to wearing time? Is the pain relieved by removal of the lens?

2. In noninfectious conditions, while the contact lens is still in the eye, evaluate its fit and examine its surface for deposits and defects at the slit lamp.

3. Remove lens and examine the eye with fluorescein. Evert the upper eyelids of both eyes and inspect the superior tarsal conjunctiva for papillae.

4. Smears and cultures are taken when an infectious corneal ulcer is suspected with infiltrate >1 mm or when an unusual organism is suspected (i.e., *Acanthamoeba* or fungus). See 4.11, *Bacterial Keratitis,* 4.12, *Fungal Keratitis,* 4.13, *Acanthamoeba Keratitis,* and Appendix 8, *Corneal Culture Procedure.*

5. The contact lenses and lens case are also cultured occasionally.

Treatment

When the diagnosis of infection is suspected:

1. Discontinue contact lens wear.

2. Antibiotic treatment regimen varies with diagnosis as follows.

Possible Corneal Ulcer (Corneal Infiltrate, Epithelial Defect, Anterior Chamber Reaction, Pain)

a. Obtain appropriate smears and cultures. See Appendix 8, *Corneal Culture Procedure.*

b. Start intensive topical antibiotics, fortified or a fluoroquinolone (given every 30 minutes initially), and a cycloplegic. See 4.11, *Bacterial Keratitis.*

Small Subepithelial Infiltrates, Corneal Abrasion, or Diffuse SPK

a. Topical antibiotic (e.g., fluoroquinolone) drops four to eight times per day and a cycloplegic.

b. Can also add tobramycin or bacitracin/polymyxin B ointment q.h.s. Beware of toxicity with long-term use (especially tobramycin).

c. For an abrasion, use tobramycin, bacitracin/polymyxin B, or ciprofloxacin ointment four to eight times per day. Avoid steroids.

NOTE: Never pressure patch a contact lens wearer because of the risk of rapid development of Pseudomonas infection.

When a specific contact lens problem is suspected, it may be treated as follows:

Giant Papillary Conjunctivitis (see 4.22, *Contact Lens-Induced Giant Papillary Conjunctivitis*)

Hypersensitivity/Toxicity Reaction

a. Discontinue contact lens wear.

b. Preservative-free artificial tears four to six times per day.

c. On resolution of the condition, the patient may return to new contact lenses, preferably daily disposable lenses. If the patient desires frequent-replacement or conventional lenses, hydrogen peroxide-based systems are recommended, and appropriate lens hygiene is reviewed.

Contact Lens Deposits

a. Discontinue contact lens wear.

b. Replace with a new contact lens once the symptoms resolve. Consider changing the brand of contact lens, or change to daily disposable or frequent replacement lens.

c. Teach proper contact lens care, stressing weekly enzyme treatments for lenses replaced less frequently than every 2 weeks.

Tight Lens Syndrome

a. Discontinue contact lens wear.

b. Consider a topical cycloplegic (e.g., scopolamine 0.25% b.i.d.) in the presence of an anterior chamber reaction.

c. Once resolved, refit patients with a flatter and more oxygen-permeable contact lens. Discontinue extended-wear contact lenses.

d. If a soft lens has dried out, discard and refit.

NOTE: Patients with hypopyon do not need to be cultured when tight lens syndrome is highly suspected (i.e., if surface intact, with edema but no infiltrate).

Corneal Warpage

a. Discontinue contact lens wear. Explain to patients that vision may be poor for the following 2 to 6 weeks, and they may require a change in spectacle prescription. May need to discontinue lenses one eye at a time so patient can function.

b. A gas-permeable hard contact lens should be refitted when the refraction and keratometric readings have stabilized.

Corneal Neovascularization

a. Discontinue contact lens wear.

b. Consider a topical steroid (e.g., prednisolone 1% q.i.d. or loteprednol 0.5% q.i.d.) for extensive deep neovascularization (rarely necessary).

c. Refit carefully with a highly oxygen-transmissible daily-wear disposable contact lens that moves adequately over the cornea.

Corneal Epithelial Changes

a. Discontinue contact lens wear.

b. Use preservative-free artificial tears.

c. Consider a new contact lens when the epithelial changes resolve, which may take weeks or months.

d. Consider daily disposable lenses and preservative-free solutions.

e. Refit with thinner RGP lenses if there is dryness at 3- and 9-o'clock.

Inadequate/Incomplete Blinking

a. Frequent preservative-free artificial tears.

b. Consider punctal plugs or cyclosporine 0.05% drops in dry-eye syndrome.

Pseudosuperior Limbic Keratoconjunctivitis

a. Treat as described for hypersensitivity/toxicity reactions. Use unit dose preservative-free tear. Consider bandage contact lens if needed to improve vision. When a large subepithelial opacity extends toward the visual axis, topical steroids may be added cautiously (e.g., loteprednol 0.5% q.i.d.), but they are often ineffective. Steroid use in contact lens-related problems should have concomitant antibiotic coverage.

Displaced Lens

a. Inspect lens carefully for damage. If undamaged, clean, and disinfect lens, then recheck fit when symptoms have resolved. If damaged, discard and replace.

Follow-Up

1. Next day if infection cannot be ruled out. Treatment is maintained until the condition clears.

2. In noninfectious conditions, reevaluate in 1 to 4 weeks, depending on the clinical situation. Contact lens wear is resumed when the condition resolves. Patients using topical steroids should be followed up more closely and their IOP monitored.

The following regimen for contact lens care is one we recommend if single-use daily disposable lenses are not possible.

1. Daily cleaning and disinfection with removal of lenses while sleeping for all lens types, including those approved for "extended wear" and "overnight wear." We prefer standard rather than hyperoxygen-transmissible lenses for frequent replacement, as the latter may allow greater adherence for organisms.

2. Daily cleaning regimen for soft contact lenses:

—Preservative-free daily cleaner.

—Preservative-free saline.

—Disinfectant, preferably hydrogen peroxide type.

—Disinfection solutions need to be used for recommended time (hours) prior to lens reinsertion.

—Weekly treatment with enzyme tablets (not necessary in disposable lenses replaced every 2 to 4 weeks or less).

3. RGP lenses: Cleaning/soaking/rinsing all in one solution. Lenses can be reinserted soon after the removal from disinfecting solution.

4.22 CONTACT LENS-INDUCED GIANT PAPILLARY CONJUNCTIVITIS

Symptoms

Itching, mucous discharge, decreased lens-wearing time, increased lens awareness, excessive lens movement.

Signs

Critical. Giant papillae on the superior tarsal conjunctiva (see Figure 4.22.1).

NOTE: The upper eyelid must be everted to make the diagnosis. Upper eyelid eversion should be part of the routine eye examination in any patient who wears contact lenses.

Other. Contact lens coatings, high-riding lens, mild conjunctival injection, ptosis (usually a late sign).

Work-Up

1. History: Details of contact lens use, including the age of lenses, daily or extended wear, the frequency of replacement, and the cleaning and enzyme treatment regimen.

2. Slit-lamp examination: Evert the upper eyelids and examine for large papillae (≥1 mm).

Treatment

1. Modify contact lens regimen as follows:

Mild-to-Moderate Giant Papillary Conjunctivitis

a. Replace and refit the contact lens. Consider planned replacement or daily disposable lenses (daily disposable lenses are preferred).

b. Reduce contact lens-wearing time (switch from extended-wear contact lens to daily-wear).

c. Have the patient clean the lenses more thoroughly, preferably by using preservative-free solutions, preservative-free saline, and a hydrogen peroxide-based disinfection system.

d. Increase enzyme use (use at least every week).

Severe Giant Papillary Conjunctivitis

a. Suspend contact lens wear.

b. Restart with a new contact lens when the symptoms and signs clear (usually 1 to 4 months), preferably with daily disposable soft contact lenses.

c. Careful lens hygiene as described earlier.

2. Start a topical mast cell stabilizer (e.g., pemirolast q.i.d., nedocromil b.i.d., lodox-

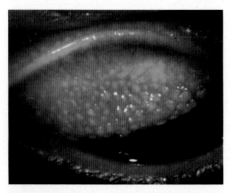

FIGURE 4.22.1. Giant papillary conjunctivitis.

amide q.i.d., or cromolyn sodium q.i.d.) or a combination antihistamine/mast cell stabilizer (e.g., olopatadine b.i.d., epinastine b.i.d.). Some patients use both types of drops.

3. In unusually severe cases, short-term use of a low-dose topical steroid may be considered (e.g., loteprednol 0.2% to 0.5% q.i.d.). Contact lenses should not be worn while using a topical steroid.

Follow-Up

In 2 to 4 weeks. The patient may resume contact lens wear once the symptoms are resolved.

Symptoms may improve before papillae resolve. Mast cell stabilizers are continued while the signs remain, and they may need to be used chronically to maintain contact lens tolerance.

NOTE: Giant papillary conjunctivitis can also result from atopic/vernal conjunctivitis, an exposed suture, or an ocular prosthesis. Exposed sutures are removed. Prostheses should be cleaned and polished. A coating can be placed on the prosthesis to reduce giant papillary conjunctivitis. Otherwise, these entities are treated as described earlier.

4.23 PERIPHERAL CORNEAL THINNING/ULCERATION

Symptoms

Pain, photophobia, red eye; may be asymptomatic.

Signs

Peripheral corneal thinning (best seen with a narrow slit beam), may have a sterile infiltrate or ulcer.

Differential Diagnosis

Infectious infiltrate or ulcer. Lesions are often treated as infectious until cultures come back negative. See 4.11, *Bacterial Keratitis*.

Etiology

■ Connective tissue disease (e.g., rheumatoid arthritis, Wegener granulomatosis, relapsing polychondritis, polyarteritis nodosa, systemic lupus erythematosus, others). Peripheral (unilateral or bilateral) corneal thinning/ulcers may be associated with inflammatory infiltrates. May progress circumferentially to involve the entire peripheral cornea. Perforation may occur. This may be the first manifestation of systemic disease (see Figure 4.23.1).

■ Terrien marginal degeneration: Often asymptomatic; usually bilateral; slowly progressive thinning of the peripheral cornea; typically

superior; more often in men. The anterior chamber is quiet, and the eye is typically not injected. A yellow line (lipid) may appear, with a fine pannus over the thinned areas of involvement. The thinning may slowly spread circumferentially. Irregular and against-the-rule astigmatism is often present. The epithelium usually remains intact, but perforation may occur with minor trauma.

■ Mooren ulcer: Unilateral or bilateral; idiopathic (autoimmunity may play a key role); diagnosis of exclusion. Painful corneal thinning and ulceration with inflammation; initially starts as a focal area in the peripheral cornea nasally or temporally without limbal sparing with subsequent extension circumferentially or centrally. An epithelial defect,

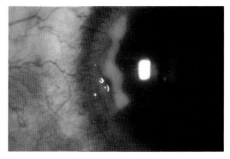

FIGURE 4.23.1. Peripheral ulcerative keratitis.

stromal thinning, and a leading undermined edge are present. Limbal blood vessels may grow into the ulcer, and perforation can occur. Mooren-like ulcer has been associated with systemic hepatitis C virus infection.

- Pellucid marginal degeneration: Painless, bilateral asymmetric corneal thinning of the inferior peripheral cornea (usually from the 4- to 8-o'clock portions). There is no anterior chamber reaction, conjunctival injection, lipid deposition, or vascularization. The epithelium is intact. Corneal protrusion may be seen above the area of thinning. The thinning may slowly progress.

- Furrow degeneration: Painless corneal thinning just peripheral to an arcus senilis, typically in the elderly. Noninflammatory without vascularization. Perforation is rare. Usually nonprogressive and does not require treatment.

- Delle: Painless oval corneal thinning resulting from corneal drying and stromal dehydration adjacent to an abnormal conjunctival or corneal elevation. The epithelium is usually intact. See 4.24, *Dellen*.

- Staphylococcal hypersensitivity/marginal keratitis: Peripheral, white corneal infiltrate(s) with limbal clearing that may have an epithelial defect and mild thinning. See 4.19, *Staphylococcal Hypersensitivity*.

- Dry-eye syndrome: Peripheral (or central) sterile corneal melts may result from severe cases of dry eye. See 4.3, *Dry-Eye Syndrome*.

- Exposure/neurotrophic keratopathy: Typically, a sterile oval ulcer develops inferiorly on the cornea without signs of significant inflammation. May be associated with an eyelid abnormality, a fifth or seventh cranial nerve defect, or proptosis. The ulcer may become superinfected. See 4.5, *Exposure Keratopathy*, and 4.6, *Neurotrophic Keratopathy*.

- Sclerokeratitis: Corneal ulceration is associated with severe radiating ocular pain because of accompanying scleritis. The sclera develops a blue hue, scleral vessels are engorged, and scleral edema with or without nodules is present. An underlying connective tissue disease, especially Wegener granulomatosis, must be ruled out. See 5.7, *Scleritis*.

- Vernal keratoconjunctivitis: Superior, shallow, shield-shaped, sterile corneal infiltrate/ulcer, accompanied by giant papillae on the superior tarsal conjunctiva or limbus, with or without degenerated limbal eosinophils (Horner–Trantas dots). The conjunctivitis is usually bilateral, often occurs in children, and recurs during the summer months, but it can occur anytime in warm climates. See 5.1, *Acute Conjunctivitis*.

- Ocular rosacea: Typically affects the inferior cornea in middle-aged patients. Erythema and telangiectasia of the eyelid margins, corneal neovascularization. See 5.9, *Ocular Rosacea*.

- Others: Cataract surgery, inflammatory bowel disease, previous HSV or VZV infections, and leukemia can rarely cause peripheral corneal thinning/ulceration.

Work-Up

1. History: Contact lens wearer or previous HSV or VZV keratitis? Connective tissue disease or inflammatory bowel disease? Other systemic symptoms? Seasonal conjunctivitis with itching (vernal)? Prior ocular surgery?

2. External examination: Old facial scars of VZV? Eyelid-closure problem causing exposure? Blue tinge to the sclera? Rosacea facies?

3. Slit-lamp examination: Look for infiltrate, corneal ulcer, hypopyon, uveitis, scleritis, old herpetic corneal scarring, poor tear lake, SPK, blepharitis. Look for giant papillae on the superior tarsal conjunctiva or limbal papillae. Measure IOP.

4. Schirmer test (see 4.3, *Dry-Eye Syndrome*).

5. Dilated fundus examination: Look for cotton-wool spots consistent with connective tissue disease or evidence of posterior scleritis (e.g., vitritis, subretinal fluid, chorioretinal folds, exudative retinal detachment).

6. Corneal scrapings and cultures when infection is suspected. See Appendix 8, *Corneal Culture Procedure*.

7. Systemic work-up including serum anti-nuclear antibody, rheumatoid factor, erythrocyte sedimentation rate, antineutrophilic cytoplasmic antibody levels, complement CH50, C3, C4, angiotension-converting enzyme, chest x-ray, and complete blood count with differential to rule out connective tissue disease and leukemia.

8. Scleritis work-up, when present (see 5.7, *Scleritis*).

9. Refer to an internist (or rheumatologist) when connective tissue disease is suspected.

Treatment

See sections on dellen, staphylococcal hypersensitivity, dry-eye syndrome, exposure and neurotrophic keratopathies, scleritis, vernal conjunctivitis, and ocular rosacea.

1. Corneal thinning due to connective tissue disease: Management is usually coordinated with a rheumatologist or internist.

—Antibiotic ointment (e.g., erythromycin ointment q2h) or preservative-free ointment.

—Cycloplegic drops (e.g., scopolamine 0.25% or atropine 1% b.i.d. to t.i.d.) when an anterior chamber reaction or pain is present.

—Consider doxycycline 100 mg p.o. b.i.d. because of its metalloproteinase inhibition properties.

—Systemic steroids (e.g., prednisone 60 to 100 mg p.o. q.d.; the dosage is adjusted according to the response) and a histamine type 2 receptor (H2) blocker (e.g., ranitidine 150 mg p.o. b.i.d.) are used for significant and progressive corneal thinning, but not for perforation.

—An immunosuppressive agent (e.g., methotrexate, mycophenolate mofetil, infliximab, azathioprine, cyclophosphamide) is often required, especially for Wegener granulomatosis. This should be done in coordination with the patient's internist or rheumatologist.

—Excision of adjacent inflamed conjunctiva is occasionally helpful when the condition progresses despite treatment.

—Punctal occlusion if dry-eye syndrome is present. Typical cyclosporine 0.05% to 2% b.i.d. to q.i.d. also may be helpful. Experimental research suggests benefits of oral omega-3 fatty acids for severe dry-eye syndrome.

—Consider cyanoacrylate tissue adhesive or corneal transplantation surgery for an impending or actual corneal perforation. A conjunctival flap or amniotic membrane graft can also be used for an impending corneal perforation.

—Patients with significant corneal thinning should wear their glasses [or protective glasses (e.g., polycarbonate lens)] during the day and an eye shield at night.

NOTE: Topical steroids are usually not used in the presence of significant corneal thinning because of the risk of perforation. Gradually taper topical steroids if the patient is already taking them. Corneal thinning due to relapsing polychondritis, however, seems to improve with topical steroids (e.g., prednisolone acetate 1% q1–2h).

---

2. Terrien marginal degeneration: Correct astigmatism with glasses or contact lenses if possible. Protective eyewear should be worn if significant thinning is present. Lamellar grafts can be used if thinning is extreme.

3. Mooren ulcer: Underlying systemic diseases must be ruled out before this diagnosis can be made. Topical corticosteroids, topical cyclosporine 0.05% to 2%, limbal conjunctival excision, corneal gluing, and lamellar keratoplasty may be beneficial. Systemic immunosuppressants (e.g., oral corticosteroids, methotrexate, cyclophosphamide, and cyclosporine) are indicated and may be lifesaving. See treatment for corneal thinning secondary to connective tissue disease above.

4. Pellucid marginal degeneration: See 4.25, *Keratoconus*.

5. Furrow degeneration: No treatment is required.

NOTE: If systemic steroid therapy is to be instituted, obtain a steroid work-up as indicated and involve the patient's primary medical doctor.

Follow-Up

Patients with severe disease are examined daily; those with milder conditions are checked less frequently. Watch carefully for signs of superinfection (e.g., increased pain, stromal infiltration, anterior chamber cells and flare, conjunctival injection), increased IOP, and progressive corneal thinning. Treatment is maintained until the epithelial defect over the ulcer heals and is then gradually tapered. As long as an epithelial defect is present, there is risk of progressive thinning and perforation.

4.24   DELLEN

Symptoms

Usually asymptomatic; irritation, foreign body sensation.

Signs

Critical. Corneal thinning, usually at the limbus, often in the shape of an ellipse, accompanied by an adjacent focal conjunctival or corneal elevation.

Other. Fluorescein pooling in the area, but minimal staining. No infiltrate, no anterior chamber reaction, minimal-to-moderate hyperemia.

Differential Diagnosis

See 4.23, *Peripheral Corneal Thinning/Ulceration.*

Etiology

Poor spread of the tear film over a focal area of cornea (with resultant stromal dehydration) due to an adjacent surface elevation (e.g., chemosis, conjunctival hemorrhage, filtering bleb, pterygium, tumor, and poststrabismus surgery).

Work-Up

1. History: Previous eye surgery?

2. Slit-lamp examination with fluorescein staining: Look for an adjacent area of elevation.

Treatment

1. Lubricating or antibiotic ointment every 2 to 4 hours and q.h.s. Maintain the ointment at least q.h.s. until the adjacent elevation is eliminated.

2. If the cause cannot be removed (e.g., filtering bleb), lubricating ointment should be applied nightly, and viscous artificial tear drops should be used four to eight times per day. If drops are needed more than four times per day, a preservative-free drop should be used.

Follow-Up

Unless there is severe thinning, reexamination can be performed in 1 to 7 days, at which time the cornea can be expected to be of normal thickness. If it is not, full-time patching and lubrication should again be instituted.

4.25   KERATOCONUS

Symptoms

Progressive decreased vision, usually beginning in adolescence and continuing into middle age. Acute corneal hydrops can cause a sudden decrease in vision, pain, red eye, photophobia, and profuse tearing.

Signs

(See Figure 4.25.1.)

Critical. Slowly progressive irregular astigmatism resulting from paracentral thinning and bulging of the cornea (maximal thinning near the apex of the protrusion), vertical tension lines in the posterior cornea (Vogt striae), an irregular corneal retinoscopic reflex (scissor reflex), and egg-shaped mires on keratometry. Inferior steepening is seen on corneal topographic evaluation. Usually bilateral but often asymmetric.

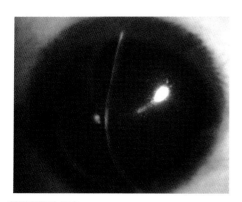

FIGURE 4.25.1. Keratoconus.

Other. Fleischer ring (epithelial iron deposits at the base of the cone), bulging of the lower eyelid when looking downward (Munson sign), superficial corneal scarring. Corneal hydrops (sudden development of corneal edema) results from a rupture in Descemet membrane (see Figure 4.25.2).

Associations

Keratoconus is associated with Down syndrome, atopic disease, Turner syndrome, Leber congenital amaurosis, mitral valve prolapse, retinitis pigmentosa, and Marfan syndrome. It is related to chronic eye rubbing. Family history of keratoconus is also a risk factor.

Differential Diagnosis

- Pellucid marginal degeneration: Corneal thinning in the inferior periphery, 1 to 2 mm from the limbus. The cornea protrudes superior to the band of thinning.

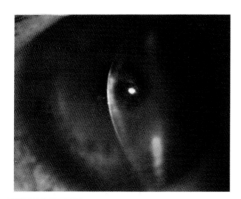

FIGURE 4.25.2. Acute corneal hydrops.

- Keratoglobus: Rare, congenital, nonprogressive. Uniform circularly thinned cornea with maximal thinning in the mid-periphery of the cornea. The cornea protrudes central to the area of maximal thinning.

NOTE: Treatment for pellucid marginal degeneration is the same as for keratoconus, except corneal transplantation is technically more difficult due to peripheral thinning and has a higher failure rate because larger grafts are necessary.

- Postrefractive surgery ectasia: After lamellar refractive surgery such as LASIK, and rarely surface ablation, a condition very similar to keratoconus can develop. It is treated in the same manner as keratoconus.

Work-Up

1. History: Duration and rate of decreased vision? Frequent change in eyeglass prescriptions? History of eye rubbing? Medical problems? Allergies? Family history? Previous refractive surgery?

2. Slit-lamp examination with close attention to location and characteristics of corneal thinning, Vogt striae, and a Fleischer ring (may be best appreciated with cobalt blue light).

3. Retinoscopy and refraction. Look for irregular astigmatism and a waterdrop or scissors red reflex.

4. Corneal topography (can show central and inferior steepening) and keratometry (irregular mires and steepening).

Treatment

1. Patients are instructed not to rub their eyes.

2. Correct refractive errors with glasses or soft contact lenses (for mild cases) or RGP contact lenses (successful in most cases). Occasionally, hybrid contact lenses are required.

3. Partial thickness or full-thickness corneal transplantation surgery is usually indicated when contact lenses cannot be tolerated or no longer produce satisfactory vision.

4. Intracorneal ring segments have been successful in getting some patients back into

contact lenses, especially in mild-to-moderate keratoconus.

5. Corneal collagen cross-linking: A surgical procedure where typically a large corneal epithelial defect is created, riboflavin drops are placed on the cornea for 30 minutes and then ultraviolet light is shined on the cornea for another 30 minutes. The goal is to "cross-link" collagen bonds in the cornea to strengthen it and slow down (ideally eliminate) the progression of keratoconus. It is not currently FDA approved.

6. Acute corneal hydrops:

   —Cycloplegic agent (e.g., cyclopentolate 1%), bacitracin ointment q.i.d., and consider brimonidine 0.1% b.i.d. to t.i.d.

—Start sodium chloride 5% ointment b.i.d. until resolved (usually several weeks to months).

—Glasses or a shield should be worn by patients at risk for trauma or by those who rub their eyes.

NOTE: Acute hydrops is not an indication for emergency corneal transplantation, except in the extremely rare case of corneal perforation (which is first treated medically and sometimes with tissue adhesives).

Follow-Up

Every 3 to 12 months, depending on the progression of symptoms. After an episode of hydrops, examine the patient every 1 to 4 weeks until resolved (which can take several months).

4.26   CORNEAL DYSTROPHIES

Bilateral, inherited, progressive corneal disorders without inflammation or corneal neovascularization. Most are autosomal dominant disorders, except macular dystrophy and type 3 lattice dystrophy (autosomal recessive).

ANTERIOR CORNEAL DYSTROPHIES

Epithelial Basement Membrane Dystrophy (Map–Dot–Fingerprint Dystrophy)

Most common anterior dystrophy. Diffuse gray patches (maps), creamy white cysts (dots), or fine refractile lines (fingerprints) in the corneal epithelium, best seen with retroillumination or a broad slit-lamp beam angled from the side. Spontaneous painful corneal erosions may develop, particularly on opening the eyes after sleep. May cause decreased vision, monocular diplopia, and shadow images. See 4.2, *Recurrent Corneal Erosion,* for treatment.

Meesmann Dystrophy

Rare, epithelial dystrophy that is seen in the first years of life, but is usually asymptomatic until middle age. Retroillumination shows discrete, tiny epithelial vesicles diffusely involving the cornea but concentrated in the palpebral fissure. Although treatment is usually not required, bandage soft contact lenses or superficial keratectomy may be beneficial if significant photophobia is present or if visual acuity is severely affected.

Corneal Dystrophy of Bowman Layer Type I (Reis–Bücklers) and Type II (Thiel–Behnke)

Appears early in life. Subepithelial, gray reticular opacities are seen primarily in the central cornea. Painful episodes from recurrent erosions are relatively common and require treatment. Corneal transplantation surgery may be necessary to improve vision, but the dystrophy often recurs in the graft. Excimer laser PTK or superficial lamellar keratectomy may be adequate treatment in many cases.

CORNEAL STROMAL DYSTROPHIES

When these conditions cause reduced vision, patients usually benefit from a corneal transplant or PTK.

Lattice Dystrophy

Four clinical forms. Type 1 (Biber–Haab–Dimmer, most common): refractile branching lines, white subepithelial dots, and scarring of the corneal stroma centrally, best seen with retroillumination. Recurrent erosions are common (see 4.2, *Recurrent Corneal Erosion*). The corneal periphery is typically clear. Tends to recur within 3 to 5 years after PTK or corneal transplantation. Type 2 (Meretoja syndrome): associated with systemic amyloidosis, facial mask, ear abnormalities, cranial and peripheral nerve palsies, dry and lax skin). Type 3 and 4: Symptoms delayed until fifth to seventh decades.

Granular Dystrophy

White anterior stromal deposits in the central cornea, separated by discrete clear intervening spaces ("bread-crumb-like" opacities). The corneal periphery is spared. Appears in the first decade of life but rarely becomes symptomatic before adulthood. Erosions are uncommon. Also may recur after PTK or corneal transplantation within 3 to 5 years.

Macular Dystrophy

Gray-white stromal opacities with ill-defined edges extending from limbus to limbus with cloudy intervening spaces. Can involve the full thickness of the stroma, more superficial centrally and deeper peripherally. Causes late decreased vision more commonly than recurrent erosions. May recur many years after corneal transplantation.

Schnyder Crystalline Dystrophy

Fine, yellow-white anterior stromal crystals located in the central cornea. Later develop full-thickness central haze and a dense arcus senilis. Work-up includes fasting serum cholesterol and triglyceride levels due to association with systemic lipid abnormalities. Rarely compromises vision enough to require PTK or corneal transplantation. See 4.14, *Crystalline Keratopathy.*

CORNEAL ENDOTHELIAL DYSTROPHIES

Fuchs Dystrophy

See 4.27, *Fuchs Endothelial Dystrophy.*

Posterior Polymorphous Dystrophy

Changes at the level of Descemet membrane, including vesicles arranged in a linear or grouped pattern, gray haze, or broad bands with irregular, scalloped edges. Iris abnormalities, including iridocorneal adhesions and corectopia (a decentered pupil), may be present and are occasionally associated with corneal edema. Glaucoma may occur. See 8.12, *Developmental Anterior Segment and Lens Anomalies/Dysgenesis,* for differential diagnosis. Treatment includes management of corneal edema and corneal transplantation for severe cases.

Congenital Hereditary Endothelial Dystrophy

Bilateral corneal edema with normal corneal diameter, normal IOP, and no cornea guttata (see 8.11, *Congenital/Infantile Glaucoma,* for differential diagnosis). Rare. Two distinct types distinguished by clinical presentation and genetics:

■ Autosomal recessive: Present at birth, non-progressive, nystagmus present. Pain or photophobia uncommon.

■ Autosomal dominant: Is first seen during childhood, slowly progressive, no nystagmus. Pain, tearing, and photophobia are common.

Treatment

Some patients may benefit from a corneal transplant.

4.27   FUCHS ENDOTHELIAL DYSTROPHY

Symptoms

Glare and blurred vision, worse on awakening. May progress to severe pain due to ruptured bullae. Symptoms rarely develop before age 50.

Signs

(See Figure 4.27.1.)

Critical. Cornea guttata with stromal edema. Bilateral, but may be asymmetric.

NOTE: Central cornea guttata without stromal edema is called endothelial dystrophy. This condition may progress to Fuchs dystrophy over years.

Other. Fine pigment dusting on the endothelium, central epithelial edema and bullae, folds in Descemet membrane, subepithelial haze, or scarring.

Differential Diagnosis

- Aphakic or pseudophakic bullous keratopathy: History of cataract surgery, unilateral. See 4.28, *Aphakic Bullous Keratopathy/Pseudophakic Bullous Keratopathy.*

- Congenital hereditary endothelial dystrophy: Bilateral corneal edema at birth. See 4.26, *Corneal Dystrophies.*

- Posterior polymorphous dystrophy: Seen early in life. Corneal endothelium shows either grouped vesicles, geographic gray lesions, or broad bands. Occasionally corneal edema. See 4.26, *Corneal Dystrophies.*

- Iridocorneal endothelial (ICE) syndrome: "Beaten metal" corneal endothelial appearance, with corneal edema, increased IOP, variable iris thinning, and pupil distortion. Typically unilateral, in young to middle-aged adults. See 9.15, *Iridocorneal Endothelial Syndrome.*

Work-Up

1. History: Previous cataract surgery?

2. Slit-lamp examination: Cornea guttata are best seen with retroillumination. Fluorescein staining may demonstrate intact or ruptured bullae.

3. Measure IOP.

4. Consider specular microscopy to evaluate the endothelial cells and corneal pachymetry to determine the central corneal thickness.

Treatment

1. Topical sodium chloride 5% drops q.i.d. and ointment q.h.s.

2. May gently blow warm air from a hair dryer at arm's length toward the eyes for a few minutes every morning to dehydrate the cornea.

3. IOP reduction if needed.

4. Ruptured corneal bullae are painful and should be treated as recurrent erosions (see 4.2, *Recurrent Corneal Erosion*).

5. Endothelial keratoplasty such as Descemet stripping endothelial keratoplasty (DSEK) is usually indicated when visual acuity decreases due to corneal edema, or penetrating keratoplasty (PK) if anterior stromal scarring is present.

Follow-Up

Every 3 to 12 months to check IOP and assess corneal edema. The condition progresses very slowly, and visual acuity typically remains good until significant stromal edema or any epithelial edema develop.

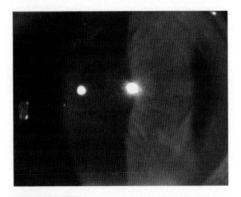

FIGURE 4.27.1. Fuchs endothelial dystrophy.

4.28 APHAKIC BULLOUS KERATOPATHY/ PSEUDOPHAKIC BULLOUS KERATOPATHY

Symptoms

Decreased vision, pain, tearing, foreign body sensation, photophobia, red eye; history of cataract surgery in the involved eye.

Signs

(See Figure 4.28.1.)

Critical. Corneal edema in an eye in which the native lens has been removed.

Other. Corneal bullae, Descemet folds, subepithalial haze or scarring, corneal neovascularization, with or without preexisting guttata. Cystoid macular edema (CME) may be present.

Etiology

Multifactorial: Corneal endothelial damage, intraocular inflammation, vitreous or subluxed intraocular lens or tube shunt touching (or intermittently touching) the cornea, preexisting endothelial dysfunction.

Work-Up

1. Slit-lamp examination: Stain the cornea with fluorescein to check for denuded epithelium, check the position of the intraocular lens if present, determine whether vitreous is touching the corneal endothelium, and evaluate the eye for inflammation. Check for subepithelial haze or scarring. Evaluate the fellow eye for endothelial dystrophy.

2. Check IOP.

3. Dilated fundus examination: Look for CME.

4. Consider a fluorescein angiogram or optical coherence tomography to help detect CME.

Treatment

1. Topical sodium chloride 5% drops q.i.d. and ointment q.h.s., if epithelial edema is present.

2. Reduce IOP with medications if increased. Avoid epinephrine derivatives and prostaglandin analogs, if possible, because of the risk of CME (see 9.1, *Primary Open-Angle Glaucoma*).

3. Ruptured epithelial bullae (producing corneal epithelial defects) may be treated with:

   a. An antibiotic ointment (e.g., erythromycin), a cycloplegic (e.g., scopolamine 0.25%). The antibiotic ointment can be used frequently (e.g., q2h) without patching.

   b. Alternatively, sodium chloride 5% ointment q.i.d., a bandage soft contact lens, or, in patients with limited visual potential, anterior stromal micropuncture or PTK can be used for recurrent ruptured epithelial bullae (see 4.2, *Recurrent Corneal Erosion*).

4. Full-thickness corneal transplant or endothelial keratoplasty such as DSEK (in patients with posterior chamber intraocular lenses), combined with possible intraocular lens repositioning, replacement, or removal and/or vitrectomy, is indicated when vision fails or when the disease becomes advanced and painful. Conjunctival flap or amniotic membrane graft surgery may be indicated for a painful eye with poor visual potential.

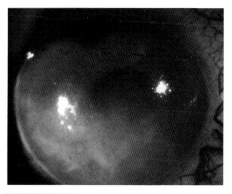

FIGURE 4.28.1. Pseudophakic bullous keratopathy.

5. See 11.14, *Cystoid Macular Edema,* for treatment of CME.

NOTE: Although both CME and corneal disease may contribute to decreased vision, the precise role of each is often difficult to determine preoperatively. CME is less likely with a posterior chamber intraocular

lens than a closed-loop anterior chamber intraocular lens.

Follow-Up

In 24 to 48 hours, for ruptured bullae until the epithelial defect heals. Otherwise, every 1 to 6 months, depending on the symptoms.

4.29 CORNEAL GRAFT REJECTION

Symptoms

Decreased vision, mild pain, redness, and photophobia with prior corneal transplantation, usually several weeks to years previously. Posterior lamellar grafts [e.g., DSEK (Descemet stripping endothelial keratoplasty) and DLEK (deep lamellar endothelial keratoplasty)] are also at risk for endothelial rejection. Often asymptomatic and diagnosed on routine follow-up examination.

Signs

(See Figure 4.29.1.)

Critical. New keratic precipitates localized to the donor endothelium associated with stromal edema, a line of keratic precipitates on the corneal endothelium (endothelial rejection line or Khodadoust line), subepithelial infiltrates (early rejection), an irregularly elevated

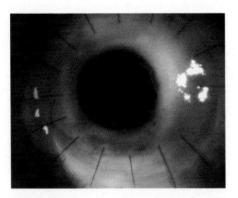

FIGURE 4.29.1. Corneal graft rejection with endothelial rejection line and keratic precipitates.

epithelial line (epithelial rejection line—early in post-op course), or localized stromal neovascularization and infiltrate.

Other. Conjunctival injection (particularly circumcorneal), anterior chamber inflammation, neovascularization growing up to or extending onto the graft, broken graft suture. Tearing may occur, but discharge is not present.

Differential Diagnosis

- Suture abscess or corneal infection: May have a corneal infiltrate, hypopyon, or a purulent discharge. Remove the suture (by pulling the contaminated portion through the shortest track possible) and obtain smears and cultures, including a culture of the suture. Steroid frequency is usually reduced slowly. Treat with intensive topical fluoroquinolone or fortified antibiotics and monitor closely, sometimes in the hospital. See 4.11, *Bacterial Keratitis.*

- Uveitis: Anterior chamber cells and flare with keratic precipitates. Often, a previous history of uveitis is obtained, but it is best to treat as if it were a graft rejection. See Chapter 12, *Uveitis.*

- Increased IOP: A markedly increased IOP may produce epithelial corneal edema without other graft rejection signs. Edema clears after the IOP is reduced.

- Other causes of graft failure: Corneal endothelial decompensation in the graft, recurrent disease in the graft (e.g., herpes keratitis, corneal dystrophy).

Work-Up

1. History: Time since corneal transplantation? Current eye medications? Recent change in topical steroid regimen? Indication for corneal transplantation (e.g., HSV)?

2. Slit-lamp examination, with careful inspection for endothelial rejection line, keratic precipitates, subepithelial infiltrates, and other signs listed above.

Treatment

Endothelial Rejection (Endothelial Rejection Line, Corneal Edema, and/or Keratic Precipitates):

1. Topical steroids (e.g., prednisolone acetate 1% q1h or difluprednate 0.05% q2h while awake and dexamethasone 0.1% ointment q.h.s.).

2. If rejection is severe, recurrent, or recalcitrant, consider systemic steroids (e.g., prednisone 40 to 80 mg p.o. q.d.) or, rarely, subconjunctival steroids (e.g., betamethasone 3 mg in 0.5 mL). In high-risk patients with severe rejection, consider hospitalization and single-pulse or three-pulse treatment with methylprednisolone 500 mg i.v.

3. In select cases, other systemic immunosuppressives may be considered including cyclosporine and rarely tacrolimus.

4. Cycloplegic agent (e.g., scopolamine 0.25% b.i.d. to t.i.d.).

5. Control IOP if increased. See 9.7, *Inflammatory Open-Angle Glaucoma*.

6. Topical cyclosporine 0.05% to 2% b.i.d. to q.i.d. may be helpful in the treatment and prevention of graft rejection.

Epithelial and Stromal Rejection (Subepithelial Infiltrates or Epithelial Rejection Line):

1. Double the current level of topical steroids or use prednisolone acetate 1% q.i.d. (whichever is more).

2. Cycloplegic agent, topical cyclosporine, and IOP control as above.

Follow-Up

Institute treatment immediately to maximize the likelihood of graft survival. Examine the patient every 3 to 7 days. Once improvement is noted, the steroids are tapered very slowly and may need to be maintained at low doses for months to years. IOP must be checked regularly in patients taking topical steroids.

4.30 CORNEAL REFRACTIVE SURGERY COMPLICATIONS

The basic principle of corneal refractive surgery is to induce a change in the curvature of the cornea to correct a preexisting refractive error.

COMPLICATIONS OF SURFACE ABLATION PROCEDURES (PHOTOREFRACTIVE KERATECTOMY, LASER SUBEPITHELIAL KERATECTOMY, AND EPITHELIAL-LASER IN SITU KERATOMILEUSIS)

In photorefractive keratectomy (PRK), the corneal epithelium is removed and the corneal stroma is ablated using an argon–fluoride excimer laser (193 nm, ultraviolet) to correct a refractive error. In laser subepithelial keratectomy (LASEK), the epithelium is chemically separated from the Bowman layer, moved to the side before laser ablation of the stroma, and then repositioned centrally. In epithelial-laser in situ keratomileusis (epi-LASIK), the epithelium is mechanically separated from the Bowman layer, moved to the side before laser ablation of the stroma, and then repositioned centrally or discarded (see Table 4.30.1).

Symptoms

Early (1 to 14 days). Decreasing visual acuity, increased pain.

NOTE: The induced epithelial defect at surgery, which usually takes a few days to heal, normally will cause a certain amount of postoperative pain.

TABLE **4.30.1** Refractive Surgery Characteristics				
	PRK	**LASEK**	**Epi-LASIK**	**LASIK**
Epithelial flap or method of stromal exposure	No flap. Epithelium removed by blade, spatula, brush, excimer laser, or dilute absolute alcohol.	Epithelial flap created by 20% absolute alcohol concentrated on epithelium by marker well.	Epithelial flap created by a blunt blade epi-keratome. Epithelial flap may be replaced (epi-on) or discarded (epi-off).	Epithelial and stromal flap created by sharp microkeratome or femtosecond laser.
Depth of exposure	Bowman membrane	Bowman membrane	Bowman membrane	Anterior stroma (sub-Bowman keratomileusis provides more superficial stromal exposure)
Typical refractive limitations	Spherical range –8.0D to +4.0D, Cylinder range up to 4.0D	Spherical range –8.0D to +4.0D, Cylinder range up to 4.0D	Spherical range –8.0D to +4.0D, Cylinder range up to 4.0D	Spherical range –10.0D to +4.0D, Cylinder range up to 4.0D
Advantages	Useful in thin corneas, epithelial pathology. No stromal flap healing issues.	Useful in thin corneas, epithelial pathology. No stromal flap healing issues.	Useful in thin corneas, epithelial pathology. No stromal flap healing issues.	Minimal pain, rapid visual recovery, minimal stromal haze.
Disadvantages	Postoperative pain, slower visual recovery, higher risk of subepithelial haze.	Postoperative pain, slower visual recovery, higher risk of subepithelial haze. Presence of flap with possible complications (see text).	Postoperative pain, slower visual recovery, higher risk of subepithelial haze. Not ideal with significant glaucoma. Presence of flap with possible complications (see text).	Not ideal for thin corneas, epithelial dystrophies, severe dry eyes, significant glaucoma. Presence of flap with possible complications (see text).

Later (2 weeks to several months). Decreasing visual acuity, severe glare, monocular diplopia.

Signs

Corneal infiltrate, central corneal scar.

Etiology

Early

- Dislocated bandage soft contact lens (see 4.21, *Contact Lens-Related Problems*).

- Nonhealing epithelial defect (see 3.2, *Corneal Abrasion*).

- Corneal ulcer (see 4.11, *Bacterial Keratitis*). Mycobacterial infections are more common after refractive surgery.

- Medication allergy (see 5.1, *Acute Conjunctivitis*).

Later

- Corneal haze (scarring) noted in anterior corneal stroma.

- Irregular astigmatism (e.g., central island, decentered ablation).

- Regression or progression of refractive error (under- or overcorrection).

- Steroid-induced glaucoma (see 9.9, *Steroid-Response Glaucoma*).

Work-Up

1. Complete ophthalmic examination, including IOP measurement by Tono-Pen and applanation. IOP may be underestimated given decreased corneal thickness.

2. Refraction if change in refractive error suspected. Hard contact lens overrefraction corrects irregular astigmatism.

3. Corneal topography if irregular astigmatism is suspected.

Treatment and Follow-Up

1. Epithelial defect (see 3.2, *Corneal Abrasion*).

2. Corneal infiltrate (see 4.11, *Bacterial Keratitis*).

3. Corneal haze: Increase steroid drop frequency. Follow-up in 1 to 2 weeks. Cases of severe haze may respond to PTK with mitomycin C.

4. Refractive error or irregular astigmatism: Consider surface ablation enhancement. If irregular astigmatism present, custom surface ablation, PTK, or hard contact lens may be needed.

5. Steroid-induced glaucoma. See 9.9, *Steroid-Response Glaucoma.*

COMPLICATIONS OF LASER IN SITU KERATOMILEUSIS

In LASIK, a hinged, partial-thickness corneal flap is created using a microkeratome or femtosecond laser, and then the underlying stroma is ablated with an excimer laser to correct refractive error. The corneal flap is repositioned over the stroma without sutures.

Symptoms

Early (1 to 14 days). Decreasing visual acuity, increased pain.

Later (2 weeks to several months). Decreasing visual acuity, severe glare, monocular diplopia, dry-eye symptoms.

Signs

Severe conjunctival injection, corneal infiltrate, large fluorescein-staining epithelial defect, dislocated corneal flap, interface inflammation, epithelial ingrowth under the flap, central corneal scar, SPK.

Etiology

Early

- Flap folds, dislocation, or lost corneal flap.

- Large epithelial defect.

- Diffuse lamellar keratitis (DLK). Also known as "sands of the Sahara" because of its appearance (multiple fine inflammatory infiltrates in the flap interface). Usually occurs within 5 days of surgery (see Figure 4.30.1).

- Corneal ulcer and/or infection in flap interface. See 4.11, *Bacterial Keratitis.*

- Medication allergy. See 5.1, *Acute Conjunctivitis.*

NOTE: Patients after LASIK have reduced corneal sensation in the area of the flap for at least 3 months (returns to essentially normal in 6 to 12 months).

Later

- Epithelial ingrowth into flap interface.

- Corneal haze (scarring): Less common than after surface ablation procedures.

- Irregular astigmatism (e.g., decentered ablation, central island, flap irregularity, ectasia).

- Regression or progression of refractive error.

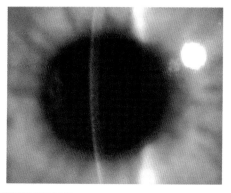

FIGURE 4.30.1. Diffuse lamellar keratitis.

- Dry-eye syndrome/neurotrophic keratopathy.

- DLK can occur weeks to years after LASIK in response to a corneal insult such as corneal abrasion, recurrent erosion, or viral keratitis.

Work-Up

1. Complete slit-lamp examination, including fluorescein staining and IOP measurement by Tono-Pen and applanation. IOP may be underestimated given flap creation and decreased corneal thickness.

2. Schirmer test, as needed.

3. Refraction if irregular astigmatism or change in refractive error is suspected. Refraction with hard contact lens for irregular astigmatism.

4. Corneal topography for suspected irregular astigmatism.

Treatment and Follow-Up

1. Visually significant stromal folds: Lift flap and refloat within 24 hours. Flap dislocation: Requires urgent surgical repositioning. Persistent symptomatic flap striae may require flap lifting and suturing.

2. Lost corneal flap: Treat as epithelial defect. See 3.2, *Corneal Abrasion*.

3. Epithelial defect. See 3.2, *Corneal Abrasion*.

4. SPK. See 4.1, *Superficial Punctate Keratopathy*, and 4.3, *Dry-Eye Syndrome*.

5. DLK: Aggressive treatment with frequent topical steroids (e.g., prednisolone acetate 1% q1h). If severe, may also require lifting of flap and irrigation of interface. Treat any underlying cause, such as an epithelial defect.

6. Corneal infiltrate. See 4.11, *Bacterial Keratitis*, and Appendix 8, *Corneal Culture Procedure*. The flap may need to be lifted to obtain the best culture results.

7. Epithelial ingrowth: Observation if very peripheral and not affecting vision. Surgical debridement if dense, affecting the health of flap, approaching visual axis, or affecting vision.

8. Corneal haze: Increase steroid drop frequency. Follow-up in 1 to 2 weeks.

9. Refractive error or irregular astigmatism: Appropriate refraction. Consider repositioning flap or LASIK enhancement. If irregular astigmatism, may need surface ablation, LASIK enhancement, or hard contact lens.

COMPLICATIONS OF RADIAL KERATOTOMY

In radial keratotomy (RK), partial-thickness, spokelike cuts are made in the peripheral cornea using a diamond blade (often 90% to 95% depth), which results in a flattening of the central cornea and correction of myopia. Astigmatic keratotomy (AK) is a similar procedure in which arcuate or tangential relaxing incisions are made to correct astigmatism.

Symptoms

Early (1 to 14 days).   Decreasing visual acuity, increased pain.

Later (2 weeks to years).   Decreasing visual acuity, severe glare, monocular diplopia.

NOTE: RK weakens the corneal integrity placing patients at higher risk for rupture after trauma.

Signs

Corneal infiltrate, large fluorescein-staining epithelial defect, rupture at RK incision site after trauma, anterior chamber reaction.

Etiology

Early

- Large epithelial defect. See 3.2, *Corneal Abrasion*.

- Corneal ulcer/infection in RK incision. See 4.11, *Bacterial Keratitis*.

- Medication allergy. See 5.1, *Acute Conjunctivitis*.

- Very rarely, endophthalmitis. See 12.13, *Postoperative Endophthalmitis*.

Later

- RK incisions approaching the visual axis causing glare and starbursts.

- Irregular astigmatism.

- Regression of refractive error; common in first few months after surgery.

- Progression of refractive error; common after first few years after surgery.

- Ruptured globe at RK incision site after trauma. See 3.14, *Ruptured Globe and Penetrating Ocular Injury.*

Work-Up

1. Complete slit-lamp examination, including IOP measurement and fluorescein staining.

2. Refraction if change in refractive error is suspected. Refraction with hard contact lens for irregular astigmatism.

3. Corneal topography if irregular astigmatism suspected.

Treatment and Follow-Up

1. Corneal infiltrate: See 4.11, *Bacterial Keratitis,* and Appendix 8, *Corneal Culture Procedure.*

2. Epithelial defect: See 3.2, *Corneal Abrasion.*

3. Endophthalmitis: See 12.13, *Postoperative Endophthalmitis.*

4. Refractive error or irregular astigmatism. Appropriate refraction. Consider enhancement of RK incisions or AK. Rarely, surface laser ablation with mitomycin C can be used. Irregular astigmatism may require a hard contact lens.

5. Ruptured globe at RK incision. Requires surgical repair. See 3.14, *Ruptured Globe and Penetrating Ocular Injury.*

4

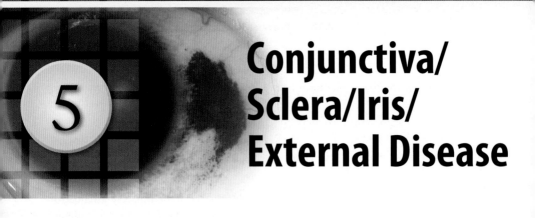

Conjunctiva/ Sclera/Iris/ External Disease

5

5.1 ACUTE CONJUNCTIVITIS

Symptoms

"Red eye" (conjunctival hyperemia), discharge, eyelids sticking or crusting (worse in the morning), foreign body sensation, <4-week duration of symptoms (otherwise, see 5.2, *Chronic Conjunctivitis*) (see Figure 5.1.1).

See 8.9, *Ophthalmia Neonatorum (Newborn Conjunctivitis),* for detailed discussion of acute conjunctivitis in the newborn.

VIRAL CONJUNCTIVITIS/EPIDEMIC KERATOCONJUNCTIVITIS

Symptoms

Itching, burning, tearing, gritty, or foreign body sensation; history of recent upper respiratory tract infection or sick contact. Often

starts in one eye and involves the fellow eye a few days later.

Signs

(See Figure 5.1.2.)

Critical. Inferior palpebral conjunctival follicles (see Figure 5.1.3), tender palpable preauricular lymph node.

Other. Watery discharge, red and edematous eyelids, pinpoint subconjunctival hemorrhages, punctate keratopathy (epithelial erosion in severe cases), membrane/pseudomembrane (see Figure 5.1.4). Intraepithelial microcysts are an early corneal finding which, if present, can be helpful in diagnosis. Subepithelial infiltrates (SEIs) can

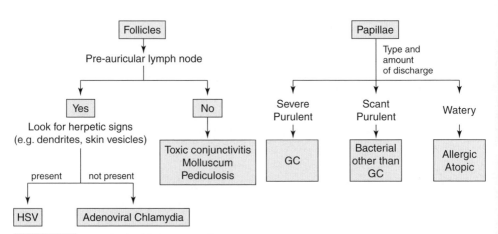

FIGURE 5.1.1. Algorithm for follicles and papillae.

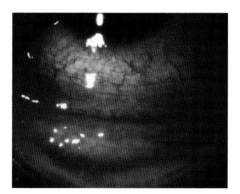

FIGURE 5.1.2. Viral conjunctivitis.

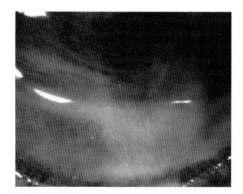

FIGURE 5.1.4. Viral conjunctivitis with pseudomembranes.

5

develop several weeks after the onset of the conjunctivitis.

Etiology and Variants of Viral Conjunctivitis

▪ Most commonly adenovirus.

▪ Pharyngoconjunctival fever: Associated with pharyngitis and fever; usually in children.

▪ Acute hemorrhagic conjunctivitis: Associated with a large subconjunctival hemorrhage, coxsackie and enterovirus, 1 to 2 weeks duration. Tends to occur in tropical regions.

NOTE: Many systemic viral syndromes (e.g., measles, mumps, influenza) can cause a nonspecific conjunctivitis. The underlying condition should be managed appropriately; the eyes are treated with artificial tears four to eight times per day. If tears are used greater than four times daily, preservative-free unit-dose tears should be used.

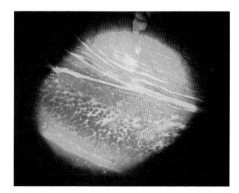

FIGURE 5.1.3. Follicles on the inferior palpebral conjunctiva.

Work-Up

No conjunctival cultures/swabs are indicated unless discharge is excessive or the condition becomes chronic (see 5.2, *Chronic Conjunctivitis*).

Treatment

1. Counsel the patient that viral conjunctivitis is a self-limited condition that typically gets worse for the first 4 to 7 days after onset and may not resolve for 2 to 3 weeks or longer with corneal involvement.

2. Viral conjunctivitis is highly contagious, usually for 10 to 12 days from onset, as long as the eyes are red (when not on steroids). Patients should avoid touching their eyes, shaking hands, sharing towels or pillows, etc. Restrict work and school for patients with significant exposure to others while the eyes are red and weeping.

3. Frequent handwashing.

4. Preservative-free artificial tears four to eight times per day for 1 to 3 weeks. Use single-use vials to limit tip contamination and spread of the condition.

5. Cool compresses several times per day.

6. Antihistamine drops (e.g., epinastine 0.05% b.i.d.) if itching is severe.

7. If a membrane/pseudomembrane present, it may be gently peeled or left.

8. If a membrane/pseudomembrane is acutely present or if SEIs reduce vision later, use

topical steroids. For membranes/pseudo-membranes, use a more frequent steroid dose or stronger steroid (e.g., loteprednol 0.5% q.i.d.) and consider a steroid ointment (e.g., fluorometholone 0.1% ointment q.i.d. or dexamethasone/tobramycin 0.1%/0.3% ointment q.i.d.) in the presence of significant tearing to maintain longer medication exposure. For SEIs, a weaker steroid with less frequent dosing is usually sufficient (e.g., loteprednol 0.2% b.i.d.). Given the possible side effects, prescription of topical steroids is cautionary in the emergency room setting or in patients with questionable follow-up. Steroids may hasten the resolution of the symptoms but prolong the infectious period. Steroid treatment is maintained for 1 week and then slowly tapered. SEIs can recur during or after tapering.

NOTE: Routine use of topical antibiotics for viral conjunctivitis is discouraged unless erosions are present or in severe cases.

Follow-Up

In 2 to 3 weeks, but sooner if the condition worsens significantly or if topical steroids are prescribed.

HERPES SIMPLEX VIRUS CONJUNCTIVITIS

See 4.15, *Herpes Simplex Virus,* for a detailed discussion. Patients may have a history of perioral cold sores. Manifests with a unilateral (sometimes recurrent) follicular conjunctival reaction, palpable preauricular node, and, occasionally, concurrent herpetic skin vesicles along the eyelid margin or periocular skin. Treat with antiviral therapy (e.g., trifluridine 1% drops or ganciclovir 0.05% gel five times per day) and cool compresses. Steroids are contraindicated.

ALLERGIC CONJUNCTIVITIS

Symptoms

Itching, watery discharge, and a history of allergies are typical. Usually bilateral.

Signs

(See Figure 5.1.5.)

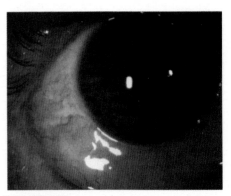

FIGURE 5.1.5. Allergic conjunctivitis.

Chemosis, red and edematous eyelids, conjunctival papillae, no preauricular node.

Treatment

1. Eliminate the inciting agent. Frequent washing of hair and clothes may be helpful.

2. Cool compresses several times per day.

3. Topical drops, depending on the severity.

   —Mild: Artificial tears four to eight times per day.

   —Moderate: Use olopatadine 0.1% to 0.2%, epinastine 0.05%, nedocromil 2%, bepotastine 1.5%, or ketotifen 0.025% (over-the-counter) b.i.d. to help relieve itching. Ketorolac 0.5%, pemirolast 0.1%, and lodoxamide 0.1% q.i.d. can also reduce symptoms.

   —Severe: Mild topical steroid (e.g., loteprednol 0.2% or fluorometholone 0.1% q.i.d. for 1 to 2 weeks) in addition to the preceding medications.

4. Oral antihistamine (e.g., diphenhydramine 25 mg p.o. t.i.d. to q.i.d. or loratadine 10 mg p.o. q.d.) in moderate-to-severe cases can be very helpful.

NOTE: Routine use of topical antibiotics or steroids for allergic conjunctivitis is discouraged.

Follow-Up

Two weeks. If topical steroids are used, tapering is required and patients should be monitored for side effects.

VERNAL/ATOPIC CONJUNCTIVITIS

Symptoms

Usually bilateral but possibly asymmetric itching, thick, ropy discharge, especially in boys. Seasonal (spring/ summer) recurrences in vernal, history of atopy in atopic conjunctivitis. Vernal conjunctivitis is usually seen in younger patients.

Signs

Critical. Large conjunctival papillae seen under the upper eyelid or along the limbus (limbal vernal) (see Figure 5.1.6).

Other. Superior corneal "shield" ulcer (a well-delineated, sterile, gray-white infiltrate), limbal raised white dots (Horner–Trantas dots) of degenerated eosinophils (see Figure 5.1.7), superficial punctate keratopathy (SPK).

Treatment

1. Treat as for allergic except prophylactically use a mast cell stabilizer (e.g., lodoxamide 0.1% q.i.d. or pemirolast 0.1% q.i.d.), or a mast cell stabilizer and/or antihistamine (e.g., nedocromil 2% b.i.d., olopatadine 0.1% b.i.d., ketotifen 0.025%, bepotastine 1.5%, or azelastine 0.05%) for 2 to 3 weeks before the allergy season starts.

2. If a shield ulcer is present, add:

   —Topical steroid (e.g., loteprednol 0.5% or prednisolone 1% drops, dexamethasone 0.1% ointment) four to six times per day.

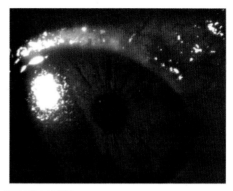

FIGURE 5.1.7. Vernal/atopic conjunctivitis with raised white dots of eosinophils along limbus.

5

   —Topical antibiotic (e.g., erythromycin ointment q.i.d., polymyxin B/bacitracin q.i.d.).

   —Cycloplegic agent (e.g., scopolamine 0.25% t.i.d.).

NOTE: Shield ulcers may need to be scraped to remove superficial plaque-like material before re-epithelialization will occur.

---

3. Cool compresses q.i.d.

4. Consider cyclosporine 0.05% to 2% b.i.d. to q.i.d. if not responding to the preceding treatment. Maximal effect not seen for several weeks.

5. If associated with atopic dermatitis of eyelids, consider tacrolimus 0.03% to 0.1% q.h.s. or b.i.d. (preferred), pimecrolimus 1% b.i.d., or topical steroid ophthalmic ointment (e.g., fluorometholone 0.1% q.i.d.) to the affected skin.

Follow-Up

Every 1 to 3 days in the presence of a shield ulcer; otherwise, every few weeks. Topical medications are tapered slowly as improvement is noted. Antiallergy drops are maintained for the duration of the season and are often reinitiated a few weeks before the next spring. Patients on topical steroids should be monitored regularly, including IOP monitoring, even if used only on the skin.

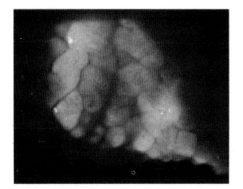

FIGURE 5.1.6. Vernal/atopic conjunctivitis with large superior tarsal papillae.

BACTERIAL CONJUNCTIVITIS (NONGONOCOCCAL)

Symptoms

Redness, foreign body sensation, discharge; itching is much less prominent.

Signs

Critical. Purulent white-yellow discharge of mild-to-moderate degree.

Other. Conjunctival papillae, chemosis, preauricular node typically absent but is often present in gonococcal conjunctivitis.

Etiology

Commonly, *Staphylococcus aureus* (associated with blepharitis, phlyctenules, and marginal sterile infiltrates), *Staphylococcus epidermidis, Haemophilus influenzae* (especially in children and commonly associated with otitis media), *Streptococcus pneumoniae,* and *Moraxella catarrhalis.*

NOTE: Suspect gonococcus if onset is hyperacute with significant discharge, see this chapter *Gonococcal Conjunctivitis.*

Work-Up

If severe, recurrent, or recalcitrant, conjunctival swab for routine cultures and sensitivities (blood and chocolate agar) and immediate Gram stain to evaluate for gonococcus.

Treatment

1. Use topical antibiotic therapy (e.g., trimethoprim/polymyxin B or fluoroquinolone drops q.i.d.) for 5 to 7 days.

2. *H. influenzae* conjunctivitis should be treated with oral amoxicillin/clavulanate (20 to 40 mg/kg/day in three divided doses) because of occasional extraocular involvement (e.g., otitis media, pneumonia, and meningitis).

3. If associated with dacryocystitis, systemic antibiotics are necessary. See 6.9, *Dacryocystitis/Inflammation of the Lacrimal Sac.*

Follow-Up

Every 2 to 3 days initially, then every 5 to 7 days until resolved. Antibiotic therapy is adjusted according to culture and sensitivity results.

GONOCOCCAL CONJUNCTIVITIS

Signs

Critical. Severe purulent discharge, hyperacute onset (within 12 to 24 hours).

Other. Conjunctival papillae, marked chemosis, preauricular adenopathy, eyelid swelling. See 8.9, *Ophthalmia Neonatorum (Newborn Conjunctivitis),* for a detailed discussion of gonococcal conjunctivitis in the newborn.

Work-Up

1. Examine the entire cornea for peripheral ulcers (especially superiorly) because of the risk for rapid progression to perforation. (see Figure 5.1.8).

2. Conjunctival scrapings for immediate Gram stain and for culture and sensitivities (e.g., blood agar and chocolate agar).

Treatment

Initiated if the Gram stain shows Gram-negative intracellular diplococci or there is a high clinical suspicion of gonococcal conjunctivitis.

1. Ceftriaxone 1 g intramuscularly (i.m.) in a single dose. If corneal involvement exists, or cannot be excluded because of chemosis and eyelid swelling, hospitalize the patient and treat with ceftriaxone 1 g intravenously (i.v.) every 12 to 24 hours. The duration of treatment depends on the clinical response. In penicillin-allergic patients, consider an

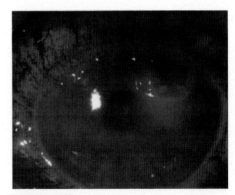

FIGURE 5.1.8. Gonococcal conjunctivitis with corneal involvement.

oral fluoroquinolone (e.g., ciprofloxacin 500 mg p.o. b.i.d. for 5 days) and consider consulting an infectious disease specialist (fluoroquinolones are contraindicated in pregnant women and children). Additionally, due to increased resistance, fluoroquinolones should not be used to treat gonococcal infections in men who have sex with men, in areas of high endemic resistance, and in patients with a recent foreign travel history. For penicillin-allergic patients with the above characteristics, one possible treatment alternative is a single dose of azithromycin 1 g p.o. An infectious disease consultation should be considered.

2. Topical ciprofloxacin ointment q.i.d. or ciprofloxacin drops q2h. If the cornea is involved, use a fluoroquinolone drop q1h (e.g., gatifloxacin, moxifloxacin, besifloxacin, levofloxacin, or ciprofloxacin).

3. Saline irrigation q.i.d. until the discharge resolves.

4. Treat for possible chlamydial coinfection (e.g., azithromycin 1 g p.o. single dose or doxycycline 100 mg p.o. b.i.d. for 7 days).

5. Treat sexual partners with oral antibiotics for both gonorrhea and chlamydia as described previously.

Follow-Up

Daily until consistent improvement is noted and then every 2 to 3 days until the condition resolves. The patient and sexual partners should be evaluated by their medical doctors for other sexually transmitted diseases.

PEDICULOSIS (LICE, CRABS)

Typically develops from contact with pubic lice (usually sexually transmitted). Can be unilateral or bilateral.

Symptoms

Itching, mild conjunctival injection.

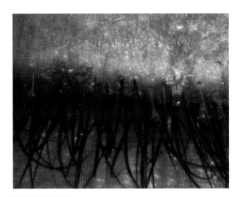

FIGURE 5.1.9. Pediculosis.

Signs

(See Figure 5.1.9.)

Critical. Adult lice, nits, and blood-tinged debris on the eyelids and eyelashes.

Other. Follicular conjunctivitis.

Treatment

1. Mechanical removal of lice and eggs with jeweler's forceps.

2. Any bland ophthalmic ointment (e.g., erythromycin) to the eyelids t.i.d. for 10 days to smother the lice and nits.

3. Antilice lotion and shampoo as directed to nonocular areas for patient and close contacts.

4. Thoroughly wash and dry all clothes and linens.

NOTE: In children, pediculosis is suspicious for possible sexual abuse and involvement of social services and/or child protection agency is recommended.

For chlamydial, toxic, and molluscum contagiosum-related conjunctivitis, see 5.2, *Chronic Conjunctivitis.*

Also see related sections: 8.9, *Ophthalmia Neonatorum (Newborn Conjunctivitis);* 13.6, *Stevens–Johnson Syndrome (Erythema Multiforme Major);* and 5.10, *Ocular Cicatricial Pemphigoid.*

5

5.2   CHRONIC CONJUNCTIVITIS

Symptoms

"Red eye" (conjunctival hyperemia), conjunctival discharge, eyelids sticking (worse in morning), foreign body sensation, duration >4 weeks (otherwise see 5.1, *Acute Conjunctivitis*).

Differential Diagnosis

- Parinaud oculoglandular conjunctivitis (see 5.3, *Parinaud Oculoglandular Conjunctivitis*).

- Silent dacryocystitis (see 6.9, *Dacryocystitis/ Inflammation of the Lacrimal Sac*).

- Contact lens-related (see 4.21, *Contact Lens-Related Problems*).

- Conjunctival tumors (see 5.12, *Conjunctival Tumors*).

- Autoimmune disease (e.g., reactive arthritis, sarcoidosis, discoid lupus, others).

CHLAMYDIAL INCLUSION CONJUNCTIVITIS

Sexually transmitted, typically found in young adults. A history of vaginitis, cervicitis, or urethritis may be present.

Signs

Inferior tarsal or bulbar conjunctival follicles, superior corneal pannus, palpable preauricular node, or peripheral SEIs. A stringy, mucous discharge may be present.

Work-Up

1. History: Determine the duration of red eye, any prior treatment, concomitant vaginitis, cervicitis, or urethritis. Sexually active?

2. Slit-lamp examination.

3. In adults, direct chlamydial immunofluorescence test, DNA probe, chlamydial culture of conjunctiva, or polymerase chain reaction when available.

NOTE: Topical fluorescein can interfere with immunofluorescence test results.

---

4. Consider conjunctival scraping for Giemsa stain: Shows basophilic intracytoplasmic inclusion bodies in epithelial cells, polymorphonuclear leukocytes, and lymphocytes in newborns.

Treatment

1. Azithromycin 1 g p.o. single dose, doxycycline 100 mg p.o. b.i.d., or erythromycin 500 mg p.o. q.i.d. for 7 days is given to the patient and sexual partners.

2. Topical erythromycin or tetracycline ointment b.i.d. to t.i.d. for 2 to 3 weeks.

Follow-Up

In 2 to 3 weeks, depending on the severity. The patient and sexual partners should be evaluated by their medical doctors for other sexually transmitted diseases. Occasionally a 6-week course of doxycycline may be required.

TRACHOMA

Principally occurs in developing countries in areas of poor sanitation and crowded conditions.

Signs

(See Figure 5.2.1.)

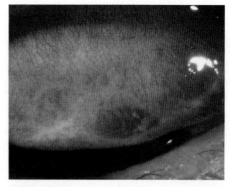

FIGURE 5.2.1.   Trachoma showing Arlt line, or scarring, of the surgery tarsal conjunctiva.

MacCallan Classification

- Stage 1: Superior tarsal follicles, mild superior SPK, and pannus, often preceded by purulent discharge and tender preauricular node.

- Stage 2: Florid superior tarsal follicular reaction (2a) or papillary hypertrophy (2b) associated with superior corneal SEIs, pannus, and limbal follicles.

- Stage 3: Follicles and scarring of superior tarsal conjunctiva.

- Stage 4: No follicles, extensive conjunctival scarring.

- Late complications: Severe dry eyes, trichiasis, entropion, keratitis, corneal scarring, superficial fibrovascular pannus, Herbert pits (scarred limbal follicles), corneal bacterial superinfection, and ulceration.

World Health Organization Classification

- TF (trachomatous inflammation: follicular): More than five follicles on the upper tarsus.

- TI (trachomatous inflammation: intense): Inflammation with thickening obscuring >50% of the tarsal vessels.

- TS (trachomatous scarring): Cicatrization of tarsal conjunctiva with fibrous white bands.

- TT (trachomatous trichiasis): Trichiasis of at least one eyelash.

- CO (corneal opacity): Corneal opacity involving at least part of the pupillary margin.

Work-Up

1. History of exposure to endemic areas (e.g., North Africa, Middle East, India, Southeast Asia).

2. Examination and diagnostic studies as above (chlamydial inclusion conjunctivitis).

Treatment

1. Azithromycin 20 mg/kg p.o. single dose, doxycycline 100 mg p.o. b.i.d., erythromycin 500 mg p.o. q.i.d., or tetracycline 250 mg p.o. q.i.d. for 2 weeks.

2. Tetracycline, erythromycin, or sulfacetamide ointment b.i.d. to q.i.d. for 3 to 4 weeks.

NOTE: Tetracyclines are contraindicated in children younger than 8 years, pregnant women, and nursing mothers.

Follow-Up

Every 2 to 3 weeks initially, then as needed. Although treatment is usually curative, reinfection is common if hygienic conditions do not improve.

NOTE: Currently, the World Health Organization is conducting a large-scale program to eradicate trachoma through intermittent widespread distribution of azithromycin as well as information on facial cleanliness and water sanitation to endemic areas. The aim is global elimination of blindness caused by trachoma by the year 2020.

MOLLUSCUM CONTAGIOSUM

Signs

Critical. Dome shaped, usually multiple, umbilicated shiny nodules on the eyelid or eyelid margin.

Other. Follicular conjunctival response from toxic viral products, corneal pannus. Immunocompromised patients may have more lesions and less conjunctival reaction.

Treatment

Removal of lesions by simple excision, incision and curettage, or cryosurgery.

Follow-Up

Every 2 to 4 weeks until the conjunctivitis resolves, which often takes 4 to 6 weeks. If many lesions are present, consider human immunodeficiency virus (HIV) testing.

MICROSPORIDIAL KERATOCONJUNCTIVITIS

Signs

Chronic superficial punctate keratitis and conjunctival injection not responsive to conservative treatment. Diagnosed with Giemsa stain of corneal or conjunctival scraping.

5

Treatment

Topical fumagillin and/or oral itraconazole 200 mg p.o. q.d. Epithelial debridement followed by antibiotic ointment (e.g., erythromycin or bacitracin/polymyxin B t.i.d.) may be useful for mild cases. Treat underlying disease. Consider HIV testing.

TOXIC CONJUNCTIVITIS/MEDICAMENTOSA

Signs

Inferior papillary reaction and/or inferior conjunctival staining with fluorescein from topical eye drops. Most notably from aminogly-

cosides, antivirals, and preserved drops. With long-term use, usually more than 1 month, a follicular response can be seen with other medications including atropine, brimonidine, miotics, epinephrine agents, antibiotics, and antivirals. Inferior SPK and scant discharge may be noted.

Treatment

Usually sufficient to discontinue the offending eye drop. Can add preservative-free artificial tears four to eight times per day.

Follow-Up

In 1 to 4 weeks, as needed.

5.3 PARINAUD OCULOGLANDULAR CONJUNCTIVITIS

Symptoms

Red eye, mucopurulent discharge, foreign body sensation.

Signs

Critical. Granulomatous nodule(s) on the palpebral conjunctiva; visibly swollen ipsilateral, preauricular, or submandibular lymph nodes.

Other. Fever, rash, follicular conjunctivitis.

Etiology

■ Cat-scratch disease from *Bartonella henselae* (most common cause): Often a history of being scratched or licked by a kitten within 2 weeks of symptoms.

■ Tularemia: History of contact with rabbits, other small wild animals, or ticks. Patients have severe headache, fever, and other systemic manifestations.

■ Tuberculosis and other mycobacteria.

■ Rare causes: Syphilis, leukemia, lymphoma, mumps, Epstein–Barr virus, fungi, sarcoidosis, listeria, and others.

Work-Up

Initiated when etiology is unknown (e.g., no recent cat scratch).

1. Conjunctival biopsy with scrapings for Gram, Giemsa, and acid-fast stains.

2. Conjunctival cultures on blood, Löwenstein–Jensen, Sabouraud, and thioglycolate media.

3. Complete blood count, rapid plasma reagin (RPR), fluorescent treponemal antibody-absorbed (FTA-ABS), angiotensin converting enzyme (ACE), and, if the patient is febrile, blood cultures.

4. Chest radiograph, purified protein derivative (PPD), and anergy panel.

5. If tularemia is suspected, serologic titers are necessary.

6. If diagnosis of cat-scratch disease is uncertain, cat-scratch serology, and cat-scratch skin test (Hanger–Rose) can be performed.

Treatment

1. Warm compresses for tender lymph nodes.

2. Antipyretics as needed.

3. Disease specific:

—Cat-scratch disease: Generally resolves spontaneously in 6 weeks. Consider azithromycin 500 mg p.o. q.i.d., then 250 mg daily for four doses (for children, 10 mg/kg q.i.d., then 5 mg/kg daily for four doses); alternatives include trimethoprim/sulfamethoxazole DS p.o. b.i.d.; or ciprofloxacin 500 mg p.o. b.i.d. Duration should be individualized. Use a topical antibiotic (e.g., bacitracin/polymyxin B ointment or gentamicin drops q.i.d.). The cat does not need to be removed.

—Tularemia: Tobramycin 5 mg/kg/day in three divided doses q8h or gentamicin (same dosing) for 7 to 14 days. Gentamicin drops q2h for 1 week, and then five times per day until resolved. Often patients are systemically ill and under the care of a medical internist for tularemia; if not, refer to a medical internist for systemic management.

—Tuberculosis: Refer to an internist for antituberculosis medication.

—Syphilis: Systemic penicillin (dose depends on the stage of the syphilis) and topical tetracycline ointment (see 12.12, *Syphilis*).

Follow-Up

Repeat the ocular examination in 1 to 2 weeks. Conjunctival granulomas and lymphadenopathy can take 4 to 6 weeks to resolve for cat-scratch disease.

5

5.4 SUPERIOR LIMBIC KERATOCONJUNCTIVITIS

Symptoms

Red eye, burning, foreign body sensation, pain, tearing, mild photophobia, frequent blinking. The course can be chronic with exacerbations and remissions.

Signs

(See Figure 5.4.1.)

Critical. Thickening, inflammation, and radial injection of the superior bulbar conjunctiva, especially at the limbus.

Other. Fine papillae on the superior palpebral conjunctiva; fine punctate fluorescein staining on the superior cornea, limbus, and conjunctiva; superior corneal micropannus and filaments. Usually bilateral.

Work-Up

1. History: Recurrent episodes? Thyroid disease?

2. Slit-lamp examination with fluorescein staining, particularly of the superior cornea and adjacent conjunctiva. Lift the upper eyelid to see the superior limbal area and then evert to visualize the tarsus. Sometimes the localized hyperemia is best appreciated by direct inspection by raising the eyelids of the patient on downgaze.

3. Thyroid function tests (50% prevalence of thyroid disease in patients with superior limbic keratoconjunctivitis).

Treatment

Mild

1. Aggressive lubrication with preservative-free artificial tears four to eight times per day and artificial tear ointment q.h.s.

2. Consider punctal occlusion with plugs or cautery.

3. Treat any concurrent blepharitis.

4. Consider treatment with cyclosporine 0.05% b.i.d. if not responding to lubrication.

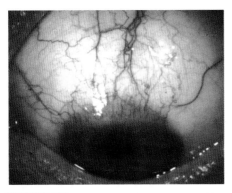
FIGURE 5.4.1. Superior limbic keratoconjunctivitis.

Moderate to Severe (in Addition to Preceding)

1. Silver nitrate 0.5% solution applied on a cotton-tipped applicator for 10 to 20 seconds to the superior tarsal and superior bulbar conjunctiva after topical anesthesia (e.g., proparacaine). Then irrigation with saline and antibiotic ointment (e.g., erythromycin) q.h.s. for 1 week.

NOTE: Do not use silver nitrate cautery sticks, which cause severe ocular burns.

---

2. In the absence of dry eyes, a bandage or daily disposable soft contact lens can be tried.

3. If significant amount of mucus or filaments is present, then add acetylcysteine 10% drops three to six times per day.

4. If two to three separate silver nitrate solution applications are unsuccessful, consider cautery, surgical resection, or recession of the superior bulbar conjunctiva.

Follow-Up

Every 2 to 4 weeks during an exacerbation. If signs and symptoms persist, a reapplication of silver nitrate solution, as described previously, can be performed at the weekly follow-up visit.

5.5   SUBCONJUNCTIVAL HEMORRHAGE

Symptoms

Red eye, usually asymptomatic.

Signs

(See Figure 5.5.1.)
Blood underneath the conjunctiva, often in one sector of the eye. The entire view of the sclera can be obstructed by blood.

Differential Diagnosis

- Kaposi sarcoma: Red or purple lesion beneath the conjunctiva, usually elevated slightly. HIV/AIDS testing should be performed.

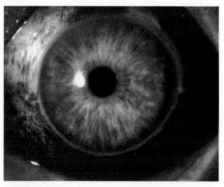

FIGURE 5.5.1. Subconjunctival hemorrhage.

- Other conjunctival lesions (e.g., lymphoma or amyloid) with secondary hemorrhage.

Etiology

- Valsalva (e.g., coughing, sneezing, constipation, or other forms of straining).

- Traumatic: Can be isolated or associated with a retrobulbar hemorrhage or ruptured globe.

- Hypertension.

- Bleeding disorder.

- Antiplatelet or anticoagulant medications (e.g., aspirin, clopidogrel, warfarin).

- Hemorrhage due to orbital mass (rare).

- Idiopathic.

Work-Up

1. History: Bleeding or clotting problems? Medications? Eye rubbing, trauma, heavy lifting, or valsalva? Recurrent subconjunctival hemorrhage? Acute or chronic cough?

2. Ocular examination: If recurrent, rule out a conjunctival lesion when resolved. If severe, check extraocular motility, resistance to retropulsion, and IOP. In traumatic cases, rule out other ocular injuries [e.g., a ruptured globe (signs may include reduced visual acuity, abnormally deep

anterior chamber, severe bullous subconjunctival hemorrhage, hyphema, vitreous hemorrhage, or uveal prolapse), retrobulbar hemorrhage (associated with proptosis and increased IOP), or orbital fracture]. See 3.14, *Ruptured Globe And Penetrating Ocular Injury,* 3.10, *Traumatic Retrobulbar Hemorrhage,* 3.9, *Orbital Blow-out Fracture.*

3. Check blood pressure.

4. If the patient has recurrent subconjunctival hemorrhages or a history of bleeding problems, a bleeding time, prothrombin time, partial thromboplastin time, complete blood count with differential (to evaluate for leukemia), liver function tests, and protein C and S should be obtained.

5. If orbital signs are present (proptosis, decreased extraocular motility, elevated IOP) in atraumatic cases, perform axial and coronal computed tomographic scanning of the orbits with and without contrast to evaluate for an orbital mass (e.g., neuroblastoma in children or lymphangioma in adults). In traumatic cases, image as appropriate (see 3.9, *Orbital Blow-Out Fracture*).

Treatment

None required. Artificial tear drops q.i.d. can be given if mild ocular irritation is present. In addition, elective use of aspirin products and nonsteroidal anti-inflammatory drugs (NSAIDs) should be discouraged if possible in the context of coexisting medical conditions.

Follow-Up

Usually clears spontaneously within 2 to 3 weeks. Patients are told to return if the blood does not fully resolve or if they experience a recurrence. Referral to an internist or family physician should be made as indicated for hypertension or a bleeding diathesis.

5.6   EPISCLERITIS

Symptoms

Acute onset of redness and mild pain in one or both eyes, typically in young adults; a history of recurrent episodes is common. No discharge.

Signs

(See Figure 5.6.1.)

Critical. Sectoral (and, less commonly, diffuse) redness of one or both eyes, mostly due to engorgement of the episcleral vessels. These vessels are large and run in a radial direction beneath the conjunctiva.

Other. Mild-to-moderate tenderness over the area of episcleral injection or a nodule that can be moved slightly over the underlying sclera may be seen. Fluorescein staining can sometimes be seen over the nodule. Associated anterior uveitis and corneal involvement are rare. Vision is normal.

Differential Diagnosis

- Scleritis: Typically older patient. May have known underlying immune-mediated disease (e.g., collagen vascular disease). Pain is deep, severe, and often radiates to the ipsilateral side of the head or face. The sclera may have a bluish hue when observed in natural light. Scleral (and deep episcleral) vessels, as well as conjunctival and superficial episcleral vessels, are injected. The scleral vessels do not blanch on application of topical phenylephrine 2.5%. Possible

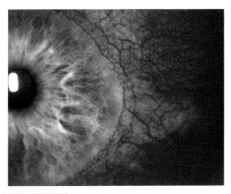

FIGURE 5.6.1. Episcleritis.

corneal involvement with adjacent stromal keratitis. See 5.7, *Scleritis*.

■ Iritis: Cells and flare in the anterior chamber. May be present with scleritis. See 3.5, *Traumatic Iritis* and 12.1, *Anterior Uveitis (Iritis/ Iridocyclitis)*.

■ Conjunctivitis: Diffuse redness and discharge with follicles or papillae. See 5.1 *Acute Conjunctivitis,* and 5.2, *Chronic Conjunctivitis.*

■ Contact lens overwear or tight contact lens syndrome. May be reaction to contact lens solution. Must be considered in all contact lens wearers. See 4.21, *Contact Lens-Related Problems.*

Etiology

■ Idiopathic: Most common.

■ Infectious: Herpes zoster virus (scars from an old facial rash may be present, may cause episcleritis or scleritis) and others.

■ Others: Rosacea, atopy, collagen vascular diseases, gout, and thyroid disease.

Work-Up

1. History: Assess for a history of rash, arthritis, venereal disease, recent viral illness, other medical problems.

2. External examination in natural light: Look for the bluish hue of scleritis.

3. Slit-lamp examination: Anesthetize (e.g., topical proparacaine) and move the conjunctiva with a cotton-tipped applicator to determine the depth of the injected blood vessels. Evaluate for any corneal or anterior chamber involvement. Check IOP.

4. Place a drop of phenylephrine 2.5% in the affected eye and reexamine the vascular

pattern 10 to 15 minutes later. Episcleral vessels should blanch, highlighting any underlying scleral vascular engorgement.

5. If the history suggests an underlying etiology, or in cases with multiple recurrences, the appropriate laboratory tests should be obtained [e.g., antinuclear antibody (ANA), rheumatoid factor, erythrocyte sedimentation rate (ESR), serum uric acid level, RPR, FTA-ABS, antineutrophil cytoplasmic antibody (ANCA)].

Treatment

1. If mild, treat with artificial tears q.i.d.

2. If moderate to severe, a mild topical steroid (e.g., fluorometholone 0.1% or loteprednol 0.5% q.i.d.) often relieves the discomfort. Occasionally, more potent or frequent topical steroid application is necessary.

3. Oral NSAIDs may be used as an alternate steroid-sparing initial therapy (e.g., ibuprofen 200 to 600 mg p.o. t.i.d. to q.i.d., or naproxen 250 to 500 mg p.o. b.i.d. with food or antacids).

NOTE: Many physicians prefer oral NSAIDs to topical steroids as initial therapy.

Follow-Up

Patients treated with artificial tears need not be seen for several weeks unless discomfort worsens or persists. If topical steroids are used, recheck every 2 to 3 weeks until symptoms resolve. The frequency of steroid administration is then tapered. Patients are informed that episcleritis may recur in the same or contralateral eye.

5.7 | SCLERITIS

Symptoms

Severe and boring eye pain (most prominent feature), which may radiate to the forehead, brow, or jaw, and may awaken the patient at

night. Gradual or acute onset with red eye and decrease in vision. Recurrent episodes are common. Scleromalacia perforans may have minimal symptoms.

Signs

Critical. Inflammation of scleral, episcleral, and conjunctival vessels (scleral vessels are large, deep vessels that cannot be moved with a cotton swab and do not blanch with topical phenylephrine) can be sectoral or diffuse. Characteristic bluish scleral hue (best seen in natural light by gross inspection). Scleral thinning or edema may be present.

Other. Scleral nodules, corneal changes (peripheral keratitis, limbal guttering, or keratolysis), glaucoma, uveitis, or cataract.

Signs of Posterior Scleritis. Subretinal granuloma, exudative retinal detachment, proptosis, or rapid-onset hyperopia.

Differential Diagnosis

- Episcleritis: Sclera not involved. Blood vessels blanch with topical phenylephrine. More acute onset than scleritis. Patients tend to be younger and have very mild symptoms, if any. See 5.6, *Episcleritis*.

Etiology

Fifty percent of patients with scleritis have an associated systemic disease. Work-up indicated if no known underlying disease is present.

More Common. Connective tissue disease (e.g., rheumatoid arthritis, Wegener granulomatosis, relapsing polychondritis, systemic lupus erythematosus, reactive arthritis, polyarteritis nodosa, ankylosing spondylitis, inflammatory bowel disease), herpes zoster ophthalmicus, syphilis, status-post ocular surgery, gout.

Less Common. Tuberculosis, other bacteria (e.g., *Pseudomonas* species with scleral ulceration, *Proteus* species associated with scleral buckle), Lyme disease, sarcoidosis, hypertension, foreign body, parasite.

Classification

1. Diffuse anterior scleritis: Widespread inflammation of the anterior segment.

2. Nodular anterior scleritis: Immovable inflamed nodule(s) (see Figure 5.7.1).

3. Necrotizing anterior scleritis with inflammation (see Figure 5.7.2): Extreme pain. The sclera becomes transparent (choroidal

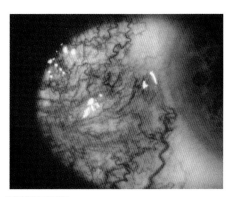

FIGURE 5.7.1. Nodular scleritis.

5

pigment visible) because of necrosis. High association with systemic inflammatory diseases.

4. Necrotizing anterior scleritis without inflammation (scleromalacia perforans): Typically asymptomatic. Seen most often in long-standing rheumatoid arthritis.

5. Posterior scleritis: May start posteriorly, or rarely be an extension of anterior scleritis, or simulate an amelanotic choroidal mass. Associated with exudative retinal detachment, disc swelling, retinal hemorrhage, choroidal folds, choroidal detachment, restricted motility, proptosis, pain, tenderness. Usually unrelated to systemic disease.

Work-Up

1. History: Previous episodes? Medical problems?

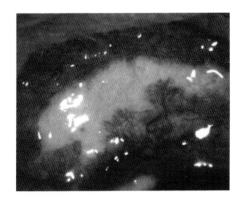

FIGURE 5.7.2. Necrotizing scleritis with thin, bluish sclera.

2. Examine the sclera in all directions of gaze by gross inspection in natural light or adequate room light.

3. Slit-lamp examination with a red-free filter (green light) to determine whether avascular areas of the sclera exist. Check for corneal or anterior chamber involvement.

4. Dilated fundus examination to rule out posterior involvement.

5. Complete physical examination (especially joints, skin, cardiovascular and respiratory systems) by an internist or a rheumatologist.

6. Complete blood count, ESR, uric acid, RPR, FTA-ABS, rheumatoid factor, ANA, fasting blood sugar, ACE, CH 50 (total complement activity assay), C3, C4, and serum ANCA.

7. Other tests if clinical suspicion warrants additional work-up: PPD with anergy panel, chest radiograph, radiograph of sacroiliac joints, B-scan ultrasonography to detect posterior scleritis (e.g., T-sign), and magnetic resonance imaging (MRI) or computed tomographic (CT) scan if indicated.

Treatment

1. Diffuse and nodular scleritis: One or more of the following may be required. Concurrent antacid or histamine type 2 receptor blocker (e.g., ranitidine 150 mg p.o. b.i.d.) is advisable.

   —NSAIDs (e.g., ibuprofen 400 to 600 mg p.o. q.i.d.; naproxen 250 to 500 mg p.o. b.i.d.; indomethacin 25 mg p.o. t.i.d.): Three separate NSAIDs may be tried before therapy is considered a failure. If still no improvement, consider systemic steroids.

   —Systemic steroids: Prednisone 60 to 100 mg p.o. q.d. for 1 week, followed by a taper to 20 mg q.d. over the next 2 to 6 weeks, followed by a slower taper. An oral NSAID often facilitates the tapering of the steroid. If unsuccessful, consider immunosuppressive therapy.

   —Immunosuppressive therapy (e.g., cyclophosphamide, methotrexate, cyclosporine, azathioprine, anti-TNFα agents): If one drug is ineffective or not tolerated, additional agents should be tried. Systemic steroids may be used in conjunction. Immunosuppressive therapy should be coordinated with an internist or a rheumatologist. The role of topical cyclosporine drops is unclear.

2. Necrotizing scleritis:

   —Systemic steroid and immunosuppressive therapies are used as above.

   —Scleral patch grafting may be necessary if there is significant risk of perforation.

3. Posterior scleritis: Therapy is controversial and may include systemic aspirin, NSAIDs, steroids, or immunosuppressive therapy as described previously. Consult a retina specialist.

4. Infectious etiologies: Treat with appropriate topical and systemic antimicrobials. Oral fluoroquinolones have good tissue penetration. If a foreign body [e.g., scleral buckle (associated with *Proteus*)] is present, surgical removal is indicated.

5. Glasses or eye shield should be worn at all times if there is significant thinning and perforation risk.

NOTE: Topical steroids are not effective in scleritis. Although controversial, periocular steroids are usually contraindicated, especially in necrotizing scleritis, and may lead to scleral thinning and perforation.

Follow-Up

Depends on the severity of the symptoms and the degree of scleral thinning. Decreased pain is a sign of response to treatment, even if inflammation appears unchanged.

5.8 · BLEPHARITIS/MEIBOMITIS

Symptoms

Itching, burning, mild pain, foreign body sensation, tearing, and crusting around the eyes on awakening. This is in contrast to dry-eye syndrome in which, symptoms are usually worse later in the day.

Signs

Critical. Crusty, red, thickened eyelid margins with prominent blood vessels (see Figure 5.8.1) or inspissated oil glands at the eyelid margins (see Figure 5.8.2).

Other. Conjunctival injection, swollen eyelids, mild mucous discharge, and SPK. Rosacea may be present. Corneal infiltrates and phlyctenules may be present.

Differential Diagnosis

- Pediculosis. See 5.1, *Acute Conjunctivitis.*

Treatment

See 5.9, *Ocular Rosacea,* for treatment options in the presence of acne rosacea.

1. Scrub the eyelid margins twice a day with a commercial eyelid scrub or mild shampoo on a wash cloth.
2. Warm compresses for 10 to 15 minutes b.i.d. to q.i.d.
3. If associated with dry eyes, use artificial tears four to eight times per day.
4. If moderately severe, add erythromycin ointment or azithromycin gel to the eyelids q.h.s.
5. Consider cyclosporine 0.05% drops b.i.d., especially for meibomitis.
6. Unresponsive meibomitis can be treated with tetracycline 250 mg p.o. q.i.d. or doxycycline 100 mg p.o. q.d. for 1 to 2 weeks, then taper slowly to one-fourth full dose for 3 to 6 months.

NOTE: Tetracycline and doxycycline should not be used in pregnant women, nursing mothers, or children ≤8 years. Erythromycin 200 mg p.o. b.i.d. can be used instead.

Follow-Up

Three to four weeks. Eyelid scrubs and warm compresses may be reduced to q.d. as the condition improves. They often need to be maintained indefinitely.

NOTE: Rarely, intractable, unilateral, or asymmetric blepharitis is a manifestation of sebaceous carcinoma of the eyelid. See 6.11, *Malignant Tumors of the Eyelid.*

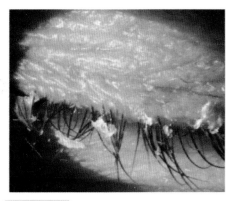

FIGURE 5.8.1. Blepharitis with lash collarettes.

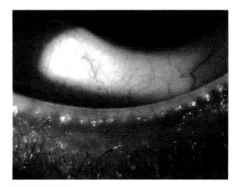

FIGURE 5.8.2. Meibomitis with inspissated meibomian glands.

5.9	OCULAR ROSACEA

Symptoms

Bilateral chronic ocular irritation, redness, burning, photophobia, and foreign body sensation. Typically middle-aged adults, but it can be found in children. More common in women.

Signs

Critical. Telangiectasias, pustules, papules, or erythema of the cheeks, forehead, and nose. Findings may be subtle, often best seen in natural light. Superficial or deep corneal vascularization, particularly in the inferior cornea, is sometimes seen and may extend into a stromal infiltrate.

Other. Rhinophyma of the nose occurs in the late stages of the disease, especially in men. Blepharitis (telangiectasias of the eyelid margin with inflammation) and a history of chalazia are common. Conjunctival injection, SPK, phlyctenules, perilimbal infiltrates of staphylococcal hypersensitivity, iritis, or even corneal perforation may occur.

Differential Diagnosis

- Herpes simplex keratitis: Usually unilateral. Stromal keratitis with neovascularization may appear similar. See 4.15, *Herpes Simplex Virus.*

- See 4.1, *Superficial Punctate Keratopathy,* for additional differential diagnoses.

Etiology

Unknown, but signs and symptoms are often induced by certain environmental/local factors, including coffee, tea, and alcohol.

Work-Up

1. External examination: Look at the face for the characteristic skin findings.

2. Slit-lamp examination: Look for telangiectasias and meibomitis on the eyelids, conjunctival injection, and corneal scarring and vascularization.

Treatment

1. Warm compresses and eyelid hygiene for blepharitis or meibomitis (see 5.8, *Blepharitis/ Meibomitis*). Treat dry eyes if present (see 4.3, *Dry-Eye Syndrome*).

2. Avoidance of exacerbating foods, beverages, and environmental factors.

3. Tetracycline 250 mg p.o. q.i.d. or doxycycline 100 mg p.o. b.i.d. for 1 to 2 weeks then daily; taper the dose slowly once relief from symptoms is obtained. Some patients are maintained on low-dose tetracycline (e.g., 250 mg p.o. q.d.) or doxycycline (e.g., 40 to 100 mg p.o. q.d. or less than daily) indefinitely, if active disease recurs when the patient is off medication. Erythromycin 250 mg q.i.d. may be substituted if tetracycline or doxycycline is contraindicated.

NOTE: Tetracycline and doxycycline should not be given to pregnant women, nursing women, or children ≤8 years. Patients should be told to take the tetracycline on an empty stomach and should be warned of susceptibility to sunburn while taking tetracycline and doxycycline.

NOTE: Asymptomatic ocular rosacea without progressively worsening eye disease does not require oral antibiotics.

---

4. Facial lesions can be treated with metronidazole gel (0.75%) application b.i.d.

5. Treat chalazia as needed (see 6.2, *Chalazion/ Hordeolum*).

6. Cyclosporine 0.05% drops b.i.d. is often helpful for chronic rosacea-related ocular and eyelid inflammation.

7. Corneal perforations may be treated with cyanoacrylate tissue adhesive if small, whereas larger perforations may require surgical correction. Tetracycline is usually

given for treatment of underlying blepharitis and for its antimelting properties.

8. If infiltrates stain with fluorescein, an infectious corneal ulcer may be present. Smears, cultures, and antibiotic treatment may be necessary. See 4.11, *Bacterial Keratitis,* and Appendix 8, *Corneal Culture Procedure.*

Follow-Up

Variable; depends on the severity of disease. Patients without corneal involvement are seen weeks to months later. Those with corneal disease are examined more often. Patients with moderate-to-severe facial disease should also seek dermatologic consultation.

5.10 OCULAR CICATRICIAL PEMPHIGOID

Symptoms

Insidious onset of dryness, redness, foreign body sensation, tearing, and photophobia. Bilateral involvement. The course is characterized by remissions and exacerbations. Usually occurs in patients older than 55 years.

Signs

(See Figure 5.10.1.)

Critical. Inferior symblepharon (linear folds of conjunctiva connecting the palpebral conjunctiva of the lower eyelid to the inferior bulbar conjunctiva), foreshortening, and tightness of the lower fornix.

Other. Secondary bacterial conjunctivitis, SPK, corneal ulcer. Later, poor tear film, resulting in severe dry-eye syndrome; entropion; trichiasis (if present, carefully examine fornices for symblepharon); corneal opacification with pannus and keratinization; obliteration of the fornices, with eventual limitation of ocular motility; and ankyloblepharon may occur.

Systemic. Mucous membrane (e.g., oropharynx, esophagus, anus, vagina, urethra) vesicles; scarring or strictures; ruptured or formed bullae; denuded epithelium. Desquamative gingivitis is common. Cutaneous vesicles and bullae may occur, sometimes with erythematous plaques or scars near affected mucous membranes.

Differential Diagnosis

- Stevens–Johnson syndrome (erythema multiforme major) and toxic epidermal necrolysis (TEN): Acute onset, but similar ocular involvement as ocular pemphigoid. Often precipitated by drugs (e.g., sulfa, penicillin, other antibiotics, phenytoin) or infections (e.g., herpes and mycoplasma). See 13.6, *Stevens–Johnson Syndrome (Erythema Multiforme Major).*

- History of membranous conjunctivitis with scarring: Usually adenovirus or beta-hemolytic *Streptococcus.* Symblepharon can follow any severe membranous/pseudomembranous conjunctivitis. See 5.1, *Acute Conjunctivitis* and 5.2, *Chronic Conjunctivitis.*

- Severe chemical burn: See 3.1, *Chemical Burn.*

- Chronic topical medicine: e.g., glaucoma medications (especially pilocarpine and phospholine iodide), antiviral agents.

- Others: Atopic keratoconjunctivitis, radiation treatment, squamous cell carcinoma.

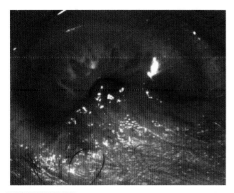

FIGURE 5.10.1. Ocular cicatricial pemphigoid with symblepharon.

Work-Up

1. History: Long-term topical medications? Acute onset of severe systemic illness in the past? Recent systemic medications?

2. Skin and mucous membrane examination.

3. Slit-lamp examination: Especially for inferior symblepharon, by pulling down the lower eyelid during upgaze. Check IOP.

4. Gram stain and culture of the cornea or conjunctiva if secondary bacterial infection is suspected. See Appendix 8, *Corneal Culture Procedure*.

5. Consider a biopsy of the conjunctiva or other involved mucous membrane for direct immunofluorescence studies, or indirect immunofluorescence for the presence of antibodies.

6. Obtain appropriate consults, as below.

Treatment

Multidisciplinary approach often needed, including dermatology, oculoplastics, cornea, otolaryngology, gastroenterology, and pulmonology. Early diagnosis of the ocular involvement is critical for optimal management.

1. Preservative-free artificial tears four to ten times per day. Can add an artificial tear ointment b.i.d. to q.i.d. and q.h.s.

2. Treat blepharitis vigorously with eyelid hygiene, warm compresses, and antibiotic ointment (e.g., erythromycin t.i.d.). Oral tetracycline/doxycycline can be used if blepharitis is present (particularly given its anti-inflammatory properties). See 5.8, *Blepharitis/Meibomitis.*

3. Goggles or glasses with sides to provide a moist environment for the eyes.

4. Punctal occlusion if puncta are not already closed by scarring.

5. Topical steroids may rarely help in suppressing acute exacerbations, but be cautious of corneal melting.

6. Systemic steroids (e.g., prednisone 60 mg p.o. q.d.) may also help in suppressing acute exacerbations but are most effective when used with other immune modulators.

7. Immunosuppressive agents (e.g., mycophenolate mofetil, methotrexate, or cyclophosphamide) are typically used for progressive disease.

8. Dapsone is occasionally used for progressive disease. Starting dose is 25 mg p.o. for 3 to 7 days; increase by 25 mg every 4 to 7 days until the desired result is achieved (usually 100 to 150 mg p.o. q.d.). Dapsone is maintained for several months and tapered slowly.

NOTE: Dapsone can cause a dose-related hemolysis. A complete blood count and glucose-6-phosphate dehydrogenase (G-6-PD) must be checked before administration. Dapsone should be avoided in patients with G-6-PD deficiency. A complete blood count with reticulocyte count is obtained weekly as the dose is increased every 3 to 4 weeks until blood counts are stable and then every few months.

---

9. Consider surgical correction of entropion and cryotherapy or electrolysis of trichiasis. Surgery carries risk of further scarring and is best performed when inflammation is absent.

10. Mucous membrane grafts (e.g., buccal or amniotic membrane graft) can be used to reconstruct the fornices if needed.

11. Consider a keratoprosthesis in an end-stage eye with good macular and optic nerve function if the inflammation and IOP are controlled.

Follow-Up

Every 1 to 2 weeks during acute exacerbations, and every 1 to 6 months during remissions.

5.11   CONTACT DERMATITIS

Symptoms

Sudden onset of a periorbital rash or eyelid swelling, mild watery discharge.

Signs

(See Figure 5.11.1.)

Critical. Periorbital edema, erythema, vesicles, lichenification of the skin. Conjunctival chemosis out of proportion to injection and papillary response.

Other. Watery discharge; crusting of the skin may develop.

Differential Diagnosis

- Varicella zoster virus (shingles): Dermatomal pattern with severe pain. See 4.16, *Herpes Zoster Ophthalmicus/Varicella Zoster Virus.*

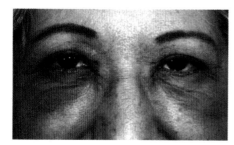

FIGURE 5.11.1.   Contact dermatitis.

- Eczema: Recurrent in nature and is markedly pruritic.

- Impetigo: Pruritic with honey-colored crusts.

- Orbital cellulitis or preseptal cellulites: See 7.3.1, *Orbital Cellulitis,* and 6.10, *Preseptal Cellulitis.*

Etiology

Most commonly, eye drops and cosmetics.

Treatment

1. Avoid the offending agent(s).

2. Cool compresses four to six times per day.

3. Preservative-free artificial tears four to eight times per day and topical antihistamines (e.g., levocabastine 0.05% q.i.d.).

4. Consider tacrolimus 0.03% to 0.1% q.h.s. or b.i.d. (preferred).

5. Consider a mild steroid cream (e.g., fluorometholone 0.1%) applied to the periocular area b.i.d. to t.i.d. for 4 to 5 days for skin involvement.

6. Consider an oral antihistamine (e.g., diphenhydramine 25 to 50 mg p.o. t.i.d. to q.i.d.) for several days.

Follow-Up

Re-examine within 1 week.

5.12   CONJUNCTIVAL TUMORS

The following are the most common and important conjunctival tumors. Phlyctenulosis and Pterygium/Pinguecula are discussed in 4.20 and 4.9, respectively.

AMELANOTIC LESIONS

Limbal Dermoid

Congenital benign tumor, usually located in the inferotemporal quadrant of the limbus, can involve the cornea. Lesions are white, solid, fairly well circumscribed, elevated, and can have hair arising from their surface. May enlarge, particularly at puberty. Associated with eyelid colobomas, preauricular skin tags, and vertebral abnormalities (Goldenhar syndrome). Surgical removal may be performed for cosmetic purposes or if they are affecting the visual axis, although a white corneal scar may persist postoperatively and cause astigmatism if a patch penetrating keratoplasty is needed.

NOTE: The cornea or sclera underlying a dermoid can be very thin or even absent. Penetration of the eye can occur with surgical resection. Ultrasound biomicroscopy may be helpful to determine depth.

Dermolipoma

Congenital benign tumor, usually occurring under the bulbar conjunctiva temporally, often superotemporally. Yellow-white, solid tumor. Can have hair arising from its surface. High association with Goldenhar syndrome. Surgical removal is avoided because of the frequent posterior extension of this tumor into the orbit. If necessary, partial resection of the anterior portion can usually be done without difficulty.

Pyogenic Granuloma

Benign, deep-red, pedunculated mass. Typically develops at a site of prior surgery, trauma, or chalazion. This lesion consists of exuberant granulation tissue. May respond to topical steroids. A topical steroid–antibiotic combination (e.g., dexamethasone/tobramycin 0.1%/0.3% q.i.d. for 1 to 2 weeks) can be helpful because infection can be present. Excision required if it persists.

Lymphangioma

Probably congenital but often not detected until years after birth. Slowly progressive benign lesion that appears as a diffuse, multiloculated, cystic mass. Seen most commonly between birth and young adulthood, often before 6 years of age. Hemorrhage into the cystic spaces can produce a "chocolate cyst." Can enlarge, sometimes due to an upper respiratory tract infection. Concomitant eyelid, orbital, facial, nasal, or oropharyngeal lymphangiomas can be present. Surgical excision may be performed for cosmetic or functional purposes, but it often must be repeated because it is difficult to remove the entire tumor with one surgical procedure. Lesions often stabilize in early adulthood. These lesions do not regress like the capillary hemangiomas.

Granuloma

Can occur at any age, predominantly on the tarsal conjunctiva. No distinct clinical appearance, but patients can have an associated embedded foreign body, sarcoidosis, tuberculosis, or another granulomatous disease. For systemic granulomatous diseases (e.g., sarcoidosis), conjunctival granulomas can be an excellent source of tissue. Management often includes a course of topical corticosteroids or excisional biopsy.

Papilloma

1. Viral: Frequently multiple pedunculated or sessile lesions in children and young adults. May occur on palpebral or bulbar conjunctiva. They are benign and are usually left untreated because of their high recurrence rate (which is often multiple) and their tendency for spontaneous resolution. They can also be treated with oral cimetidine 30 mg/kg/day in children or 150 mg p.o. b.i.d. in adults, because of the drug's immune-stimulating properties.

2. Nonviral: Typically, a single sessile or pedunculated lesion found in older patients. These are located more commonly near the limbus and can represent precancerous lesions with malignant potential. Complete wide excisional biopsy with cryotherapy at the conjunctival margin is the preferred treatment since it may be difficult to differentiate from squamous cell carcinoma.

NOTE: In dark-skinned individuals, papillomas can appear pigmented and can be mistaken for malignant melanoma.

Kaposi Sarcoma

Malignant, nontender subconjunctival nodule, usually red. May simulate a conjunctival hemorrhage. Perform HIV/AIDS testing. Kaposi sarcoma lesions may resolve when patients are placed on highly active antiretroviral therapy (HAART). Other treatments include vinblastine, vincristine, excision, cryotherapy, or irradiation.

Conjunctival Intraepithelial Neoplasia (Dysplasia and Carcinoma in Situ)

Typically occurs in middle-aged to elderly people. Leukoplakic or gray-white, gelatinous lesion that usually begins at the limbus. Occasionally, a papillomatous, fernlike appearance develops. Usually unilateral and unifocal. Can evolve into invasive

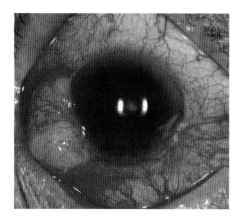

FIGURE 5.12.1. Conjunctival squamous cell carcinoma.

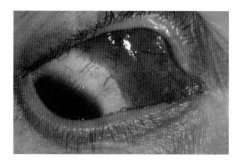

FIGURE 5.12.2. Conjunctival lymphoma (salmon patch).

squamous cell carcinoma (see Figure 5.12.1) if not treated early and successfully. Can spread over the cornea or, less commonly, invade the eye or metastasize. Preferred treatment is a complete excisional biopsy followed by supplemental cryotherapy to the remaining adjacent conjunctiva. Excision may require lamellar dissection into the corneal stroma and sclera in recurrent or long-standing lesions. Topical forms of mitomycin C, 5-fluorouracil, and interferon have also been used. Periodic follow-up examinations are required to detect recurrences.

Lymphoid Tumors (Range from Benign Reactive Lymphoid Hyperplasia to Lymphoma)

Can occur in young- to middle-aged adults, but mean age of diagnosis is 61 years. Usually appears as a light pink, salmon-colored lesion. Can appear in the bulbar conjunctiva, where it is typically oval, or in the fornix, where it is usually horizontal, conforming to the contour of the fornix (see Figure 5.12.2). Excisional or incisional biopsy is performed for immunohistochemical studies (require fresh non-fixed tissue). Symptomatic benign reactive lymphoid hyperplasia can be treated by excisional biopsy or topical steroid drops. Lymphomas should be completely excised when possible, without damage to the extraocular muscles or excessive sacrifice of conjunctiva. If not possible, an incisional biopsy is justified. Refer to an internist or oncologist for systemic evaluation. Systemic lymphoma may develop, if it is not already present.

Epibulbar Osseous Choristoma

Congenital, benign, hard, bony mass, usually on the superotemporal bulbar conjunctiva. Surgical removal can be performed for cosmetic purposes.

Amyloid

(See Figure 5.12.3.)

Smooth, waxy, yellow-pink masses seen especially in the lower fornix when the conjunctiva is involved. Often there are associated small hemorrhages. Definitive diagnosis is made with biopsy. Consider work-up for systemic amyloidosis, although most cases in the conjunctiva are localized and solitary.

Amelanotic Melanoma

Pigmentation of conjunctival melanoma is variable. Look for bulbar or limbal lesions with significant vascularity to help make this difficult diagnosis.

Sebaceous Carcinoma

Although usually involving the palpebral conjunctiva, this tumor can involve the bulbar

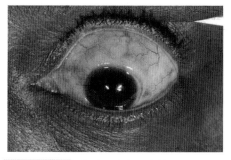

FIGURE 5.12.3. Conjunctival amyloid.

conjunctiva (when there is pagetoid invasion of the conjunctiva). This diagnosis should always be considered in older patients with refractory unilateral blepharoconjunctivitis.

(See 6.11, *Malignant Tumors of the Eyelid,* for a detailed discussion of sebaceous carcinoma.)

MELANOTIC LESIONS

Nevus

(See Figure 5.12.4.)
Commonly develops during puberty, most often within the palpebral fissure on the bulbar conjunctiva. Usually well demarcated with variable pigmentation. The degree of pigmentation can also change with time. A key sign in the diagnosis is the presence of small cysts in the lesion. Benign nevi can enlarge; however, a melanoma can occasionally develop from a nevus, and enlargement can be an early sign of malignant transformation. Nevi of the palpebral conjunctiva are rare, and primary acquired melanosis and malignant melanoma must be considered in such lesions. A baseline photograph of the nevus should be taken, and the patient should be observed every 6 to 12 months. Surgical excision is elective. Nevi may be amelanotic.

Ocular or Oculodermal Melanocytosis

Congenital episcleral (not conjunctival) lesion, as demonstrated (after topical anesthesia) by moving the conjunctiva back and forth over the area of pigmentation with a cotton-tipped swab (conjunctival pigmentation will move with the conjunctiva). Typically, the lesion is unilateral, blue-gray, and often accompanied by a darker ipsilateral iris and choroid. In oculodermal melanocytosis, also called nevus of Ota, the periocular skin is also pigmented. These lesions can become pigmented at puberty. Both conditions predispose to melanoma of the uveal tract, orbit, and brain (most commonly in whites) and glaucoma.

Primary Acquired Melanosis

Flat, brown patches of pigmentation, without cysts, in the conjunctiva. Usually arise during or after middle age and almost always occur in whites. Classically, approximately 30% of these lesions develop into melanoma. More recent studies suggest the true incidence is much lower. Malignant transformation should be suspected when an elevation or increase in vascularity in one of these areas develops. Management options include careful observation with photographic comparison for any change and incisional or excisional biopsy followed by cryotherapy for suggestive lesions.

Malignant Melanoma

(See Figure 5.12.5.)
Typically occurs in middle-aged to elderly patients. The lesion is a nodular brown mass. Well vascularized. Often a large conjunctival feeding vessel present. May develop de novo, from a nevus, or from primary acquired melanosis. Check for an underlying ciliary body

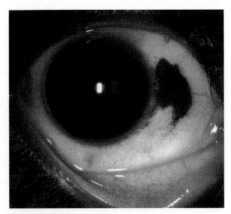

FIGURE 5.12.4. Conjunctival nevus.

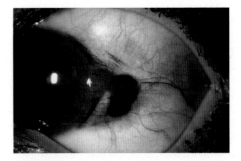

FIGURE 5.12.5. Conjunctival melanoma.

melanoma (dilated fundus examination, transillumination, and ultrasonographic biomicroscopy). Intraocular and orbital extension can occur. Excisional biopsy (often with supplemental cryotherapy) is performed unless intraocular or orbital involvement is present. In advanced cases, orbital exenteration is necessary. Sentinel lymph node biopsy is advised to detect early metastatic disease.

Less Common Causes of Conjunctival Pigmentation

1. Ochronosis with alkaptonuria: Autosomal recessive enzyme deficiency. Occurs in young adults with arthritis and dark urine.

Pigment is at the level of the sclera. "Pigmented pinguecula."

2. Argyrosis: Silver deposition causes black discoloration. Patients have a history of long-term use of silver nitrate drops.

3. Hemochromatosis: Bronze diabetes.

4. Ciliary staphyloma: Scleral thinning with uveal show.

5. Adrenochrome deposits: Long-term epinephrine or dipivefrin use.

6. Mascara deposits: Usually occurs in the inferior fornix and becomes entrapped in epithelium or cysts.

5

5.13 MALIGNANT MELANOMA OF THE IRIS

Malignant melanoma of the iris can occur as a localized or diffuse pigmented (melanotic) or nonpigmented (amelanotic) lesion.

Signs

(See Figure 5.13.1.)

Critical. Unilateral brown or translucent iris mass lesion exhibiting slow growth. It is more common in the inferior half of the iris and in light-skinned individuals. Rare in blacks.

Other. A localized melanoma is usually >3 mm in diameter at the base and >1 mm in depth with a variable prominent feeder vessel. Can produce a sector cortical cataract, ectropion iridis, spontaneous hyphema,

seeding of tumor cells into the anterior chamber, or direct invasion of tumor into the trabecular meshwork and secondary glaucoma. A diffuse melanoma causes progressive darkening of the involved iris, loss of iris crypts, and increased IOP. Focal iris nodules can be present.

Differential Diagnosis

Melanotic Masses

- Nevi: Typically become clinically apparent at puberty, usually flat or minimally elevated (i.e., <1 mm) and uncommonly exceed 3 mm in diameter. Can cause ectropion iridis, sector cortical cataract, or secondary glaucoma. Usually not vascular. More common in the inferior half of the iris. Nevi do not usually grow.

- Tumors of the iris pigment epithelium: Usually black in contrast to melanomas, which are often brown or amelanotic.

Amelanotic Masses

- Metastasis: Grows rapidly. More likely to be multiple or bilateral than is melanoma. Frequently liberates cells and produces a pseudohypopyon. Involves the superior and inferior halves of the iris equally.

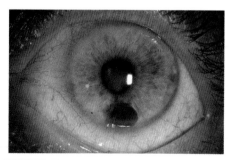

FIGURE 5.13.1. Iris melanoma.

5

- Leiomyoma: Transparent and vascular. Difficult to distinguish from an amelanotic melanoma.

- Iris cyst: Unlike melanoma, most transmit light with transillumination. Can arise from the iris pigment epithelium or within the iris stroma. Each with very different clinical features.

- Inflammatory granuloma: Sarcoidosis, tuberculosis, juvenile xanthogranuloma, others. Often have other signs of inflammation such as keratic precipitates, synechiae, and posterior subcapsular cataracts. A history of iritis or a systemic inflammatory disease may be elicited. See Chapter 12, *Uveitis*.

Diffuse Lesions

- Congenital iris heterochromia: The darker iris is present at birth or in early childhood. It is nonprogressive and usually is not associated with glaucoma. The iris has a smooth appearance.

- Fuchs heterochromic iridocyclitis: Asymmetry of iris color, mild iritis in the eye with the lighter-colored iris, usually unilateral. Often associated with a cataract or glaucoma. See 12.1, *Anterior Uveitis (Iritis/Iridocyclitis)*.

- Iris nevus syndrome: Corneal edema, peripheral anterior synechiae, iris atrophy, or an irregular pupil can be present along with multiple iris nodules and glaucoma.

- Pigment dispersion: Usually bilateral. The iris is rarely heavily pigmented (although the trabecular meshwork can be), and iris transillumination defects are often present. See 9.10, *Pigment Dispersion Syndrome/Pigmentary Glaucoma*.

- Hemosiderosis: A dark iris can result after iron breakdown products from old blood deposit on the iris surface. Patients have a history of a traumatic hyphema or vitreous hemorrhage.

- Siderosis from a retained metallic foreign body.

Work-Up

1. History: Previous cancer, ocular surgery, or trauma? Weight loss? Anorexia?

2. Slit-lamp examination: Carefully evaluate the irides. Check IOP.

3. Gonioscopy.

4. Dilated fundus examination using indirect ophthalmoscopy.

5. Transillumination of iris mass (helps differentiate epithelial cysts that transmit light from pigmented lesions that do not).

6. Photograph the lesion and accurately draw it in the chart, including dimensions. Ultrasonographic biomicroscopy and anterior segment optical coherence tomography can be helpful.

Treatment/Follow-Up

1. Observe the patient with periodic examinations and photographs every 3 to 12 months, depending on the suspicion of malignancy.

2. Surgical resection is indicated if growth is documented, the tumor interferes with vision, or it produces intractable glaucoma.

3. Diffuse iris melanoma with secondary glaucoma may require enucleation.

NOTE: Avoid filtering surgery for glaucoma associated with possible melanoma because of the risk of tumor dissemination.

Eyelid 6

6.1 PTOSIS

Symptoms

Drooping upper eyelid, visual loss often worse with reading and at night.

Signs

(See Figure 6.1.1.)

Critical. Drooping upper eyelid.

Other. Concerning associated signs include anisocoria, diplopia, ocular motility defects, headache, or neck pain. See individual entities.

Etiology

NOTE: Although the vast majority of ptosis is of benign etiology, five entities must be ruled out in every single case by careful examination.

1. Horner syndrome.

2. Third cranial nerve (CN) palsy (complete, partial, or aberrant CN III regeneration).

3. Myasthenia gravis.

4. Superior eyelid or orbital malignancy.

5. Chronic progressive external ophthalmoplegia (CPEO) (particularly Kearns–Sayre syndrome. See 10.12, *Chronic Progressive External Ophthalmoplegia*).

- Myogenic: Congenital myogenic ptosis is present at birth with poor levator function and a poor or absent lid crease due to dysgenesis of the levator muscle, fibrosis, and its replacement with adipose tissue. A poor Bell phenomenon, lagophthalmos in downgaze, and upgaze limitation may

indicate a double elevator palsy. Acquired myogenic ptosis is uncommon and may be seen with muscular dystrophy and CPEO.

- Aponeurotic: This is characterized by a high or absent eyelid crease, moderate degree of ptosis, good levator function (10 to 15 mm). May worsen in downgaze. Levator stretching or dehiscence can be due to normal aging, repetitive eye rubbing, use of rigid contact lenses, or previous intraocular surgery.

- Neurogenic: Third cranial nerve palsy (often complete ptosis, never an isolated abnormality; congenital, compressive, vasculopathic, see 10.5, *Isolated Third Nerve Palsy*); Horner syndrome (subtle upper and lower eyelid ptosis, see 10.2, *Horner Syndrome*); myasthenia gravis (variable ptosis, worsens with fatigue, see 10.11, *Myasthenia Gravis*); Marcus Gunn jaw-winking syndrome (ptotic eyelid elevates with jaw movement); ophthalmoplegic migraine; multiple sclerosis.

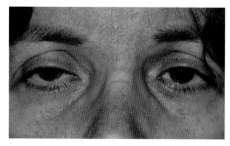

FIGURE 6.1.1. Ptosis.

135

- Mechanical: Retained contact lens in upper fornix; upper eyelid inflammation (chalazion, giant papillary conjunctivitis, posttraumatic or postsurgical edema) or neoplasm.

- Traumatic: History of eyelid laceration with levator transection, contusion injury to the levator, tethering or ischemia within an orbital roof fracture, late dehiscence or cicatricial changes.

- Pseudoptosis: Contralateral eyelid retraction or proptosis, ipsilateral enophthalmos, hypertropia, microphthalmia, phthisis bulbi, dermatochalasis, brow ptosis, chalazion or other eyelid tumor, eyelid edema, blepharospasm, Duane syndrome.

Work-Up

1. History: Determine the onset and duration of ptosis. Present since birth? Acute onset? Old photographs (e.g., driver's license) and family members' opinions are useful adjuncts to the history. History of surgery in either eye? Orbital or eyelid trauma (orbital blow-out fractures resulting in enophthalmos can mimic ptosis)? Variability with fatigue? Associated with headache or neck pain? Any history of autoimmune disease (lupus, Sjogren syndrome) or corneal abnormalities (may predispose the patient to postoperative exposure keratopathy)?

2. Mandatory documentation: Must carefully check and document pupillary size and extraocular motility, even if normal. If anisocoria is present, measurements should be documented under light and dark conditions. Additional pharmacologic testing may be indicated (see 10.1, *Anisocoria*). If extraocular muscle dysfunction is noted, additional testing with prism bars may be indicated.

3. Complete orbital examination of both eyes: Measure and compare margin–reflex distance, levator function (full upper eyelid excursion while preventing frontalis muscle assistance), upper eyelid crease position of both eyes. Is there lagophthalmos? Associated lower eyelid "ptosis" (elevation of ipsilateral lower eyelid) is often seen in

Horner syndrome. Proptosis or eyelid lag may masquerade as contralateral ptosis. Exophthalmometry measurements are useful. Any sign of aberrant eyelid movements like jaw-winking, variability and/or fatigue, orbicularis weakness, eyelid retraction with adduction and/or infraduction? Palpate the superior orbit to rule out a mass or superior orbital rim deformity.

4. Complete ocular examination: Determine if there are associated pupillary or extraocular motility abnormalities. Flip upper eyelid to examine conjunctival surface and superior fornix. Dilated fundus examination to look for pigmentary changes in adolescents and young adults who present with ptosis, poor levator function, and external ophthalmoplegia (possible Kearns–Sayre syndrome).

5. Corneal protective mechanisms. Document the presence or absence of preoperative lagophthalmos, orbicularis function, Bell phenomenon, and tear production. Check the cornea carefully for any abnormalities or dystrophies, which may predispose the patient to postoperative keratopathy.

6. Other tests

—Ice test: Apply ice pack to ptotic eye for 2 minutes and reassess the degree of ptosis. Improvement with ice is highly suggestive of myasthenia gravis.

—Neosynephrine test: Instill one drop of 2.5% phenylephrine in the ptotic eye(s) and reassess the degree of ptosis. Patients with improvement of ptosis after 5 to 7 minutes may be good candidates for ptosis correction by an internal approach.

—Cocaine, apraclonidine, and hydroxyamphetamine tests. See 10.2, *Horner Syndrome.*

7. Imaging studies: In very select cases where a systemic or neurologic cause is suspected:

—Computed tomography (CT) or magnetic resonance imaging (MRI) of orbit if a superior orbital mass is suspected.

—Emergent CT/computed tomography angiogram (CTA) or MRI/magnetic resonance angiogram (MRA) of the head and neck if carotid artery dissection is suspected in a patient with a painful Horner syndrome. Imaging of the head alone is inadequate. See 10.2, *Horner Syndrome.*

—Emergent CT/CTA, MRI/MRA, or conventional angiography if intracranial aneurysm causing a third cranial nerve palsy with pupillary involvement or a partial third cranial nerve palsy is suspected. See 10.5, *Isolated Third Nerve Palsy.*

—Chest CT if myasthenia gravis is suspected to rule out thymoma. See 10.11, *Myasthenia Gravis.*

8. Ancillary studies:

—Urgent ECG and cardiology consult if Kearns–Sayre syndrome is suspected. These patients can have heart block, resulting in sudden death.

—If myasthenia gravis is suspected, acetylcholine receptor antibody testing, single-fiber electromyography (including the orbicularis muscle), and/or edrophonium chloride testing under monitored conditions may be indicated. See 10.11, *Myasthenia Gravis.*

—If severe dry eye is found, consider an autoimmune work-up to rule out lupus and Sjogren syndrome.

Treatment

1. Depends on the underlying etiology (see 10.2, *Horner Syndrome;* 10.5, *Isolated Third Nerve Palsy;* 10.11, *Myasthenia Gravis*).

2. Nonsurgical options: Observation. Taping upper lids open and eyelid crutches attached to glasses in neurogenic and myogenic ptosis. Management of chalazion with warm compresses and/or excision, eyelid and/or orbital neoplasms with excision.

3. Surgical options: Transcutaneous levator advancement, transconjunctival levator advancement, frontalis muscle suspension, Müller muscle resection. Surgical approach depends on preoperative evaluation and the underlying etiology of ptosis.

Follow-Up

1. Congenital: Close follow-up is required to monitor for the presence of amblyopia, caused either by occlusion or by refractive error secondary to induced corneal astigmatism, abnormal head positioning, and exposure keratopathy.

2. Traumatic: Observation for 6 months before considering surgical intervention.

3. Neurologic: Reevaluate based on particular entity.

4. Postoperative (after ptosis repair).
Acute: Monitor for infection and hemorrhage.
Subacute: Monitor for exposure keratopathy and for asymmetry that may require postoperative readjustment. Mild lagophthalmos is common for 2 to 3 weeks after surgical repair and usually resolves.
Chronic: Monitor for ptosis recurrence and exposure keratopathy.

6.2 CHALAZION/HORDEOLUM

Symptoms

Acute or chronic eyelid lump, eyelid swelling, tenderness.

Signs

(See Figure 6.2.1.)

Critical. Visible, or palpable, well-defined subcutaneous nodule in the eyelid. In some cases, a nodule cannot be identified.

Other. Blocked meibomian orifice, eyelid swelling and erythema, localized eyelid tenderness, associated blepharitis or acne rosacea. May also note "pointing" of mucopurulent material.

Definitions

Chalazion: Area of focal inflammation within the eyelid secondary to the obstruction of a meibomian gland or gland of Zeis.

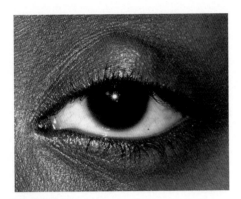

FIGURE 6.2.1. Chalazion.

Hordeolum: Acute infection; can be external (stye: abscess of gland of Zeis on lid margin) or internal (abscess of meibomian gland). Usually involves *Staphylococcus* species and occasionally evolves into a preseptal cellulitis.

Differential Diagnosis

- Preseptal cellulitis: Eyelid and periorbital erythema, edema, and warmth. See 6.10, *Preseptal Cellulitis.*

- Sebaceous carcinoma: Suspect in older patients with recurrent chalazia, eyelid thickening, or chronic unilateral blepharitis. See 6.11, *Malignant Tumors of the Eyelid.*

- Pyogenic granuloma: Benign, deep-red, pedunculated lesion often associated with chalazia, hordeola, trauma, or surgery. May be excised or treated with a topical antibiotic–steroid combination such as neomycin/polymixin B/dexamethasone q.i.d. for 1 to 2 weeks. Intraocular pressure must be monitored if topical steroids are used.

Work-Up

1. History: Previous ocular surgery or trauma? Previous chalazia or eyelid lesions?

2. External examination: Palpate the involved eyelid for a nodule.

3. Slit-lamp examination: Evaluate the meibomian glands for inspissation and evert the eyelid to rule out other etiologies.

Treatment

1. Warm compresses for 10 minutes q.i.d. with light massage over the lesion.

2. Consider a topical antibiotic if lesion is draining or for associated blepharitis (e.g., bacitracin or erythromycin ointment b.i.d.). Consider systemic therapy with doxycycline 100 mg b.i.d. for its antibacterial and anti-inflammatory actions.

3. If a hordeola worsens, consider incision and drainage and management as per preseptal cellulitis (see 6.10, *Preseptal Cellulitis*).

4. If the chalazion fails to resolve after 3 to 4 weeks of appropriate medical therapy and the patient wishes to have it removed, incision and curettage are performed. Occasionally, an injection of steroid (e.g., 0.2 to 1.0 mL of triamcinolone 40 mg/mL usually mixed 1:1 with 2% lidocaine with epinephrine) into the lesion is performed instead of minor surgery, especially if the chalazion is near the lacrimal apparatus. The total dosage depends on the size of the lesion. All recurrent or atypical chalazia must be sent for pathology.

NOTE: A steroid injection can lead to permanent depigmentation or atrophy of the skin at the injection site. The manufacturer of triamcinolone has recently recommended against its use intraocularly and in the periocular region. Vigorous injection can rarely result in retrograde intraarterial injection with resultant central retinal artery occlusion. Use of triamcinolone injection for chalazion treatment must include a detailed discussion between physician and patient, as well as adequate documentation in the patient's record.

Follow-Up

Patients are not seen after instituting medical therapy unless the lesion persists beyond 3 to 4 weeks. Patients who have incision and curettage are reexamined in 1 week or as needed.

6.3 ECTROPION

Symptoms

Tearing, eye or eyelid irritation. May be asymptomatic.

Signs

(See Figure 6.3.1.)

Critical. Outward turning of the eyelid margin.

Other. Superficial punctate keratopathy (SPK) from corneal exposure; conjunctival injection, thickening, and eventual keratinization from chronic conjunctival dryness. Scarring of skin may be seen in cicatricial cases. Facial hemiparesis and lagophthalmos may be seen in paralytic cases.

Etiology

- Involutional: Aging.

- Paralytic: Seventh cranial nerve palsy.

- Cicatricial: Due to chemical burn, surgery, eyelid laceration scar, skin diseases (e.g., eczema, ichthyosis), and others.

- Mechanical: Due to herniated orbital fat, eyelid tumor, and others.

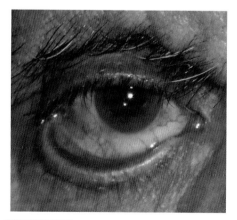

FIGURE 6.3.1. Ectropion.

- Allergic: Contact dermatitis.

- Congenital: Facial dysmorphic syndromes (e.g., Treacher–Collins syndrome) or isolated abnormality.

Work-Up

1. History: Previous surgery, trauma, chemical burn, or seventh nerve palsy?

2. External examination: Check orbicularis oculi function, look for an eyelid tumor, eyelid scarring, herniated orbital fat, and other causes.

3. Slit-lamp examination: Check for SPK due to exposure and evaluate conjunctival integrity.

Treatment

1. Treat exposure keratopathy with lubricating agents. See 4.5, *Exposure Keratopathy.*

2. Treat an inflamed, exposed eyelid margin with warm compresses and antibiotic ointment (e.g., bacitracin or erythromycin t.i.d.). A short course of combination antibiotic–steroid ointment (e.g., neomycin/polymixin B/dexamethasone) may be helpful if close follow-up is ensured.

3. Taping the eyelids into position may be a temporizing measure.

4. Definitive treatment usually requires surgery. Surgery is delayed for 3 to 6 months in patients with a seventh nerve palsy because the ectropion may resolve spontaneously (see 10.9, *Isolated Seventh Nerve Palsy*). Corneal exposure may make repair more urgent.

Follow-Up

Patients with signs of corneal or conjunctival exposure are examined every 1 to 2 weeks to evaluate the integrity of the ocular surface. Otherwise, follow-up is not urgent.

6

6.4   ENTROPION

Symptoms

Ocular irritation, foreign-body sensation, tearing, redness.

Signs

(See Figure 6.4.1.)

Critical. Inward turning of the eyelid margin that pushes otherwise normal lashes onto the globe.

Other. SPK from eyelashes contacting the cornea, conjunctival injection. In severe cases, corneal thinning and ulceration are possible.

Etiology

- Involutional: Aging.

- Cicatricial: Due to conjunctival scarring in ocular cicatricial pemphigoid, Stevens–Johnson syndrome, chemical burns, trauma, trachoma, and others.

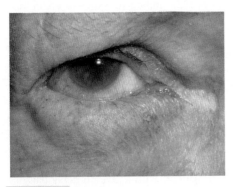

FIGURE 6.4.1. Entropion.

- Spastic: Due to surgical trauma, ocular irritation, or blepharospasm.

- Congenital.

Work-Up

1. History: Previous surgery, trauma, chemical burn, or infection (trachoma, herpes simplex, and varicella zoster)?

2. Slit-lamp examination: Check for corneal involvement as well as conjunctival and eyelid scarring.

Treatment

If blepharospasm is present, see 6.7, *Blepharospasm.*

1. Antibiotic ointment (e.g., erythromycin or bacitracin ophthalmic t.i.d.) for SPK.

2. Everting the eyelid margin away from the globe and taping it in place with adhesive tape may be a temporizing measure.

3. For spastic entropion, a Quickert suture placed at the bedside or in the office can temporarily resolve the eyelid malposition.

4. Surgery is often required for permanent correction.

Follow-Up

If the cornea is relatively healthy, the condition does not require urgent attention or follow-up. If the cornea is significantly damaged, aggressive treatment is indicated (see 4.1, *Superficial Punctate Keratopathy*). Follow-up is determined by the severity of corneal involvement.

6.5   TRICHIASIS

Symptoms

Ocular irritation, foreign-body sensation, tearing, redness.

Signs

Critical. Misdirected eyelashes rubbing against the globe.

Other. SPK, conjunctival injection.

Differential Diagnosis

- Entropion: Inward turning of eyelid pushing normal lashes onto cornea. See 6.4, *Entropion.*

- Epiblepharon: Congenital or familial condition in which an extra lower eyelid skin fold redirects lashes into a vertical position, where they may contact the globe. Most common in Asian individuals, especially children.

- Distichiasis: An aberrant second row of lashes that emanates from meibomian gland openings. Most commonly acquired in the setting of trauma or chronic inflammation (e.g., blepharitis). Congenital distichiasis is a rare, sometimes hereditary condition in which the meibomian glands are replaced by an extra row of eyelashes.

Etiology

- Idiopathic.
- Chronic blepharitis: Inflamed eyelid margin. See 5.8, *Blepharitis/Meibomitis*.
- Cicatricial: Eyelid scarring from trauma, surgery, ocular cicatricial pemphigoid (see 5.10, *Ocular Cicatricial Pemphigoid*), trachoma, and others.

Work-Up

1. History: Recurrent episodes? Severe systemic illness in the past? Previous trauma?
2. Slit-lamp examination: Evert the eyelids and inspect the palpebral conjunctiva for scarring and symblepharon. Check the cornea for abrasions and SPK.

Treatment

1. Epilation: Remove the misdirected lashes.

   —A few misdirected lashes: Remove them at the slit lamp with fine forceps. Recurrence is common.

   —Diffuse, severe, or recurrent trichiasis: Can attempt to epilate as described; definitive therapy usually requires electrolysis, cryotherapy, radiofrequency epilation, or eyelid surgery.

2. Treat SPK with antibiotic ointment (e.g., erythromycin or bacitracin t.i.d.).
3. Treat any underlying blepharitis. See 5.8, *Blepharitis/Meibomitis*.

Follow-Up

As needed based on the symptoms and integrity of the cornea. Closer follow-up is needed if evidence of SPK or corneal abrasion.

6

6.6 FLOPPY EYELID SYNDROME

Symptoms

Chronically red, irritated eye with mild mucous discharge, often worst on awakening from sleep due to eyelid eversion during the night. Usually bilateral but may be asymmetric. Typically seen in obese males. Strongly associated with sleep apnea.

Signs

Critical. Upper eyelids are easily everted without an accessory finger or cotton-tipped applicator exerting counterpressure.

Other. Soft and rubbery superior tarsal plate, superior tarsal papillary conjunctivitis, SPK, ptosis. Associated with keratoconus, obesity, hyperglycemia, and sleep apnea.

Differential Diagnosis

Key differentiating factor is laxity and spontaneous eversion of the upper eyelids.

- Vernal conjunctivitis: Seasonal, itching, and giant papillary reaction. See 5.2, *Chronic Conjunctivitis*.
- Giant papillary conjunctivitis: Often related to contact lens wear or an exposed suture. See 4.22, *Contact Lens-Induced Giant Papillary Conjunctivitis*.
- Superior limbic keratoconjunctivitis: Hyperemia and thickening of the superior bulbar conjunctiva. See 5.4, *Superior Limbic Keratoconjunctivitis*.
- Toxic keratoconjunctivitis: Papillae or follicles are usually more abundant on the inferior tarsal conjunctiva in a patient using eye drops. See 5.2, *Chronic Conjunctivitis*.

Etiology

The underlying defect is not definitively known. Studies have suggested an abnormality of collagen and elastin fibers. The symptoms are thought to result from spontaneous eversion of the upper eyelid during sleep, allowing the superior palpebral conjunctiva to rub against a pillow or sheets. Unilateral symptoms are often on the side on which the patient predominantly sleeps.

Work-Up

1. Pull the upper eyelid toward the patient's forehead to determine if it spontaneously everts or is abnormally lax.

2. Conduct slit-lamp examination of the cornea and conjunctiva with fluorescein staining, looking for upper palpebral conjunctival papillae and SPK.

3. Ask family members whether patient snores severely or if the patient has a history of sleep apnea.

Treatment

1. Topical antibiotic ointment for any mild corneal or conjunctival abnormality (e.g.,

erythromycin ointment b.i.d. to t.i.d.). May change to artificial tear ointment when lesions resolve.

2. The eyelids may be taped closed during sleep, or a shield may be worn to protect the eyelid from rubbing against the pillow or bed. Patients are asked to refrain from sleeping face down. Asking patients to sleep on their contralateral side may be therapeutic as well as diagnostic.

3. Surgical horizontal tightening of the eyelid is often required for definitive treatment.

Follow-Up

1. Every 2 to 7 days initially and then every few weeks to months as the condition stabilizes.

2. Refer to an internist, otolaryngologist, or pulmonologist for evaluation and management of possible obstructive sleep apnea. Evaluation is important because of the systemic sequelae of untreated sleep apnea and for anesthesia risk assessment before eyelid surgery.

6.7   BLEPHAROSPASM

Symptoms

Uncontrolled blinking, twitching, or closure of the eyelids. Always bilateral, but may briefly be unilateral at first onset.

Signs

Critical. Bilateral, episodic, involuntary contractions of the orbicularis oculi muscles.

Other. Disappears during sleep. May have uncontrolled orofacial, head, and neck movements (Meige syndrome).

Differential Diagnosis

- Hemifacial spasm: Unilateral contractures of the entire side of the face that do not disappear during sleep. Usually idiopathic but may be related to prior cranial nerve VII palsy, injury at the level of the brainstem, or compression of cranial nerve VII by a blood vessel or tumor. MRI of the cerebellopontine angle should be obtained in all patients to rule out tumor. Treatment

options include observation, botulinum toxin injections, or neurosurgical decompression of cranial nerve VII.

- Ocular irritation (e.g., corneal or conjunctival foreign body, trichiasis, blepharitis, dry eye).

- Eyelid myokymia: Subtle eyelid twitch felt by the patient but difficult to observe, commonly brought on by stress, caffeine, alcohol, or ocular irritation. Usually unilateral lower eyelid involvement. Typically self-limited and can be treated by avoiding precipitating factors.

- Tourette syndrome: Multiple compulsive muscle spasms associated with utterances of bizarre sounds or obscenities.

- Tic douloureux (trigeminal neuralgia): Acute episodes of pain in the distribution of the fifth cranial nerve, often causing a wince or tic.

- Tardive dyskinesia: Orofacial dyskinesia, often with dystonic movements of the trunk and limbs, typically from long-term use of antipsychotic medications.

- Apraxia of eyelid opening. Usually associated with Parkinson disease. Unlike blepharospasm, apraxia of eyelid opening does not feature orbicularis spasm. Instead, apraxic patients simply cannot voluntarily open the eyelids.

Etiology

- Idiopathic and likely multifactorial, possibly involving dopaminergic pathways within the basal ganglia.

Work-Up

1. History: Unilateral or bilateral? Are the eyelids alone involved or are the facial and limb muscles also involved? Medications?

2. Slit-lamp examination: Examination for ocular disorders such as dry eyes, blepharitis, or a foreign body.

3. Neuro-ophthalmic examination to rule out other accompanying abnormalities.

4. Typical blepharospasm does not require CNS imaging as part of the work-up. MRI of the brain with attention to the posterior fossa is reserved for atypical cases or other diagnoses (e.g., hemifacial spasm).

Treatment

1. Treat any underlying eye disorder causing ocular irritation. See 4.3, *Dry-Eye Syndrome*, and 5.8, *Blepharitis/Meibomitis*.

2. Consider botulinum toxin injections into the orbicularis muscles around the eyelids if the blepharospasm is severe.

3. If the spasm is not relieved with botulinum toxin injections, consider surgical excision of the orbicularis muscle from the upper eyelids and brow (e.g., limited myectomy).

4. Muscle relaxants and sedatives are rarely of value but can be helpful in some patients. Oral medications such as lorazepam can help but their use is often limited by their sedative qualities.

Follow-Up

Not an urgent condition, but with severe blepharospasm, patients can be functionally blind.

6.8   CANALICULITIS

Symptoms

Tearing or discharge, red eye, mild tenderness over the nasal aspect of the lower or upper eyelid.

Signs

(See Figure 6.8.1.)

Critical. Erythematous pouting of the punctum and erythema of the surrounding skin. Expression of mucopurulent discharge or concretions from the punctum is diagnostic.

Other. Recurrent conjunctivitis confined to the nasal aspect of the eye, gritty sensation on probing of the canaliculus, and focal injection of the nasal conjunctiva.

Differential Diagnosis

- Dacryocystitis: Infection of the lacrimal sac with more lacrimal sac swelling, tenderness, and pain than canaliculitis. See 6.9, *Dacryocystitis/Inflammation of the Lacrimal Sac.*

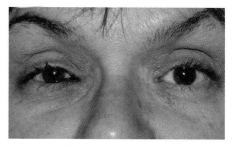

FIGURE 6.8.1. Canaliculitis.

- Chalazion: Focal inflammatory eyelid nodule without discharge from punctum. See 6.2, *Chalazion/Hordeolum.*

- Nasolacrimal duct obstruction: Tearing, minimal-to-no erythema or tenderness around the punctum. See 8.10, *Congenital Nasolacrimal Duct Obstruction.*

Etiology

- *Actinomyces israelii* (streptothrix): Most common. Gram-positive rod with fine, branching filaments.

- Other bacteria (e.g., *Fusobacterium* and *Nocardia* species).

- Fungal (e.g., *Candida, Fusarium,* and *Aspergillus* species).

- Viral (e.g., herpes simplex and varicella zoster).

- Retained punctal plug or foreign body.

Work-Up

1. Apply gentle pressure over the lacrimal sac with a cotton-tipped swab and roll it toward the punctum while observing for mucopurulent discharge or concretions.

2. Smears and cultures of the material expressed from the punctum, including slides for Gram stain and Giemsa stain. Consider thioglycolate and Sabouraud cultures.

3. Ask about a history of punctal plug placement in the past.

Treatment

1. Remove obstructing concretions or retained plug. Concretions may be expressed through the punctum at the slit lamp. A canaliculotomy is usually required for complete removal or in the setting of a retained punctual plug. If necessary, marsupialize the horizontal canaliculus from a conjunctival approach and allow incision to heal by secondary intention.

2. If concretions are removed, consider irrigating the canaliculus with an antibiotic solution (e.g., trimethoprim sulfate/polymyxin B, moxifloxacin, penicillin G solution 100,000 units/mL, iodine 1% solution). The patient is irrigated while in the upright position, so the solution drains out of the nose and not into the nasopharynx.

3. Treat the patient with antibiotic drops (e.g., trimethoprim sulfate/polymyxin B, moxifloxacin) q.i.d. and oral antibiotics for 1 to 2 weeks (e.g., doxycycline 100 mg b.i.d.).

4. If a fungus is found on smears and cultures, nystatin 1:20,000 drops t.i.d. and nystatin 1:20,000 solution irrigation several times per week may be effective. If evidence of herpes virus is found on smears, treat with trifluridine 1% drops five times per day. Silicone intubation along with appropriate antiviral therapy is sometimes required in viral canaliculitis.

5. Apply warm compresses to the punctal area q.i.d.

Follow-Up

Five to 7 days depending on severity. This is usually not an urgent condition.

6.9 DACRYOCYSTITIS/INFLAMMATION OF THE LACRIMAL SAC

Symptoms

Pain, redness, and swelling over the lacrimal sac in the innermost aspect of the lower eyelid. Also tearing, discharge, or fever. Symptoms may be recurrent.

Signs

(See Figure 6.9.1.)

Critical. Erythematous, tender, tense swelling over the nasal aspect of the lower eyelid and extending around the periorbital area

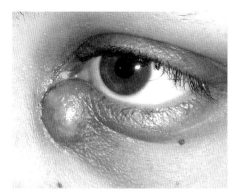

FIGURE 6.9.1. Dacryocystitis.

nasally. A mucoid or purulent discharge can be expressed from the punctum when pressure is applied over the lacrimal sac.

NOTE: Swelling in dacryocystitis is below the medial canthal tendon. Suspect lacrimal sac tumor (rare) if mass is above the medial canthal tendon.

Other. Fistula formation from the skin beneath the medial canthal tendon. A lacrimal sac cyst or mucocele can occur in chronic cases. Progression to a lacrimal sac abscess, and rarely, orbital or facial cellulitis may occur.

Differential Diagnosis

- Facial cellulitis involving the medial canthus: No discharge from punctum with pressure over the lacrimal sac. The lacrimal drainage system is patent on irrigation. See 6.10, *Preseptal Cellulitis.*

- Dacryocystocele: Mild enlargement of a non-inflamed lacrimal sac in an infant. Present at birth but may not be detected until later. Caused by nasolacrimal duct obstruction or entrapment of mucus or amniotic fluid in the lacrimal sac and is usually unilateral. If bilateral, assess breathing to rule out nasal obstruction. Conservative therapy with antibiotic ointment and warm compresses is usually sufficient for nonobstructive cases.

- Acute ethmoid sinusitis: Pain, tenderness, nasal obstruction, and erythema over the nasal bone, just medial to the inner canthus. Patients may be febrile. Imaging is diagnostic.

- Frontal sinus mucocele/mucopyocele: The swelling typically occurs well above the medial canthal tendon. Proptosis and external ophthalmoplegia are often present. Imaging is diagnostic.

Etiology

- Almost always related to nasolacrimal duct obstruction.

- Uncommon causes include diverticula of the lacrimal sac, dacryoliths, nasal or sinus surgery, trauma, and rarely a lacrimal sac tumor.

- Gram-positive bacteria are the most common pathogens; however, Gram-negative and atypical organisms are seen more commonly in diabetics, immunocompromised, and nursing home patients.

Work-Up

1. History: Previous episodes? Concomitant ear, nose, or throat infection?

2. External examination: Apply gentle pressure to the lacrimal sac in the nasal corner of the lower eyelid with a cotton-tipped swab in an attempt to express discharge from the punctum. Perform bilaterally to uncover subtle contralateral dacryocystitis.

3. Ocular examination: Assess extraocular motility both for proptosis, and for other evidence of orbital cellulitis.

4. Obtain a Gram stain and blood agar culture (and chocolate agar culture in children) of any discharge expressed from the punctum.

5. Consider a CT scan of the orbits and paranasal sinuses in atypical cases, severe cases, and those that do not respond to appropriate antibiotics.

NOTE: Do not attempt to probe or irrigate the lacrimal system during the acute infection.

Treatment

1. Systemic antibiotics in the following regimen:

   Children older than 5 years and <40 kg:

   —Afebrile, systemically well, mild case, and reliable parent: Amoxicillin/clavulanate: 25 to 45 mg/kg/day p.o. in two divided doses

6

6

for children, maximum daily dose of 90 mg/kg/day.

—Alternative treatment: Cefpodoxime: 10 mg/kg/day p.o. in two divided doses for children, maximum daily dose of 400 mg.

—Febrile, acutely ill, moderate-to-severe case, or unreliable parent: Hospitalize and treat with cefuroxime, 50 to 100 mg/kg/day intravenously (i.v.) in three divided doses in consultation with infectious disease specialist.

Adults:

—Afebrile, systemically well, mild case, and reliable patient: Cephalexin 500 mg p.o. q6h.

—Alternative treatment: Amoxicillin/ clavulanate 500 mg p.o. q8h.

—Febrile, acutely ill, or unreliable: Hospitalize and treat with cefazolin 1 g i.v. q8h. See 7.3.1, *Orbital Cellulitis.*

The antibiotic regimen is adjusted according to the clinical response and the culture/ sensitivity results. The i.v. antibiotics can be changed to comparable p.o. antibiotics depending on the rate of improvement, but systemic antibiotic therapy should be continued for a full 10- to 14-day course.

2. Topical antibiotic drops (e.g., trimethoprim/polymyxin B q.i.d.) may be used in addition to systemic therapy. Topical therapy alone is not adequate.

3. Apply warm compresses and gentle massage to the inner canthal region q.i.d.

4. Administer pain medication (e.g., acetaminophen with or without codeine) p.r.n.

5. Consider incision and drainage of a pointing abscess.

6. Consider surgical correction (e.g., dacryocystorhinostomy with silicone intubation) only after the acute episode has resolved, particularly with chronic dacryocystitis.

Follow-Up

Daily until improvement confirmed. If the condition of an outpatient worsens, hospitalization and i.v. antibiotics are recommended.

6.10 PRESEPTAL CELLULITIS

Symptoms

Tenderness, redness, and swelling of the eyelid and periorbital area. Often history of sinusitis, local skin abrasions, hordeolum, or insect bites. May be a mild fever.

Signs

(See Figures 6.10.1 and 6.10.2.)

Critical. Eyelid erythema, tense edema, warmth, tenderness. No proptosis, no optic neuropathy, no restriction of extraocular motility, usually little conjunctival injection, and no pain with eye movement (unlike orbital cellulitis). The patient may not be able to open the eye because of the eyelid edema.

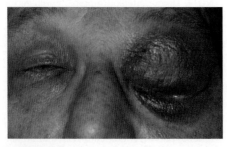

FIGURE 6.10.1. Preseptal cellulitis.

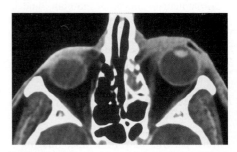

FIGURE 6.10.2. CT of preseptal cellulitis.

Other. Tightness of the eyelid skin or fluctuant lymphedema of the eyelids. The eye itself may be slightly injected but is relatively uninvolved.

Differential Diagnosis

- Orbital cellulitis: Proptosis, pain with eye movement, restricted motility. See 7.3.1, *Orbital Cellulitis.*

- Chalazion: Focal inflammatory eyelid nodule. See 6.2, *Chalazion/Hordeolum.*

- Allergic: Sudden onset, nontender itchy, swollen eyelids. See 5.11, *Contact Dermatitis.*

- Erysipelas: Rapidly advancing streptococcal cellulitis, often with a clear demarcation line, high fever, and chills.

- Necrotizing fasciitis: Severe bacterial infection involving the subcutaneous soft tissue and deep fascia. Typically due to group A beta-hemolytic streptococci and *Staphylococcus aureus.* Grayish-purplish skin discoloration with local hypesthesia characteristic. Patients are often septic and may rapidly deteriorate. This potentially fatal condition requires emergent surgical debridement with i.v. antibiotic treatment.

- Viral conjunctivitis with secondary eyelid swelling: Follicular conjunctivitis present. See 5.1, *Acute Conjunctivitis.*

- Cavernous sinus thrombosis: Proptosis with multiple cranial neuropathies. See 10.10, *Cavernous Sinus and Associated Syndromes (Multiple Ocular Motor Nerve Palsies).*

- Varicella zoster virus: Vesicular rash that respects midline. See 4.16, *Herpes Zoster Ophthalmicus/Varicella Zoster Virus.*

- Other orbital disorders: Proptosis, globe displacement, or restricted ocular motility. See 7.1, *Orbital Disease.*

- Others: Insect bite, angioedema, trauma, maxillary osteomyelitis, ocular vaccinia (see 4.17, *Ocular Vaccinia*), and others.

Etiology

- Adjacent infection (e.g., hordeolum or dacryocystitis).

- Trauma (e.g., puncture wound, laceration, insect bite).

Organisms

S. aureus and *Streptococcus* are most common, but *Haemophilus influenzae* should be considered in nonimmunized children. Suspect anaerobes if a foul-smelling discharge or necrosis is present or if there is a history of an animal or a human bite. Consider a viral cause if preseptal cellulitis is associated with a vesicular skin rash (e.g., herpes simplex or varicella zoster).

Work-Up

1. History: Pain with eye movements? Prior trauma or cancer? Sinus congestion or purulent nasal discharge? Recent smallpox vaccine?

2. Complete ocular examination: Look carefully for restriction of ocular motility or proptosis. An eyelid speculum or Desmarres eyelid retractor may facilitate the ocular examination if the eyelids are excessively swollen.

3. Check facial sensation in the distribution of first and second divisions of the trigeminal nerve.

4. Palpate the periorbital area and the head and neck lymph nodes for a mass.

5. Check vital signs.

6. Obtain Gram stain and culture of any open wound or drainage.

7. Perform CT scan of the brain and orbits (axial and coronal views) with contrast if there is a history of significant trauma or a concern about the possibility of an orbital or intraocular foreign body, orbital cellulitis, a subperiosteal abscess, paranasal sinusitis, cavernous sinus thrombosis, or malignancy.

8. Consider obtaining a complete blood count with differential and blood cultures in severe cases or when a fever is present.

Treatment

1. Antibiotic therapy

   a. Mild preseptal cellulitis, older than 5 years (<40 kg), afebrile, reliable patient/parent:

6

—Amoxicillin/clavulanate: 25 to 45 mg/kg/day p.o. in two divided doses for children, maximum daily dose of 90 mg/kg/day; 875 mg p.o. q12h for adults.

or

—Cefpodoxime: 10 mg/kg/day p.o. in two divided doses for children, maximum daily dose of 400 mg; 200 mg p.o. q12h for adults.

or

—Cefdinir: 14 mg/mg/day p.o. in two divided doses for children with maximum daily dose of 600 mg; 600 mg p.o. once daily for adults.

If the patient is allergic to penicillin, then

—Trimethoprim/sulfamethoxazole: 8 to 12 mg/kg/day trimethoprim with 40 to 60 mg/kg/day sulfamethoxazole p.o. in two divided doses for children; 160 to 320 mg trimethoprim with 800 to 1,600 mg sulfamethoxazole (one to two double-strength tablets) p.o. b.i.d. for adults.

or

—Moxifloxacin 400 mg p.o. daily (contraindicated in children).

If exposure to methicillin-resistant Staphylococcus aureus (MRSA) is suspected, then

—Trimethoprim/sulfamethoxazole: 8 to 12 mg/kg/day trimethoprim with 40 to 60 mg/kg/day sulfamethoxazole p.o. in two divided doses for children; 160 to 320 mg trimethoprim with 800 to 1,600 mg sulfamethoxazole (one to two double-strength tablets) p.o. b.i.d. for adults.

or

—Doxycycline: 100 mg p.o. b.i.d (contraindicated in children, pregnant women, and nursing mothers).

or

—Clindamycin: 10 to 30 mg/kg/day p.o. in three to four divided doses for children; 450 mg p.o. t.i.d. for adults. In addition to covering MRSA, this antibiotic also gives good coverage for streptococci and methicillin-sensitive *Staphylococcus aureus*.

NOTE: Patients with the following risk factors should be covered for MRSA: history of MRSA infection or colonization, recurrent skin infections, contact with someone known to have MRSA, admission to a health care or long-term care facility within the past year, placement of a permanent indwelling catheter, on hemodialysis, i.v. drug use, incarceration within the last 12 months, participation in sports that include skin-to-skin contact or sharing of equipment and clothing, poor personal hygiene.

NOTE: Oral antibiotics are maintained for 10 days.

---

b. Moderate-to-severe preseptal cellulitis, or any one of the following:

—Patient appears toxic.

—Patient may be noncompliant with outpatient treatment and follow-up.

—Child 5 years or younger.

—No noticeable improvement or worsening after 24 to 48 hours of oral antibiotics.

Admit to the hospital for i.v. antibiotics as follows:

—Vancomycin: 10 to 15 mg/kg i.v. every 6 hours in children; 0.5 to 1 g i.v. q12h for adults. (Dose adjustment is needed in cases of impaired renal function.)

Plus one of the following:

—Ampicillin/sulbactam: 300 mg/kg/day i.v. in four divided doses for children; 3.0 g i.v. q6h for adults.

—Ceftriaxone: 80 to 100 mg/kg/day i.v. in two divided doses for children with maximum of 4 g/day; 2 g i.v. q12h for adults.

—Piperacillin-tazobactam: 240 mg/kg/day i.v. in three divided doses for children; 4.5 g i.v. q6h adults.

—Cefotaxime: 150 to 200 mg/kg/day in three to four divided doses in children; 2 g i.v. q4h in adults.

If the patient is allergic to penicillin, see 7.3.1, Orbital Cellulitis, for alternatives.

NOTE: Intravenous antibiotics can be changed to comparable oral antibiotics after significant improvement is observed. Systemic antibiotics are maintained for a complete 10- to 14-day course. See 7.3.1, *Orbital Cellulitis,* for alternative treatment. In complicated cases or patients with multiple allergies, consider consultation with infectious disease specialist for antibiotic management.

---

2. Warm compresses to the inflamed area t.i.d. p.r.n.

3. Polymyxin B/bacitracin ointment to the eye q.i.d. if secondary conjunctivitis is present.

4. Tetanus toxoid if needed. See Appendix 2, *Tetanus Prophylaxis.*

5. Nasal decongestants if sinusitis is present.

6. Orbital exploration and debridement is warranted if a fluctuant mass or abscess is present, or if a retained foreign body is suspected. Obtain Gram stain and culture of any drainage. Avoid the orbital septum if possible. A drain may need to be placed.

7. Consider an Infectious Disease consult in patients who have failed oral antibiotics and require i.v. treatment.

Follow-Up

Daily until clear and consistent improvement is demonstrated, then every 2 to 7 days until the condition has totally resolved. If a preseptal cellulitis progresses despite antibiotic therapy, the patient is admitted to the hospital and a repeat (or initial) orbital CT scan is obtained. For patients already on p.o. antibiotics, switch to i.v. antibiotics (see 7.3.1, *Orbital Cellulitis*).

6.11 MALIGNANT TUMORS OF THE EYELID

Symptoms

Asymptomatic or mildly irritating eyelid lump.

Signs

Skin ulceration and inflammation with distortion of the normal eyelid anatomy. Abnormal color, texture, or persistent bleeding. Loss of eyelashes (madarosis) or whitening of eyelashes (poliosis) over the lesion. Sentinel vessels may be seen. Diplopia or external ophthalmoplegia are ominous and signs of possible orbital invasion.

Differential Diagnosis of Benign Eyelid Tumors

- Seborrheic keratosis: Middle-aged or elderly patients. Brown-black, well-circumscribed, crust-like lesion, usually slightly elevated, with or without surrounding inflammation. May be removed by shave biopsy.

- Chalazion/Hordeolum: Acute, erythematous, tender, well-circumscribed lesion. See 6.2, *Chalazion/Hordeolum.*

- Cysts: Well-circumscribed white or yellow lesions on the eyelid margin or underneath the skin. Epidermal inclusion cysts, sebaceous cysts, and eccrine and apocrine hydrocystomas may be excised.

- Molluscum contagiosum: A viral infection of the epidermis, typically seen in children. Multiple small papules characterized by a central umbilication. Can be severe in HIV-positive patients. May produce a chronic follicular conjunctivitis. Treat lesions by unroofing and curettage. While some recommend curettage until bleeding occurs, there is no clear evidence that this is more effective. A variety of other therapies (e.g., cryotherapy, cautery, chemical, laser) are used for lesions found elsewhere on the body but are typically not necessary for periocular regions and may cause injury to the ocular surfaces. See 5.2, *Chronic Conjunctivitis.*

- Nevus: Incompletely differentiated melanocytes that can clump at the epidermis, dermis, or the junction of the two layers.

Congenital nevi may be present at, or shortly after, birth; however, most nevi appear during childhood and may enlarge during puberty. Nevi are well-circumscribed lesions, usually round or oval, with uniform pigmentation. Melanomas may develop within preexisting nevi and may manifest as a changing pigmented lesion and/or as a pigmented lesion with asymmetry of shape, irregular borders, color variegation, and possibly pruritus or bleeding. Suspicious lesions should be biopsied, preferably with removal of the entire lesion to the subcutaneous fat.

- Xanthelasma: Multiple, often bilateral, soft yellow plaques of lipid-laden macrophages in the upper and sometimes lower eyelids. Patients 40 years and younger should have a serum cholesterol and lipid profile evaluation to rule out hypercholesterolemia. Surgical excision can be performed for cosmesis; however, recurrence is possible.

- Squamous papilloma: Soft, skin-colored lesions that may be smooth, rounded, or pedunculated. May enlarge slowly over time. Often spontaneously regress. Occasionally squamous carcinomas can appear papillomatous. Therefore, excisional biopsy should be performed for suspicious lesions.

- Actinic keratosis: Round, erythematous, premalignant lesion with scaly surface. Found in sun-exposed areas of skin. Treat with excisional biopsy.

- Inflammatory conditions: Blepharitis, blepharoconjunctivitis.

- Allergic conditions: Chronic contact dermatitis can appear unilateral, cause cilia loss, and simulate malignancy.

- Others: Verrucae from human papillomavirus, benign tumors of hair follicles or sweat glands, inverted follicular keratosis, neurofibroma, neurilemmoma, capillary hemangioma, cavernous hemangioma, and pseudoepitheliomatous hyperplasia. Necrobiotic xanthogranuloma nodules of multiple myeloma appear as yellow plaques or nodules are often mistaken for xanthelasma.

Etiology

- Basal cell carcinoma: Most common malignant eyelid tumor, usually on the lower eyelid or medial canthus of middle-aged or elderly patients. Rarely metastasizes but may be locally invasive, particularly when it is present in the medial canthal region. There are two forms:

—Nodular: Indurated, firm mass, commonly with telangiectases over the tumor margins. Sometimes the center of the lesion is ulcerated (see Figure 6.11.1). On rare occasions, a cystic variant is seen.

—Morpheaform: Firm, flat, subcutaneous lesion with indistinct borders. More difficult to excise and may result in a large eyelid defect.

- Sebaceous gland carcinoma: Usually in middle-aged or elderly patients. Most common on the upper eyelid but may be multifocal, involving both the upper and the lower eyelids. Often confused with recurrent chalazia or intractable blepharitis. Loss of eyelashes and destruction of the meibomian gland orifices in the region of the tumor may occur. Regional and systemic metastasis or orbital extension is possible. Can follow many decades after radiation exposure to the eyelids (see Figure 6.11.2).

- Squamous cell carcinoma: Variable presentation, often appearing similar to a basal

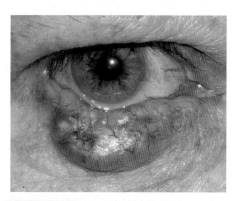

FIGURE 6.11.1. Basal cell carcinoma.

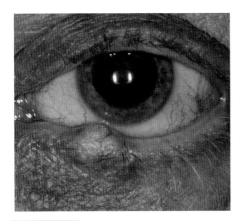

FIGURE 6.11.2. Sebaceous cell carcinoma.

cell carcinoma. Regional metastasis may occur and can be extensive with a propensity for perineural invasion. A premalignant lesion, actinic keratosis, may appear either as a scaly, erythematous flat lesion or as a cutaneous horn.

■ Keratoacanthoma: This lesion was previously considered to be benign and self-limiting; however, it is now regarded as a low-grade squamous cell carcinoma. Clinically may resemble basal and squamous cell carcinomas. Typically, the lesion is elevated with rolled margins and a large central ulcer filled with keratin. Rapid growth with slow regression and even spontaneous resolution have been observed. Lesions usually involve the lower eyelid and can be destructive. Complete excision is recommended.

■ Others: Malignant melanoma, lymphoma; sweat gland carcinoma, metastasis (usually breast or lung), Merkel cell tumor, Kaposi sarcoma, and others.

Work-Up

1. History: Duration? Rapid or slow growth? Previous malignant skin lesion or other malignancies? Previous treatment of inflammatory or allergic condition? Previous radiation therapy?

2. External examination: Check the skin for additional lesions, palpate the preauricular, submaxillary, and cervical nodes for metastasis.

3. Slit-lamp examination: Look for telangiectases on nodular tumors, loss of eyelashes in the region of the tumor, meibomian orifice destruction. Evert eyelids of all patients with eyelid complaints.

4. Photograph or draw the lesion and its location for documentation.

5. Perform a biopsy of the lesion. An incisional biopsy is commonly performed when a malignancy is suspected. Depending on the depth of invasion, sentinel node biopsy may be indicated with eyelid melanoma. Histopathologic confirmation must precede any extensive procedures.

6. Sebaceous gland carcinoma may be difficult to diagnose histopathologically. In the past, fresh tissue with oil red-O staining was recommended. This is no longer necessary if the pathologist is experienced with this malignancy.

7. For lymphoma, the pathologist would prefer the tissue to be sent fresh for flow cytometry. Contact the pathologist first. If confirmed, a systemic work-up is indicated. See 7.4.2, *Orbital Tumors in Adults.*

Treatment

1. Basal cell carcinoma: Surgical excision with histologic evaluation of the tumor margins either by frozen sections or by Mohs techniques. The entire tumor should be excised with clean margins. Cryotherapy and radiation are used rarely. Topical imiquimod, an immune modulator, is a newer treatment that might be beneficial but could be toxic to the surface of the eye. Patients are informed about the etiologic role of the sun and are advised to avoid sunlight when possible and to use protective sunscreens.

2. Sebaceous gland carcinoma: Poorly responsive to radiation. Excision requires the use of permanent sectioning for negative margins prior to attempted reconstruction. Map biopsies of the bulbar and palpebral conjunctiva should be performed in all cases because of the propensity for skip lesions. Close follow-up of regional nodes is indicated. Exenteration is often required when orbital invasion is present. Referral to

6

oncologist or internist for systemic work-up and surveillance is important with attention to the lymph nodes, lungs, brain, liver, and bone.

3. Squamous cell carcinoma: Same as for basal cell carcinoma. Radiation therapy is the second-best treatment after surgical excision. Patients are informed about the etiologic role of the sun. Referral to an oncologist or internist for regional and/or systemic work-up and surveillance is important.

4. Malignant melanoma: Treatment requires wide surgical excision. The margins must be free of tumor and require permanent sections. Sentinel lymph node biopsy may be required depending on the depth of the tumor. Referral to an oncologist or internist for regional and/or systemic work-up and surveillance is important.

NOTE: Because both melanoma and sebaceous gland carcinoma are difficult to diagnose by frozen section, multiple excisions utilizing permanent sectioning may be necessary until all surgical margins are free of tumor. The cornea and globe must be protected during this interim time with lubrication or temporary tarsorrhaphies.

Follow-Up

Initial follow-up is every 1 to 4 weeks to ensure proper healing of the surgical site. Patients are then reevaluated every 6 to 12 months, or more frequently, for more aggressive lesions. Patients who have had one skin malignancy are at greater risk for additional malignancies.

6

Orbit

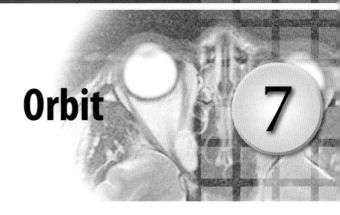

7

ORBITAL DISEASE

This section provides a framework to evaluate a variety of orbital diseases.

Symptoms

Eyelid swelling, bulging eye(s), and double vision are common. Pain and decreased vision can occur.

Signs

Critical. Proptosis and restriction of ocular motility, which can be confirmed by forced-duction testing (see Appendix 6, *Forced-Duction Test and Active Force Generation Test*). Resistance to retropulsion of the globe is common.

Differential Diagnosis of Pseudoproptosis

- Enlarged globe (e.g., myopia). Large, myopic eyes frequently have tilted discs and peripapillary crescents, and ultrasonography (US) reveals a long axial length.

- Enophthalmos of the fellow eye (e.g., after an orbital floor fracture).

- Asymmetric eyelid position: Unilateral upper and/or lower eyelid retraction, or contralateral upper eyelid ptosis.

Etiology

Rarely, specific signs of orbital disease are diagnostic. Otherwise, orbital disease can be grouped into five broad categories to help tailor the necessary work-up:

1. Inflammatory: Thyroid eye disease (TED), idiopathic orbital inflammatory syndrome (IOIS), sarcoidosis, Wegener granulomatosis, etc.

2. Infectious: Orbital cellulitis, subperiosteal abscess, etc.

3. Neoplastic (benign and malignant): Dermoid cyst, capillary hemangioma, rhabdomyosarcoma, metastasis, lymphangioma, optic nerve glioma, neurofibroma, leukemia, lymphoproliferation (including lymphoma), neurilemmoma, mucocele, etc.

4. Trauma: Orbital fracture, retrobulbar hemorrhage, orbital foreign body, carotid-cavernous fistula, etc.

5. Malformation: Congenital, vascular, etc.

Work-Up

1. History: Rapid or slow onset? Pain? Ocular bruit and/or pulsation? Fever, chills, systemic symptoms? History of cancer, diabetes, pulmonary disease, or renal disease? Skin rash? Trauma?

2. Vital signs, particularly temperature.

3. External examination:

—In addition to classic axial exophthalmos, also look for nonaxial displacement of the globe (e.g., hypoglobus, hyperglobus).

—Test for resistance to retropulsion by gently pushing each globe into the orbit with your thumbs.

—Feel along the orbital rim for a mass. Check the conjunctival cul-de-sacs carefully and evert the upper eyelid.

—Check extraocular movements. Measure any ocular misalignment with prisms (see

Appendix 3, *Cover/Uncover and Alternate Cover Tests*).

—To examine for proptosis, tilt the patient's head back and look from below ("ant's-eye view"). Measure with a Hertel exophthalmometer. Position the exophthalmometer against the lateral orbital rims, not the lateral canthi. Upper limits of normal are approximately 22 and 24 mm in white people and black people, respectively. A difference between the two eyes of more than 2 mm is considered abnormal. Can be used in conjunction with a Valsalva maneuver if a venous malformation is suspected.

4. Ocular examination: Specifically check the size and reactivity of the pupils, visual fields, color vision (by color plates), intraocular pressure (IOP), optic nerves (pallor, swelling), posterior pole (especially for chorioretinal folds), and peripheral retina.

5. Imaging studies: Orbital computed tomography (CT) (axial and coronal views) or magnetic resonance imaging (MRI) with gadolinium and fat suppression, depending on suspected etiology. Orbital US with or without color Doppler imaging is useful if the diagnosis is uncertain or when a cystic or vascular lesion is suspected. See Chapter 14, *Imaging Modalities in Ophthalmology.*

6. Laboratory tests when appropriate: Triiodothyronine (T3), thyroxine (T4), selective thyroid-stimulating hormone (TSH), thyroid-stimulating immunoglobulin, complete blood count (CBC) with differential, Westergren erythrocyte sedimentation rate (ESR), antinuclear antibody (ANA), blood urea nitrogen (BUN)/creatinine (if CT contrast or gadolinium are indicated in at-risk individuals), fasting blood sugar, blood cultures, angiotensin-converting enzyme (ACE), cytoplasmic antineutrophil cytoplasmic antibody (cANCA), prostate-specific antigen, lactate dehydrogenase, etc.

7. Consider a forced-duction test in select cases. See Appendix 6, *Forced-Duction Test and Active Force Generation Test.*

8. Consider an excisional or incisional biopsy, as dictated by the working diagnosis. Fine-needle aspiration biopsy has a limited role in orbital diagnosis.

Additional work-up, treatment, and follow-up vary according to the suspected diagnosis. See individual sections.

7.2 INFLAMMATORY ORBITAL DISEASE

7.2.1. THYROID EYE DISEASE

Synonyms: THYROID-RELATED ORBITOPATHY OR GRAVES DISEASE

Ocular Symptoms

Early: Nonspecific complaints including foreign-body sensation, redness, tearing, photophobia, and morning puffiness of the eyelids. Early symptoms are often nonspecific and may mimic allergy, blepharoconjunctivitis, chronic conjunctivitis, etc.

Late: Eyelid and orbital symptoms including eyelid retraction, prominent eyes, persistent eyelid swelling, double vision, "pressure" behind the eyes, and decreased vision in one or both eyes.

Signs

(See Figure 7.2.1.1.)

Critical. Retraction of the upper eyelids (highly specific) with lateral flare and eyelid lag on downward gaze (von Graefe sign), lagophthalmos. Lower lid retraction is less specific for TED. Unilateral or bilateral axial proptosis with variable resistance to retropulsion. When extraocular muscles are involved, elevation and abduction are commonly restricted and there is resistance on forced-duction testing. Although often bilateral, unilateral or asymmetric TED is also frequently seen.

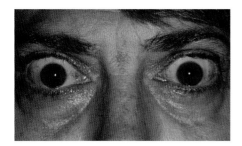

FIGURE 7.2.1.1. Thyroid-related orbitopathy with eyelid retraction and proptosis of the right eye.

Thickening of the extraocular muscles (inferior, medial, superior, and lateral, in order of frequency) without involvement of the associated tendons may be noted on orbital imaging. Isolated enlargement of the superior or lateral recti muscles is highly atypical of TED and requires further work-up.

NOTE: Optic nerve compression caused by thickened extraocular muscles at the orbital apex can produce an afferent pupillary defect, reduced color vision, visual field, and visual acuity loss. Compressive optic neuropathy occurs in a minority of patients (5%) with TED but must be ruled out in every patient at every visit. Optic neuropathy in the setting of TED almost invariably occurs in the setting of restrictive strabismus and increased resistance to retropulsion. Counterintuitively, in cases of compressive optic neuropathy from TED, axial proptosis is usually either absent or mild.

Other. Reduced frequency of blinking, inferior chemosis, significantly elevated IOP (especially in upgaze), injection of the blood vessels over the insertion sites of horizontal rectus muscles, superior limbic keratoconjunctivitis, superficial punctate keratopathy, or infiltrate or ulceration from exposure keratopathy.

Systemic Signs

Hyperthyroidism is common. Symptoms include a rapid pulse, hot and dry skin, diffusely enlarged thyroid gland (goiter), weight loss, muscle wasting with proximal muscle weakness, hand tremor, pretibial dermopathy or myxedema, cardiac arrhythmias. Some patients are hypo- or euthyroid. Euthyroid patients should undergo thyroid function testing every

6 to 12 months; a significant proportion will develop thyroid abnormalities. Concomitant myasthenia gravis with fluctuating double vision and ptosis may occur in a minority of patients. TED does not necessarily follow the associated thyroid dysfunction and may occur months to years before or after the thyroid dysfunction. The clinical progression of TED also has only minimal correlation to control of the thyroid dysfunction.

Differential Diagnosis of Eyelid Retraction

- Previous eyelid surgery may produce eyelid retraction or eyelid lag.

- Severe contralateral ptosis may produce eyelid retraction because of Hering Law, especially if the nonptotic eye is amblyopic.

- Third cranial nerve palsy with aberrant regeneration: The upper eyelid may elevate with downward gaze, simulating eyelid lag (pseudo-von Graefe sign). Ocular motility may be limited, but results of forced-duction testing and orbital imaging are normal. Eyelid retraction is typically accentuated in adduction or in downgaze. See 10.6, *Aberrant Regeneration of the Third Nerve.*

- Parinaud syndrome: Eyelid retraction and limitation of upward gaze may accompany convergence-retraction nystagmus and mildly dilated pupils that react poorly to light with an intact near response (light-near dissociation).

Work-Up

1. History: Duration of symptoms? Pain? Change in vision? Known thyroid disease or cancer? Smoker?

2. Complete ocular examination to establish the diagnosis and to determine whether the patient is developing exposure keratopathy (slit-lamp examination with fluorescein staining) or optic nerve compression (afferent pupillary defect, color plate deficiency, optic nerve edema). Diplopia is measured with prisms (see Appendix 3, *Cover/Uncover and Alternate Cover Tests*) and proptosis is measured with a Hertel exophthalmometer. Check IOP in both primary and upgaze (increase in upgaze correlated with severity

of inferior rectus muscle enlargement). Dilated fundus examination with optic nerve assessment.

3. CT of the orbit (axial and coronal views without contrast) is performed when presentation is atypical (e.g., all cases of unilateral proptosis or any bilateral proptosis without upper eyelid retraction), or in the presence of severe congestive orbitopathy or optic neuropathy. CT in TED varies from patient to patient. In patients with restrictive strabismus and minimal proptosis ("myogenic variant"), imaging may show thickened extraocular muscles without the involvement of the associated tendons. In patients with full or nearly full extraocular motility, severe proptosis, and exposure keratopathy ("lipogenic variant"), increased fat volume with minimal muscle involvement is typical.

4. Formal visual field testing when signs or symptoms of optic nerve compression are present.

5. Thyroid function tests (T3, T4, selective TSH). These may be normal. Thyroid-stimulating immunoglobulin is sometimes ordered, but the clinical significance of this test is still unclear.

6. Work-up for suspected myasthenia gravis is necessary in selected cases. See 10.11, *Myasthenia Gravis.*

Treatment

1. Smoking cessation: All patients with TED who smoke must be explicitly told that continued tobacco use increases the risk of progression and the severity of the orbitopathy. This conversation should be clearly documented in the medical record.

2. Refer the patient to a medical internist or endocrinologist for management of systemic thyroid disease, if present. If TFTs are normal, the patient's TFTs should be checked every 6 to 12 months.

3. Treat exposure keratopathy with artificial tears and lubrication or by taping eyelids closed at night (see 4.5, *Exposure Keratopathy*). Swimmer's goggles at night may be helpful. The use of topical cyclosporine drops for the treatment of ocular surface inflammation in TED is still under investigation, but is a reasonable long-term treatment option if dry-eye syndrome is present.

4. Treat eyelid edema with cold compresses in the morning and head elevation at night. The use of systemic diuretics for eyelid edema is controversial and is usually not recommended.

5. Indications for orbital decompression surgery include: Optic neuropathy, worsening or severe exposure keratopathy despite adequate treatment, globe luxation, uncontrollably high IOP, cosmesis.

6. A stepwise approach is used for surgical treatment, starting with orbital decompression (if needed), followed by strabismus surgery (for significant strabismus, if present), followed by eyelid surgery. Alteration of this sequence may lead to unpredictable results.

The following recommendations are somewhat controversial:

▪ Corticosteroids: During the acute inflammatory phase, prednisone 1 mg/kg p.o. q.d., tapered over 4 to 6 weeks, is a reasonable temporizing measure to improve proptosis and diplopia in preparation for orbital decompression surgery. Recently, pulse intravenous corticosteroids have been recommended in the European literature to arrest the progression of the orbitopathy. The dosing schedule is still under investigation, but is being used more frequently by clinicians. Corticosteroid injection into the orbital fat for local control of orbitopathy has also been described, but at present the efficacy of this modality remains unclear. Chronic systemic corticosteroids for long-term management have been advocated by some, but in general should be avoided because of the systemic side effects.

▪ Orbital irradiation: The use of orbital radiation in the management of TED is still under active debate. It may be used as a modality in the acute inflammatory phase of TED. Irradiation may have a limited benefit for the management of diplopia and compressive optic neuropathy, but does not improve proptosis in TED. It may, however, prevent the progression of disease and provide long-term control. Should be used with caution in patients with diabetes, as it may worsen diabetic retinopathy, and in vasculopaths, as it may increase the risk of radiation retinopathy or optic neuropathy. As a result, all patients offered radiation therapy should be informed of the potential risks.

Radiation is best performed according to strict protocols with carefully controlled dosage and shielding, under the supervision of a radiation oncologist familiar with the technique. Typically, a total dose of 2,000 cGy is administered in 10 fractions over 2 weeks.

Treatment may transiently exacerbate inflammatory changes, and a methylprednisolone dose pack may mitigate these symptoms. Improvement is often seen within a few weeks of treatment, but may take several months to attain maximal effect. It is unusual for radiation to succeed if a trial of corticosteroids has failed.

- Biologics: Limited data are available on the use of biologic agents (rituximab, infliximab) for the treatment of TED that is progressing despite the use of more conventional therapy. At present, small series have shown promise, but the use of such agents is off-label and should be considered experimental.

- Visual loss from optic neuropathy: Treat immediately with prednisone 100 mg p.o. q.d with close monitoring. Radiation therapy may be offered for mild-to-moderate optic neuropathy, with the understanding that there is typically a lag in the treatment effect. Posterior orbital decompression surgery (for mild-to-severe optic neuropathy) is usually effective in rapidly reversing or stabilizing the optic neuropathy. The role of anterior or soft-tissue (fat) decompression for compressive optic neuropathy is controversial and in all likelihood has a very limited effect. Decompression of the medial orbital apex typically results in the reversal of the optic neuropathy, but recurrence is possible if orbital inflammation progresses. Isolated deep lateral wall decompression has also been advocated by some specialists.

Follow-Up

1. Optic nerve compression requires immediate attention and close follow-up.

2. Patients with advanced exposure keratopathy and severe proptosis also require prompt attention and close follow-up.

3. Patients with minimal-to-no exposure problems and mild-to-moderate proptosis are reevaluated every 3 to 6 months. Because of the potential risk of optic neuropathy, patients with restrictive strabismus may be followed more frequently and are instructed to check for red desaturation on a weekly basis.

4. Patients with fluctuating diplopia or ptosis should be evaluated for myasthenia gravis.

5. All patients with TED are instructed to return immediately with any new visual problems, worsening diplopia, or significant ocular irritation.

7.2.2. IDIOPATHIC ORBITAL INFLAMMATORY SYNDROME

Synonyms: INFLAMMATORY ORBITAL PSEUDOTUMOR

Symptoms

May be acute, recurrent, or chronic. An explosive, painful onset is the hallmark of idiopathic orbital inflammatory syndrome (IOIS). Pain, prominent red eye, "boggy" pink eyelid edema, double vision, or decreased vision. Children may have concomitant constitutional symptoms (fever, headache, vomiting, abdominal pain, lethargy) and bilateral presentation, which are not typical in adults.

Signs

Critical. Proptosis and/or restriction of ocular motility, usually unilateral, typically of explosive onset. On imaging studies, soft-tissue anatomy is involved in varying degrees. The extraocular muscles are thickened in cases of myositis, with involvement of the associated tendons. The sclera (in posterior scleritis), Tenon capsule (in tenonitis), orbital fat, or lacrimal gland (in dacryoadenitis) may be involved. The paranasal sinuses are usually clear.

Other. Boggy, pink eyelid erythema and edema, conjunctival injection and chemosis, lacrimal gland enlargement or a palpable orbital mass, decreased vision, uveitis, increased IOP, hyperopic shift, optic nerve swelling or atrophy (uncommon).

NOTE: Bilateral IOIS in adults can occur, but should prompt a careful evaluation to rule out a systemic cause (e.g., sarcoidosis, Wegener granulomatosis, metastases, lymphoma). Children may have bilateral disease in one-third of the cases and may have associated systemic disorders.

Differential Diagnosis

- Orbital cellulitis and/or abscess.
- TED.
- Other inflammatory conditions (e.g., sarcoidosis, Wegener granulomatosis).
- Lymphoproliferative disease (including lymphoma).
- Primary orbital malignancy.
- Metastasis.
- Rhabdomyosarcoma.
- Leaking dermoid cyst.
- Lymphangioma with acute hemorrhage.
- Spontaneous orbital hemorrhage.
- Necrotic choroidal melanoma.

Work-Up

See 7.1, *Orbital Disease,* for general orbital work-up.

1. History: Previous episodes? Any other systemic symptoms or diseases? History of cancer? Smoking? Last mammogram, chest X-ray, colonoscopy, prostate examination? History of breathing problems? A careful review of systems is warranted.

2. Complete ocular examination, including ocular motility, exophthalmometry, IOP, and optic nerve evaluation.

3. Vital signs, particularly temperature.

4. Orbital CT (axial and coronal views) with contrast: may show a thickened posterior sclera (the "ring sign" of 360 degrees of scleral thickening), orbital fat or lacrimal gland involvement, or thickening of the extraocular muscles (including their tendons). Bony erosion is very rare in IOIS and warrants further work-up.

5. Blood tests as needed (e.g., bilateral or atypical cases): ESR, CBC with differential, ANA, BUN, creatinine, and fasting blood sugar (before instituting systemic steroids). Consider checking ACE levels and a chest X-ray if sarcoidosis is suspected and cANCA if Wegener granulomatosis is suspected. Mammography, chest imaging, and prostate evaluation are warranted in specific or atypical cases.

6. Consider incisional biopsy when the diagnosis is uncertain, the case is atypical or recurrent, the patient has a history of cancer, or a patient with an acute presentation does not respond to adequate systemic steroids within a few days. Also consider biopsy in cases of presumed inflammatory dacryoadenitis, because this procedure carries a low morbidity, and the use of corticosteroids may mask the true pathology on future biopsy.

Treatment

1. Prednisone 80 to 100 mg p.o. q.d. as an initial dose in an adult, along with gastric prophylaxis (e.g., ranitidine 150 mg p.o. b.i.d.). Pediatric dosages typically begin with 1 mg/kg/day of prednisone. All patients are warned about potential systemic side effects and are instructed to follow up with their primary physicians to monitor blood sugar and electrolytes.

2. Low-dose radiation therapy may be used when the patient does not respond to systemic corticosteroids, when disease recurs as corticosteroids are tapered, or when corticosteroids pose a significant risk to the patient. Radiation therapy should only be used once orbital biopsy has excluded other etiologies.

Follow-Up

Reevaluate in 1 to 2 days. Patients who respond to steroids are maintained at the initial dose for 3 to 5 days, followed by a slow taper to 40 mg/day over 2 weeks, and an even slower taper below 20 mg/day, usually over several weeks. If the patient does not respond dramatically to appropriate corticosteroid doses, biopsy should be strongly considered.

7.3   INFECTIOUS ORBITAL DISEASE

7.3.1. ORBITAL CELLULITIS

Symptoms

Red eye, pain, blurred vision, double vision, eyelid swelling, nasal congestion/discharge, sinus headache/pressure/congestion, tooth pain, infra- and/or supraorbital pain, or hypesthesia.

Signs

(See Figures 7.3.1.1 and 7.3.1.2.)

Critical. Eyelid edema, erythema, warmth, and tenderness. Conjunctival chemosis and injection, proptosis, and restricted ocular motility with pain on attempted eye movement are usually present. Signs of optic neuropathy (e.g., afferent pupillary defect, dyschromatopsia) may be present in severe cases.

Other. Decreased vision, retinal venous congestion, optic disc edema, purulent discharge, decreased periorbital sensation, fever. CT scan usually shows an adjacent sinusitis (typically an ethmoid sinusitis), possibly a subperiosteal orbital collection.

Differential Diagnosis

See 7.1, *Orbital Disease.*

Etiology

- Direct extension from a paranasal sinus infection (especially ethmoiditis), focal periorbital infection (e.g., dacryoadenitis, dacryocystitis, panophthalmitis), or dental infection.

- Sequela of orbital trauma (e.g., orbital fracture, penetrating trauma, retained intraorbital foreign body).

- Sequela of orbital surgery or paranasal sinus surgery.

- Sequela of other ocular surgery (less common).

- Vascular extension (e.g., seeding from a systemic bacteremia or locally from facial cellulitis via venous anastomoses).

- Secondary orbital venous stasis and inflammation from a septic cavernous sinus thrombosis.

7

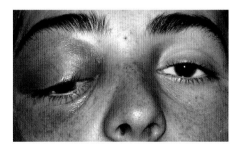

FIGURE 7.3.1.1. Orbital cellulitis.

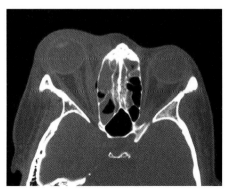

FIGURE 7.3.1.2. CT of right orbital cellulitis showing fat stranding and right ethmoiditis.

NOTE: In cases of unsuspected retained foreign body, cellulitis may develop months after injury (see 3.12, *Intraorbital Foreign Body*).

Organisms

- Adult: Staphylococcus species, Streptococcus species, Bacteroides.

- Children: *Haemophilus influenzae* (rarely in vaccinated children).

- Following trauma: Gram-negative rods.

- Dental abscess: Mixed, aggressive aerobes and anaerobes.

- Immunocompromised patients (diabetes, chemotherapy, HIV infection): Fungi (Mucormycosis/Zygomycosis, Aspergillus).

Work-Up

See 7.1, *Orbital Disease,* for a nonspecific orbital work-up.

1. History: Trauma or surgery? Ear, nose, throat, or systemic infection? Tooth pain or recent dental abscess? Stiff neck or mental status changes? Diabetes or an immunosuppressive illness?

2. Complete ophthalmic examination: Look for an afferent pupillary defect, limitation of or pain with eye movements, proptosis, increased resistance to retropulsion, elevated IOP, decreased color vision, decreased skin sensation, or an optic nerve or fundus abnormality.

3. Check vital signs, mental status, and neck flexibility.

4. CT scan of the orbits and paranasal sinuses (axial and coronal views, with contrast if possible) to confirm the diagnosis and to rule out a retained foreign body, orbital or subperiosteal abscess, paranasal sinus disease, or cavernous sinus thrombosis.

5. CBC with differential.

6. Blood cultures (especially helpful in pediatric cases).

7. Explore and debride any penetrating wound, if present, and obtain a Gram stain and culture of any drainage (e.g., blood and

chocolate agars, Sabouraud dextrose agar, thioglycolate broth).

8. Consult Neurology or Neurosurgery for suspected meningitis for management and possible lumbar puncture. If paranasal sinusitis is present, consider consultation with Otorhinolaryngology for possible surgical drainage. Consider an Infectious Disease consultation in atypical, severe, or unresponsive cases. If a dental source is suspected, Oral Maxillofacial Surgery should be consulted for assessment, since infections from this area tend to be aggressive, potentially vision threatening, and may spread into the cavernous sinus.

NOTE: Mucormycosis/zygomycosis is an orbital, nasal, and sinus disease occurring in diabetic or otherwise immunocompromised patients. Typically associated with severe pain and external ophthalmoplegia. Profound visual loss may rapidly occur. Metabolic acidosis may be present. Sinoorbital mucormycosis/zygomycosis is rapidly progressive and life-threatening. See 10.10, *Cavernous Sinus and Associated Syndromes (Multiple Ocular Motor Nerve Palsies).*

Treatment

1. Admit the patient to the hospital and consider consultation with Infectious Disease and Otorhinolaryngology.

2. Broad-spectrum intravenous antibiotics to cover Gram-positive, Gram-negative, and anaerobic organisms are recommended for 48 to 72 hours, followed by oral medication for at least 1 week. The specific antibiotic agents vary. In patients from the community with no recent history of hospitalization, nursing home stay, or institutional stay, we currently recommend:

—Ampicillin-sulbactam 3 g i.v. q6h in adults; 300 mg/kg per day in four divided doses in children, maximum daily dose 12 g ampicillin-sulbactam (8 g ampicillin component).

or

—Piperacillin-tazobactam 4.5 g i.v. q8h or 3.375 g q6h in adults; 240 mg of piperacillin component/kg/day in three divided doses in children, maximum daily dose 18 g piperacillin.

■ For adults who are allergic to penicillin but can tolerate cephalosporins, use vancomycin as dosed below plus:

—Ceftriaxone 2 g i.v. q.d. and metronidazole 500 mg i.v. q6–8h (not to exceed 4 g per day).

■ For adults who are allergic to penicillin/cephalosporin, treat with a combination of a fluoroquinolone (for patients >17 years of age, moxifloxacin 400 mg i.v. daily or ciprofloxacin 400 mg i.v. q12h or levofloxacin 750 mg i.v. q.d.) and metronidazole 500 mg i.v. q6–8h.

■ Given the prevalence of community-associated methicillin-resistant *Staphylococcus aureus* (CA-MRSA), treatment with trimethoprim-sulfamethoxazole, tetracycline derivatives, vancomycin, or clindamycin may also be started initially. Some clinicians prefer to save these antibiotics and institute them only if the patient fails to improve or worsens over the first 48 hours of intravenous therapy. In patients suspected of harboring hospital-associated MRSA or in those suspected of meningitis, intravenous vancomycin is started at 15 mg/kg q12–24h in adults with normal renal function and 40 mg/kg per day in two or three divided doses in children, with a maximum daily dose of 2 g.

NOTE: Antibiotic dosages may need to be reduced in the presence of renal insufficiency or failure. Peak and trough levels of vancomycin are usually monitored, and dosages are adjusted as needed. BUN and creatinine levels are monitored closely.

---

3. Nasal decongestant spray as needed for up to 3 days. Nasal corticosteroid spray may also be added to quicken the resolution of sinusitis.

4. Erythromycin ointment q.i.d. for corneal exposure and chemosis if needed.

5. If the orbit is tight, an optic neuropathy is present, or the IOP is severely elevated,

immediate canthotomy/cantholysis may be needed. See 3.10, *Traumatic Retrobulbar Hemorrhage,* for technique.

6. The use of systemic corticosteroids in the management of orbital cellulitis remains controversial. If systemic corticosteroids are considered, it is probably safest to wait 24 to 48 hours until an adequate intravenous antibiotic load has been given (three to four doses).

Follow-Up

Reevaluate at least twice daily in the hospital for the first 48 hours. Severe infections may require multiple daily examinations. Clinical improvement may take 24 to 36 hours.

1. Progress is monitored by:

—Patient's symptoms.

—Temperature and white blood cell count (WBC).

—Visual acuity and evaluation of optic nerve function.

—Ocular motility.

—Degree of proptosis and any displacement of the globe (significant displacement may indicate an abscess).

NOTE: If clinical deterioration is noted after an adequate antibiotic load (three to four doses), a CT scan of the orbit and brain with contrast should be repeated to look for abscess formation (see 7.3.2, *Subperiosteal Abscess*). If an abscess is found, surgical drainage may be required. Radiographic findings may lag behind the clinical examination, and so clinical deterioration itself may be an indication for surgical drainage. Other conditions that should be considered when the patient is not improving include cavernous sinus thrombosis, meningitis, or a noninfectious etiology.

---

2. Evaluate the cornea for signs of exposure.

3. Check IOP.

4. Examine the retina and optic nerve for signs of posterior compression (e.g., chorioretinal folds), inflammation, or exudative retinal detachment.

7

5. When orbital cellulitis is clearly and consistently improving, then the regimen can be changed to oral antibiotics (depending on the culture and sensitivity results) to complete a 10- to 14-day course. We often use:

—Amoxicillin/clavulanate: 25 to 45 mg/kg/day p.o. in two divided doses for children, maximum daily dose of 90 mg/kg/day; 875 mg p.o. q12h for adults.

or

—Cefpodoxime: 10 mg/kg/day p.o. in two divided doses for children, maximum daily dose of 400 mg; 200 mg p.o. q12h for adults.

Doxycycline or trimethoprim-sulfamethoxazole are also reasonable alternatives, especially if CA-MRSA is suspected.

The patient is examined every few days as an outpatient until the condition resolves and instructed to return immediately with worsening signs or symptoms.

NOTE: Medication noncompliance is an extremely common reason for recurrence or failure to Improve. The oral antibiotic regimen should be individualized for ease of use and affordability. Effective generic alternatives include doxycycline and trimethoprim/sulfamethoxazole.

7.3.2. SUBPERIOSTEAL ABSCESS

Signs and Symptoms

Similar to orbital cellulitis, though may be magnified in scale. Suspect an abscess if a patient with orbital cellulitis fails to improve or deteriorates after 48 to 72 hours of intravenous antibiotics.

Differential Diagnosis

■ Intraorbital abscess: Rare, because periosteum is an excellent barrier to intraorbital spread. May be seen following penetrating trauma, previous surgery, retained foreign body, extrascleral extension of endophthalmitis, extension of subperiosteal abscess (SPA), or from endogenous seeding. Treatment is surgical drainage and intravenous antibiotics. Drainage may be difficult because of several isolated loculations.

■ Cavernous sinus thrombosis: Rare in era of antibiotics. Most commonly seen with Mucormycosis/Zygomycosis [see 10.10, *Cavernous Sinus and Associated Syndromes (Multiple Ocular Motor Nerve Palsies)*]. In bacterial cases, the patient is usually also septic and may be obtunded and hemodynamically unstable. Prognosis is guarded in all cases. Manage with hemodynamic support (usually in intensive care unit), broad-spectrum antibiotics, and surgical drainage if an infectious nidus is identified (e.g., paranasal sinuses, orbit). Anticoagulation can be considered.

Work-Up

See 7.3.1, *Orbital Cellulitis*, for work-up. In addition:

1. Obtain CT with contrast, which allows for easier identification and extent of abscess. In cases of suspected cavernous sinus thrombosis, discuss with the radiologist before CT, since special CT techniques and windows may help with diagnosis. MRI may also be indicated.

NOTE: All orbital cellulitis patients who do not improve after 48 to 72 hours of intravenous antibiotic therapy should undergo repeat imaging.

Treatment

1. Microbes involved in SPA formation are related to the age of the patient. The causative microbes influence response to intravenous antibiotics and the need for surgical drainage. See Table 7.3.2.1.

NOTE: These are guidelines only. Any patient with an optic neuropathy should be drained urgently, regardless of age. All patients with SPA should be followed closely, regardless of age.

---

2. If there is an optic neuropathy, emergent drainage of abscess is required. Drainage is usually managed as a combined approach with Otorhinolaryngology. Unless the SPA is very medial and isolated, drainage

TABLE 7.3.2.1	Age and Subperiosteal Abscess	
Age (y)	**Cultures**	**Need to Drain**
<9	Sterile (58%) or single aerobe	No in 93%
9 to 14	Mixed aerobe and anaerobe	+/−
>14	Mixed, anaerobes in all	Yes

Harris GJ. Subperiosteal abscess of the orbit: older children and adults require aggressive treatment. *Ophthal Plast Reconstr Surg.* 2001;17(6):395–397.

typically necessitates an external incision for adequate orbital exploration. Occasionally, small medial abscesses may be drained by an endoscopic approach alone.

3. Leave a drain in place for 24 to 48 hours to prevent abscess reformation.

4. Intracranial extension necessitates neurosurgical involvement.

5. Expect dramatic and rapid improvement after adequate drainage. Additional imaging, exploration, and drainage may be indicated if improvement does not occur rapidly.

6. Do not reimage immediately unless patient is deteriorating postoperatively. Imaging usually lags behind clinical response by at least 48 to 72 hours.

7.3.3. ACUTE DACRYOADENITIS: INFECTION/ INFLAMMATION OF THE LACRIMAL GLAND

Symptoms

Unilateral pain, redness, and swelling over the outer one-third of the upper eyelid, often with tearing or discharge. Typically occurs in children and young adults.

Signs

(See Figures 7.3.3.1 and 7.3.3.2.)

Critical. Erythema, swelling, and tenderness over the outer one-third of the upper eyelid. May be associated with hyperemia of the palpebral lobe of the lacrimal gland, S-shaped upper eyelid.

Other. Ipsilateral preauricular lymphadenopathy, ipsilateral conjunctival chemosis temporally, fever, elevated WBC.

Differential Diagnosis

■ Chalazion: Tender inflammatory eyelid nodule. See 6.2, *Chalazion/Hordeolum.*

■ Preseptal cellulitis: Erythema and warmth of the eyelids and the surrounding soft tissue. See 6.10, *Preseptal Cellulitis.*

■ Orbital cellulitis: Proptosis and limitation of ocular motility often accompany eyelid erythema and swelling. See 7.3.1, *Orbital Cellulitis.*

7

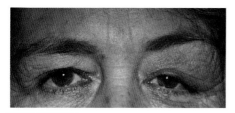

FIGURE 7.3.3.1. Dacryoadenitis.

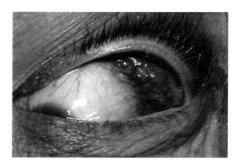

FIGURE 7.3.3.2. Dacryoadenitis.

7

■ IOIS involving more than just the lacrimal gland: May have concomitant proptosis, downward displacement of the globe, or limitation of ocular motility. Typically afebrile with a normal WBC. Does not respond to antibiotics but improves dramatically with systemic steroids. See 7.2.2, *Idiopathic Orbital Inflammatory Syndrome*.

■ Leaking dermoid cyst: Dermoid cysts often occur either superomedially or superolaterally. Leakage causes an intense and acute inflammatory reaction.

■ Rhabdomyosarcoma: Most common pediatric orbital malignancy. Rapid presentation, but pain and erythema occur in only a minority of cases. See 7.4.1, *Orbital Tumors in Children*.

■ Primary malignant lacrimal gland tumor or lacrimal gland metastasis: Commonly produces displacement of the globe or proptosis. May present with an acute inflammatory clinical picture. Often palpable, evident on CT scan. See 7.6, *Lacrimal Gland Mass/Chronic Dacryoadenitis*.

■ Retained foreign body, with secondary infectious or inflammatory process: The patient may not remember any history of penetrating trauma.

Etiology

■ Inflammatory, noninfectious: By far the most common. More indolent and painless course in lymphoproliferation and sarcoidosis. More acute presentation in IOIS.

■ Bacterial: Rare. Usually due to *Staphylococcus aureus, Neisseria gonorrhoeae,* or streptococci.

■ Viral: Seen in mumps, infectious mononucleosis, influenza, and varicella zoster. May result in severe dry eye due to lacrimal gland fibrosis.

Work-Up

The following is performed when an acute etiology is suspected. When the disease does not respond to medical therapy or another etiology is being considered, see 7.6, *Lacrimal Gland Mass/Chronic Dacryoadenitis*.

1. History: Acute or chronic? Fever? Discharge? Systemic infection or viral syndrome?

2. Palpate the eyelid and the orbital rim for a mass.

3. Evaluate the resistance of each globe to retropulsion.

4. Look for proptosis by Hertel exophthalmometry.

5. Complete ocular examination, particularly extraocular motility assessment.

6. Obtain smears and bacterial cultures of any discharge.

7. Examine the parotid glands (often enlarged in mumps, sarcoidosis, tuberculosis, lymphoma, and syphilis).

8. Perform CT scan of the orbit (axial and coronal views), preferably with contrast (see Figure 7.3.3.3). CT is preferable to MRI in assessment of the lacrimal gland because of better detail of the adjacent bony anatomy.

9. If the patient is febrile, a CBC with differential and sometimes blood cultures are obtained.

Treatment

If the specific etiology is unclear, it is best to empirically treat the patient with systemic antibiotics (see bacterial etiology below) for 24 hours with careful clinical reassessment. The clinical response to antibiotics can guide further

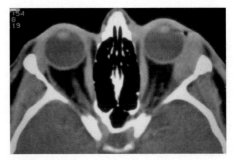

FIGURE 7.3.3.3. CT of dacryoadenitis.

management and direct one toward a specific etiology.

1. Inflammatory:

—For treatment, see 7.2.2, *Idiopathic Orbital Inflammatory Syndrome.*

—Analgesic as needed.

2. Viral (e.g., mumps, infectious mononucleosis):

—Cool compresses to the area of swelling and tenderness.

—Analgesic as needed (e.g., acetaminophen 650 mg p.o. q4h p.r.n.).

NOTE: Aspirin is contraindicated in children with a viral syndrome because of the risk of Reye syndrome.

---

3. Bacterial or infectious (but unidentified) etiology:

a. If mild-to-moderate:

—Amoxicillin/clavulanate: 25 to 45 mg/kg/day p.o. in two divided doses for children, maximum daily dose of 90 mg/kg/day; 875 mg p.o. q12h for adults.

or

—Cephalexin 25 to 50 mg/kg/day p.o. in four divided doses for children; 250 to 500 mg p.o. q6h for adults.

b. If moderate-to-severe, hospitalize and treat as per 7.3.1, *Orbital Cellulitis.*

Follow-Up

Daily until improvement confirmed. In patients who fail to respond to antibiotic therapy, judicious use of oral prednisone (see 7.2.2, *Idiopathic Orbital Inflammatory Syndrome*) is reasonable, as long as close follow-up is maintained. Inflammatory dacryoadenitis should respond to oral corticosteroid therapy within 48 hours. Watch for signs of orbital involvement, such as decreased motility or proptosis, which requires hospital admission for i.v. antibiotic therapy and close monitoring. Patients who fail to respond to medical therapy are managed similarly to those with chronic dacryoadenitis, and biopsy is usually needed. See 7.6, *Lacrimal Gland Mass/Chronic Dacryoadenitis.*

7

| 7.4 | **ORBITAL TUMORS** |

7.4.1. ORBITAL TUMORS IN CHILDREN

Signs

Critical. Proptosis or globe displacement.

Other. See the specific etiologies for additional presenting signs. See Tables 7.4.1.1 and 7.4.1.2 for imaging characteristics.

Differential Diagnosis

■ Orbital cellulitis from adjacent ethmoiditis: Most common cause of proptosis in children. It is of paramount importance to efficiently rule out this etiology. See 7.3.1, *Orbital Cellulitis.*

■ Dermoid and epidermoid cysts: Manifest clinically from birth to young adulthood and enlarge slowly. Preseptal dermoid cysts may become symptomatic in childhood and are most commonly found in the temporal upper eyelid or brow, and less often in the medial upper eyelid. The palpable, smooth mass may be mobile or fixed to the periosteum. Posterior dermoids typically become symptomatic in adulthood and may cause proptosis or globe displacement. Dermoid cyst rupture may mimic orbital cellulitis. B-scan US, when used, reveals a cystic lesion with good transmission of echoes.

TABLE 7.4.1.1	Childhood Orbital Lesions
Well circumscribed	Dermoid cyst, rhabdomyosarcoma, optic nerve glioma, plexiform neurofibroma, capillary hemangioma
Diffuse and/or infiltrating	Lymphangioma, leukemia, IOIS, capillary hemangioma, rhabdomyosarcoma, neuroblastoma, teratoma

TABLE 7.4.1.2   CT and MRI Characteristics of Pediatric Orbital Lesions

Lesion	CT Characteristics	MRI Features	
		T1 Sequence	**T2 Sequence**
Dermoid or epidermoid cyst	Well-defined lesion that may mold the bone of the orbital walls	Hypointense to fat, only capsule enhances with gadolinium. Signal may increase if a large amount of viscous mucus is present within the lesion	Iso- or hypointense to fat
Capillary hemangioma	Irregular, contrast enhancing	Well defined, hypointense to fat, hyperintense to muscle	Hyperintense to fat and muscle
Rhabdomyosarcoma	Irregular, well-defined lesion with possible bone destruction	Isointense to muscle	Hyperintense to muscle
Metastatic neuroblastoma	Poorly defined mass with bony destruction		
Lymphangioma	Nonencapsulated irregular mass, "crabgrass of the orbit"	Cystic, possibly multiloculated, heterogeneous mass Hypointense to fat, hyperintense to muscle, diffuse enhancement May show signal of either acute and subacute hemorrhage	Markedly hyperintense to fat and muscle
Optic nerve glioma	Fusiform enlargement of the optic nerve	Tubular or fusiform mass, hypointense to gray matter	Homogenous hyperintensity
Plexiform neurofibroma	Diffuse, irregular soft-tissue mass, possible defect in orbital roof	Iso- or slightly hyperintense to muscle	Hyperintense to fat and muscle
Leukemia (granulocytic sarcoma)	Irregular mass with occasional bony erosion		

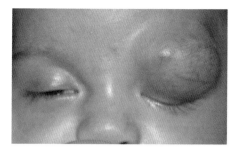

FIGURE 7.4.1.1. Capillary hemangioma.

- Capillary hemangioma: Seen from birth to 2 years, may be slowly progressive with sudden rapid expansion. May be observed through the eyelid as a bluish mass or be accompanied by a red hemangioma of the skin (strawberry nevus, stork bite), which blanches with pressure. Proptosis may be exacerbated by crying. It can enlarge over 6 to 12 months, but spontaneously regresses over the following several years. Not to be confused with the unrelated cavernous hemangioma of the orbit, typically seen in adults (see Figure 7.4.1.1).

- Rhabdomyosarcoma: Average age of presentation is 8 to 10 years, but may occur from infancy to adulthood. May have explosive proptosis, edema of the eyelids, a palpable superonasal eyelid or subconjunctival mass, new-onset ptosis or strabismus, or a history of nosebleeds. Malignant and may metastasize. Hallmarks are rapid onset and progression. Urgent biopsy if suspected.

- Metastatic neuroblastoma: Seen during the first few years of life. Abrupt presentation with unilateral or bilateral proptosis, eyelid ecchymosis, and globe displacement. The child is usually systemically ill, and 80% to 90% of patients presenting with orbital involvement already have a known history of neuroblastoma.

- Lymphangioma: Usually seen in the first two decades of life with a slowly progressive course but may abruptly worsen if the tumor bleeds. Proptosis may be intermittent and exacerbated by upper respiratory tract infections. This mass may present as atraumatic eyelid or orbital ecchymosis. Concomitant conjunctival, eyelid, or oropharyngeal

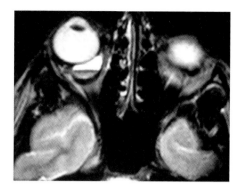

FIGURE 7.4.1.2. T-2-weighted MRI of orbital lymphangioma with subacute blood cyst.

lymphangiomas may be noted (a conjunctival lesion appears as a multicystic mass). MRI is often diagnostic. B-scan US, when used, often reveals cystic spaces. Surgical extirpation is difficult (see Figure 7.4.1.2).

- Optic nerve glioma (juvenile pilocytic astrocytoma): Usually first seen at age 2 to 6 years and is slowly progressive. Painless axial proptosis with decreased visual acuity and a relative afferent pupillary defect. Optic atrophy or optic nerve swelling may be present. May be associated with neurofibromatosis (types I and II), in which case it may be bilateral. See 13.13, *Phakomatoses*.

- Plexiform neurofibroma: First seen in the first decade of life and is pathognomonic of neurofibromatosis type I. Ptosis, eyelid hypertrophy, S-shaped deformity of the upper eyelid, or pulsating proptosis (from absence of the greater sphenoid wing) may be present. Facial asymmetry and a palpable anterior orbital mass may also be evident. See 13.13, *Phakomatoses*.

- Leukemia (granulocytic sarcoma): Seen in the first decade of life with rapidly evolving unilateral or bilateral proptosis and, occasionally, swelling of the temporal fossa area due to a mass. Typically, these lesions precede blood or bone marrow signs of leukemia, usually acute myelogenous leukemia, by several months. Any patient with a biopsy-proven granulocytic sarcoma of the orbit must be closely followed by an oncologist for leukemia.

7

NOTE: Acute lymphoblastic leukemia also can produce unilateral or bilateral proptosis.

Work-Up

1. History: Determine the age of onset and the rate of progression. Does the proptosis vary (e.g., with crying)? Nosebleeds? Systemic illness? Fever? Recent URI? Purulent nasal discharge?

2. External examination: Look for an anterior orbital mass, a skin hemangioma, or a temporal fossa lesion. Measure any proptosis (Hertel exophthalmometer) or globe displacement. Refer to a pediatrician for abdominal examination to rule out mass or organomegaly.

3. Complete ocular examination, including visual acuity, pupillary assessment, color vision, IOP, refraction, and optic nerve evaluation.

4. CT (axial and coronal views) of the orbit and brain. If neoplasia is suspected, orbital MRI (with gadolinium-DTPA and fat suppression). Imaging may be performed urgently to rule out true pediatric orbital emergencies such as infection and rhabdomyosarcoma.

5. If paranasal sinus opacification is noted in the clinical setting of orbital inflammation, initiate immediate systemic antibiotic therapy (see 7.3.1, *Orbital Cellulitis*).

6. In cases of acute onset and rapid progression with evidence of mass on imaging, an emergency incisional biopsy for frozen and permanent microscopic evaluation is indicated to rule out an aggressive malignancy (e.g., rhabdomyosarcoma).

7. Other tests as determined by the working diagnosis (usually performed in conjunction with a pediatric oncologist):

—Rhabdomyosarcoma: Physical examination (look especially for enlarged lymph nodes), chest and bone radiographs, bone marrow aspiration, lumbar puncture, liver function studies.

—Leukemia: CBC with differential, bone marrow studies, others.

—Neuroblastoma: Abdominal CT scan, urine for vanillylmandelic acid.

Treatment

1. Dermoid and epidermoid cysts: Complete surgical excision with the capsule intact. If the cyst ruptures, the contents can incite an acute inflammatory response.

2. Capillary hemangioma: Observe if not causing visual obstruction, astigmatism, and amblyopia. All capillary hemangiomas will eventually involute. In the presence of visual compromise (e.g., amblyopia, optic neuropathy) several treatment options exist:

a. Oral corticosteroids may be used: 2 to 3 mg/kg, tapered over 6 weeks. IOP must be monitored, and patients should be placed on GI prophylaxis.

b. A local corticosteroid injection (e.g., betamethasone 6 mg/mL and triamcinolone 40 mg/mL) may be given to shrink the lesion if necessary. Care should be taken to avoid orbital hemorrhage and central retinal artery occlusion (CRAO) during injection. Skin atrophy and depigmentation are other potential complications. Periocular injection of triamcinolone is not recommended by the manufacturer because of the potential risk of embolic infarction. See note in 6.2, *Chalazion/Hordeolum*.

c. Systemic beta blockers: While the exact mechanism remains unclear and its use is off label, case reports and small case series have shown propranolol to be a viable option in the treatment of refractory capillary hemangiomas. Some nonophthalmic studies recommend this as first-line treatment if the hemangioma is rapidly proliferating. Side effects of propranolol include hypoglycemia, hypotension, and bradycardia. Asthmatics and those with reactive airway disease are at risk of bronchospasm. Therefore, patients should be evaluated by a pediatrician pretreatment and monitored throughout the course of treatment.

d. Surgical excision.

e. Interferon therapy: Usually reserved for large or systemic lesions which may be associated with a consumptive coagulopathy or high-output congestive heart failure (Kasabach–Merritt syndrome). There is a risk of spastic diplegia with this therapy. This therapy is not used frequently because of other viable alternatives, including propranolol.

3. Rhabdomyosarcoma: Managed by urgent biopsy and referral to a pediatric oncologist in most cases. Local radiation therapy and systemic chemotherapy are given once the diagnosis is confirmed by biopsy and the patient has been appropriately staged. Significant orbital and ocular complications are common even with prompt and aggressive management. Overall, the long-term prognosis for orbital rhabdomyosarcoma is good in the absence of extraorbital extension.

4. Lymphangioma: Most are managed by observation. Surgical debulking is performed for a significant cosmetic deformity, ocular dysfunction (e.g., strabismus and amblyopia), or compressive optic neuropathy from acute orbital hemorrhage. Incidence of hemorrhage into the lesion is increased after surgery. May recur after excision. Aspiration drainage of hemorrhagic cysts ("chocolate cysts") may temporarily improve symptoms.

5. Optic nerve glioma: Controversial. Observation, surgery, and radiation are used variably on a case-by-case basis.

6. Leukemia: Managed by a pediatric oncologist. Systemic chemotherapy for the leukemia. Some physicians administer orbital radiation therapy alone in isolated orbital lesions (chloromas), when systemic leukemia cannot be confirmed on bone marrow studies. However, patients need to be monitored closely for eventual systemic involvement.

7. Metastatic neuroblastoma: Managed by a pediatric oncologist in most cases. Local radiation and systemic chemotherapy.

8. Plexiform neurofibroma: Surgical excision is reserved for patients with significant symptoms or disfigurement. The lesions tend to be vascular.

Follow-Up

1. Tumors with rapid onset and progression require urgent attention.

2. Tumors that progress more slowly may be managed less urgently.

7.4.2. ORBITAL TUMORS IN ADULTS

Symptoms

Prominent eye, double vision, decreased vision, may be asymptomatic.

Signs

Critical. Proptosis, pain, displacement of the globe away from the location of the tumor, orbital mass on palpation, mass found with neuroimaging. Specific tumors may cause enophthalmos secondary to orbital fibrosis.

Other. A palpable mass, limitation of ocular motility, orbital inflammation, optic disc edema, or choroidal folds may be present. See the individual etiologies for more specific findings. See Tables 7.4.2.1 and 7.4.2.2 for imaging characteristics.

Etiology

■ Primarily Intraconal:

1. Cavernous hemangioma: Most common benign orbital mass in adults. Middle-age women most commonly affected, with a slow onset of orbital signs. Growth may accelerate during pregnancy (see Figure 7.4.2.1).

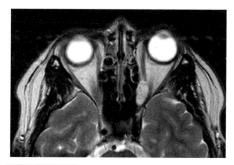

FIGURE 7.4.2.1. T-2-weighted MRI of cavernous hemangioma.

TABLE 7.4.2.1	CT and MRI Characteristics of Selected Adult Orbital Lesions		
		MRI Features	
Lesion	**CT Characteristics**	**T1 Sequence**	**T2 Sequence**
Metastasis	Poorly defined mass conforming to orbital structure, possible bony erosion	Infiltrating mass, hypointense to fat, isointense to muscle, moderate-to-marked enhancement	Hyperintense to fat and muscle
Well-Circumscribed Intraconal Tumors			
Cavernous hemangioma	Encapsulated mass typically within muscle cone	Iso- or hyperintense to muscle. Heterogeneous, diffuse enhancement	Hyperintense to muscle and fat
Fibrous histiocytoma	Well-defined mass anywhere in the orbit	Heterogeneous mass, hypointense to fat, hyper- or isointense to muscle. Irregular enhancement	Similar to T1
Neurilemmoma	Fusiform or ovoid mass often in the superior orbit	Iso- or hyperintense to muscle with variable enhancement	Variable intensity
Hemangiopericytoma	Similar to cavernous hemangioma and fibrous histiocytoma	Hypointense to fat, isointense to muscle. Moderate diffuse contrast enhancement	Variable
Neurofibroma	Diffuse, irregular soft-tissue mass, possible defect in orbital roof	Iso- or slightly hyperintense to muscle	Hyperintense to fat and muscle

2. Solitary fibrous tumor: A compendium for mesenchymal lesions with varying degrees of aggressive behavior. Occurs at any age. Includes fibrous histiocytoma and hemangiopericytoma, which cannot be distinguished without biopsy.

3. Neurilemmoma (benign schwannoma): Progressive, painless proptosis. Rarely associated with neurofibromatosis type II.

4. Neurofibroma: See 7.4.1, *Orbital Tumors in Children*.

5. Meningioma: Optic nerve sheath meningioma (ONSM) typically occurs in middle-aged women with painless, slowly progressive visual loss, often with mild proptosis. An afferent pupillary defect develops. Ophthalmoscopy can reveal optic nerve swelling, optic atrophy, or

TABLE 7.4.2.2 **CT and MRI Characteristics of Select Adult Extraconal Orbital Lesions**

		MRI Features	
Lesion	**CT Characteristics**	**T1 Sequence**	**T2 Sequence**
Mucocele	Frontal or ethmoid sinus cyst that extends into orbit	Variable from hypo- to hyperintense, depending on the protein content/viscosity of the lesion	Hyperintense to fat
Lymphoid tumors	Irregular mass molding to the shape of orbital bones or globe. Bone destruction possible in aggressive lesions and HIV	Irregular mass Hypointense to fat Iso- or hyperintense to muscle. Moderate-to-marked enhancement	Hyperintense to muscle
Localized neurofibroma	Well-defined mass in superior orbit	Well-circumscribed, heterogeneous. Iso- or hyperintense to muscle	Hyperintense to fat and muscle
Optic nerve sheath meningioma	Tubular enhancement of the optic nerve, "railroad track" appearance, possible calcification	Variable intensity lesion around optic nerve with marked enhancement Optic nerve tissue should not enhance	

7

abnormal collateral vessels around the optic nerve head.

6. Other neurogenic tumors: optic nerve glioma, optic nerve sarcoid, malignant optic nerve glioma of adulthood.

7. Lymphangioma: Usually discovered in childhood. See 7.4.1, *Orbital Tumors in Children.*

■ Primarily Extraconal:

1. Mucocele: Often a frontal headache and a history of chronic sinusitis or sinus trauma. Usually nasally or superonasally located, emanating from the frontal and ethmoid sinuses.

2. Localized neurofibroma: Occurs in young-to middle-aged adults with slow development of orbital signs. Eyelid infiltration results in an S-shaped upper eyelid. Some have neurofibromatosis type I, but most do not.

3. SPA or hematoma: See 7.3.2, *Subperiosteal Abscess.*

4. Dermoid cyst: See 7.4.2, *Orbital Tumors in Adults.*

5. Others: Tumors of the lacrimal gland [(pleomorphic adenoma (well circumscribed), adenoid cystic carcinoma (variably circumscribed)], sphenoid wing meningiomas, secondary tumors extending from the brain or paranasal sinuses, primary osseous tumors, and vascular lesions (e.g., varix, arteriovenous malformation).

■ Intraconal or Extraconal:

1. Lymphoproliferative disease (lymphoid hyperplasia and lymphoma): More commonly extraconal. About 50% are well circumscribed on imaging, 50% are infiltrative. Usually occurs in middle-aged to elderly adults. Slow onset and progression. Typically develops superiorly in the anterior aspect of the orbit. May be accompanied by a subconjunctival, salmon-colored lesion. More indolent clinically and less responsive to systemic steroids than IOIS. Can occur without evidence of systemic lymphoma.

2. Metastatic: Usually occurs in middle-aged to elderly people with a variable onset of orbital signs. Common primary sources include the breast (most

common in women), lung (most common in men), genitourinary tract (especially prostate), and gastrointestinal tract. Twenty percent of orbital breast cancer metastases are bilateral and frequently involve extraocular muscles. Enophthalmos (not proptosis) may be seen with scirrhous breast carcinoma. Uveal metastases are far more common, outpacing orbital lesions by 10:1.

3. Others: Mesenchymal tumors and other malignancies.

Work-Up

1. History: Determine the age of onset and rate of progression. Headache or chronic sinusitis? History of cancer? Trauma (e.g., mucocele, hematocele, orbital foreign body, ruptured dermoid)?

2. Complete ocular examination, particularly visual acuity, pupillary response, ocular motility, color vision and visual field of each eye, measurement of globe displacement (from the bridge of the nose with a ruler) and proptosis (Hertel exophthalmometer), IOP, and optic nerve evaluation. Examine conjunctival surface and cul-de-sacs carefully for salmon patches if lymphoma suspected.

3. CT (axial and coronal views) of the orbit and brain or orbital MRI with fat suppression/gadolinium-DPTA, depending on suspected etiology and age. See 14.2, *Computed Tomography.*

4. Orbital US with color Doppler imaging as needed to define the vascularity of the lesion. Conventional B-scan has a limited role in the diagnosis of orbital pathology because of the availability and resolution of CT and MRI.

5. When a metastasis is suspected and primary tumor is unknown, the following should be performed:

—Incisional biopsy to confirm the diagnosis, with estrogen receptor assay if breast carcinoma is suspected.

—Breast examination and palpation of axillary lymph nodes by the primary physician.

—Medical work-up (e.g., chest radiograph, mammogram, prostate examination).

6. If lymphoproliferative disease (lymphoma or lymphoid hyperplasia) is suspected, biopsy for definitive diagnosis is indicated. Include adequate fixed tissue for immunohistochemistry and fresh tissue for flow cytometry. If lymphoproliferative disease is confirmed, the systemic work-up is almost identical for polyclonal (lymphoid hyperplasia) and monoclonal (lymphoma) lesions [e.g., CBC with differential, serum protein electrophoresis, lactate dehydrogenase, and whole-body imaging (CT/MRI or positron emission tomography/CT)]. Bone marrow biopsy may be indicated in certain forms of lymphoma. Close surveillance with repeat testing is indicated over several years in all patients with lymphoproliferative disease, regardless of clonality. A significant percentage of patients initially diagnosed with orbital lymphoid hyperplasia will eventually develop systemic lymphoma.

Treatment

1. Metastatic disease: Systemic chemotherapy as required for the primary malignancy. Radiation therapy is often used palliatively for the orbital mass; high-dose radiation therapy may result in ocular and optic nerve damage. Hormonal therapy may be indicated in certain cases (e.g., breast, prostate carcinoma). Carcinoid tumors are occasionally resected.

2. Well-circumscribed lesions: Complete surgical excision is performed when there is compromised visual function, diplopia, rapid growth, or high suspicion of malignancy. Excision for cosmesis can be offered if the patient is willing to accept the surgical risks. An asymptomatic patient can be followed every 6 to 12 months with serial examinations and imaging. Progression of symptoms and increasing size on serial imaging are indications for exploration and biopsy/excision.

3. Mucocele: Systemic antibiotics (e.g., ampicillin/sulbactam 3 g i.v. q6h) followed by surgical drainage of the mucocele and possible exenteration of the involved sinus.

4. Lymphoid tumors: Lymphoid hyperplasia and lymphoma without systemic involvement are treated almost identically. With few exceptions, orbital lymphoproliferations respond dramatically to relatively low doses of radiation; ocular and optic nerve complications are therefore much rarer than with other malignancies. Systemic lymphoma is treated with chemotherapy and in many cases with biologics (e.g., rituximab). The majority of orbital lymphoma is of B-cell origin, and most are of the mucosa-associated lymphoid tissue subtype, presently called extranodal marginal zone lymphoma (EMZL). In older individuals with few symptoms and indolent lesions, more conservative measures may be indicated, including observation alone or brief courses of corticosteroids. To date, there is no clear role for the use of systemic antibiotics in the treatment of orbital lymphoproliferative disease. There is also no clear evidence that orbital EMZL is in any way related to *Helicobacter pylori*-associated gastric EMZL.

5. ONSM: The diagnosis is usually based on slow progression and typical MRI findings. MRI with gadolinium is the preferred imaging modality. CT is occasionally helpful in demonstrating intralesional calcifications. Stereotactic radiation therapy is usually indicated when the tumor is growing and causing significant visual loss. Otherwise, the patient may be followed every 3 to 6 months with serial clinical examinations and imaging studies as needed. Recent studies have shown significant efficacy of stereotactic radiotherapy in decreasing tumor growth and in visual preservation. Stereotactic radio-therapy is not equivalent to gamma knife therapy ("radiosurgery"). Empiric stereotactic radiotherapy (i.e., without confirmatory biopsy) is a reasonable treatment option but is reserved for typical cases of ONSM. Atypical or rapidly progressive lesions still require biopsy.

6. Localized neurofibroma: Surgical removal is performed for symptomatic and enlarging tumors.

7. Neurilemmoma: Same as for cavernous hemangioma (see above).

8. Solitary fibrous tumor (including fibrous histiocytoma and hemangiopericytoma): Complete excision when possible. The lesion may be fixed to the surrounding normal anatomy and abut critical structures. In such cases, debulking is reasonable, with long-term follow-up and serial imaging to rule out aggressive recurrence or potential malignant transformation.

Follow-Up

1. In cases of isolated lesions that can be completely excised (e.g., cavernous hemangioma), routine ophthalmologic follow-up is all that is necessary.

2. Other etiologies require long-term follow-up at variable intervals.

3. Metastatic disease requires work-up without delay.

NOTE: See 7.6, *Lacrimal Gland Mass/Chronic Dacryoadenitis,* especially if the mass is in the outer one-third of the upper eyelid, and 7.4.1, *Orbital Tumors in Children.*

7.5   TRAUMATIC ORBITAL DISEASE

ORBITAL BLOW-OUT FRACTURE

(See 3.9, *Orbital Blow-Out Fracture.*)

TRAUMATIC RETROBULBAR HEMORRHAGE

(See 3.10, *Traumatic Retrobulbar Hemorrhage.*)

7.6 LACRIMAL GLAND MASS/CHRONIC DACRYOADENITIS

Symptoms

Persistent or progressive swelling of the outer one-third of the upper eyelid. Pain or double vision may be present.

Signs

Critical. Chronic eyelid swelling, predominantly in the outer one-third of the upper eyelid, with or without proptosis and displacement of the globe inferiorly and medially. Erythema is less common.

Other. A palpable mass may be present in the outer one-third of the upper eyelid. Extraocular motility may be restricted. May have conjunctival injection.

Etiology

- Sarcoidosis: May be bilateral. May have concomitant lung, skin, or ocular disease. Lymphadenopathy, parotid gland enlargement, or seventh nerve palsy may be present. More common in American blacks and white Northern Europeans.

- IOIS: See 7.2.2, *Idiopathic Orbital Inflammatory Syndrome.* Chronic, painless lacrimal gland enlargement is atypical for IOIS.

- Infectious: Enlarged palpebral lobe with surrounding conjunctival injection. Purulent discharge with bacterial dacryoadenitis. Bilateral lacrimal gland enlargement may be seen in patients with viral illnesses. CT scan may show fat stranding, abscess.

- Benign mixed epithelial tumor (pleomorphic adenoma): Slowly progressive, painless proptosis or displacement of the globe in middle-aged adults. Usually involves orbital lobe of lacrimal gland. CT may show a well-circumscribed mass with pressure-induced remodeling and enlargement of the lacrimal gland fossa. No bony erosion occurs.

- Dermoid cyst: Typically a painless, subcutaneous cystic mass that enlarges slowly. Anterior lesions manifest in childhood, while more posterior lesions hide effectively into adulthood. May rarely rupture, causing acute swelling and inflammation. Well-defined, cystic, extraconal mass noted on CT.

- Lymphoproliferative tumor: Slowly progressive proptosis and globe displacement in a middle-aged or elderly patient. May have a pink "salmon-patch" area of subconjunctival extension. CT usually shows a lacrimal gland lesion that conforms to the native anatomy and does not erode bone. About 50% of lesions will be well circumscribed. Bony erosion may be seen in aggressive histopathology.

- Adenoid cystic carcinoma: Subacute onset of pain over 1 to 3 months, proptosis, and diplopia, with variable progression. Globe displacement, ptosis, and a motility disturbance are common. This malignant lesion often exhibits perineural invasion, resulting in significant pain and intracranial extension. CT shows an irregular mass, often with bony erosion (see Figure 7.6.1).

- Malignant mixed epithelial tumor (pleomorphic adenocarcinoma): Occurs primarily in elderly patients, acutely producing pain and progressing rapidly. Usually develops within a long-standing benign mixed epithelial

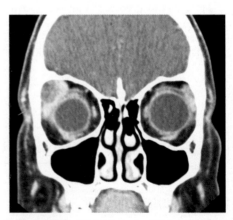

FIGURE 7.6.1. CT of right lacrimal gland adenoid cystic carcinoma.

tumor (pleomorphic adenoma), or secondarily, as a recurrence of a previously resected benign mixed tumor. CT findings are similar to those for adenoid cystic carcinoma.

■ Lacrimal gland cyst (dacryops): Usually an asymptomatic mass that may fluctuate in size. Typically occurs in a young adult or middle-aged patient.

■ Others: Tuberculosis, syphilis, leukemia, mumps, mucoepidermoid carcinoma, plasmacytoma, metastasis.

NOTE: Primary neoplasms (except lymphoma) are almost always unilateral; inflammatory disease may be bilateral. Lymphoma is more commonly unilateral, but may be bilateral.

Work-Up

1. History: Determine the duration of the abnormality and rate of progression. Associated pain, tenderness, double vision? Weakness, weight loss, fever, or other signs of systemic malignancy? Breathing difficulty, skin rash, or history of uveitis (sarcoidosis)? Any known medical problems? Prior lacrimal gland biopsy or surgery?

2. Complete ocular examination: Specifically look for keratic precipitates, iris nodules, posterior synechiae, and old retinal periphlebitis from sarcoidosis.

3. Orbital CT (axial and coronal views): MRI is rarely required unless intracranial extension is suspected. CT is helpful in defining bony anatomy and abnormality.

4. Consider a chest radiograph or chest CT, which may diagnose sarcoidosis, primary malignancy, lymphoproliferative disease, metastatic disease, and, rarely, tuberculosis.

5. Consider CBC with differential, ACE, cANCA, SPEP, RPR, FTA-ABS, and PPD with anergy panel if clinical history suggests a specific etiology. In most cases, ACE level suffices.

6. Lacrimal gland biopsy is indicated when a malignant tumor is suspected, or if the diagnosis is uncertain.

7. Systemic work-up by an internist or hematologist/oncologist when lymphoma is suspected (e.g., abdominal and head CT scan, possible bone marrow biopsy).

NOTE: Do not perform an incisional biopsy on lesions thought to be benign mixed tumors or dermoid cysts. Incomplete excision of a benign mixed tumor may lead to a recurrence with or without malignant transformation. Rupture of a dermoid cyst may lead to a severe inflammatory reaction. These two lesions must be completely excised without rupturing the capsule or pseudocapsule.

Treatment

1. Sarcoidosis: Systemic corticosteroids or low-dose antimetabolite therapy. See 12.6, *Sarcoidosis*.

2. IOIS: Systemic corticosteroids. See 7.2.2, *Idiopathic Orbital Inflammatory Syndrome*.

3. Benign mixed epithelial tumor: Complete surgical removal.

4. Dermoid cyst: Complete surgical removal.

5. Lymphoma:
   —Confined to the orbit: Orbital irradiation, corticosteroids in indolent cases, systemic surveillance.

   —Systemic involvement: Chemotherapy. Orbital irradiation is usually withheld until the response of the orbital lesion to chemotherapy can be evaluated.

6. Adenoid cystic carcinoma: Consider orbital exenteration with irradiation. Systemic chemotherapy is used. Consider pretreatment with intraarterial cisplatinum, followed by wide excision, including exenteration and possible craniectomy. Proton beam radiotherapy is offered by some centers. Regardless of the treatment regimen, prognosis is guarded and recurrence is the rule. There is no clear evidence that wide craniofacial resection improves survival. Survival appears to be most dependent on specific tumor subtype.

7. Malignant mixed epithelial tumor: Same as for adenoid cystic carcinoma.

8. Lacrimal gland cyst: Excise if symptomatic.

Follow-Up

Depends on the specific cause.

7

7.7	**MISCELLANEOUS ORBITAL DISEASES**

1. Intracranial disease. Extension of intracranial tumors, usually frontal lobe or sphenoid wing meningiomas, may present with proptosis in addition to cranial neuropathy and decreased vision. Imaging, preferably with MRI, is indicated.

2. Arteriovenous fistula (AVF) (e.g., carotid–cavernous or dural sinus fistula): AVF is either spontaneous (usually in older patients) or post-traumatic (in younger patients). A bruit is sometimes heard by the patient and may be detected if ocular auscultation is performed. Pulsating proptosis, arterialized "corkscrew" conjunctival vessels, increased IOP, retinal venous congestion, and chemosis may be present. May mimic orbital disease, including TED and IOS. In early stages, often misdiagnosed as conjunctivitis, asymmetric glaucoma, etc. CT scan reveals enlarged superior ophthalmic vein, sometimes accompanied by enlarged extraocular muscles. Orbital color Doppler US shows reversed, arterialized flow in superior ophthalmic vein. MRA or CTA may reveal AVF but definitive diagnosis usually requires arteriography. Evidence of posterior cortical venous outflow on arteriography increases the risk of hemorrhagic stroke.

3. Septic cavernous sinus thrombosis: Orbital cellulitis signs, plus dilated and sluggish pupils as well as palsies of the third, fourth, fifth, and sixth cranial nerves out of proportion to the degree of orbital edema. Decreasing level of consciousness, nausea, vomiting, and fevers may be seen. May be bilateral with rapid progression.

4. Orbital vasculitis (e.g., Wegener granulomatosis, polyarteritis nodosa): Systemic signs and symptoms of vasculitis (especially sinus, renal, pulmonary, and skin disease), fever, markedly increased ESR, positive cANCA, or pANCA. cANCA may be normal in one-third of patients with limited sino-orbital Wegener granulomatosis.

5. Varix: A large, dilated vein in the orbit that produces proptosis when it fills and dilates (e.g., during a Valsalva maneuver or with the head in a dependent position). When the vein is not engorged, the proptosis disappears. CT demonstrates the dilated vein if an enhanced scan is performed during a Valsalva maneuver. Calcification may be seen in long-standing lesions.

6. Poorly understood processes:

   ▪ Tolosa Hunt syndrome: NOT equivalent to orbital apical IOIS. Histopathologically, a granulomatous inflammation of the orbital apex and/or carotid siphon within the cavernous sinus. Presents with acute pain, cranial neuropathy, and sometimes proptosis. A diagnosis of exclusion. Difficult to diagnose with CT. MRI shows isolated ipsilateral enlargement of the cavernous sinus. Usually sensitive to corticosteroid therapy, but may not respond as rapidly as IOIS. Because confirmatory biopsy is usually not feasible, every patient with presumed Tolosa Hunt syndrome must be followed long term, even after rapid response to corticosteroids, to rule out other etiologies. Repeat imaging is usually indicated several months after the initial event to rule out progression. Presumed Tolosa Hunt syndrome recurs in a minority of patients.

   ▪ Sclerosing orbital pseudotumor: Likely not a true orbital inflammation and certainly not a subtype of IOIS. Presents with chronic pain, external ophthalmoplegia, and possibly optic neuropathy. Diagnosis requires biopsy. Histopathology shows wide swaths of monotonous fibrous tissue interspersed with mild inflammation. Treatment is difficult and may necessitate antimetabolite therapy, debulking, and in severe cases, exenteration.

   ▪ Orbital amyloid: May be primary (isolated) or secondary to systemic disease. All patients require a systemic work-up, including a cardiology consult to rule out cardiomyopathy. Diagnosis is made by judicious orbital biopsy (this lesion is highly vascular and hemostasis is often difficult to obtain). Treatment is highly variable.

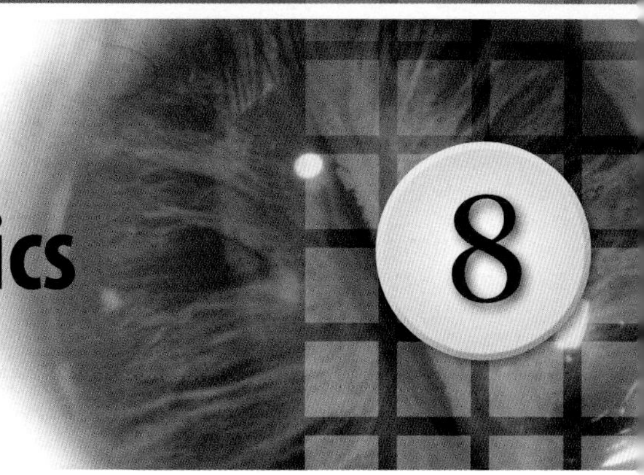

Pediatrics 8

8.1   LEUKOCORIA

Definition

A white pupillary reflex (see Figure 8.1.1).

Etiology

- Retinoblastoma: A malignant tumor of the retina that appears as a white, nodular mass that breaks through the internal limiting membrane into the vitreous (endophytic), as a yellowish subretinal mass lesion often underlying a serous retinal detachment (exophytic), or as a diffusely spreading lesion simulating uveitis (diffuse infiltrating). Iris neovascularization is common. Pseudohypopyon and vitreous seeding may occur. Cataract is uncommon, and the eye is normal in size. May be bilateral, unilateral, or multifocal. Diagnosis is usually made between 12 and 24 months of age. A family history may be elicited in about 10%.

- Toxocariasis: A nematode infection that may appear as a localized, white, elevated granuloma in the retina or as a diffuse endophthalmitis. Associated with localized inflammation of ocular structures, vitreous traction bands and related macular dragging, traction retinal detachment, and cataract. It is rarely bilateral and is usually diagnosed between 6 months and 10 years of age. Paracentesis of the anterior chamber may reveal eosinophils; serum enzyme-linked immunosorbent assay (ELISA) test for Toxocara organisms is positive. The patient may have a history of contact with puppies or eating dirt. Toxocariasis may also be acquired prenatally and present as a congenital infection.

- Coats disease (see Figure 8.1.2): A retinal vascular abnormality resulting in small multifocal outpouchings of the retinal vessels. Leukocoria may develop secondary to an exudative retinal detachment or to extensive yellow intraretinal and subretinal exudate. Usually develops in boys during the first decade of life; more severe cases

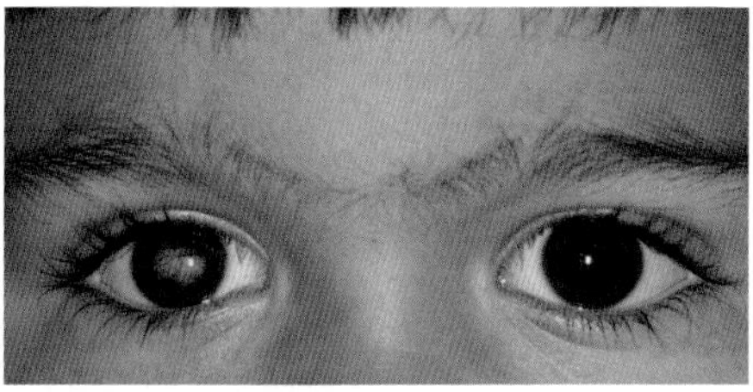

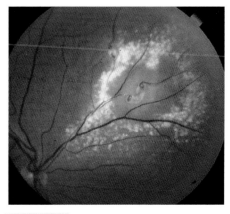

FIGURE 8.1.1. Leukocoria.

FIGURE 8.1.2. Coats disease.

occur in early childhood. Coats disease is rarely bilateral. No family history.

■ Persistent fetal vasculature (PFV)/persistent hyperplastic primary vitreous (PHPV): A developmental ocular abnormality consisting of a varied degree of glial and vascular proliferation in the vitreous cavity. It is usually associated with a slightly small eye. Typically there is a membrane behind the lens that may place traction on the ciliary processes. This is a progressive condition with a cataract present at birth or early in life. The membrane and lens may rotate anteriorly, shallowing the anterior chamber and resulting in secondary glaucoma. Retinal detachments may be seen. Rarely bilateral. No family history.

■ Congenital cataract: Opacity of the lens present at birth; may be unilateral or bilateral. There may be a family history or an associated systemic disorder. See 8.8, *Congenital Cataract.*

■ Retinal astrocytoma: A sessile to slightly elevated, yellow-white retinal mass that may be calcified and is often associated with tuberous sclerosis and rarely neurofibromatosis. May occur on the optic nerve head (giant drusen) in patients with tuberous sclerosis.

■ Retinopathy of prematurity (ROP): Predominantly occurs in premature children. Leukocoria is usually the result of a retinal detachment. See 8.2, *Retinopathy of Prematurity.*

■ Others: Retinochoroidal coloboma, retinal detachment, familial exudative vitreoretinopathy (FEVR), myelinated nerve fibers, uveitis, incontinentia pigmenti, toxoplasmosis.

Work-Up

1. History: Age at onset? Family history of one of the conditions mentioned? Prematurity? Contact with puppies or habit of eating dirt?

2. Complete ocular examination, including a measurement of corneal diameters (look for a small eye), an examination of the iris (look for neovascularization), and an inspection of the lens (look for a cataract). A dilated fundus examination and anterior vitreous examination are essential.

3. Any or all of the following may be helpful in diagnosis and planning treatment:

—B-scan ultrasonography (US), especially if there is no view of the fundus. This can be used to look for calcification within a suspected lesion.

—Intravenous fluorescein angiogram (Coats disease, ROP, retinoblastoma).

—Computed tomographic (CT) scan or magnetic resonance imaging (MRI) of the orbit and brain (retinoblastoma), particularly for bilateral cases or those with a family history, as well as for cases of advanced Coats disease.

—Serum ELISA test for Toxocara (positive at 1:8 in the vast majority of infected patients).

—Systemic examination (retinal astrocytoma, retinoblastoma) by pediatrician.

—Anterior chamber paracentesis (toxocariasis). See Appendix 13, *Anterior Chamber Paracentesis.*

NOTE: Anterior chamber paracentesis in a patient with a retinoblastoma can possibly lead to tumor cell dissemination.

---

4. Consider examination under anesthesia (EUA) in young or uncooperative children, particularly when retinoblastoma, toxocariasis, Coats disease, or ROP is being considered as a diagnosis. See 8.8, *Congenital Cataract,* for a more specific cataract work-up.

Treatment

1. **Retinoblastoma:** Chemoreduction, intraarterial chemotherapy, cryotherapy, thermotherapy, laser photocoagulation, or plaque radiotherapy. These treatment modalities are typically used in combination. Enucleation is now reserved for cases not amenable to the above treatment options. Systemic chemotherapy is used in metastatic disease.

Irradiation is no longer used as it is associated with a high incidence of secondary tumors later in life.

2. **Toxocariasis:**

—Steroids (topical, periocular, or systemic routes may be used, depending on the severity of the inflammation).

—Consider a surgical vitrectomy when vitreoretinal traction bands form or when the condition does not improve or worsens with medical therapy.

—Consider laser photocoagulation of the nematode if it is visible.

3. **Coats disease:** Laser photocoagulation or cryotherapy to leaking vessels. Though associated with a poor outcome, surgery may be required for a retinal detachment.

4. **PFV/PHPV:**

—Cataract and retrolental glial membrane extraction.

—Treat any amblyopia, though visual outcome is often poor secondary to foveal hypoplasia associated with PFV.

5. **Congenital cataract:** See 8.8, *Congenital Cataract.*

6. **Retinal astrocytoma:** Observation.

7. **ROP:** See 8.2, *Retinopathy of Prematurity.*

Follow-Up

Variable, depending on the diagnosis.

8.2 RETINOPATHY OF PREMATURITY

Risk Factors

■ Prematurity, especially <32 weeks of gestation.

■ Birthweight <1,500 g (3 lb, 5 oz), especially <1,250 g (2 lb, 12 oz).

■ Supplemental oxygen therapy, neonatal sepsis, hypoxemia, hypercarbia, and concurrent illness.

■ Risk factors mentioned above, when present concurrently, have an additive effect on the risk for development of ROP.

Signs

Critical. Avascular peripheral retina. Demarcation line between vascular and avascular retina.

Other. Extraretinal fibrovascular proliferation, vitreous hemorrhage, retinal detachment, or leukocoria, sometimes bilateral. Engorgement and tortuosity of the vessels in the posterior pole and/or iris in plus disease. Poor pupillary dilation despite mydriatic drops. In older children and adults, decreased visual acuity, amblyopia, myopia, strabismus, macular dragging, lattice-like vitreoretinal degeneration, or retinal detachment may occur.

Differential Diagnosis

■ FEVR: Appears similar to ROP, except FEVR is most commonly autosomal dominant (though family members may be asymptomatic); asymptomatic family members often show peripheral retinal vascular abnormalities. There usually is no history of prematurity or oxygen therapy. See 8.3, *Familial Exudative Vitreoretinopathy.*

■ Incontinentia pigmenti: X-linked dominant condition that only occurs in girls. Lethal in males. Characterized by skin changes including erythematous macular papular lesions, vesicles, hypopigmented patches, and alopecia. Central nervous system and dental abnormalities may be seen.

■ See 8.1, *Leukocoria,* for additional differential diagnoses.

Classification

Location

■ **Zone I: Posterior pole:** Twice the disc–fovea distance, centered around the disc (poorest prognosis).

8

NOTE: With the nasal edge of the optic disc at one edge of the field of view with a 28D lens, the limit of Zone I is at the temporal field of view.

- **Zone II:** From zone I to the nasal ora serrata; temporally equidistant from the disc.

NOTE: ROP should not be considered zone III until one is sure the nasal side is vascularized to the ora serrata.

- **Zone III:** The remaining temporal periphery.

Extent
- Number of clock hours (30-degree sectors) involved.

Severity
- **Stage 1:** Flat demarcation line separating the vascular posterior retina from the avascular peripheral retina (see Figure 8.2.1).
- **Stage 2:** Ridged demarcation line.
- **Stage 3:** Ridged demarcation line with fibrovascular proliferation or neovascularization extending from the ridge into the vitreous (see Figure 8.2.2).
- **Stage 4A:** Extrafoveal partial retinal detachment.

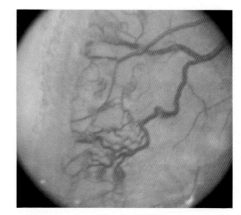

FIGURE 8.2.2. Retinopathy of prematurity: Stage 3.

- **Stage 4B:** Foveal partial retinal detachment.
- **Stage 5:** Total retinal detachment.

NOTE: The overall stage is determined by the most severe manifestation, however, it is recommended to define each stage and record its extent.

"Plus" Disease
(See Figure 8.2.3.)
At least two quadrants of engorged veins and tortuous arteries in the posterior pole; iris vascular engorgement, poor pupil dilatation, and vitreous haze with more advanced plus disease. If plus disease is present, a "+" is placed

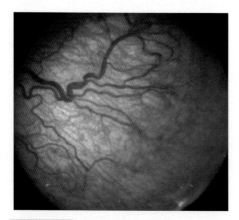

FIGURE 8.2.1. Retinopathy of prematurity: Stage 1.

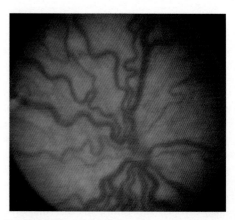

FIGURE 8.2.3. Retinopathy of prematurity: Plus disease.

after the stage (e.g., stage 3+). If vascular dilatation and tortuosity are present but inadequate to diagnose plus disease, it is called "pre-plus" disease and noted after the stage (e.g., stage 3 with pre-plus disease). Posterior ROP (usually Zone I) with plus disease out of proportion to the peripheral retinopathy, or so-called "rush" disease (also known as aggressive posterior disease), may progress rapidly to stage 5 ROP without passing through the other stages. This aggressive ROP may also show hemorrhages at the junction between vascular and avascular retina.

Threshold Disease

Defines high-risk eyes that meet the criteria for treatment:

—Zone I, any stage with plus disease.

—Zone I, stage 3, no plus disease.

—Zone II, stage 2 or 3 with plus disease.

Prethreshold Disease

Defines less severely advanced eyes that should be monitored closely for progression to threshold disease:

—Zone I, stage 1 and 2 without plus disease.

—Zone II, stage 3 without plus disease.

Screening Recommendations

■ Birth weight <1,500 g.

■ Gestational age ≤32 weeks.

■ Selected infants with birth weight of 1,500 to 2,000 g or gestational age ≥32 weeks with unstable clinical course thought to be at high risk.

■ Timing of first eye examination is based on gestational age at birth.

Work-Up

1. Dilated retinal examination with scleral depression at 31 to 32 weeks after date of mother's last menstrual period, or 4 weeks after birth, whichever is later.

2. Can dilate with combination phenylephrine 1.0% and cyclopentolate 0.2%.

Treatment

Based on severity. The presence of plus disease is typically an indication for early treatment.

1. Prethreshold disease: Close observation.

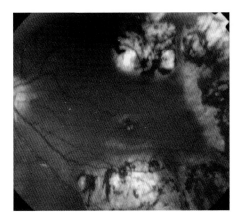

FIGURE 8.2.4. Retinopathy of prematurity after laser treatment.

2. Threshold disease: Ablative treatment of avascular zone of retina. Laser photocoagulation is preferred over cryotherapy. Treatment should be instituted within 72 hours (see Figure 8.2.4).

3. Stages 4 and 5: Surgical repair of retinal detachment by scleral buckling, vitrectomy surgery, or both.

Follow-Up

■ One week or less: Zone I, stage 1 or 2; or zone II, stage 3.

■ One to 2 weeks: Immature vascularization, zone I; or zone II, stage 2; or zone I, regressing ROP.

■ Two weeks: Zone II, stage 1; or zone II, regressing ROP.

■ Two to 3 weeks: Immature vascularization, zone II, no ROP; or zone III, stage 1 or 2; or zone III, regressing ROP.

1. Children who have had ROP have a higher incidence of myopia, strabismus, amblyopia, macular dragging, cataracts, glaucoma, and retinal detachment. An untreated fully vascularized fundus needs examination at age 6 months to rule out these complications.

NOTE: Because of the possibility of late retinal detachments and other ocular complications, ROP patients should be followed at yearly intervals for life.

8

2. Acute-phase ROP screening can be discontinued when any of the following signs is present, indicating that the risk of visual loss from ROP is minimal or passed:

—Zone III retinal vascularization attained without previous zone I or II ROP. If there is doubt about the zone or if the postmenstrual age is unexpectedly young, confirmatory examinations may be warranted.

—Full retinal vascularization.

—Postmenstrual age of 45 weeks and no prethreshold or worse ROP.

8.3 FAMILIAL EXUDATIVE VITREORETINOPATHY

Symptoms

Majority are asymptomatic, but patients may report decreased vision.

Signs

(See Figure 8.3.1.)

Critical. Peripheral retinal capillary nonperfusion, most prominently temporally, and may be present for 360 degrees. Bilateral but may be asymmetric. Peripheral retinal vessels have a fimbriated border. Present at birth.

Other. Peripheral neovascularization and/or fibrovascular proliferation at the border of vascular and avascular retina; temporal dragging of macula through contraction of fibrovascular tissue; vitreous hemorrhage; tractional, exudative, or rhegmatogenous retinal detachment; peripheral intraretinal and subretinal lipid exudation. May present with strabismus or leukocoria in childhood. Cataract, band keratopathy, neovascular glaucoma, or phthisis possible.

Differential Diagnosis

■ Retinopathy of prematurity: Appears similar to FEVR, but there should be no family history, and there should be a history of prematurity. See 8.2, *Retinopathy of Prematurity.*

■ See 8.1, *Leukocoria,* for additional differential diagnosis, e.g., retinoblastoma, Coats, PFV/PHPV, incontinentia pigmenti, Norrie disease, X-linked retinoschisis, and peripheral retinal nonperfusion. Positive family history and bilaterality can help distinguish from others.

Etiology

Due to defects in the Wnt signaling pathway. Usually autosomal dominant, though autosomal recessive, and X-linked cases have been reported. No history of prematurity or oxygen therapy. FEVR is similar to ROP, histologically.

Work-Up

1. History: Positive family history? No history of prematurity or oxygen therapy?

2. Complete ocular examination, including dilated retinal examination with a slit lamp and a 60- or 90-diopter lens looking for temporal dragging of the macula. Indirect ophthalmoscopy looking for peripheral nonperfusion, fibrovascular membranes, tractional retinal detachment. All family members should also have dilated retinal examinations.

Treatment

Laser of peripheral nonperfused retina is sometimes considered if there is documented

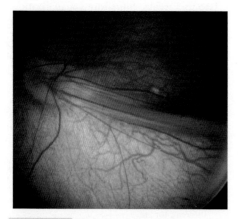

FIGURE 8.3.1. FEVR with a falciform fold.

progression. Small, stable tufts of neovascularization can be observed. Scleral buckling and vitrectomy can be considered for retinal detachments. Often complicated by proliferative vitreoretinopathy. Treat amblyopia as needed.

Follow-Up

Asymptomatic patients should be followed every 6 to 12 months throughout life to monitor for progression.

8.4   ESODEVIATIONS IN CHILDREN

Signs

(See Figure 8.4.1.)

Critical. Either eye is turned inward. The nonfixating eye turns outward to fixate straight ahead when the previously fixating eye is covered during the cover–uncover test. See Appendix 3, *Cover/Uncover and Alternate Cover Tests.*

Other. Amblyopia, overaction of the inferior oblique muscles.

Differential Diagnosis

- Pseudoesotropia: The eyes appear esotropic; however, there is no ocular misalignment detected during cover–uncover testing. Usually, the child has a wide nasal bridge, prominent epicanthal folds, or a small interpupillary distance (see Figure 8.4.2).

- See 8.6, *Strabismus Syndromes.*

Types

Comitant or Concomitant Esotropic Deviations

A manifest convergent misalignment of the eyes in which the measured angle of esodeviation is nearly constant in all fields of gaze at distance fixation.

1. **Congenital (infantile) esotropia:** Manifests by age 6 months, the angle of esodeviation is usually large (>40 to 50 prism diopters) and mostly equal at distance and near fixation. Refractive error is usually normal for age (slightly hyperopic). Amblyopia is uncommon but may be present in those who do not cross-fixate. Family history may be present but is not mandatory. Latent nystagmus, inferior oblique overaction, and dissociated vertical deviation may develop as late findings. Congenital esotropia can occur in up to 30% of children with neurological and developmental disorders (e.g., cerebral palsy, hydrocephalus).

2. **Accommodative esotropia:** Convergent misalignment of the eyes associated with activation of the accommodative reflex. Average age of onset is 2.5 years.

Subtypes of accommodative esotropia:

—Refractive accommodative esotropia: These children are hyperopic in the range of +3.00 to +10.00 diopters (average, +4.75). The measured angle of esodeviation is usually moderate (20- to 30-prism diopters) and is relatively equal at distance and near

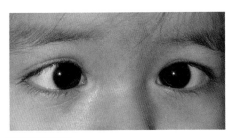

FIGURE 8.4.1. Esotropia.

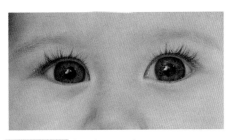

FIGURE 8.4.2. Pseudoesotropia.

fixation. Full hyperopic correction elimi-nates the esodeviation. The accommoda-tive convergence–accommodation angle ratio (AC/A) is normal. Amblyopia is com-mon at presentation.

—Nonrefractive accommodative esotropia (high AC/A ratio): The measured angle of esodeviation is greater at near fixation than at distance fixation. The refractive error may range from normal for age (slight hyperopia) to high hyperopia (may be seen in conjunc-tion with refractive-type accommodative esotropia) or even myopia. Amblyopia is common.

—Partial or decompensated accommoda-tive esotropia: Refractive and nonrefrac-tive accommodative esotropias that have a reduction in the esodeviation when given full hyperopic correction, but still have a residual esodeviation. The residual esodeviation is the nonaccommodative component.

3. **Sensory-deprivation esotropia:** An esode-viation that occurs in a patient with a mon-ocular or binocular condition that prevents good vision.

4. **Divergence insufficiency:** A convergent ocular misalignment that is greater at dis-tance fixation than at near fixation. This is a diagnosis of exclusion and must be differ-entiated from divergence paralysis, which, when sudden in onset, can be associated with pontine tumors, neurologic trauma, and elevated intracranial pressure. See 10.8, *Isolated Sixth Nerve Palsy.*

Incomitant Esodeviations

The measured angle of esodeviation increases in lateral gaze at distance fixation.

1. Central nervous system pathology caus-ing increased intracranial pressure: Acute and new onset of diplopia secondary to an acquired sixth nerve palsy, which may be accompanied by nystagmus, headache, or other focal neurologic deficits depending on etiology.

2. Medial rectus restriction (e.g., thyroid disease, medial orbital wall fracture with entrapment).

3. Lateral rectus weakness (e.g., isolated sixth cranial nerve palsy, slipped or detached lat-eral rectus from trauma or previous surgery).

4. See 8.6, *Strabismus Syndromes,* and 10.8, *Isolated Sixth Nerve Palsy,* for additional etiologies.

Other

1. Esophoria: Latent esodeviation controlled by fusion. Eyes are aligned under binocular conditions.

2. Intermittent esotropia: Esodeviation that is intermittently controlled by fusion. Becomes manifest spontaneously, especial-ly with fatigue or illness.

Work-Up

1. History: Age of onset, frequency of cross-ing, prior therapy (e.g., glasses, patching).

2. Visual acuity of each eye, with best correction and pinhole. Color vision and stereopsis.

3. Ocular motility examination; observe for restricted movements or oblique overactions.

4. Measure the distance deviation in all fields of gaze and the near deviation in the pri-mary position (straight ahead) using prisms (see Appendix 3, *Cover/Uncover and Alter-nate Cover Tests*). Look specifically for an esotropia increasing in either side gaze.

5. Manifest and cycloplegic refractions espe-cially if <7 years of age.

6. Complete eye examination. Look for any cranial nerve abnormalities and causes of sensory deprivation.

7. If acute-onset non-accommodative esotro-pia, divergence insufficiency or paralysis, paralysis, or incomitant esotropia is pres-ent, a head CT scan (axial and coronal views) and/or an MRI is necessary to rule out an intracranial or orbital process, extra-ocular muscle pathology, or bony lesion.

8. With incomitant esodeviation greater in side gaze, determine whether the lateral rectus function is deficient or the medial rectus is restricted. Forced-duction testing may be necessary for that distinction (see Appendix 6, *Forced-Duction Test and Active*

Force Generation Test). This may need to be done under anesthesia for children. Consider thyroid function tests or a work-up for myasthenia gravis, or look for characteristics of strabismus syndromes (see 8.6, *Strabismus Syndromes*).

Treatment

In all cases, correct refractive errors of +2.00 diopters or more, and in children treat any amblyopia (see 8.7, *Amblyopia*).

1. Congenital esotropia: When equal vision is obtained in the two eyes, strabismus surgery is indicated.

2. Accommodative esotropia: Glasses must be worn full time.

   a. If the patient is <6 years, correct the hyperopia with the full cycloplegic refraction.

   b. If the patient is >6 years, attempts should be made to give as close to the full-plus refraction as possible, knowing that some may not tolerate the full prescription. Attempts to push plus lenses during the manifest (noncycloplegic) refraction until distance vision blurs may be tried to give the most plus lenses without blurring distance vision. The goal of refractive correction should be straight alignment without sacrificing visual acuity.

   c. If the patient's eyes are straight at distance with full correction, but still esotropic at near fixation (high AC/A ratio), treatment options include the following:

      • Bifocals (executive type) +2.50 or +3.00 diopter add, with top of the bifocal at the lower pupillary border.

      • Extraocular muscle surgery targeting the near deviation only may be indicated. This typically requires posterior fixation sutures to the muscle to modify the surgical effect for near only.

      • Wearing full-plus distance glasses only.

      NOTE: There is no universal agreement on the treatment of patients with excess crossing at near only.
      ---

3. Non-accommodative, partially accommodative, or decompensated accommodative esotropia: Muscle surgery is usually performed to correct only the significant residual esotropia that remains when glasses are worn.

4. Sensory-deprivation esotropia:

   • Attempt to identify and correct the cause of poor vision.

   • Amblyopia treatment.

   • Give the full cycloplegic correction (in fixing eye) if the patient is <6 years of age, otherwise give the full manifest refraction.

   • Muscle surgery to correct the manifest esotropia.

   • All patients with very poor vision in one eye need to wear protective polycarbonate lens glasses at all times.

Follow-Up

At each visit, evaluate for amblyopia and measure the degree of deviation with prisms (with glasses worn).

1. If amblyopia is present, see 8.7, *Amblyopia*, for management.

2. In the absence of amblyopia, the child is reevaluated in 3 to 6 weeks after a new prescription is given. If no changes are made and the eyes are straight, the patient should be followed several times a year when young, decreasing to annually when stable.

3. When a residual esotropia is present while the patient wears glasses, an attempt is made to add more plus power to the current prescription. Children <6 years should receive a new cycloplegic refraction; plus lenses are pushed without cycloplegia in older children. The maximal additional plus lens that does not blur distance vision is prescribed. If the eyes cannot be straightened with more plus power, then a decompensated accommodative esotropia has developed (see preceding).

4. Hyperopia often decreases slowly after age 5 to 7 years, and the strength of the glasses may need to be reduced so as not to blur distance vision. If the strength of the glasses must be reduced to improve visual acuity and the esotropia returns, then this is a decompensated accommodative esotropia (see preceding).

8

8.5   EXODEVIATIONS IN CHILDREN

Signs

(See Figure 8.5.1.)

Critical.   Either eye is constantly or intermittently turned outward. On the cover–uncover test, the uncovered eye moves from the outturned position to the midline to fixate when the previously fixating eye is covered (see Appendix 3, *Cover/Uncover and Alternate Cover Tests*).

Other.   Amblyopia, "A" pattern deviation (superior oblique overaction producing an increased deviation in downgaze compared to upgaze), "V" pattern deviation (inferior oblique overaction producing an increased deviation in upgaze compared to downgaze), vertical deviation.

Differential Diagnosis

Pseudoexotropia: The patient appears to have an exodeviation, but no movement is noted on cover–uncover testing despite good vision in each eye. A wide interpupillary distance, a naturally large angle κ (angle between the pupil and the visual axis), or temporal dragging of the macula (e.g., from ROP, FEVR, toxocariasis, or other retinal disorders) may be responsible.

Types

1. Exophoria: Exodeviation controlled by fusion under conditions of normal binocular vision. Usually asymptomatic, but prolonged strenuous visual activity may cause asthenopia.

2. Intermittent exotropia: The most common type of exodeviation in children. Onset is usually before age 5. Frequency often increases over time. Amblyopia is rare.

A. There are three phases:

—Phase 1: One eye turns out at distance fixation, spontaneously or when it is covered. Usually occurs when the patient is fatigued, sick, or not attentive. The eyes become straight within one to two blinks or when the cover is removed. The eyes are straight at near fixation. Patient often closes one eye or squints in bright sunlight. This is likely due to dissociation and breakdown of their binocular alignment.

—Phase 2: Increasing frequency of exotropia at distance fixation. Exophoria begins to occur at near fixation.

—Phase 3: There is a constant exotropia at distance and near fixations.

B. These phases can be seen in all four types of intermittent exotropia:

—Basic: Exodeviation is approximately the same with distance and near fixation.

—True divergence excess: Exodeviation that remains greater at distance than near after a period of monocular occlusion.

—Simulated divergence excess: Exodeviation that is initially greater with distance fixation than near that becomes approximately the same after an interval of monocular occlusion.

—Convergence insufficiency: Exodeviation is greater at near than distance. Distinct from isolated convergence insufficiency. See 13.4, *Convergence Insufficiency*.

3. Constant exotropia: Encountered more often in older children. There are three types:

—Congenital exotropia: presents before age 6 months with a large angle deviation.

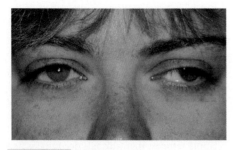

FIGURE 8.5.1. Exotropia.

Uncommon in otherwise healthy infants and may be associated with a central nervous system or craniofacial disorder.

—Sensory-deprivation exotropia: An eye that does not see well for any reason may turn outward.

—Consecutive exotropia: Follows previous surgery for esotropia.

4. Duane syndrome, type 2: Limitation of adduction of one eye, with globe retraction and narrowing of the palpebral fissure on attempted adduction. Rarely bilateral. See 8.6, *Strabismus Syndromes.*

5. Neuromuscular abnormalities:

—Third nerve palsy: See 10.5, *Isolated Third Nerve Palsy.*

—Myasthenia gravis: See 10.11, *Myasthenia Gravis.*

—Internuclear ophthalmoplegia: See 10.13, *Internuclear Ophthalmoplegia.*

6. Dissociated Horizontal Deviation: A change in horizontal ocular alignment caused by a change in the balance of visual input from the two eyes. Not related to accommodation. Seen clinically as a spontaneous unilateral exodeviation or an exodeviation of greater magnitude in one eye during prism and alternate cover testing.

7. Orbital disease (e.g., tumor, idiopathic orbital inflammatory syndrome): Proptosis and restriction of ocular motility are usually evident. See 7.1, *Orbital Disease.*

8. Isolated convergence insufficiency: Usually occurs in patients >10 years. Blurred near vision, asthenopia, or diplopia when reading. An exophoria at near fixation, but straight or small exophoria at distance fixation. Must be differentiated from convergence paralysis. See 13.4, *Convergence Insufficiency.*

9. Convergence paralysis: Similar to convergence insufficiency, but with a relatively acute onset, an exotropia at near, and an inability to overcome base out prism. Often secondary to an intracranial lesion.

Work-Up

1. Evaluate visual acuity of each eye, with correction and pinhole, to evaluate for amblyopia. Color vision and stereopsis.

2. Perform motility examination; observing for restricted eye movements or signs of Duane syndrome.

3. Measure the exodeviation in all cardinal fields of gaze at distance and in primary position (straight ahead) at near, using prisms. See Appendix 3, *Cover/Uncover and Alternate Cover Tests.*

4. Perform pupillary, slit-lamp, and fundus examinations; check for causes of sensory deprivation (if poor vision).

5. Refraction (cycloplegic or manifest depending on age of the patient).

6. Consider work-up for myasthenia gravis when suspected by evidence of fatigability. See 10.11, *Myasthenia Gravis.*

7. Consider a CT scan (axial and coronal views) or an MRI of the orbit and brain, when orbital or neurologic disease is suspected.

Treatment

In all cases, correct significant refractive errors and treat amblyopia. See 8.7, *Amblyopia.*

1. Exophoria:

—No treatment necessary unless it progresses to intermittent exotropia.

2. Intermittent exotropia:

—Phase 1: Follow patient closely.

—Phase 2: Muscle surgery may be considered to maintain normal binocular vision.

—Phase 3: Muscle surgery is often indicated at this point. Bifixation or peripheral fusion can occasionally be attained.

3. Sensory-deprivation exotropia:

—Correct the underlying cause, if possible.

—Treat any amblyopia.

—Muscle surgery may be performed for manifest exotropia.

8

—When one eye has very poor vision, protective glasses (polycarbonate lens glasses) should be worn at all times to protect the good eye.

4. Congenital exotropia:

—Muscle surgery early in life, as in patients with congenital esotropia.

5. Consecutive exotropia:

—Additional muscle surgery may be considered.

—Prism correction in glasses can be used.

—Over-minus or under-plus correction can stimulate accommodative convergence.

6. Dissociated horizontal deviation:

—Muscle surgery may be considered.

7. Duane syndrome: See 8.6, *Strabismus Syndromes*.

8. Third nerve palsy: See 10.5, *Isolated Third Nerve Palsy*.

9. Convergence insufficiency: See 13.4, *Convergence Insufficiency*.

10. Convergence paralysis:

—Base-in prisms at near to alleviate diplopia.

—Plus lenses if accommodation is also weakened.

Follow-Up

1. If amblyopia is present, see 8.7, *Amblyopia*.

2. If no amblyopia is present, then reexamine every 4 to 6 months. The parents and patient are asked to return sooner if the deviation increases, becomes more frequent, stays out longer, or patient begins to close one eye.

---

8 | **8.6** | **STRABISMUS SYNDROMES**

Motility disorders that demonstrate typical features of a particular syndrome.

Syndromes

■ Duane syndrome: A congenital motility disorder, usually unilateral (85%), characterized by limited abduction, limited adduction, or both. The globe retracts and the eyelid fissure narrows on adduction. In unilateral cases, the strabismus will be incomitant and the patient will often adopt a face-turn to allow them to use both eyes together. Classified into three types:

—Type 1 (most common): Limited abduction. Primary position frequently esotropia. In unilateral cases, nearly always with face turn toward affected side.

—Type 2: Limited adduction. Primary position usually exotropia. In unilateral cases, often with face turn away from affected side.

—Type 3: Limited abduction and adduction. Esotropia, exotropia, or no primary position deviation. Significant globe retraction.

■ Brown syndrome: A motility disorder characterized by limitation of elevation in adduction. Elevation in abduction is normal. Typically, eyes are aligned in primary gaze. Usually congenital, but may be acquired secondary to trauma, surgery, or inflammation in the area of the trochlea, or idiopathic. Bilateral in 10% of patients.

■ Monocular elevation deficiency (double-elevator palsy): Congenital. Unilateral limitation of elevation in all fields of gaze secondary to restriction of the inferior rectus or paresis of the inferior oblique and/ or superior rectus. There may be hypotropia of the involved eye that increases in upgaze. Ptosis or pseudoptosis may be present in primary gaze. The patient may assume a chin-up position to maintain fusion if a hypotropia in primary gaze is present.

■ Möbius syndrome: Rare congenital condition associated with both sixth and seventh nerve palsies. Esotropia is usually present.

Limitation of abduction and/or adduction, with a unilateral or bilateral, partial or complete facial nerve palsy. Other cranial nerve palsies as well as deformities of the limbs, chest, and tongue may occur.

- Congenital fibrosis syndrome: Congenital group of disorders with restriction and fibrous replacement of the extraocular muscles. Usually involves all of the extraocular muscles with total external ophthalmoplegia and ptosis. Usually both eyes are directed downward, so the patient assumes a chin-up position to see. Often autosomal dominant.

Work-Up

1. History: Age of onset? History of trauma? Family history? History of other ocular or systemic diseases?

2. Complete ophthalmic examination, including alignment in all fields of gaze. Note head position. Look for retraction of globe and narrowing of interpalpebral fissure in adduction (common in Duane syndrome).

3. Pertinent physical examination, including cranial nerve evaluation.

4. Radiologic studies (e.g., MRI or CT scan) may be indicated for acquired, atypical, or progressive motility disturbances.

5. Forced-duction testing is used to differentiate the two etiologies of monocular elevation deficiency (test will be positive with inferior rectus fibrosis and negative with superior rectus and inferior oblique paresis). Forced ductions can also confirm the diagnosis of Brown syndrome.

Treatment

1. Treatment is usually indicated for a cosmetically significant abnormal head position, or if a significant horizontal or vertical deviation exists in primary gaze.

2. Surgery, when indicated, depends on the particular motility disorder, extraocular muscle function, and the degree of abnormal head position.

Follow-Up

Follow-up depends on the condition or conditions being treated.

8

8.7 AMBLYOPIA

Symptoms

Usually none. Usually found when decreased vision is detected by vision testing in each eye. A history of patching, strabismus, or muscle surgery as a child may be elicited.

NOTE: Amblyopia occasionally occurs bilaterally as a result of bilateral visual deprivation (e.g., congenital cataracts not treated within the first months of life).

Signs

Critical. Poorer vision in one eye that is not improved with refraction and not entirely explained by an organic lesion. The involved eye nearly always has a higher refractive error. The decrease in vision develops during the first several years of life. Central vision is primarily affected, while the peripheral visual field usually remains normal.

Other. Individual letters are more easily read than a full line (crowding phenomenon). In reduced illumination, the visual acuity of an amblyopic eye is reduced much less than an organically diseased eye (neutral-density filter effect).

NOTE: Amblyopia, when severe, may cause a trace relative afferent pupillary defect. Care must be taken to be sure that the light is directed along the same axis in each eye, particularly in patients with strabismus. Directing the light off-axis may result in a false-positive result.

Etiology

- Strabismus: Most common form (along with anisometropia). The eyes are misaligned. Vision is worse in the consistently deviating, nonfixating eye. Strabismus can lead to or be the result of amblyopia.

- Anisometropia: Most common form (along with strabismus). A large difference in refractive error (usually ≥1.50 diopters) between the two eyes. Can be seen in cases of eyelid hemangioma or congenital ptosis inducing astigmatism.

- Media opacity: A unilateral cataract, corneal scar, or PFV/PHPV may cause a preference for the other eye and thereby cause amblyopia.

- Occlusion: Amblyopia that occurs in the fellow eye as a result of too much patching or excessive use of atropine. Prevented by examining at appropriate intervals (1 week per year of age), patching part-time, or using the full cycloplegic refraction when using atropine.

Work-Up

1. History: Eye problem in childhood, such as misaligned eyes, patching, or muscle surgery?

2. Ocular examination to rule out an organic cause for the reduced vision.

3. Cover–uncover test to evaluate eye alignment. See Appendix 3, *Cover/Uncover and Alternate Cover Tests.*

4. Refraction; cycloplegic in children too young to cooperate.

Treatment

1. Patients younger than 12 years:

   —Appropriate spectacle correction (full cycloplegic refraction or reduce the hyperopia in both eyes symmetrically ≥1.50 diopters). If vision remains reduced after period of refractive adaptation (6 to 12 weeks), begin patching or penalization of fellow eye.

   —Patching: Patch the eye with better corrected vision 2 to 6 hours/day for 1 week per year of age (e.g., 3 weeks for a 3-year-old), with at least 1 hour of near activity. Adhesive patches placed directly over the eye are most effective. A patch can be worn over the glasses as long as the child does not peek around the patch. If a patch causes local irritation, use tincture of benzoin on the skin before applying the patch and use warm water compresses on the patch before removal.

   —Penalization with atropine: Atropine 1% once daily (used with glasses) has been shown to be equally effective as patching in mild-to-moderate amblyopia (20/100 or better). If vision does not improve, the effect of the atropine can be increased by removing the hyperopic lens from the glasses of the nonamblyopic eye. If the child is experiencing difficulty with school work with the use of atropine, he/she can wear full hyperopic correction with a +2.50 bifocal during school.

   —Optical degradation: Use a high plus lens (e.g., +9.00 diopters or an aphakic contact lens) to blur the image. If the child is highly myopic, may remove the minus lens from the preferred eye.

   • Continue patching until the vision is equalized or shows no improvement after three compliant cycles of patching. If a recurrence of amblyopia is likely, use part-time patching to maintain improved vision.

   • If occlusion amblyopia (a decrease in vision in the patched eye) develops, patch the opposite eye for a short period (e.g., 1 day per year of age), and repeat the examination.

   —In strabismic amblyopia, delay strabismus surgery until the vision in the two eyes is equal, or maximal vision has been obtained in the amblyopic eye.

2. If treatment of amblyopia fails or patient presents outside of treatment age range, protective glasses should be worn to prevent accidental injury to the nonamblyopic eye. Any child who does not have vision improved to at least 20/40 needs to wear eye protection during sports (one-eyed athlete rule).

3. Treatment of media opacity: Remove the media opacity and begin patching the nonamblyopic eye.

4. Treatment of anisometropic amblyopia: Give the appropriate spectacle correction at the youngest age possible. If vision remains reduced after period of refractive adaptation (6 to 12 weeks), begin patching or penalization of fellow eye.

8.8 CONGENITAL CATARACT

Signs

(See Figure 8.8.1.)

Critical. Opacity of the lens at birth.

Other. A white fundus reflex (leukocoria), absent red pupillary reflex, abnormal eye movements (nystagmus) in one or both eyes, and strabismus. Infants with bilateral cataracts may be noted to be visually inattentive. In patients with a monocular cataract, the involved eye may be smaller. A cataract alone does not cause a relative afferent pupillary defect.

Differential Diagnosis

See 8.1, *Leukocoria.*

Etiology

- Idiopathic (most common).

- Familial, autosomal dominant.

- Galactosemia: Cataract may be the sole manifestation when galactokinase deficiency is responsible. A deficiency of galactose-1-phosphate uridyl transferase may produce mental retardation and symptomatic cirrhosis along with cataracts. The typical oil-droplet opacity may or may not be seen. Cataract may be reversible with appropriate dietary modifications.

- PFV/PHPV: Unilateral. The involved eye is usually slightly smaller than the normal fellow eye. Examination after pupil dilation may reveal a plaque of fibrovascular tissue behind the lens with elongated ciliary processes extending to it. Progression of the lens opacity often leads to angle-closure glaucoma.

- Rubella: "Pearly white" nuclear cataract, "salt-and-pepper" chorioretinitis, microphthalmos, corneal clouding, and poorly dilating pupils. Glaucoma may occur with congenital rubella but usually does not occur in the presence of a rubella cataract. Associated hearing defects and heart abnormalities are common.

- Lowe syndrome (oculocerebrorenal syndrome): Opaque lens, congenital glaucoma, renal disease, and mental retardation. X-linked recessive. Patients' mothers may have small cataracts.

- Others: Chromosomal disorders, systemic syndromes, other intrauterine infections, trauma, drugs, other metabolic abnormalities, aniridia, anterior segment dysgenesis, radiation.

Types

1. Zonular (lamellar): Most common type of congenital cataract. White opacities that surround the nucleus with alternating clear and white cortical lamella like an onion skin.

2. Polar: Small opacities of the lens capsule and adjacent cortex on the anterior or posterior pole of the lens. Anterior polar cataracts usually have little effect on vision and tend to grow very little over time. Posterior polar cataracts are variable and may grow significantly, causing decreased vision.

3. Nuclear: Opacity within the embryonic/ fetal nucleus.

4. Posterior lenticonus: A posterior protrusion, usually opacified, in the posterior capsule.

Work-Up

1. History: Maternal illness or drug ingestion during pregnancy? Systemic or ocular

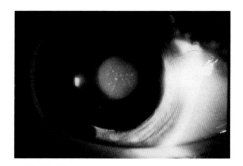

FIGURE 8.8.1. Congenital nuclear cataract.

8

disease in the infant or child? Radiation exposure or trauma? Family history of congenital cataracts?

2. Visual assessment of each eye individually by using techniques for non-verbal children (tumbling E's, pictures, Teller cards, or by following small toys or a light).

3. Ocular examination: Attempt to determine the visual significance of the cataract by evaluating the size and location of the cataract and whether the retina can be seen with a direct ophthalmoscope or retinoscope when looking through an undilated pupil. A blunted retinoscopic reflex suggests the cataract is visually significant. Cataracts ≥3 mm in diameter usually but not always affect vision. Cataracts ≤3 mm may not be visually significant but have been associated with amblyopia secondary to induced anisometropia. Check for signs of associated glaucoma (see 8.11, *Congenital/Infantile Glaucoma*) and examine the optic nerve and retina for abnormalities, if possible.

4. Cycloplegic refraction.

5. B-scan US may be helpful when the fundus view is obscured.

6. Bilateral cataracts suggest a genetic or metabolic etiology; medical examination by a pediatrician looking for associated abnormalities.

7. Red blood cell (RBC) galactokinase activity (galactokinase levels) with or without RBC galactose-1-phosphate uridyl transferase activity to rule out galactosemia. The latter test is performed routinely on all infants in the United States as part of the newborn screen.

8. Other tests as suggested by the systemic or ocular examination. The chance that one of these conditions is present in a healthy child is remote.

—Urine: Amino acid quantitation (Alport syndrome), amino acid content (Lowe syndrome).

—Antibody titers for rubella.

Treatment

1. Referral to a pediatrician to treat any underlying disorder.

2. Treat associated ocular diseases.

3. Cataract extraction, usually within days to weeks of discovery to prevent irreversible amblyopia, is performed in the following circumstances:

—Vision is obstructed, and the eye's visual development is at risk.

—Cataract progression threatens the health of the eye (e.g., in PFV/PHPV).

4. After cataract extraction, treat amblyopia (see 8.7, *Amblyopia*).

5. A dilating agent (e.g., phenylephrine 2.5%, t.i.d., homatropine 2% t.i.d., or scopolamine 0.25% q.d.) may be used as a temporizing measure, allowing peripheral light rays to pass around the lens opacity and reach the retina. This rarely is successful long term.

6. Unilateral cataracts that are not large enough to obscure the visual axis and thus require removal may still result in amblyopia. Treat amblyopia as above.

Follow-Up

1. Infants and young children who do not undergo surgery are monitored closely for cataract progression and amblyopia.

2. Amblyopia is less likely to develop in older children even if the cataract progresses. Therefore, this age group is followed less frequently.

NOTE: Children with rubella must be isolated from pregnant women.

8.9 — OPHTHALMIA NEONATORUM (NEWBORN CONJUNCTIVITIS)

Signs

Critical. Purulent, mucopurulent, or mucoid discharge from one or both eyes in the first month of life with diffuse conjunctival injection.

Other. Eyelid edema, chemosis.

Differential Diagnosis

- Dacryocystitis: Swelling and erythema just below the inner canthus. See 6.9, *Dacryocystitis/Inflammation of the Lacrimal Sac.*

- Nasolacrimal duct obstruction: See 8.10, *Congenital Nasolacrimal Duct Obstruction.*

- Congenital glaucoma: See 8.11, *Congenital/Infantile Glaucoma.*

Etiology

- Chemical: Seen within a few hours of instilling a prophylactic agent (e.g., silver nitrate). Lasts no more than 24 to 36 hours. Rarely seen now that erythromycin is used routinely. Gentamicin should be avoided since it may be associated with a toxic reaction.

- *Neisseria gonorrhoeae:* Usually seen within 3 to 4 days after birth. May present as mild conjunctival hyperemia to severe chemosis, copious discharge, rapid corneal ulceration, or corneal perforation. Gram-negative intracellular diplococci seen on Gram stain.

- *Chlamydia trachomatis:* Usually presents within first week or two of birth with mild swelling, hyperemia, tearing, and primarily a mucoid discharge. May see basophilic intracytoplasmic inclusion bodies in conjunctival epithelial cells, polymorphonuclear leukocytes, or lymphocytes on Giemsa stain. Diagnosis usually made with various molecular tests including immunoassay (e.g., ELISA, EIA, direct antibody tests), PCR, or DNA-hybridization probe.

- Bacteria: Staphylococci (including MRSA), streptococci, and Gram-negative species may be seen on Gram stain.

- Herpes simplex virus: May have typical herpetic vesicles on the eyelid margins. Can see multinucleated giant cells on Giemsa stain.

Work-Up

1. History: Previous or concurrent venereal disease in the mother? Were cervical cultures performed during pregnancy?

2. Ocular examination with a penlight and then a blue light after fluorescein instillation; look for corneal involvement.

3. Conjunctival scrapings for two slides: Gram and Giemsa stain.

   —Technique: Irrigate the discharge out of the fornices, place a drop of topical anesthetic (e.g., proparacaine) in the eye, and scrape the palpebral conjunctiva of the lower eyelid with a flame-sterilized spatula after it cools off, or use a calcium alginate swab. Place the scrapings on the slides.

4. Conjunctival cultures with blood and chocolate agars: Chocolate agar should be placed in an atmosphere of 2% to 10% carbon dioxide immediately after being plated.

   —Technique: Anesthetize the eye. Moisten a calcium alginate swab (a cotton-tipped applicator is a less desirable alternative) with liquid broth media and vigorously rub it along the inferior palpebral conjunctiva. Plate it directly on the culture dish. Repeat for additional cultures.

5. Scrape the conjunctiva for the chlamydial immunofluorescent antibody test or polymerase chain reaction, if available.

6. Viral culture: Moisten another cotton-tipped applicator and roll it along the palpebral conjunctiva. Break off the end of the applicator and place it into the viral transport medium.

7. Systemic evaluation by primary care provider.

Treatment

Initial therapy is based on the results of the Gram and Giemsa stains if they can be

8

examined immediately. Therapy is then modified according to the culture results and the clinical response.

1. No information from stains, no particular organism suspected: Erythromycin ointment q.i.d. plus erythromycin elixir 50 mg/kg/day in four divided doses for 2 to 3 weeks.

2. Suspect chemical (e.g., silver nitrate) toxicity: Discontinue offending agent. No treatment or preservative-free artificial tears q.i.d. Reevaluate in 24 hours.

3. Suspect chlamydial infection: Erythromycin elixir 50 mg/kg/day for 14 days, plus erythromycin ointment q.i.d. If confirmed by culture or immunofluorescent stain, treat the mother and her sexual partners with one of the following:

—Tetracycline 250 to 500 mg p.o. q.i.d. or doxycycline 100 mg p.o. b.i.d. for 7 days (for mothers who are neither breast-feeding nor pregnant, or for men) or azithromycin 1 g as a single dose or erythromycin 250 to 500 mg p.o. q.i.d. for 7 days (for breast-feeding or pregnant women).

NOTE: Inadequately treated chlamydial conjunctivitis in a neonate can lead to chlamydial otitis or pneumonia.

---

4. Suspect *N. gonorrhoeae:*

—Saline irrigation of the conjunctiva and fornices until discharge gone.

—Hospitalize and evaluate for disseminated gonococcal infection with careful physical examination (especially of joints). Blood and cerebrospinal fluid cultures are obtained if a culture-proven infection is present.

—Ceftriaxone 25 to 50 mg/kg intravenously (i.v.) or intramuscularly (i.m.) (not to exceed 125 mg), as a single dose or cefotaxime 100 mg/kg i.v. or i.m. as a single dose. In penicillin- or cephalosporin-allergic patients, an Infectious Disease consult is obtained. Systemic antibiotics sufficiently treat gonococcal conjunctivitis, and topical antibiotics are not necessary.

—If diagnosis is unclear, bacitracin ointment or ciprofloxacin ointment can be used

in addition to systemic antibiotics based on the Gram stain as outlined below.

—Topical saline lavage q.i.d. to remove any discharge.

—All neonates with gonorrhea should also be treated for chlamydial infection with erythromycin elixir 50 mg/kg/day in four divided doses for 14 days.

NOTE: If confirmed by culture, the mother and her sexual partners should be treated for 7 days. If sensitivities are not initially available, ceftriaxone is the first choice. In addition, chlamydial infection should be treated as outlined earlier.

---

5. Gram-positive bacteria with no suspicion of gonorrhea and no corneal involvement: Bacitracin ointment q.i.d. for 2 weeks.

6. Gram-negative bacteria with no suspicion of gonorrhea and no corneal involvement: Gentamicin, tobramycin, or ciprofloxacin ointment q.i.d. for 2 weeks.

7. Bacteria on Gram stain and corneal involvement: Hospitalize, work-up, and treat as discussed in 4.11, *Bacterial Keratitis*.

8. Suspect herpes simplex virus: The neonate, regardless of the presenting ocular findings, should be treated with acyclovir intravenously as well as with vidarabine 3% ointment five times per day, or trifluridine drops nine times per day. Topical therapy is optional when systemic therapy is instituted. In full-term infants, the dosage for acyclovir is 45 to 60 mg/kg/day divided in three divided doses, given intravenously for 14 days if limited to the skin, eye, and mouth, and for 21 days if the disease is disseminated or involves the central nervous system. For children with recurrent ocular lesions, oral suppressive therapy with acyclovir (20 mg/kg q6h) may be of benefit.

Follow-Up

1. Initially, examine daily as an inpatient or outpatient.

2. If the condition worsens (e.g., corneal involvement develops), reculture and hospitalize. Therapy and follow-up are tailored according to the clinical response and the culture results.

| 8.10 | CONGENITAL NASOLACRIMAL DUCT OBSTRUCTION |

Signs

Critical. Wet-looking eye or tears flowing over the eyelid; moist or dried mucopurulent material on the eyelashes (predominantly medially), and reflux of mucoid or mucopurulent material from the punctum when pressure is applied over the lacrimal sac (where the lower eyelid abuts the nose). The eye is otherwise white. Symptoms usually appear in the first 1 to 2 months of life.

Other. Erythema of the surrounding skin; redness and swelling of the medial canthus. May become infected and occasionally spread from the nasolacrimal duct, resulting in conjunctivitis. Therefore, recurrent conjunctivitis may be another sign. Preseptal cellulitis or dacryocystitis may rarely develop.

Differential Diagnosis

- Conjunctivitis: See 5.1, *Acute Conjunctivitis.*

- Congenital anomalies of the upper lacrimal drainage system: Atresia of the lacrimal puncta or canaliculus.

- Dacryocele: Bluish, cystic, firm mass located just below the medial canthal angle. Caused by both a distal and proximal obstruction of the nasolacrimal apparatus. Most often presents within the first week of life.

- Congenital glaucoma: Classic findings are tearing, light sensitivity (possibly associated with blepharospasm), corneal clouding, and a large eye (buphthalmos). See 8.11, *Congenital/Infantile Glaucoma.*

- Other causes of tearing: Entropion/trichiasis, corneal defects, foreign body under the upper eyelid.

Etiology

Usually the result of a congenitally imperforate membrane at the distal end of the nasolacrimal duct over the valve of Hasner.

Work-Up

1. Exclude other causes of tearing, particularly congenital glaucoma. See 8.11, *Congenital/Infantile Glaucoma.*

2. Palpate over the lacrimal sac; reflux of mucoid or mucopurulent discharge from the punctum confirms the diagnosis. May also use the dye disappearance test. Place fluorescein in both eyes. Check in 10 minutes; fluorescein will remain in the eye with congenital nasolacrimal duct obstruction.

Treatment

1. Digital pressure to lacrimal sac q.i.d. The parent is taught to place his or her index finger over the child's common canaliculus (inner corner of the eye) and to apply pressure in a downward fashion.

2. Topical antibiotic (e.g., polymyxin/trimethoprim q.i.d.) as needed to control mucopurulent discharge if present.

3. In the presence of acute dacryocystitis (red, swollen lacrimal sac), a systemic antibiotic is needed. See 6.9, *Dacryocystitis/Inflammation of the Lacrimal Sac.*

4. Most cases open spontaneously with this regimen by 1 year of age. Probing should be considered if the nasolacrimal duct obstruction persists beyond a year of age. Probe earlier if recurrent or persistent infections of the lacrimal system develop, or at the request of the parents. Most obstructions are corrected after the initial probing; others may require repeated probings. If primary and secondary probing fails, may use balloon dacryoplasty or silicone tubing in the nasolacrimal duct that is left in place for weeks to months. Consider dacryocystorhinostomy as a last resort.

Follow-Up

Routine follow-up unless surgery is indicated, sooner if the situation worsens or acute dacryocystitis is present.

8

8.11   CONGENITAL/INFANTILE GLAUCOMA

Signs

(See Figure 8.11.1.)

Critical. Enlarged globe and corneal diameter (horizontal corneal diameter >12 mm before 1 year of age is suggestive), corneal edema, Haab striae (linear tears in Descemet membrane of the cornea, running in any direction with scalloped edges with or without associated stromal haze), increased cup/disc ratio, axial myopia, commonly bilateral (80%). Classic findings are tearing, photophobia, blepharospasm, corneal clouding, and a large eye (buphthalmos).

Other. Corneal stromal scarring (opacification); IOP may or may not be elevated, high iris insertion on gonioscopy, and may have other signs of iris dysgenesis, including heterochromia.

Differential Diagnosis

- Congenital megalocornea: Bilateral horizontal corneal diameter usually >14 mm, with normal corneal thickness and endothelium, IOP, and cup/disc ratio. Radial iris transillumination defects may be seen. Usually X-linked recessive (boys affected, female carriers may have above normal corneal diameters) and may be associated with developmental delay (Neuhauser syndrome, autosomal recessive).

- Trauma from forceps during delivery: May produce tears in the Descemet membrane and localized corneal edema; tears are typically vertical or oblique, and the corneal diameter is normal. Always unilateral, must have history of forceps use to make diagnosis.

- Congenital hereditary endothelial dystrophy: Bilateral full-thickness corneal edema at birth with a normal corneal diameter and axial length, IOP may be artifactiously elevated by increased corneal thickness and hysteresis but true associated infantile glaucoma has been reported. See 4.26, *Corneal Dystrophies*.

- Posterior polymorphous dystrophy: Can present in infancy as bilateral but asymmetric cloudy edematous corneas with characteristic endothelial abnormalities. Normal corneal diameter, axial length, and IOP. Abnormal endothelium may be seen in one parent.

- Mucopolysaccharidoses and cystinosis: Some inborn errors of metabolism produce cloudy corneas in infancy or early childhood, usually not at birth; the corneal diameter and axial length are normal, IOP is rarely elevated and, if so, usually later in childhood. Always bilateral.

- Nasolacrimal duct obstruction: No photophobia, clear cornea, normal corneal size and axial length, normal IOP. See 8.10, *Congenital Nasolacrimal Duct Obstruction*.

- Large eye without other signs of glaucoma can be seen in overgrowth syndromes (e.g., hemihypertrophy) and phakomatoses (e.g., neurofibromatosis, Sturge–Weber) in the absence of glaucoma. May also be autosomal dominant variant without glaucoma.

Etiology

Common

- Primary congenital glaucoma: Not associated with other ocular or systemic disorders. Diagnosed after other causes of glaucoma have been ruled out. Caused by incomplete differentiation of the trabecular meshwork during embryogenesis (e.g., goniodysgenesis).

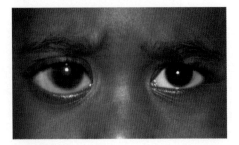

FIGURE 8.11.1. Buphthalmos of right eye in congenital glaucoma.

- Aphakic glaucoma: Most common form of pediatric glaucoma. Typically in older children. All children undergoing cataract surgery are at lifelong risk.

Less Common

- Sturge–Weber syndrome: Usually unilateral (90%); ipsilateral port-wine mark almost always involving lid(s), cerebral calcifications/atrophy, and seizures/developmental delay (central nervous system may not be involved at all); not familial. See 13.13, *Phakomatoses*.

Rare

- Other anterior segment dysgeneses: Axenfeld–Rieger spectrum, Peters anomaly, others. See 8.12, *Developmental Anterior Segment and Lens Anomalies/Dysgenesis*.

- Lowe syndrome (oculocerebrorenal syndrome): Cataract, glaucoma, developmental delay, and renal disease; X-linked recessive.

- Congenital rubella: Glaucoma, cataract, "salt-and-pepper" retinopathy, hearing and cardiac defects (usually peripheral pulmonic stenosis).

- Aniridia: Absence of almost all of the iris, often with only a rudimentary iris stub visible on gonioscopy, cataracts, glaucoma, macular hypoplasia, nystagmus. See 8.12, *Developmental Anterior Segment and Lens Anomalies/Dysgenesis*.

- Others: Neurofibromatosis, PFV/PHPV, Weill–Marchesani syndrome, Rubinstein–Taybi syndrome, covert trauma, steroid-induced infantile glaucoma, and others.

Work-Up

1. History: Other systemic abnormalities? Rubella infection during pregnancy? Birth trauma? Family history of congenital glaucoma?

2. Ocular examination, including a visual acuity assessment of each eye separately, a slit-lamp or portable slit-lamp examination to detect corneal edema and measure corneal diameter. Retinoscopy to estimate refractive error, or A-scan to measure axial length. A dilated fundus examination is performed to evaluate the optic disc and retina if able to view through cornea.

3. EUA is performed in suggestive cases and in those for whom surgical treatment is considered. The horizontal corneal diameter (measured with calipers or templates), IOP measurement, pachymetry, retinoscopy, gonioscopy, and ophthalmoscopy are performed. Axial length is measured with US. At 40 gestational weeks, the mean axial length is 17 mm. This increases to 20 mm on average by age 1 year. Axial length progression may also be monitored by successive cycloplegic refractions or serial US. Disc photos may also be taken.

NOTE: IOP may be reduced minimally by general anesthesia, particularly halothane, corneal epithelial edema, and overventilation (low end-tidal CO_2); ketamine hydrochloride, succinylcholine, endotracheal intubation (for 2 to 5 minutes), pressure from the anesthetic mask, speculum use, or inadequate ventilation with elevated end-tidal CO_2, may falsely increase IOP.

8

Treatment

Definitive treatment is usually surgical. Medical therapy is utilized as a temporizing measure before surgery and to help clear the cornea in preparation for possible goniotomy.

1. Medical:

—Oral carbonic anhydrase inhibitor (e.g., acetazolamide, 15 to 30 mg/kg/day in three or four divided doses): Most effective.

—Topical carbonic anhydrase inhibitor (e.g., dorzolamide or brinzolamide b.i.d.): Less effective; better tolerated.

—Topical beta-blocker (e.g., levobunolol or timolol, 0.25% if <1 year old or 0.5% if older b.i.d.).

—Prostaglandin analogs (e.g., latanoprost q.h.s.)

NOTE: Brimonidine is contraindicated in children under the age of 1 year because of the risk of apnea/hypotension/bradycardia/hypothermia. Caution should be used in children under 5 years old or <20 kg.

---

2. Surgical: Nasal goniotomy (incising the trabecular meshwork with a blade or needle under gonioscopic visualization) is the procedure of choice, although some surgeons initially recommend trabeculotomy. Miotics are sometimes used to constrict the pupil before a surgical goniotomy. If the cornea is not clear, trabeculotomy (opening the Schlemm canal from a scleral approach into the anterior chamber) or endoscopic goniotomy can be performed. If the initial goniotomy is unsuccessful, a temporal goniotomy may be tried. Trabeculectomy or tube shunt may be performed following failed angle-incision operations.

NOTE: Amblyopia is the most common cause of visual loss in pediatric glaucoma and should be treated appropriately. See 8.7, *Amblyopia*.

Follow-Up

1. Repeated examinations, under anesthesia as needed, to monitor corneal diameter and clarity, IOP, cup/disc ratio, and refraction/axial length.

2. These patients must be followed throughout life to monitor for progression.

3. Other forms of pediatric glaucoma in older children include uveitic glaucoma, traumatic glaucoma, juvenile open-angle glaucoma (JOAG, autosomal dominant), and others.

8.12 DEVELOPMENTAL ANTERIOR SEGMENT AND LENS ANOMALIES/DYSGENESIS

Unilateral or bilateral congenital abnormalities of the cornea, iris, anterior chamber angle, and lens.

Specific Entities

- Microcornea: Horizontal corneal diameter small for age. May be isolated or associated with microphthalmia, cataract, or nanophthalmos.

- Posterior embryotoxon: A prominent, anteriorly displaced Schwalbe ring. May be normal, or seen in association with Axenfeld–Rieger and Alagille syndrome.

- Axenfeld–Rieger spectrum: Ranges from posterior embryotoxon associated with iris strands from the periphery that span the angle to insert into the prominent Schwalbe ring to more severe iris malformations including polycoria and corectopia. Glaucoma develops in 50% to 60% of patients. Usually autosomal dominant. May be associated with abnormal teeth (e.g., microdontia, conical teeth, hypodontia), skeletal abnormalities, and redundancy of the periumbilical skin. Growth hormone deficiency, cardiac

defects, deafness, and mental retardation may be seen (see Figure 8.12.1).

- Peters anomaly: Failure of the lens to completely detach from surface epithelium during 4 to 7 weeks of gestation. Central corneal opacity, usually with iris strands that extend from the collarette to a posterior corneal defect behind the scar. The lens may be clear and normally positioned, cataractous and displaced anteriorly (making the anterior chamber shallow), or adherent to the corneal defect. "Peters plus" syndrome is characterized by an

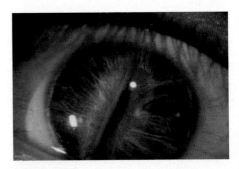

FIGURE 8.12.1. Axenfeld–Rieger anomaly.

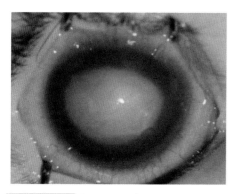

FIGURE 8.12.2. Peters anomaly.

associated skeletal dysplasia with short stature. Other malformations may also be seen (see Figure 8.12.2).

■ Microspherophakia: The lens is small and spherical in configuration. It can subluxate into the anterior chamber, causing a secondary glaucoma. Can be isolated or seen in association with Weill–Marchesani syndrome (see Figure 8.12.3).

■ Anterior and posterior lenticonus: An anterior or posterior ectasia of the lens surface, posterior occurring more commonly than anterior. Often associated with cataract. Unilateral or bilateral. Anterior lenticonus is associated with Alport syndrome. Posterior lenticonus is usually isolated and may be autosomal dominant, but can also be seen with Alport syndrome.

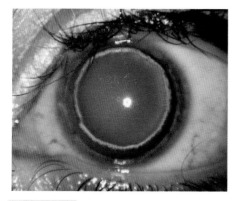

FIGURE 8.12.3. Microspherophakia.

■ Ectopia lentis: See 13.10, *Subluxed or Dislocated Crystalline Lens.*

■ Ectopia lentis et pupillae: Lens displacement associated with pupillary displacement in the opposite direction. Usually not associated with glaucoma.

■ Aniridia: Bilateral, near-total absence of the iris. Glaucoma, macular hypoplasia with poor vision, nystagmus, refractive error, and corneal pannus are common. May be part of a pan-ocular disorder due to mutations in the master control gene of the eye, PAX6. If PAX6 is deleted as part of a larger chromosomal deletion it is called WAGR syndrome (Wilms tumor, aniridia, genital abnormalities, retardation). More common in sporadic aniridia. Aniridia is autosomal dominant in two-thirds of patients, a type usually not associated with Wilms tumor.

■ Sclerocornea: Nonprogressive scleralization of the cornea. Unilateral or bilateral. May be mild and peripheral or severe and diffuse. Associated with severe anterior segment dysgenesis and risk for glaucoma. Often associated with microphthalmia.

■ Primary aphakia: Failure of lens development. Usually associated with microphthalmia and severe intraocular dysgenesis including retinal dysplasia and corneal opacity. High risk for glaucoma.

Work-Up

1. History: Family history of ocular disease? Associated systemic abnormalities?

2. Complete ophthalmic examination, including gonioscopy of the anterior chamber angle and IOP determination (may require EUA).

3. Complete physical examination by a primary care physician.

4. In patients with aniridia, obtain chromosomal karyotype with reflex microarray or PAX6 DNA analysis. Until results received, screen with renal ultrasound at diagnosis and no less than every 6 months thereafter to age 7 to 8 years old. If deletion

8

involving Wilms tumor gene is found, the frequency of ultrasound should be every 3 months.

Treatment

1. Correct refractive errors and treat amblyopia if present (see 8.7, *Amblyopia*). Children with unilateral structural abnormalities often have improved visual acuity after amblyopia therapy.

2. Treat glaucoma if present. Beta-blockers, prostaglandin analogs, and carbonic anhydrase inhibitors may be used. Pilocarpine is not effective and is not used in primary therapy (see 9.1, *Primary Open-Angle Glaucoma*).

Surgery is often used initially (see 8.11, *Congenital/Infantile Glaucoma*).

3. Consider cataract extraction if a significant cataract exists and a corneal transplant if a dense corneal opacity exists.

4. Provide genetic counseling.

5. Systemic abnormalities (e.g., Wilms tumor) are managed by pediatric specialists.

Follow-Up

1. Ophthalmic examination every 6 months throughout life, checking for increased IOP and other signs of glaucoma.

2. If amblyopia exists, follow-up may need to be more frequent (see 8.7, *Amblyopia*).

8.13   CONGENITAL PTOSIS

Signs

Critical.   Droopy eyelid(s).

Other.   Amblyopia, strabismus, telecanthus. In unilateral ptosis, the involved eye may not open for the first several days.

Differential Diagnosis

■ Simple congenital ptosis: Either unilateral or bilateral. Present at birth and stable throughout life. May have indistinct or absent upper eyelid crease. Ptosis improves with downgaze. Involved side may be higher than normal eyelid in downgaze because of levator fibrosis. May have compensatory brow elevation or chin-up head position. Coexisting motility abnormality if from a third cranial nerve palsy.

■ Blepharophimosis syndrome: Blepharophimosis, telecanthus, epicanthal folds, and ptosis. Bilateral and severe. Autosomal dominant with high penetrance (see Figure 8.13.1).

—Type I: All four eyelids phimotic with upper eyelid ptosis.

—Type II: Telecanthus, ptosis, and absent epicanthal folds.

—Type III: Telecanthus, ptosis, and present epicanthal folds. May also have flattened nasal bridge and low-set ears.

■ Marcus Gunn jaw winking: Usually unilateral. Upper eyelid movement with contraction of muscles of mastication, resulting in "winking" while chewing. Upper eyelid crease intact. The ptosis may range from none to severe, but with mastication the levator may lift the lid several millimeters above the limbus.

■ Acquired ptosis: See 6.1, *Ptosis*.

■ Horner syndrome: Usually unilateral. Typically 2 to 3 mm of ptosis, associated with anisocoria (see 10.2, *Horner Syndrome*). May be congenital (associated with iris heterochromia) or acquired. Acquired forms in children may be related to birth trauma, chest/neck trauma, or metastatic neuroblastoma.

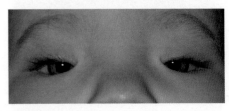

FIGURE 8.13.1. Blepharophimosis.

■ Pseudoptosis: Dermatochalasis, contralateral proptosis, enophthalmos, hypotropia. See 6.1, *Ptosis.*

Etiology

Defective function of either the levator or Müller neuromuscular complexes.

Work-Up

1. History: Age of onset? Duration? Family history? History of trauma or prior surgery? Any crossing of eyes?

2. Visual acuity for each eye separately, with correction, to evaluate for amblyopia.

3. Manifest and cycloplegic refraction checking for anisometropia.

4. Pupillary examination.

5. Ocular motility examination.

6. Measure interpalpebral fissure distance, distance between corneal light reflex and upper eyelid margin, levator function (while manually fixing eyebrow), position and depth of upper eyelid crease. Check for Bell phenomenon.

7. Slit-lamp examination; look for signs of corneal exposure.

8. Dilated fundus examination.

9. If Horner syndrome is suspected, refer to pediatrician for systemic evaluation.

Treatment

1. Observation if degree of ptosis mild, no evidence of amblyopia, and no abnormal head positioning.

2. Simple congenital ptosis: If levator function is poor, consider a frontalis suspension. If levator function is moderate or normal, consider a levator resection.

3. Blepharophimosis syndrome: Ptosis must be repaired by frontalis suspension because of poor levator function. Telecanthus often gets better with time as the head grows and the bridge of the nose grows forward. If the telecanthus is severe, it may be treated with surgery.

4. Marcus Gunn jaw winking: No treatment if mild. In general, the jaw winking gets better around school age. Any treatment for ptosis with levator resection will increase the excursion during jaw winking.

Follow-Up

1. If observing, patients should be reexamined every 3 to 12 months, depending on severity and age, to monitor for occlusion or anisometropic amblyopia.

2. After surgery, patients should be monitored for undercorrection or overcorrection and recurrence. Exposure keratopathy may be a significant problem after ptosis surgery.

8.14 THE BILATERALLY BLIND INFANT

Signs

Searching, roving movements of the eyes starting at about 4 to 6 weeks of age. Poor pupillary constriction to light in infants >31 weeks gestation is a key finding. Inability to fix or follow large, bright objects after 4 months corrected age.

Etiology with an Abnormal Ocular Exam

■ Severe ocular disease or malformation.

■ Retinopathy of prematurity. See 8.2, *Retinopathy of Prematurity.*

■ Dense bilateral cataracts in children >8 weeks of age. See 8.8, *Congenital Cataract.*

■ Aniridia and other severe anterior segment dysgenesis. See 8.12, *Developmental Anterior Segment and Lens Anomalies/Dysgenesis.*

■ Albinism: Iris transillumination defects and foveal hypoplasia. See 13.8, *Albinism.*

NOTE: Ocular abnormalities in patients with albinism and aniridia may be subtle and difficult to assess during an office evaluation.

■ Optic nerve hypoplasia: Small optic discs can be difficult to detect when bilateral. When present, a "double-ring" sign (a pigmented ring at the inner and outer edge of a peripapillary scleral ring) is diagnostic. If unilateral, may be seen with strabismus, a relative afferent pupillary defect, and unilateral poor fixation instead of searching nystagmus. Usually idiopathic.

NOTE: Bilateral optic nerve hypoplasia is occasionally associated with septooptic dysplasia (de Morsier syndrome). In contrast, unilateral optic nerve hypoplasia is only rarely associated with this syndrome. De Morsier syndrome includes midline abnormalities of the brain and growth, thyroid, and other trophic hormone deficiencies. Growth retardation, seizures as a result of hypoglycemia, and diabetes insipidus may develop. If bilateral optic nerve hypoplasia is present, obtain an MRI with attention to the hypothalamic-pituitary area. If unilateral optic nerve hypoplasia is present, imaging studies may be considered as clinically relevant.

■ Congenital optic atrophy: Rare. Pale, normal-sized optic disc, often associated with mental retardation or cerebral palsy. Normal electroretinogram (ERG). Autosomal recessive or sporadic.

■ Shaken baby syndrome: Multilayered retinal hemorrhages often associated with subdural/subarachnoid hemorrhage. See 3.20, *Shaken Baby Syndrome/Inflicted Childhood Neurotrauma.*

■ Extreme refractive error: Diagnosed on cycloplegic refraction.

■ Congenital motor nystagmus: Patients with this condition usually have a mild visual deficit (20/60 or better). Binocular conjugate horizontal nystagmus. More than one type of nystagmus may be present, including jerk, pendular, circular, or elliptical. Patients may adopt a face turn to maximize gaze in the direction of the null point. No associated central nervous system abnormalities exist.

Etiologies With a Normal Ocular Exam

■ Leber congenital amaurosis: Rod–cone disorder. May have a normal-appearing fundus initially, but by childhood ocular exam reveals narrowing of retinal blood vessels, optic disc pallor, and pigmentary changes. ERG is markedly abnormal or flat which makes diagnosis. Autosomal recessive.

■ Congenital stationary night blindness: Visual acuity may be close to normal, nystagmus less common, associated with myopia. ERG is abnormal. Autosomal dominant, recessive, and X-linked forms exist. Often have paradoxical pupillary response (pupillary constriction in dim light after exposure to bright light). Retinal pigmentary abnormalities are seen in some types of congenital stationary night blindness.

■ Achromatopsia (rod monochromatism): Vision is in the 20/200 range. Marked photophobia. Pupils react normally to light but may have paradoxical pupil response. Normal fundus, but photopic ERG is markedly attenuated. Absence of response to flicker light stimulus (25 Hz) is diagnostic. Scotopic ERG is normal.

■ Cortical visual impairment: Vision is variable. There is a normal ocular exam, but there is underlying neurologic deficiency causing decreased visual responses.

■ Diffuse cerebral dysfunction: Infants do not respond to sound or touch and are neurologically abnormal. Vision may slowly improve with time.

■ Delayed maturation of the visual system: Normal response to sound and touch and neurologically normal. The ERG is normal, and vision usually develops between age 4 and 12 months. More common in patients with some type of albinism (may have nystagmus at presentation).

Work-Up

1. History: Premature? Normal development and growth? Maternal infection, diabetes, or drug use during pregnancy? Seizures or other neurologic deficits? Family history of eye disease?

2. Evaluate the infant's ability to fixate on an object and follow it.

3. Pupillary examination, noting both equality and briskness.

4. Look carefully for nystagmus (see 10.21, *Nystagmus*).

5. Examination of the anterior segment; check especially for iris transillumination defects.

6. Dilated retinal and optic nerve evaluation.

7. Cycloplegic refraction.

8. ERG, especially if Leber congenital amaurosis is suspected.

9. Consider a CT scan or MRI of the brain in cases with other focal neurologic signs, seizures, failure to thrive, developmental delay, optic nerve hypoplasia, or neurologically localizing nystagmus (e.g., seesaw, vertical, gaze paretic, vestibular). If optic atrophy, either unilateral or bilateral, is present, obtain an MRI to evaluate for a glioma of the optic nerve or chiasm and craniopharyngioma.

10. Consider a sweep visual-evoked potential for vision measurement.

11. Consider eye movement recordings to evaluate the nystagmus wave form, if available.

Treatment

1. Correct refractive errors and treat known or suspected amblyopia.

2. Parental counseling is necessary in all of these conditions with respect to the infant's visual potential and the likelihood of visual problems in siblings, etc.

3. Referral to educational services for the visually handicapped or blind may be helpful.

4. Provide genetic counseling.

5. If neurologic or endocrine abnormalities are found or suspected, the child should be referred to a pediatrician for appropriate work-up and management.

8

Glaucoma

9.1 PRIMARY OPEN-ANGLE GLAUCOMA

Symptoms

Usually asymptomatic until the later stages. Early symptoms may include parts of a page missing. Tunnel vision and loss of central fixation typically do not occur until late in the disease.

Signs

- Intraocular pressure (IOP): Although most patients will have an elevated IOP (normal range of 10 to 21 mm Hg), nearly half have an IOP of 21 mm Hg or lower at any one screening.

- Gonioscopy: Normal-appearing, open anterior chamber angle on gonioscopic evaluation. No peripheral anterior synechiae (PAS).

- Optic nerve: See Figure 9.1.1. Characteristic appearance includes loss of rim tissue (includes notching; increased narrowing superiorly, inferiorly, or nasally more than temporally; progressive narrowing over time), regional pallor, splinter or nerve fiber layer hemorrhage that crosses the disc margin (Drance hemorrhage), acquired pit, nerve fiber layer defect, cup/disc (C/D) asymmetry >0.2 in the absence of a cause (e.g., anisometropia, different nerve sizes), bayoneting (sharp angulation of the blood vessels as they exit the nerve), enlarged C/D ratio (>0.6; less specific), progressive enlargement of the cup, greater Disc Damage Likelihood Scale (DDLS) score (see Figure 9.1.2).

- Visual fields: Characteristic visual field loss includes nasal step, paracentral scotoma, arcuate scotoma extending from the blind spot nasally (defects usually respect the horizontal midline or are greater in one hemifield than the other), altitudinal defect, or generalized depression (see Figure 9.1.3).

Other. Large fluctuations in IOP, absence of microcystic corneal edema, an uninflamed eye.

Differential Diagnosis

If Anterior Chamber Angle Open on Gonioscopy:

- Ocular hypertension: Normal optic nerve and visual field. See 9.3, *Ocular Hypertension.*

- Physiologic optic nerve cupping: Static enlarged C/D ratio without rim notching or visual field loss. Usually normal IOP and

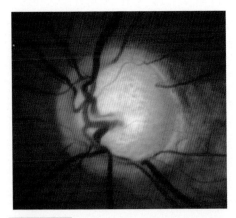

FIGURE 9.1.1. Primary open-angle glaucoma with advanced optic nerve cupping.

	DDLS Stage	Narrowest rim width (rim/disc ratio) [average disc size: 1.50 - 2.00 mm]	Example
At Risk	1	**0.4 or more**	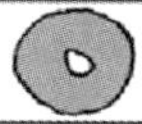
	2	**0.3 to 0.39**	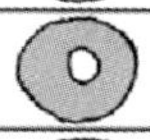
	3	**0.2 to 0.29**	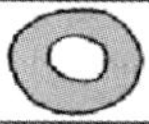
	4	**0.1 to 0.19**	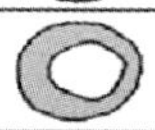
Glaucoma Damage	5	less than **0.1**	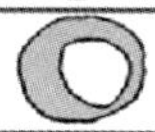
	6	**0** (*extension*: less than 45°)	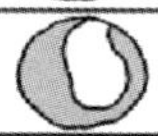
	7	**0** (*extension*: 46° to 90°)	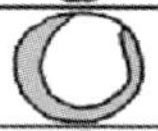
Glaucoma Disability	8	**0** (*extension*: 91° to 180°)	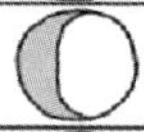
	9	**0** (*extension*: 181° to 270°)	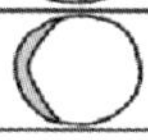
	10	**0** (*extension*: more than 270°)	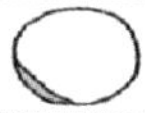

FIGURE 9.1.2. Disc Damage Likelihood Damage Scale.

large optic nerve (> about 2 mm). Often familial.

- Secondary open-angle glaucoma: Identifiable cause for open-angle glaucoma including lens-induced, inflammatory, exfoliative, pigmentary, steroid-induced, angle recession, traumatic (as a result of direct injury, blood, or debris), and glaucoma related to increased episcleral venous pressure (e.g., Sturge–Weber syndrome, carotid–cavernous fistula), intraocular tumors, degenerated red blood cells (ghost cell glaucoma), degenerated photoreceptor outer segments following chronic rhegmatogenous retinal detachment (Schwartz–Matsuo syndrome), or developmental anterior segment abnormalities. See specific sections.

- Low-pressure glaucoma: Same as primary open-angle glaucoma (POAG) except normal IOP. See 9.2, *Low-Pressure Primary Open-Angle Glaucoma (Normal Pressure Glaucoma)*.

- Previous glaucomatous damage (e.g., from steroids, uveitis, glaucomatocyclitic crisis,

trauma) in which the inciting agent has been removed. Nerve appearance now static.

- Optic atrophy: Characterized by disproportionally more optic nerve pallor than cupping. IOP usually normal unless a secondary or unrelated glaucoma is present. Color vision and central vision are often decreased. Causes include optic nerve, chiasmal, or tract tumors, syphilis, ischemic optic neuropathy, drugs, retinal vascular or degenerative disease, others. Visual field defects that respect the vertical midline are typical of intracranial lesions at or posterior to the chiasm.

- Congenital optic nerve defects (e.g., tilted discs, colobomas, optic nerve pits): Visual field defects may be present but are static.

- Optic nerve drusen: Optic nerves not usually cupped and drusen often visible. Visual field defects may remain stable or progress unrelated to IOP. The most frequent defects include arcuate defects or an enlarged blind spot. Characteristic calcified lesions can be

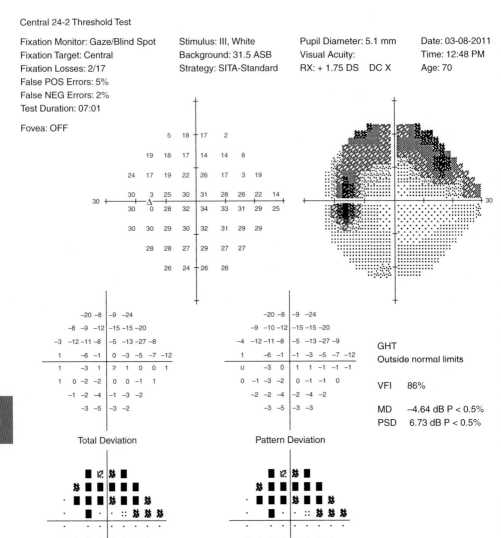

Central 24-2 Threshold Test

Fixation Monitor: Gaze/Blind Spot Stimulus: III, White Pupil Diameter: 5.1 mm Date: 03-08-2011
Fixation Target: Central Background: 31.5 ASB Visual Acuity: Time: 12:48 PM
Fixation Losses: 2/17 Strategy: SITA-Standard RX: + 1.75 DS   DC X Age: 70
False POS Errors: 5%
False NEG Errors: 2%
Test Duration: 07:01

Fovea: OFF

GHT
Outside normal limits

VFI   86%

MD   −4.64 dB P < 0.5%
PSD   6.73 dB P < 0.5%

Total Deviation   Pattern Deviation

FIGURE 9.1.3.   HVF showing a supero-nasal arcuate scotoma.

seen on B-scan ultrasonography (US) and on computed tomography (CT).

If Closed or Partially Closed Angle on Gonioscopy:

■ Chronic angle-closure glaucoma (CACG): Shallow anterior chamber, blurred vision, headache. PAS present on gonioscopy. See 9.5, *Chronic Angle-Closure Glaucoma.*

Work-Up

1. History: Presence of risk factors (family history of blindness or visual loss from glaucoma, older age, African descent, diabetes, myopia, hypertension or hypotension)? Previous history of increased IOP or chronic steroid use? Refractive surgery including laser in situ keratomileusis (LASIK) in past

(change in pachymetry)? Review of past medical history to determine appropriate therapy including asthma, chronic obstructive pulmonary disease (COPD), congestive heart failure, heart block or bradyarrhythmia, renal stones, allergies?

2. Baseline glaucoma evaluation: All patients with suspected glaucoma of any type should have the following:

—Complete ocular examination including visual acuity, pupillary assessment for a relative afferent pupillary defect, confrontational visual fields using a red object (e.g., red top of a mydriatic drop), slit-lamp examination, applanation tonometry, gonioscopy, and dilated fundus examination (if the angle is open) with special attention to the optic nerve.

—Baseline documentation of the optic nerves (e.g., stereoscopic disc photos, red-free photographs, computerized image analysis [e.g., optical coherence tomography (OCT) or Heidelberg retina tomography (HRT)], or meticulous drawings) and formal visual field testing (preferably automated, e.g., Humphrey). Goldmann visual field tests may be helpful in patients unable to take the automated tests adequately. Color vision testing indicated in those suspected of a neurologic disorder (see Figure 9.1.4).

—Measure central corneal thickness (CCT). Corneal thickness variations affect apparent IOP as measured with applanation tonometry. Average corneal thickness is 530 to 545 microns. Thinner corneas tend to underestimate IOP, whereas thicker corneas tend to overestimate IOP, although the relationship between corneal thickness and measured IOP is not exactly linear. A thin CCT is an independent risk factor for the development of POAG.

—Further evaluation for other causes of optic nerve damage should be considered when any of the following atypical features are present:

- Optic nerve pallor out of proportion to the degree of cupping.

- Visual field defects greater than expected based on amount of cupping.

- Visual field patterns not typical of glaucoma (e.g., defects respecting the vertical midline, hemianopic defects, enlarged blind spot, central scotoma).

- IOP within the average range (<21 mm Hg) or symmetric between both eyes.

- Unilateral progression despite equal IOP in both eyes.

- Decreased visual acuity out of proportion to the amount of cupping or field loss.

- Color vision loss, especially in the red–green axis.

If any of these are present, further evaluation may include:

- History: Acute episodes of eye pain or redness? Steroid use? Acute visual loss? Ocular trauma? Surgery, systemic trauma, heart attack, dialysis, or other event that may lead to hypotension?

- Diurnal IOP curve consisting of multiple IOP checks during the course of the day.

- Consider other laboratory work-up for nonglaucomatous optic neuropathy: heavy metals, angiotensin-converting enzyme, vitamin B12/folate, rapid plasma reagin, fluorescent treponemal antibody absorption, Lyme titer, antinuclear antibody. If giant cell arteritis (GCA) is a consideration, then check erythrocyte sedimentation rate, C-reactive protein, and complete blood count (CBC) with platelets [see 10.17, *Arteritic Ischemic Optic Neuropathy (Giant Cell Arteritis)*].

- In cases where a neurologic disorder is suspected, obtain magnetic resonance imaging (MRI) of the brain and orbits with gadolinium and fat suppression if no contraindications are present or CT of the head and orbits with axial and coronal views, preferably with contrast if no contraindications are present.

- Check blood pressure, fasting blood sugar, lipid panel, and CBC (screening

9

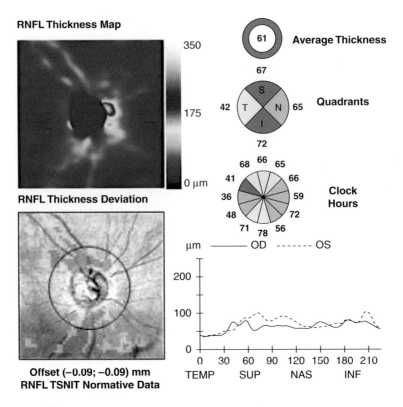

RNFL Thickness Map

350

175

0 μm

RNFL Thickness Deviation

Offset (–0.09; –0.09) mm
RNFL TSNIT Normative Data

61   **Average Thickness**

67
S
42 T   N 65   **Quadrants**
I
72

68 66 65
41   66
36   59
48   72
71 78 56

Clock
Hours

μm ——— OD ------- OS

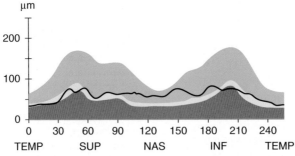

FIGURE 9.1.4. Optical coherence tomography of retinal nerve fiber layer thickness.

for anemia). Refer to an internist for a complete cardiovascular evaluation.

Treatment

General Considerations

1. Who to treat?

The decision to treat must be individualized. Some general guidelines are suggested.

Is the glaucomatous process present?
Damage is present if the DDLS score is >5, there is visual field loss, there is the pres-

ence of an acquired pit or notched rims (irregularity of rims >0.1 rim-to-disc for <2 clock hours), IOP higher than 34 mm Hg, IOP asymmetry more than 10 mm Hg, or disc is <1.5 mm with a cup-to-disc of >0.3.

Is the glaucomatous process active?
Determine the rate of damage progression by careful follow-up. Certain causes of cupping may be static (e.g., prior steroid response). Disc hemorrhages suggest active disease.

Is the glaucomatous process likely to cause disability?

Consider the patient's age, overall physical and social health, as well as an estimation of his or her life expectancy.

2. What is the treatment goal?

The goal of treatment is to enhance or maintain the patient's health by halting optic nerve damage while avoiding undue side effects of treatment. The only proven method of stopping or slowing optic nerve damage is reducing IOP. Reduction of IOP by at least 30% appears to have the best chance of preventing optic nerve damage. An optimal goal may be to reduce the IOP at least 30% below the threshold of progression. If damage is severe, greater reduction in IOP may be necessary.

3. How to treat?

The main treatment options for glaucoma include medications, laser trabeculoplasty [both argon (ALT) and selective (SLT)], and guarded filtration surgery (e.g., trabeculectomy). Typically, medications are first-line therapy. Often ALT and SLT are also appropriate initial therapies, especially in patients at risk for poor compliance, with medication side effects, and who have significant posterior trabecular meshwork pigmentation. Surgery may be appropriate initial treatment if damage is advanced in the setting of a rapid rate of progression or difficult follow-up.

Additional treatment modalities, such as tube-shunt procedures, laser cyclophotocoagulation of the ciliary body [with yttrium aluminum garnet (YAG) laser, diode laser, or endolaser], cyclocryotherapy, and cyclodialysis, are typically reserved for IOP uncontrolled by other methods. Some surgeons, however, now use tube-shunt procedures as initial surgery. Other early surgical options include canaloplasty, deep sclerectomy, and trabectome trabecular ablation.

Medications

Unless there are extreme circumstances (e.g., IOP >40 mm Hg or impending loss of central fixation), treatment is started by using one type of drop in one eye (monocular therapeutic trial) with reexamination in 3 to 6 weeks to check for effectiveness.

—Prostaglandin agonists (e.g., latanoprost 0.005% q.h.s., bimatoprost 0.03% q.h.s., travoprost 0.004% q.h.s.) are to be used with caution in patients with active uveitis or cystoid macular edema (CME) and are contraindicated in pregnant women or in women wishing to become pregnant. Inform patients of potential pigment changes in iris and periorbital skin, as well as hypertrichosis of eyelashes. Iris pigment changes rarely occur in blue or dark brown eyes. Those at highest risk for irreversible iris hyperpigmentation are hazel, grey irides.

—Beta-blockers (e.g., levobunolol or timolol 0.25% to 0.5% q.d. or b.i.d.) should be avoided in patients with asthma, COPD, heart block, bradyarrhythmia, unstable congestive heart failure, depression, or myasthenia gravis. In addition to bronchospasm and bradycardia, other side effects include hypotension, decreased libido, CNS depression, and reduced exercise tolerance.

—Selective α2-receptor agonists (brimonidine 0.1%, 0.15%, or 0.2% t.i.d. or b.i.d.) are contraindicated in patients taking monoamine oxidase inhibitors (risk of hypertensive crisis) and relatively contraindicated in children under the age of 5 (risk for cardiorespiratory and CNS depression). See 8.11, *Congenital/Infantile Glaucoma*. Apraclonidine may be used for short-term therapy (3 months), but tends to lose its effectiveness and has a high allergy rate.

—Topical carbonic anhydrase inhibitors (CAIs) (e.g., dorzolamide 2% or brinzolamide 1% t.i.d. or b.i.d.) should be avoided, but are not contraindicated, in patients with sulfa allergy. These medications theoretically could cause the same side effects as systemic CAIs, such as metabolic acidosis, hypokalemia, gastrointestinal symptoms, weight loss, paresthesias, and aplastic anemia. However, systemic symptoms from topical CAIs are extremely rare. There have been no reported cases of aplastic anemia from topical use. Corneal endothelial dysfunction may be

9

exacerbated with topical CAIs and should be used with caution in Fuchs corneal dystrophy and post keratoplasty.

—Miotics (e.g., pilocarpine q.i.d.) are usually used in low strengths initially (e.g., 0.5% to 1.0%) and then built up to higher strengths (e.g., 4%). Commonly not tolerated in patients <40 years because of accommodative spasm. Miotics are usually contraindicated in patients with retinal holes and should be used cautiously in patients at risk for retinal detachment (e.g., high myopes and aphakes).

—Sympathomimetics (dipivefrin 0.1% b.i.d. or epinephrine 0.5% to 2.0% b.i.d.) rarely reduce IOP to the degree of the other drugs, but have few systemic side effects (rarely, cardiac arrhythmias). They often cause red eyes and may cause CME in aphakic patients.

—Systemic CAIs (e.g., methazolamide 25 to 50 mg p.o. b.i.d. to t.i.d., acetazolamide 125 to 250 mg p.o. b.i.d. to q.i.d., or acetazolamide 500 mg sequel p.o. b.i.d.) should usually not be given to patients with a sulfa allergy or renal failure. Potassium levels must be monitored if the patient is taking other diuretic agents or digitalis. Side effects such as fatigue, nausea, confusion, and paresthesias are common. Rare, but severe, hematologic side effects (e.g., aplastic anemia) and Stevens–Johnson syndrome have occurred.

NOTE: Every patient should be instructed to press a tissue into the inner canthus to occlude the punctum for 10 seconds after instilling a drop. Doing so will decrease systemic absorption and reduce allergic blepharitis. If unable to perform punctal occlusion, keeping the eyelids closed without blinking for 3 minutes after drop administration also reduces systemic absorption.

Argon Laser Trabeculoplasty

In some patients, as previously defined, ALT may be used as first-line therapy. It has an initial success rate of 70% to 80%, dropping to 50% in 2 to 5 years.

Selective Laser Trabeculoplasty

The IOP-lowering effect of SLT is equivalent to ALT. SLT utilizes lower energy and causes

less tissue damage, which has led to the suggestion that it may be repeatable. This has not been proven.

Guarded Filtration Surgery

Trabeculectomy may obviate the need for medications. Adjunctive use of antimetabolites (e.g., mitomycin-C, 5-fluorouracil) may aid in the effectiveness of the surgery but increases the risk of complications (e.g., bleb leaks and hypotony).

Follow-Up

1. Patients are reexamined 4 to 6 weeks after starting a new β-blocker or prostaglandin or after ALT/SLT to evaluate efficacy. Topical CAIs, α-agonists, and miotics quickly reach a steady state, and a repeat examination may be performed at any time after 3 days.

2. Closer monitoring (e.g., 1 to 3 days) may be necessary when damage is severe and the IOP is high.

3. Once the IOP has been reduced adequately, patients are reevaluated in 3- to 6-month intervals for IOP and optic nerve checks.

4. Gonioscopy is performed yearly and after starting a new-strength cholinergic agent (e.g., pilocarpine).

5. Formal visual fields and optic nerve imaging (e.g., photographs, OCT, or HRT) are rechecked as needed, often about every 6 to 12 months. If IOP control is not thought to be adequate, visual fields may need to be repeated more often. Once stabilized, formal visual field testing can be repeated annually.

6. Dilated retinal examinations should be performed yearly.

7. If glaucomatous damage progresses, check patient compliance with medications before initiating additional therapy.

8. Patients must be questioned about side effects associated with their specific agent(s). They often do not associate eye drops with impotence, weight loss, lightheadedness, or other significant symptoms.

9.2 LOW-PRESSURE PRIMARY OPEN-ANGLE GLAUCOMA (NORMAL PRESSURE GLAUCOMA)

Definition

POAG occurring in patients without IOP elevation.

Symptoms

See 9.1, *Primary Open-Angle Glaucoma.*

Signs

Critical. See *Signs* in 9.1, *Primary Open-Angle Glaucoma,* except IOP is consistently below 22 mm Hg. There appears to be a greater likelihood of optic disc hemorrhages. Some believe visual field defects are denser, more localized, and closer to fixation. A dense nasal paracentral defect is typical. Average CCT is generally 510 to 520 microns.

Differential Diagnosis

NOTE: Determining that optic nerve changes are related to IOP and not another form of optic neuropathy is critical.

- POAG: IOP may be underestimated secondary to large diurnal fluctuations or thin corneas. See 9.1, *Primary Open-Angle Glaucoma.*

- Shock optic neuropathy from previous episode of systemic hypotension (e.g., acute blood loss, myocardial infarction, coronary artery bypass surgery, arrhythmia). Visual field loss should be nonprogressive.

- Intermittent IOP elevation (e.g. angle-closure glaucoma, glaucomatocyclitic crisis).

- Previous glaucomatous insult with severe IOP elevation that has subsequently resolved. Nonprogressive (e.g., traumatic glaucoma, steroid-induced glaucoma).

- Nonglaucomatous optic neuropathy and others. See *Differential Diagnosis* in 9.1, *Primary Open-Angle Glaucoma.*

Etiology

Controversial. Most investigators believe that IOP plays an important role in low-pressure POAG. Other proposed etiologies include vascular dysregulation (e.g., systemic or nocturnal hypotension, vasospasm, or loss of autoregulation), microischemic disease, accelerated apoptosis, and autoimmune disease.

Work-Up

See *Work-Up* in 9.1, *Primary Open-Angle Glaucoma.* Also consider:

1. History: Evidence of vasospasm (history of migraine or Raynaud phenomenon)? History of hypotensive crisis, anemia, or heart disease? Previous use of corticosteroids by any route? Trauma or uveitis in past? Has the vision loss been acute or chronic? GCA symptoms? Additional cardiovascular risk factors such as elevated cholesterol, hypertension, and systemic hypotension (including nocturnal "dippers" in the early morning hours)?

2. Check color plates.

3. Check gonioscopy to rule out angle closure, angle recession, or PAS.

4. Consider obtaining a diurnal curve of IOP measurements to help confirm the diagnosis.

5. Consider carotid dopplers to evaluate ocular blood flow. Check blood pressure (consider 24-hour automated blood pressure home monitor).

6. Consider CT or MRI to rule out compressive lesions of the optic nerve or chiasm.

Treatment

1. Research suggests that further lowering of IOP plays an important role in preventing progression of low-pressure POAG. Target IOPs are at least 30% lower than the level at which progressive damage was occurring.

9

Therapies are those for POAG. See 9.1, *Primary Open-Angle Glaucoma*, for a more in-depth discussion of these therapies.

2. Ischemia to the optic nerve head may play a role in the pathogenesis of low-pressure POAG. Modification of cardiovascular risk factors is appropriate in managing general health, but has not proven beneficial in managing glaucoma. Refer to an internist for control of blood pressure, cholesterol, and optimal management of other comorbid conditions to maximize optic nerve perfusion. Avoid use of antihypertensive drugs at bedtime and use preferentially in the morning.

3. Vasospasm may play a role in the pathogenesis of low-pressure POAG. Some investigators advocate the use of systemic calcium channel blockers in the treatment of this condition. The benefit of these medications has not been well established. Although it may improve capillary perfusion to the optic nerve head, systemic hypotension associated with this therapy may conversely have the opposite effect on ocular blood flow.

Follow-Up

See 9.1, *Primary Open-Angle Glaucoma*.

9.3 OCULAR HYPERTENSION

Signs

Critical. IOP >2 (or 3) standard deviations (approximately 3 mm Hg) above the average (15 mm Hg in most populations). Normal-appearing, open anterior chamber angle with normal anatomy on gonioscopy. Apparently normal optic nerve and visual field.

Differential Diagnosis

- POAG. See 9.1, *Primary Open-Angle Glaucoma*.

- Secondary open-angle glaucoma. See 9.1, *Primary Open-Angle Glaucoma*.

- CACG: PAS are present on gonioscopy with glaucomatous optic nerve and visual field changes. See 9.5, *Chronic Angle-Closure Glaucoma*.

Work-Up

1. See 9.1, *Primary Open-Angle Glaucoma*.

2. If any abnormalities are present on formal visual field testing, consider repeat testing in 2 to 4 weeks to exclude the possibility of learning curve artifacts. If the defects are judged to be real, the diagnosis is glaucoma or ocular hypertension along with another pathology accounting for the field loss.

3. OCT and HRT may reveal glaucomatous optic nerve defects. These objective tests may show pathology earlier than visual field testing.

Treatment

1. If there are no suggestive optic nerve or visual field changes and IOP is <24 mm Hg, no treatment other than close observation is necessary.

2. Patients with an IOP >24 to 30 mm Hg (threshold varies per glaucoma specialist), but otherwise normal examinations are candidates for IOP-lowering therapy. A decision to treat a patient should be based on the patient's choice to elect therapy and baseline risk factors such as age, CCT, initial IOP, horizontal and vertical C/D ratio, and family history. The results of the ocular hypertension treatment study (OHTS) showed that treatment reduced the development of visual field loss from 9.5% to 4.4% at 5 years, with a 20% average reduction of IOP. However, treatment also caused an increase in cataract and adverse psychological episodes. If treatment is elected, a therapeutic trial in one eye, as described for treatment of POAG, should be used. Some clinicians may elect to monitor these patients with close observation. Risk calculators have been developed to

approximate the level of risk progression to glaucoma if left untreated. These may help guide clinicians and patients as to whether treatment should be initiated. See 9.1, *Primary Open-Angle Glaucoma.*

Follow-Up

Close follow-up is required for patients being treated and observed. All patients should initially be followed similarly to POAG; see 9.1, *Primary Open-Angle Glaucoma.* If there is no progression in the first few years, monitoring frequency can be decreased to every 6 to 12 months. Stopping medication should be considered.

Reference

Kass MA, Heuer DK, Higginbotham EJ, et al. The Ocular Hypertension Treatment Study: a randomized trial determines that topical ocular hypotensive medication delays or prevents the onset of POAG. *Arch Ophthalmol* 2002;120:701–713.

9.4   ACUTE ANGLE-CLOSURE GLAUCOMA

Symptoms

Pain, blurred vision, colored halos around lights, frontal headache, nausea, and vomiting.

Signs

(See Figure 9.4.1.)

Critical. Closed angle in the involved eye, acutely increased IOP, microcystic corneal edema. Narrow or occludable angle in the fellow eye if of primary etiology.

Other. Conjunctival injection; fixed, mid-dilated pupil.

Etiology of Primary Angle Closure

—Pupillary block: Apposition of the lens and the posterior iris at the pupil leads to blockage of aqueous humor flow from the posterior chamber to the anterior chamber. This mechanism leads to increased posterior chamber pressure, forward movement of the peripheral iris, and subsequent obstruction of the trabecular meshwork (TM). Predisposed eyes have a narrow anterior chamber angle recess, anterior iris insertion of the iris root, or shorter axial length. Risk factors include increased age, East Asian descent, female gender, hyperopia, and family history. May be precipitated by topical mydriatics or, rarely, miotics, systemic anticholinergics (e.g., antihistamines and antidepressants), accommodation (e.g., reading), or dim illumination. Fellow eye has similar anatomy.

—Angle crowding as a result of an abnormal iris configuration including high peripheral iris roll or plateau iris syndrome angle closure. See 9.13, *Plateau Iris.*

Etiology of Secondary Angle Closure

- PAS pulling the angle closed: Causes include uveitis, inflammation, laser trabeculoplasty. See 9.5, *Chronic Angle-Closure Glaucoma.*

- Neovascular or fibrovascular membrane pulling the angle closed: See 9.14, *Neovascular Glaucoma.*

- Membrane obstructing the angle: Causes include endothelial membrane in irido-

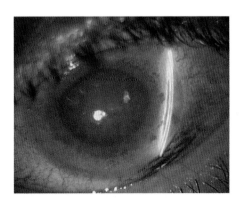

FIGURE 9.4.1. Acute angle-closure glaucoma with mid-dilated pupil and shallow anterior chamber.

9

corneal endothelial syndrome (ICE) and posterior polymorphous corneal dystrophy (PPCD), and epithelial membrane in epithelial downgrowth (often follows penetrating and nonpenetrating trauma). See 9.15, *Iridocorneal Endothelial Syndrome*.

▪ Lens-induced narrow angles: Iris–TM contact as a result of a large lens (phacomorphic), small lens with anterior prolapse (e.g., microspherophakia), small eye (nanophthalmos), or zonular loss/weakness (e.g., traumatic, advanced pseudoexfoliation, Marfan syndrome).

▪ Aphakic or pseudophakic papillary block: Iris bombe configuration secondary to occlusion of the pupil by the anterior vitreous. May also occur with anterior chamber intraocular lenses.

▪ Topiramate and sulfonamide-induced angle closure: Usually after increase in dose or within first 2 weeks of starting medication. Usually bilateral angle-closure due to supraciliary effusion and ciliary body swelling with subsequent anterior rotation of the lens–iris diaphragm. Myopia is induced secondary to anterior displacement of ciliary body and lens and lenticular swelling.

▪ Choroidal swelling: Following extensive retinal laser surgery, placement of a tight encircling scleral buckle, retinal vein occlusion, and others.

▪ Posterior segment tumor: Malignant melanoma, retinoblastoma, ciliary body tumors, and others. See 11.36, *Choroidal Nevus and Malignant Melanoma of the Choroid*.

▪ Hemorrhagic choroidal detachment: See 11.27, *Choroidal Effusion/Detachment*.

▪ Aqueous misdirection syndrome. See 9.17, *Aqueous Misdirection Syndrome/Malignant Glaucoma*.

▪ Developmental abnormalities: Axenfeld–Rieger syndrome, Peters anomaly, persistent fetal vasculature/persistent hyperplastic primary vitreous, and others. See 8.12, *Developmental Anterior Segment and Lens Anomalies/Dysgenesis*.

Differential Diagnosis of Acute IOP Increase With an Open Angle:

▪ Glaucomatocyclitic crisis (Posner–Schlossman syndrome): Recurrent IOP spikes in one eye, mild cell, and flare with or without fine keratic precipitates. See 9.8, *Glaucomatocyclitic Crisis/Posner–Schlossman Syndrome*.

▪ Inflammatory open-angle glaucoma: See 9.7, *Inflammatory Open-Angle Glaucoma*.

▪ Retrobulbar hemorrhage or inflammation. See 3.10, *Traumatic Retrobulbar Hemorrhage*.

▪ Carotid–cavernous fistula: See 7.7, *Miscellaneous Orbital Diseases*.

▪ Traumatic (hemolytic) glaucoma: Red blood cells in the anterior chamber. See 3.6, *Hyphema and Microhyphema*.

▪ Pigmentary glaucoma: Characteristic angle changes, (4+ posterior trabecular meshwork band); pigment cells floating in the anterior chamber; pigment line on the posterior lens capsule or anterior hyaloid face; radial iris transillumination defects (TIDs). See 9.10, *Pigment Dispersion Syndrome/ Pigmentary Glaucoma*.

Work-Up

1. History: Risk factors including hyperopia or family history? Precipitating events such as being in dim illumination, receiving dilating drops? Retinal problem? Recent laser treatment or surgery? Medications (e.g., topical adrenergics or anticholinergics, oral topiramate, or sulfa medications)?

2. Slit-lamp examination: Look for keratic precipitates, posterior synechiae, iris atrophy or neovascularization, a mid-dilated and sluggish pupil, a swollen lens, anterior chamber cells and flare or iridescent particles, and a shallow anterior chamber. Glaukomflecken (small anterior subcapsular lens opacities) and atrophy of the iris stroma indicate prior attacks. Always carefully examine the other eye and compare.

3. Measure IOP.

4. Gonioscopy of both anterior chamber angles. Corneal edema can be cleared by

using topical hyperosmolar agents (e.g., glycerin). Gonioscopy of the involved eye after IOP is reduced is essential in determining whether the angle has opened and whether neovascularization is present.

5. Careful examination of the fundus looking for signs of central retinal vein occlusion, hemorrhage, optic nerve cupping, or spontaneous arterial pulsations. If cupping is pronounced or if there are spontaneous arterial pulsations, treatment is more urgent.

6. When secondary angle-closure glaucoma is suspected, B-scan US or US biomicroscopy (UBM) may be helpful.

Treatment

Depends on etiology of angle closure, severity, and duration of attack. Severe, permanent damage may occur within several hours. If visual acuity is hand motions or worse, IOP reduction is usually urgent, and medications should include all topical glaucoma medications not contraindicated, intravenous acetazolamide, and in some cases intravenous osmotic (e.g., mannitol). See 9.14, *Neovascular Glaucoma,* 9.16, *Postoperative Glaucoma,* 9.17, *Aqueous Misdirection Syndrome/Malignant Glaucoma.*

1. Compression gonioscopy is essential to determine if the trabecular blockage is reversible and may break an acute attack.

2. Topical therapy with β-blockers [(e.g., timolol 0.5%) caution with asthma or COPD], α-2 agonist (e.g., brimonidine 0.15%), prostaglandin analogs (e.g., latanoprost 0.005%), and CAIs (dorzolamide 2%) should be initiated immediately. In urgent cases, three rounds of these medications may be given, with each round being separated by 15 minutes.

3. Topical steroid (e.g., prednisolone acetate 1%) may be useful.

4. Systemic carbonic anhydrase inhibitors [e.g., acetazolamide, 250 to 500 mg intravenously (i.v.), or two 250-mg tablets p.o. in one dose if unable to give i.v.] if IOP decrease is urgent or if IOP is refractory to topical therapy. Do not use in topiramate- or sulfonamide-induced angle closure.

5. Recheck the IOP and visual acuity in 1 hour. If IOP does not decrease and vision does not improve, repeat topical medications and give mannitol 1 to 2 g/kg i.v. over 45 minutes (a 500-mL bag of mannitol 20% contains 100 g of mannitol).

6. When acute angle-closure glaucoma is the result of:

a. Phakic pupillary block or angle crowding: Pilocarpine, 1% to 2%, every 15 minutes for two doses, and pilocarpine, 0.5% to 1.0%, in the contralateral eye for one dose.

b. Aphakic or pseudophakic pupillary block or secondary closure of the angle: Do not use pilocarpine. Consider a mydriatic and a cycloplegic agent (e.g., cyclopentolate, 1% to 2%, and phenylephrine 2.5% every 15 minutes for four doses) when laser or surgery cannot be performed because of corneal edema, inflammation, or both.

c. Topiramate- or sulfonamide-induced secondary angle closure: Do not use CAIs. Immediately discontinue the inciting medication. Consider cycloplegia to induce posterior rotation of the ciliary body (e.g., atropine 1% b.i.d. or t.i.d.). Consider hospitalization and treatment with intravenous hyperosmotic agents and intravenous steroids (methylprednisolone 250 mg i.v. every 6 hours) for cases of markedly elevated IOP unresponsive to other treatments. Peripheral iridectomy and miotics are not indicated.

7. In phacomorphic glaucoma, the lens should be removed as soon as the eye is quiet and the IOP controlled, if possible. See 9.12.4, *Phacomorphic Glaucoma.*

8. Address systemic problems such as pain and vomiting.

9. For pupillary block (all forms) or angle crowding: If the IOP decreases significantly (less than the fellow eye) and the angle is open by gonioscopy, definitive treatment with laser (YAG) peripheral iridotomy or surgical iridectomy is performed once the

9

cornea is clear and the anterior chamber is quiet, typically 1 to 5 days after attack. Patients are discharged on the following medications and followed daily:

- Prednisolone acetate 1% may be helpful.

- Acetazolamide 500 mg sequel p.o. b.i.d.

- Topical β-blocker b.i.d. and/or α-agonist b.i.d.

- If phakic, pilocarpine 1% to 2% q.i.d.

NOTE: Some believe that once the attack is broken, only pilocarpine and prednisolone acetate are necessary if the angle is open.

If IOP does not decrease after two courses of maximal medical therapy, a laser (YAG) PI should be considered if there is an adequate view of the iris. If IOP still does not decrease after a second attempt at a laser PI, then a laser iridoplasty or surgical PI is needed and, in some cases, a guarded filtration procedure.

NOTE: If affected eye is too inflamed initially for laser PI, perform laser PI of the fellow eye first. An untreated fellow eye has a 40% to 80% chance of acute angle closure in 5 to 10 years. Repeated angle-closure attacks with a patent PI may indicate plateau iris syndrome. See 9.13, *Plateau Iris.*

---

10. For secondary angle closure: Treat the underlying problem. Consider argon laser gonioplasty to open the angle, particularly in cases that are the result of extensive retinal laser surgery, a tight scleral buckle, or nanophthalmos. Goniosynechialysis can be performed for chronic angle closure of <6 months' duration. Systemic steroids may be required to treat serous choroidal detachments secondary to inflammation.

Follow-Up

After definitive treatment, patients are reevaluated in weeks to months initially, and then less frequently. Visual fields and stereo disc photographs are obtained for baseline purposes.

NOTE:

1. Cardiovascular status and electrolyte balance must be considered when contemplating osmotic agents, CAIs, and β-blockers.

2. The corneal appearance may worsen when the IOP decreases.

3. Worsening vision or spontaneous arterial pulsations are signs of increasing urgency for pressure reduction.

4. Since one-third to one-half of first-degree relatives may have occludable angles, patients should be counseled to alert relatives to the importance of screening.

5. Angle-closure glaucoma may be seen without an increased IOP. The diagnosis should be suspected in a patient who had pain and reduced acuity and is noted to have:

   —An edematous, thickened cornea in one eye.

   —Normal or markedly asymmetric pressure in both eyes.

   —Shallow anterior chambers in both eyes.

   —Occludable anterior chamber angle in the fellow eye.

9.5 CHRONIC ANGLE-CLOSURE GLAUCOMA

Symptoms

Usually asymptomatic, although patients with advanced disease may present with decreased vision or visual field loss. Intermittent eye pain, headaches, and blurry vision may occur.

Signs

(See Figure 9.5.1.)

Critical. Gonioscopy reveals broad bands of PAS in the angle. The PAS block visualization of the underlying structures of the angle.

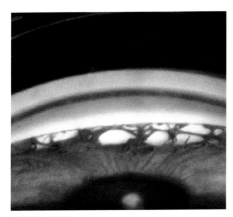

FIGURE 9.5.1. Chronic angle-closure glaucoma with peripheral anterior synechiae.

Glaucomatous optic nerve and visual field defects.

Other. Elevated IOP.

Etiology

Prolonged acute angle-closure glaucoma or multiple episodes of subclinical attacks of acute angle closure resulting in PAS, often in superior angle.

- Previous uveitic glaucoma with development of PAS, often in inferior angle.

- Regressed neovascularization of the anterior chamber angle resulting in the development of PAS.

- Previous laser to the TM, typically seen with small peaked PAS.

- Previous flat anterior chamber from surgery, trauma, or hypotony that resulted in the development of PAS.

NOTE: While acute angle closure is less common in those of African descent, chronic angle closure is more commonly seen in these patients.

Work-Up

1. History: Presence of symptoms of previous episodes of acute angle closure? History of proliferative diabetic retinopathy, retinal vascular occlusion, or ocular ischemic syndrome? History of trauma, hypotony, uveitis, or laser treatment?

2. Complete baseline glaucoma evaluation. See 9.1, *Primary Open-Angle Glaucoma.*

Treatment

See 9.1, *Primary Open-Angle Glaucoma.*

1. Laser trabeculoplasty contraindicated in CACG prior to PI and can induce greater scarring of the angle.

2. If patient has angle closure with pupillary block, perform laser peripheral iridotomy to prevent further angle-closure episodes. The TM may have sustained enough damage that the IOP will still be elevated despite a patent iridotomy, necessitating continued use of medications to lower the IOP.

3. Laser iridoplasty may be performed to attempt to decrease the formation of new PAS. This may not be effective, or may serve as a temporary measure; if successful it may be repeated. If iridoplasty fails and other medical therapy has been maximized, the patient may need additional surgery.

Follow-Up

See 9.1, *Primary Open-Angle Glaucoma.*

9

9.6 ANGLE-RECESSION GLAUCOMA

Symptoms

Usually asymptomatic. Late stages have visual field or acuity loss. A history of hyphema or trauma to the glaucomatous eye can often be elicited. Glaucoma due to the angle recession (not from the trauma that caused the angle recession) usually takes 10 to 20 years to develop. Typically unilateral.

Signs

(See Figure 9.6.1.)

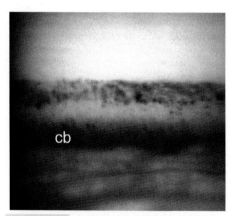

cb

FIGURE 9.6.1. Angle-recession glaucoma with increased width of the ciliary body band.

Critical. Glaucoma (see 9.1, *Primary Open-Angle Glaucoma*) in an eye with characteristic gonioscopic findings: an uneven iris insertion, an area of torn or absent iris processes, and a posteriorly recessed iris, revealing a widened ciliary band (may extend for 360 degrees). Comparison with the contralateral eye is of great help in identification of recessed areas.

Other. The scleral spur may appear abnormally white on gonioscopy because of the recessed angle; other signs of previous trauma may be present (e.g., cataract, iris sphincter tears).

Differential Diagnosis

See 9.1, *Primary Open-Angle Glaucoma.*

Work-Up

1. History: Trauma? Family history of glaucoma?

2. Complete baseline glaucoma evaluation. See 9.1, *Primary Open-Angle Glaucoma.*

Treatment

See 9.1, *Primary Open-Angle Glaucoma.* However, miotics (e.g., pilocarpine) may be ineffective or even cause increased IOP as a result of a reduction of uveoscleral outflow. ALT and SLT are rarely effective in this condition. Surgical therapy may be necessary if uncontrolled with medications.

Follow-Up

Both eyes are monitored closely because of high incidence of delayed open-angle glaucoma. Patients with angle recession without glaucoma are examined yearly. Those with glaucoma are examined according to the guidelines detailed in 9.1, *Primary Open-Angle Glaucoma.*

9

9.7 INFLAMMATORY OPEN-ANGLE GLAUCOMA

Symptoms

Pain, photophobia, decreased vision; symptoms may be minimal.

Signs

Critical. Elevated IOP with a significant amount of anterior chamber inflammation; open angle on gonioscopy. Characteristic glaucomatous optic nerve changes occur late in the disease course.

Other. Miotic pupil, PAS, keratic precipitates, conjunctival injection, ciliary flush, posterior synechiae, and increased TM pigmentation, especially inferiorly.

> **NOTE:** Acute IOP increase is distinguished from chronic IOP increase by the presence of corneal edema, pain, and visual symptoms.

Differential Diagnosis

- Glaucomatocyclitic crisis (Posner–Schlossman syndrome): Open angle and absence of synechiae on gonioscopy. Minimal to no conjunctival injection. Unilateral with recurrent attacks. See 9.8, *Glaucomatocyclitic Crisis/Posner–Schlossman Syndrome.*

- Steroid-response glaucoma: Open angle. Patient on steroid medications (including for uveitis). Can be difficult to differentiate from inflammatory open-angle glaucoma. If significant inflammation is present, it should be assumed to be inflammatory first. See 9.9, *Steroid-Response Glaucoma*.

- Pigmentary glaucoma: 3+ to 4+ trabecular pigmentation. Acute increase in IOP, often after exercise or pupillary dilatation; pigment cells in the anterior chamber. Open angle. Radial iris TIDs are common. See 9.10, *Pigment Dispersion Syndrome/Pigmentary Glaucoma*.

- Neovascular glaucoma. Nonradial, misdirected blood vessels along the pupillary margin, the TM, or both. See 9.14, *Neovascular Glaucoma*.

- Fuchs heterochromic iridocyclitis: Asymmetry of the iris color typically with mild iritis in the eye with the lighter-colored iris. Gonioscopy may reveal fine vessels that cross the TM, without PAS. Usually unilateral. See 12.1, *Anterior Uveitis (Iritis/Iridocyclitis)*.

- Pseudoexfoliation syndrome: Occasionally exfoliative material on cornea can be mistaken for keratic precipitates. See 9.11, *Pseudoexfoliation Syndrome/Exfoliative Glaucoma*.

Etiology

- Uveitis: Anterior, intermediate, posterior, or panuveitis.

- Keratouveitis.

- After trauma or intraocular surgery.

Work-Up

1. History: Previous attacks? Systemic disease [e.g., juvenile idiopathic arthritis, ankylosing spondylitis, sarcoidosis, acquired immunodeficiency syndrome (AIDS), V1 distribution varicella zoster, toxoplasmosis]? Previous corneal disease, especially herpetic keratitis?

2. Slit-lamp examination: Assess the degree of conjunctival injection and aqueous cell and flare. Posterior synechiae present?

3. Complete baseline glaucoma evaluation. See 9.1, *Primary Open-Angle Glaucoma*.

Treatment

1. Topical steroid (e.g., prednisolone acetate 1%) q1–6h, depending on the severity of the anterior chamber inflammation.

NOTE: Topical steroids are not used, or are used with extreme caution, in patients with an infectious process, particularly a fungal or herpes simplex infection.

---

2. Mydriatic/cycloplegic (e.g., scopolamine 0.25% t.i.d.).

3. One or more of the following pressure-reducing agents can be used in addition to the other treatments, depending on the IOP and the status of the optic nerve:

   a. Topical β-blocker (e.g., timolol 0.5% b.i.d.) if not contraindicated (e.g., asthma, COPD).

   b. Topical α-2 agonist (e.g., brimonidine 0.1% to 0.2% b.i.d. to t.i.d.).

   c. Topical CAI (e.g., dorzolamide 2% t.i.d.) or oral (e.g., methazolamide 25 to 50 mg p.o. b.i.d. to t.i.d., or acetazolamide 500 mg sequel p.o. b.i.d.).

   d. Anterior chamber paracentesis if IOP is believed to be causing damage (see Appendix 13, *Anterior Chamber Paracentesis*).

   e. Hyperosmotic agent when IOP is acutely increased (e.g., mannitol 20% 1 to 2 g/kg i.v. over 45 minutes).

4. Manage the underlying problem.

5. If IOP remains dangerously increased despite maximal medical therapy, glaucoma filtering surgery with adjunct antifibrosis therapy may be indicated. Trabeculectomy surgery has high rates of failure in cases of inflammatory glaucoma.

NOTE: Prostaglandin agonists (e.g., latanoprost 0.005%) and miotics (e.g., pilocarpine) should be used with caution in inflammatory glaucoma.

Follow-Up

1. Patients are seen every 1 to 7 days at first. Higher IOP and more advanced

9

glaucomatous cupping warrant more frequent follow-up.

2. Antiglaucoma medications are discontinued as IOP returns to normal. Steroid-response glaucoma should always be considered in unresponsive cases (see 9.9, *Steroid-Response Glaucoma*). IOP elevation in the presence of significant uveitis suggests the need for more, not less, steroids and additional or alternative pressure lowering therapy.

9.8 GLAUCOMATOCYCLITIC CRISIS/POSNER–SCHLOSSMAN SYNDROME

Symptoms

Mild pain, decreased vision, rainbows around lights. Often, a history of previous episodes. Usually unilateral in young to middle-aged patients.

Signs

Critical. Markedly increased IOP (usually 40 to 60 mm Hg), open angle without synechiae on gonioscopy, minimal conjunctival injection (white eye), very mild anterior chamber reaction (few aqueous cells and little flare).

Other. Corneal epithelial edema, ciliary flush, pupillary constriction, iris hypochromia, few fine keratic precipitates on the corneal endothelium or TM.

Differential Diagnosis

- Inflammatory open-angle glaucoma: Significant amount of aqueous cells and flare. Synechiae may be present. See 9.7, *Inflammatory Open-Angle Glaucoma*.

- Acute angle-closure glaucoma: Shallow anterior chamber and closed angle in the involved eye. Narrow or closed angle in the contralateral eye. See 9.4, *Acute Angle-Closure Glaucoma*.

- Pigmentary glaucoma: Acute increase in IOP, often after exercise or pupillary dilatation, with pigment cells in the anterior chamber. See 9.10, *Pigment Dispersion Syndrome/Pigmentary Glaucoma*.

- Neovascular glaucoma: Abnormal blood vessels along the pupillary margin, the TM, or both. See 9.14, *Neovascular Glaucoma*.

- Fuchs heterochromic iridocyclitis: Asymmetry of iris color, mild iritis in the eye with the lighter-colored iris. The increase in IOP is rarely as acute. See 12.1, *Anterior Uveitis (Iritis/Iridocyclitis)*.

- Others: Herpes simplex, varicella zoster keratouveitis, toxoplasmosis, and others.

Etiology

Mechanism unknown, but possible association with herpes viruses.

Work-Up

1. History: Recent dilating drops, systemic anticholinergic agents, or exercise? Previous attacks? Corneal or systemic disease? Light sensitivity? Pain?

2. Slit-lamp examination: Assess the degree of conjunctival injection and aqueous cell and flare. Careful retinal examination for vasculitis and snowbanking. Measure IOP.

3. Gonioscopy: Angle open? Synechiae, neovascular membrane, or keratic precipitates present?

4. Complete baseline glaucoma evaluation. See 9.1, *Primary Open-Angle Glaucoma*.

Treatment

1. Topical β-blocker (e.g., timolol 0.5% b.i.d.), topical α-2 agonist (e.g., brimonidine 0.1% to 0.2% b.i.d. or t.i.d.), topical CAI (e.g., dorzolamide 2% b.i.d. to t.i.d.).

2. Short course (1 week) of topical steroids (e.g., prednisolone acetate 1% q.i.d.) may decrease inflammation. Longer use may cause an elevation in IOP. Oral indomethacin (e.g., 75 to 150 mg p.o. q.d.) or topical nonsteroidal antiinflammatory drugs (NSAIDs) (e.g., ketorolac q.i.d.) may also be effective.

3. Consider a systemic CAI (e.g., acetazolamide 500 mg sequel p.o. b.i.d.) if IOP is significantly increased.

4. Anterior chamber paracentesis when the IOP is determined to be dangerously high for the involved optic nerve (see Appendix 13, *Anterior Chamber Paracentesis*). Hyperosmotic agents (e.g., mannitol 20% 1 to 2 g/kg i.v. over 45 minutes) are second line.

5. Consider a cycloplegic agent (e.g., cyclopentolate 1% t.i.d.) if the patient is symptomatic.

Follow-Up

1. Patients are seen every few days at first and then weekly until the episode resolves.

Attacks usually subside within a few hours to a few weeks.

2. Medical or surgical therapy may be required, depending on the baseline IOP between attacks.

3. If the IOP decreases to levels not associated with disc damage, no treatment is necessary.

4. Steroids are tapered rapidly if they are used for 1 week or less and slowly if they are used for longer.

5. Both eyes are at risk for the development of chronic open-angle glaucoma. Patients should be followed as if the diagnosis is POAG. See 9.1, *Primary Open-Angle Glaucoma*.

9.9 STEROID-RESPONSE GLAUCOMA

Signs

Critical. Increased IOP with the use of corticosteroids. Usually takes 2 to 4 weeks after starting topical steroids, though rarely there can be an acute rise of IOP within hours in association with systemic use of steroid or adrenocorticotropic hormone (ACTH).

Other. Signs of POAG may develop. See 9.1, *Primary Open-Angle Glaucoma.*

NOTE: Patients with POAG or a predisposition to development of glaucoma (e.g., family history, ocular trauma, diabetes, African descent, high myopia) are more likely to experience a steroid response and subsequent glaucoma.

Differential Diagnosis

- POAG. See 9.1, *Primary Open-Angle Glaucoma.*

- Exfoliative glaucoma. See 9.11, *Pseudoexfoliation Syndrome/Exfoliative Glaucoma.*

- Inflammatory open-angle glaucoma: Because steroids are used to treat ocular

inflammation, it may be difficult to determine the cause of the increased IOP. See 9.7, *Inflammatory Open-Angle Glaucoma.*

Etiology

Most commonly seen with topical, periocular, or intravitreal steroid therapy, though elevated IOP can occur with all forms of administration, including oral, intravenous, inhalational, nasal, injected, or topical skin steroids. More potent topical steroids (e.g., dexamethasone) more often cause significant rises in IOP compared to those that are less potent (e.g., fluorometholone, loteprednol). The IOP typically decreases to pretreatment levels after steroids are stopped. The rate of decrease relates to the duration of use and the severity of the pressure increase. The IOP increase is due to reduced outflow facility of the pigmented TM, and when this is severe, the IOP may remain increased for months after steroids are stopped. IOP increase may also be caused by increased inflammation in association with systemic steroid usage.

9

Work-Up

1. History: Duration of steroid use? Previous steroid use or an eye problem from steroid use? Glaucoma or family history of glaucoma? Herpetic keratouveitis? Diabetes? Myopia? Ocular trauma?

2. Complete ocular examination: Evaluate the degree of ocular inflammation and determine the presence of iris or angle neovascularization (by gonioscopy), pigment suggestive of pigment dispersion syndrome or pseudoexfoliation, blood in Schlemm canal, PAS, etc. Measure IOP and inspect the optic nerve.

3. Complete baseline glaucoma evaluation, See 9.1, *Primary Open-Angle Glaucoma*.

Treatment

Any or all of the following may be necessary to reduce IOP:

1. Determine if steroid use (in any form) is truly needed. If not needed, stop or taper steroids.

2. Reduce the concentration or dosage of the steroid.

3. Change to a steroid with lesser propensity for IOP elevation (e.g., fluorometholone, loteprednol, or rimexolone).

4. Switch to a topical NSAID (e.g., ketorolac 0.4% or 0.5%, diclofenac 0.1%).

5. Start antiglaucoma therapy. See 9.7, *Inflammatory Open-Angle Glaucoma,* for medical therapy options.

6. Consider anterior chamber paracentesis if IOP is actively causing damage (see Appendix 13, *Anterior Chamber Paracentesis*).

NOTE: For inflammatory glaucoma, if the inflammation is moderate to severe, increase the steroids initially to reduce the inflammation while initiating antiglaucoma therapy.

If a medically uncontrollable dangerously high IOP develops after a depot steroid injection, the steroid may need to be excised. After intravitreal triamcinolone, options include glaucoma filtering surgery or a pars plana vitrectomy to remove the steroid.

In general, laser trabeculoplasty is not effective for these patients.

Steroid-induced glaucoma after LASIK may be difficult to detect using applanation tonometry due to falsely low readings caused by interface fluid between the flap and the stromal bed.

Follow-Up

Dependent on the severity of pressure elevation and glaucomatous damage. Follow patients as if they have POAG. (See 9.1, *Primary Open-Angle Glaucoma*).

9.10 PIGMENT DISPERSION SYNDROME/ PIGMENTARY GLAUCOMA

Definition

Pigment dispersion refers to a pathologic increase in the TM pigment, associated with characteristic mid-peripheral, radial iris TIDs. Abnormal pigment dispersion is identified as 3+ to 4+ TM pigmentation with increasing radial TIDs or increasing corneal endothelial pigmentation. The pigment may ultimately obstruct the TM, leading to increased IOP and secondary open-angle glaucoma. Pigment on the posterior lens capsule is nearly pathognomonic and should always be looked for during examination.

Symptoms

Blurred vision, eye pain, and colored halos around lights after exercise or pupillary dilatation. May be asymptomatic. More common in young adult, myopic men (age 20 to 45 years). Usually bilateral, but asymmetric.

Signs

(See Figures 9.10.1 and 9.10.2.)

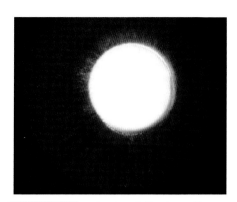

FIGURE 9.10.1. PDS with spokelike iris transillumination defects.

Critical. Mid-peripheral, spokelike iris TIDs corresponding to iridozonular contact; dense homogeneous pigmentation of the TM for 360 degrees (seen on gonioscopy) in the absence of signs of trauma or inflammation.

Other. A vertical pigment band on the corneal endothelium typically just inferior to the visual axis (Krukenberg spindle); pigment deposition on the posterior equatorial lens surface (e.g., Zentmayer line or Scheie line), on the anterior hyaloid face, on Schwalbe line, and sometimes along the iris (which can produce iris heterochromia). The angle often shows a wide ciliary body band with 3+ to 4+ pigmentation of the posterior TM at the 12-o'clock position. Pigmentary glaucoma is characterized by the pigment dispersion syndrome plus glaucomatous optic neuropathy.

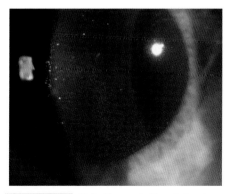

FIGURE 9.10.2. PDS with a vertical band of endothelial pigment (Krukenberg spindle).

Typically, large fluctuations in IOP can occur, during which pigment cells may be seen floating in the anterior chamber.

Differential Diagnosis

■ Exfoliative glaucoma: Iris TIDs may be present, but are near the pupillary margin and are not radial. White, flaky material may be seen on the pupillary border, anterior lens capsule, and corneal endothelium. See 9.11, *Pseudoexfoliation Syndrome/Exfoliative Glaucoma*.

■ Inflammatory open-angle glaucoma: White blood cells and flare in the anterior chamber; no radial iris TIDs; often PAS on gonioscopy. See 9.7, *Inflammatory Open-Angle Glaucoma*.

■ Iris melanoma: Pigmentation of the angular structures accompanied by either a raised, pigmented lesion on the iris or a diffusely darkened iris. No iris TIDs. See 5.13, *Malignant Melanoma of the Iris*.

■ Irradiation: Induces atrophy and depigmentation of the ciliary processes with increased TM pigment deposition.

■ Postoperative pigment liberation after posterior chamber intraocular lens implantation.

■ Siderosis.

■ Iris chafe with sulcus IOL.

Work-Up

1. History: Previous episodes of decreased vision or halos? Trauma or previous IOFB?

2. Slit-lamp examination, particularly checking for iris TIDs. Large defects may be seen by shining a small slit beam directly into the pupil to obtain a red reflex, but scleral transillumination is required if the defects are not extremely marked. Look for a Krukenberg spindle on the corneal endothelium. Look for pigment on lens equator by angling the slit beam nasally and having the patient look temporally (pathognomonic for pigment dispersion). Careful retinal examination because of increased incidence of lattice degeneration and retinal detachment.

9

3. Perform baseline glaucoma evaluation. See 9.1, *Primary Open-Angle Glaucoma.*

Treatment

Similar to POAG. Depends on the IOP, optic nerve damage, and extent of the symptoms. Usually patients with pigment dispersion without ocular hypertension, glaucoma, or symptoms are observed carefully. A stepwise approach to control IOP is usually taken when mild-to-moderate glaucomatous changes are present. When advanced glaucoma is discovered on initial examination, maximal medical therapy may be instituted initially. See 9.1, *Primary Open-Angle Glaucoma.*

1. Decrease mechanical iridozonular contact. Two methods have been proposed:

—Miotic agents: A theoretical first-line therapy because they minimize iridozonular contact. However, because most patients are young and myopic, the resulting fluctuation in myopia may not be tolerated. In addition, approximately 14% of patients have lattice retinal degeneration and are thus predisposed to retinal detachment from the use of miotics. In some cases, pilocarpine 4% gel q.h.s. may be tolerated.

—Peripheral laser iridotomy: Laser peripheral iridotomy has been recommended to reduce pigment dispersion by decreasing iridozonular contact, but it is still controversial. It may be best suited in early-stage disease and ill advised in more advanced stages.

2. Other antiglaucoma medications. See 9.1, *Primary Open-Angle Glaucoma.*

3. Patients typically respond well to SLT or ALT. Younger patients respond better than older patients, in contrast to POAG. However, there is a greater risk of post-laser IOP spikes. Lower energy should be used, and initially only 180 degrees of treatment is advised.

4. Consider guarded filtration procedure when medical and laser therapy fail. These young myopic patients are at a greater risk for the development of hypotony maculopathy, and antimetabolites should be used cautiously.

Follow-Up

Every 1 to 6 months, with a formal visual field test every 6 to 12 months, depending on the severity of the symptoms and the glaucoma.

9.11 PSEUDOEXFOLIATION SYNDROME/ EXFOLIATIVE GLAUCOMA

Definition

A systemic disease in which grayish-white material is deposited on the lens, iris, ciliary epithelium, and TM. Presence of exfoliative material increases the risk of glaucoma sixfold. Currently, the most common secondary glaucoma in those of European descent.

Symptoms

Usually asymptomatic in its early stages.

Signs

(See Figures 9.11.1 and 9.11.2.)

Critical. White, flaky material on the pupillary margin; anterior lens capsular changes (central zone of exfoliation material, often with rolled-up edges, middle clear zone, and a peripheral cloudy zone); peripupillary iris TIDs; and glaucomatous optic neuropathy. Bilateral, but often asymmetric.

Other. Irregular black pigment deposition on the TM more marked inferiorly than superiorly; black scalloped deposition of pigment anterior to Schwalbe line (Sampaolesi line) seen on gonioscopy, especially inferiorly. White, flaky material may be seen on the corneal endothelium,

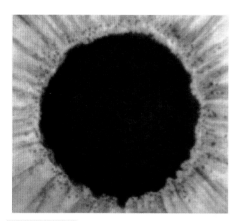

FIGURE 9.11.1. Pseudoexfoliation syndrome with white material on pupillary margin.

which often has a lower than normal endothelial cell density. Iris atrophy. Poor pupillary response to dilation (with more advanced cases, believed to be secondary to iris dilator muscle atrophy). Incidence increases with age. These patients are more prone to having narrow angles, especially inferiorly.

Differential Diagnosis

- Inflammatory glaucoma: Corneal endothelial deposits can be present in both exfoliative and uveitic glaucoma. Typically, IOP is highly unstable in both. The ragged volcano-like PAS of some inflammatory glaucomas are not seen in the exfoliation syndrome, but angle closure due to narrow angle is not rare in the exfoliation syndrome. Photophobia is common with uveitis. See 9.7, *Inflammatory Open-Angle Glaucoma.*

- Pigmentary glaucoma: Mid-peripheral iris TIDs. Pigment on the posterior equatorial lens surface. Deep anterior chamber angle. Myopia. See 9.10, *Pigment Dispersion Syndrome/Pigmentary Glaucoma.*

- Capsular delamination (true exfoliation): Trauma, exposure to intense heat (e.g., glass blower), or severe uveitis can cause a thin membrane to peel off the anterior lens capsule. Glaucoma uncommon.

- Primary amyloidosis: Amyloid material can deposit along the pupillary margin or anterior lens capsule. Glaucoma can occur.

- Uveitis, glaucoma, hyphema (UGH) syndrome: Prior surgery. See 9.16.3, *Uveitis, Glaucoma, Hyphema Syndrome.*

Work-Up

1. History: Occupational exposure to heat?

2. Slit-lamp examination with IOP measurement; look for white flaky material along the pupillary margin, often need to dilate the pupil to see the anterior lens capsular changes. Gonioscopy may reveal scattered "pepper" changes in the inferior angle, which are often the first change and are highly characteristic.

3. Perform baseline glaucoma evaluation. See 9.1, *Primary Open-Angle Glaucoma.*

Treatment

1. For medical therapy, see 9.1, *Primary Open-Angle Glaucoma.*

2. Consider SLT/ALT, which has a higher success rate in exfoliative glaucoma than in POAG, but shorter duration of effectiveness.

3. Consider guarded filtration procedure when medical or laser therapy fails.

4. The course of exfoliative glaucoma is usually not linear. Early, the condition may be relatively benign. However, the condition is associated with highly unstable IOP. Once IOP becomes difficult to control, the

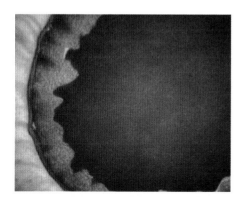

FIGURE 9.11.2. Pseudoexfoliation syndrome with white material on anterior lens capsule.

glaucoma may progress rapidly (e.g., within months).

NOTE: Cataract extraction does not eradicate the glaucoma. Cataract extraction may be complicated by weakened zonular fibers and synechiae between the iris and peripheral anterior lens capsule with increased risk of intraoperative vitreous loss and zonular dehiscence. Postoperative intraocular lens dislocation may occur with time.

Follow-Up

Every 1 to 3 months as with POAG, but with the awareness that damage can progress very rapidly.

NOTE: Many patients have pseudoexfoliation syndrome without glaucoma. These patients are reexamined every 6 to 12 months because of glaucoma risk, but they are not treated unless the IOP rises to levels considered dangerous.

9.12 LENS-INDUCED (PHACOGENIC) GLAUCOMA

9.12.1. PHACOLYTIC GLAUCOMA

Definition

Leakage of lens material through an intact lens capsule leads to TM outflow obstruction.

Symptoms

Unilateral pain, decreased vision, tearing, photophobia.

Signs

Critical. Markedly increased IOP, accompanied by iridescent particles and white material in the anterior chamber or on the anterior surface of the lens capsule. A hypermature (liquefied) or mature cataract is typical. Pain is usually severe. Vision may be light perception (LP) or no light perception (NLP).

Other. Corneal edema, anterior chamber cells and flare, pseudohypopyon, and severe conjunctival injection. Gonioscopy reveals an open anterior chamber angle. Clumps of macrophages may be seen in the inferior angle.

Differential Diagnosis

All of the following can produce an acute increase in IOP to high levels, but none displays iridescent particles and white material in the anterior chamber.

- Inflammatory glaucoma. See 9.7, *Inflammatory Open-Angle Glaucoma.*

- Glaucomatocyclitic crisis. See 9.8, *Glaucomatocyclitic Crisis/Posner–Schlossman Syndrome.*

- Acute angle-closure glaucoma. See 9.4, *Acute Angle-Closure Glaucoma.*

- Lens-particle glaucoma. See 9.12.2, *Lens-Particle Glaucoma.*

- Endophthalmitis. See 12.13, *Postoperative Endophthalmitis.*

- Glaucoma secondary to intraocular tumor: May have unilateral cataract.

- Others: Traumatic glaucoma, ghost cell glaucoma, phacomorphic glaucoma, neovascular glaucoma, and others.

Work-Up

1. History: Recent trauma or ocular surgery? Recurrent episodes? Uveitis in the past?

2. Slit-lamp examination: Look for iridescent or white particles as well as cells and flare in the anterior chamber. Check IOP. Evaluate for cataract and corneal edema.

3. Gonioscopy of the anterior chamber angles of both eyes: Topical glycerin may be placed on the cornea, after topical anesthesia, to temporarily clear any edema.

4. Retinal and optic disc examination if possible. Otherwise, B-scan US before cataract

extraction to rule out an intraocular tumor or retinal detachment.

5. If the diagnosis is in doubt, an anterior chamber paracentesis can be performed to detect macrophages bloated with lens material on microscopic examination. See Appendix 13, *Anterior Chamber Paracentesis.*

Treatment

The immediate goal of therapy is to reduce the IOP and to reduce the inflammation. The cataract should be removed promptly (within several days).

1. Topical β-blocker (e.g., timolol 0.5% b.i.d.), α-2 agonist (e.g., brimonidine 0.1% to 0.2% b.i.d. to t.i.d.), and/or topical CAI (e.g., dorzolamide 2% t.i.d.).

2. Systemic CAI (e.g., acetazolamide 500 mg sequel p.o. b.i.d.). Benefit of maintaining topical CAI in addition to a systemic agent is controversial.

3. Topical cycloplegic (e.g., scopolamine 0.25% t.i.d.).

4. Topical steroid (e.g., prednisolone acetate 1% every 15 minutes for four doses then q1h).

5. Hyperosmotic agent if necessary and no contraindications are present (e.g., mannitol, 1 to 2 g/kg i.v. over 45 minutes).

6. The IOP usually does not respond adequately to medical therapy. Although it is preferable to reduce IOP before cataract extraction, adequate IOP control may not be possible with medication alone. Cataract removal is usually performed within 24 to 48 hours. In patients who have noticed a sudden decrease in vision, the urgency of cataract surgery is increased, especially in those whose vision has progressed to NLP over a few hours. In such cases, lowering the IOP immediately with an anterior chamber paracentesis is necessary prior to cataract extraction (see Appendix 13, *Anterior Chamber Paracentesis*). Glaucoma surgery is usually not necessary at the same time as cataract surgery.

Follow-Up

1. If patients are not hospitalized, they should be reexamined the day after surgery. Patients are often hospitalized for 24 hours after cataract surgery for IOP monitoring.

2. If the IOP returns to normal, the patient should be rechecked within 1 week.

9.12.2. LENS-PARTICLE GLAUCOMA

Definition

Lens material liberated by trauma or surgery that obstructs aqueous outflow channels.

Symptoms

Pain, blurred vision, red eye, tearing, photophobia. History of recent ocular trauma or intraocular surgery.

Signs

Critical. White, fluffy pieces of lens cortical material in the anterior chamber, combined with increased IOP. A break in the lens capsule may be observed.

Other. Anterior chamber cell and flare, conjunctival injection, or corneal edema. The anterior chamber angle is open on gonioscopy.

9

Differential Diagnosis

■ See 9.12.1, *Phacolytic Glaucoma.* In phacolytic glaucoma, the cataractous lens has not been extracted or traumatized.

■ Infectious endophthalmitis: Usually a normal or low IOP. Unless lens cortical material can be unequivocally identified in the anterior chamber, and there is nothing atypical about the presentation, endophthalmitis must be excluded. See 12.13, *Postoperative Endophthalmitis,* and 12.15, *Traumatic Endophthalmitis.*

■ Phacoanaphylaxis: Follows trauma or intraocular surgery, producing anterior chamber inflammation and sometimes a high IOP. The inflammation is often granulomatous, and fluffy lens material is not present in the anterior chamber. See 9.12.3, *Phacoanaphylaxis.*

Work-Up

1. History: Recent trauma or intraocular surgery?

2. Slit-lamp examination: Search the anterior chamber for lens cortical material and measure the IOP.

3. Gonioscopy of the anterior chamber angle.

4. Optic nerve evaluation: The degree of optic nerve cupping helps determine how long the increased IOP can be tolerated.

Treatment

See 9.12.1, *Phacolytic Glaucoma,* for medical treatment. If medical therapy fails to control the IOP, the residual lens material must be removed surgically.

Follow-Up

Depending on the IOP and the health of the optic nerve, patients are reexamined in 1 to 7 days.

9.12.3. PHACOANAPHYLAXIS

Phacoanaphylaxis is a chronic granulomatous uveitis in response to lens material liberated by trauma or intraocular surgery. Phacoanaphylaxis can have an associated glaucoma, although this is very rare. After lens material is liberated, there is a latent period where an immune sensitivity develops. Inflammatory cells surround lens material, and glaucoma may result from blockage of the TM by these cells and lens particles. Other forms of uveitis should be considered, including sympathetic ophthalmia. Other forms of lens-induced glaucoma must be considered including lens particle and phacolytic glaucomas. Treatment is with topical steroids and antiglaucoma medications. The lens should be removed surgically, particularly if IOP or inflammation cannot be adequately controlled with medicine.

9.12.4. PHACOMORPHIC GLAUCOMA

Phacomorphic glaucoma is caused by closure of the anterior chamber angle by a large intumescent cataract. A pupillary block mechanism may play a role. The initial treatment includes topical antiglaucoma medication, although oral CAIs and hyperosmotics may be necessary as well (see 9.4, *Acute Angle-Closure Glaucoma*). A laser iridectomy may be effective in breaking the angle-closure attack, although this is usually unsuccessful. Cataract extraction is the definitive treatment. In cases where the lens is very dense it may be appropriate to remove the lens via a pars plana lensectomy since an extracapsular extraction may be difficult. Some have suggested treating as if for aqueous misdirection (see 9.17, *Aqueous Misdirection Syndrome/ Malignant Glaucoma*).

9.12.5. GLAUCOMA CAUSED BY LENS DISLOCATION OR SUBLUXATION

Mechanisms for glaucoma in subluxed/dislocated lenses include an inflammatory reaction caused by the lens material itself, pupillary block, or damage to the anterior chamber angle sustained during the trauma. A dislocated lens may become hypermature and cause a phacolytic glaucoma (see 9.12.1, *Phacolytic Glaucoma*). In addition, a dislocated or subluxed lens can lead to phacoanaphylaxis (see 9.12.3, *Phacoanaphylaxis*). Pupillary block is the most common mechanism and can occur secondary to anterior displacement of the lens or to vitreous plugging the pupil. Treatment is aimed at relieving the pupillary block. Iridectomy is usually indicated and necessary to prevent future attacks. Cycloplegics are helpful. IOP-lowering medications are employed. Miotics are not indicated with cycloplegics and antiglaucoma medicines. Surgical lens removal may be necessary in certain cases. See 13.10, *Subluxed or Dislocated Crystalline Lens,* for a more in-depth discussion.

9.13   PLATEAU IRIS

Symptoms

Usually asymptomatic, unless acute angle-closure glaucoma develops. See 9.4, *Acute Angle-Closure Glaucoma*.

Signs

Critical. Flat iris plane and normal anterior chamber depth centrally, sharply convex peripheral iris with an anterior iris apposition seen on gonioscopy. Hyperopia is not as common in plateau iris as it is in angle closure secondary to pupillary block. With acute angle closure associated with a plateau iris, the axial anterior chamber depth may be normal, but the peripheral iris bunches up to occlude the angle (see 9.4, *Acute Angle-Closure Glaucoma*).

Differential Diagnosis

- Acute angle-closure glaucoma associated with pupillary block: The central anterior chamber depth is decreased, and the entire iris has a convex appearance. See 9.4, *Acute Angle-Closure Glaucoma*.

- Aqueous misdirection syndrome: Marked diffuse shallowing of the anterior chamber, often after cataract extraction or glaucoma surgery. See 9.17, *Aqueous Misdirection Syndrome/Malignant Glaucoma*.

- For other disorders, see 9.4, *Acute Angle-Closure Glaucoma*.

Types

1. Plateau iris configuration: Because of the anatomic configuration of the angle, acute angle-closure glaucoma develops from only a mild degree of pupillary block. These angle-closure attacks may be treated with a laser PI.

2. Plateau iris syndrome: The peripheral iris can bunch up in the anterior chamber angle and obstruct aqueous outflow without any element of pupillary block. The plateau iris syndrome is present when the angle closes and the IOP rises after dilation, despite a patent PI, and in the absence of phacomorphic glaucoma. UBM findings are characteristic (peripheral iris cysts). See Figure 9.13.1.

Work-Up

1. Slit-lamp examination: Specifically check for the presence of a patent PI and the critical signs listed previously.

2. Measure IOP.

3. Gonioscopy of both anterior chamber angles.

4. Undilated optic nerve evaluation.

5. Can be assessed by UBM.

NOTE: If dilation must be performed in a patient suspected of having a plateau iris, warn the patient that this may provoke an acute angle-closure attack. The preferred agent is 0.5% tropicamide. Use phenylephrine 2.5% to dilate if dapiprazole 0.5% is available for reversal. If an anticholinergic is needed, use only tropicamide 0.5%. Recheck the IOP every few hours until the pupil returns to normal size. Have the patient notify you immediately if symptoms of acute angle closure develop. Dilate only one eye at a time.

Treatment

If Acute Angle Closure is Present:

1. Treat medically. See 9.4, *Acute Angle-Closure Glaucoma*.

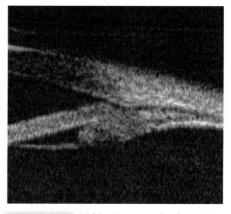

FIGURE 9.13.1. US biomicroscopy of a plateau iris.

2. A laser PI is performed within 1 to 3 days if the angle-closure attack can be broken medically. If the attack cannot be controlled, a laser or surgical PI may need to be done as an emergency procedure.

3. One week after the laser PI, gonioscopy should be repeated prior to dilating the eye with a weak mydriatic (e.g., tropicamide 0.5%). If the IOP increases or a spontaneous angle-closure episode occurs, plateau iris syndrome is diagnosed and should be treated with an iridoplasty, or as a second choice, a weak miotic (e.g., pilocarpine 0.5% to 1% t.i.d. to q.i.d.) may be used chronically.

4. Consider a laser iridoplasty to break an acute attack not responsive to medical treatment and PI.

5. If the patient's IOP does respond to a laser PI (e.g., plateau iris configuration), then a prophylactic laser PI may be indicated in the contralateral eye within 1 to 2 weeks.

If Acute Angle Closure is not Present:

1. Laser PI to relieve the pupillary block component.

2. Check gonioscopy every 4 to 6 months to evaluate the angle.

—Perform iridoplasty if new PAS or further narrowing of the angle develops.

—If the angle continues to develop new PAS or becomes narrower despite iridoplasty, then treat as CACG (see 9.5, *Chronic Angle-Closure Glaucoma*). Consider lens extraction or chronic pilocarpine therapy.

Follow-Up

1. Similar to performing a PI in acute angle closure, reevaluate in 1 week, 1 month, and 3 months, and then yearly if no problems have developed.

2. Patients with a plateau iris configuration without previous acute angle closure are examined every 6 months.

3. Every examination should include IOP measurement and gonioscopy looking for PAS formation, narrowing angle recess, or increasing angle closure. The PI should be examined for patency. Dilation should cautiously be performed periodically (approximately every 2 years) to ensure that the PI remains adequate to prevent angle closure.

4. Ophthalmoscopic disc evaluation is essential.

9.14   NEOVASCULAR GLAUCOMA

Definition

Glaucoma that is caused by a fibrovascular membrane overgrowing the anterior chamber angle structures. Initially, the angle may appear open but blocked by the membrane. The fibrovascular membrane eventually contracts, causing PAS formation and secondary angle-closure glaucoma. Rarely, may have neovascularization of the angle without neovascularization of the iris (NVI) at the pupillary margin. Ischemia-driven vascular endothelial growth factor (VEGF) release from a variety of causes results in the formation of the fibrovascular membrane.

Symptoms

May be asymptomatic or include pain, redeye, photophobia, and decreased vision.

Signs

(See Figures 9.14.1 and 9.14.2.)

Critical.

▪ Stage 1: Nonradial, misdirected blood vessels along the pupillary margin, the TM, or both. No signs of glaucoma. Normal iris blood vessels run radially and are typically symmetric.

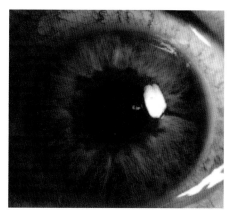

FIGURE 9.14.1. Iris neovascularization.

- Stage 2: Stage 1 plus increased IOP (open-angle neovascular glaucoma).

- Stage 3: Partial or complete angle-closure glaucoma caused by a fibrovascular membrane pulling the iris well anterior to the TM (usually at the level of Schwalbe line). NVI is common.

Other. Mild anterior chamber cells and flare, conjunctival injection, corneal edema with acute IOP increase, hyphema, eversion of the pupillary margin allowing visualization of the iris pigment epithelium (ectropion uvea), optic nerve cupping, visual field loss.

Differential Diagnosis

- Inflammatory glaucoma: Anterior chamber cells and flare, dilated normal iris blood vessels may be seen. Open angle with no neovascularization (NV). See 9.7, *Inflammatory Open-Angle Glaucoma.*

- Primary acute angle-closure glaucoma. See 9.4, *Acute Angle-Closure Glaucoma.*

Etiology

- Diabetic retinopathy with retinal ischemia. See 11.12, *Diabetic Retinopathy.*

- Central retinal vein occlusion, particularly the ischemic type. See 11.8, *Central Retinal Vein Occlusion.*

- Central retinal artery occlusion. See 11.6, *Central Retinal Artery Occlusion.*

- Ocular ischemic syndrome (carotid occlusive disease). See 11.11, *Ocular Ischemic Syndrome/Carotid Occlusive Disease.*

- Others: Branch retinal vein occlusion, chronic uveitis, chronic retinal detachment, intraocular tumors, trauma, other ocular vascular disorders, radiation therapy, chronic longstanding increased IOP (e.g., neglected angle-closure glaucoma). See specific sections.

Work-Up

1. History: Determine the underlying etiology.

2. Complete ocular examination, including IOP measurement and gonioscopy to evaluate the degree of angle closure, if any. A dilated retinal evaluation is essential in determining the etiology and for evaluating the disc.

3. Fluorescein angiography as needed to identify an underlying retinal abnormality or in preparation for panretinal photocoagulation (PRP).

4. Carotid Doppler studies to rule out stenosis when no retinal etiology is identified.

5. B-scan US is indicated when the retina cannot be visualized to rule out an intraocular tumor or retinal detachment.

Treatment

1. Reduce inflammation and pain: Topical steroid (e.g., prednisolone acetate 1%

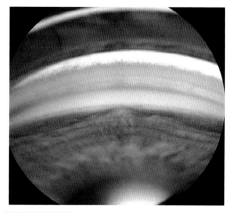

FIGURE 9.14.2. Neovascularization of the angle.

q1–6h) and a cycloplegic (e.g., atropine 1% t.i.d.). Atropine may reduce IOP when the angle is closed by increasing uveoscleral outflow.

2. Reduce the IOP if it is increased. The target IOP is around 30 mm Hg in most patients. Where visual potential is good and cupping marked, a lower target IOP may be appropriate. Any or all of the following medications are used:

—Topical β-blocker (e.g., timolol 0.5% b.i.d.).

—Topical α-2 agonists (e.g., brimonidine 0.1% to 0.2% b.i.d. to t.i.d.).

—Systemic or topical CAI (e.g., acetazolamide 500 mg sequel p.o. b.i.d. or dorzolamide 2% b.i.d. to t.i.d.).

—Prostaglandins may help lower IOP, but may increase inflammation and are usually avoided in the acute phase.

NOTE: Miotics (e.g., pilocarpine) are contraindicated because of their effects on the blood–aqueous barrier. Epinephrine compounds (e.g., dipivefrin) are usually ineffective.

---

3. If retinal ischemia is thought to be responsible for the NV, then treat with PRP. If the retina cannot be visualized, lower the IOP and treat the retina once the cornea clears. Treatment with cryotherapy can also be considered if the cornea does not clear and the retina cannot be visualized adequately. These procedures are used if the angle is open or if filtration surgery (regardless of angle status) is going to be performed.

4. Glaucoma filtration surgery may be performed when the NV is inactive and the IOP cannot be controlled with medical therapy. Tube-shunt procedures may be helpful to control IOP in some patients with active NV, but may be complicated by postoperative bleeding. They should not be performed unless there is useful vision to preserve. External or endocyclophotocoagulation is an option but should be done only with full awareness of potentially severe complications, including sympathetic ophthalmia and phthisis bulbi.

5. Intravitreal anti-VEGF agents (e.g., ranibizumab or bevacizumab) may be used to promote regression of iris neovascularization prior to, or in conjunction with, filtering surgery or PRP. Their effect is temporary, and their use for treatment of neovascularization is currently off-label. They are particularly useful in stage 1 and 2 neovascular glaucoma, where the angle is still open, to prevent angle closure during the interval required for PRP to take effect. Caution should be used when no view of the retina is possible. (See 11.12, *Diabetic Retinopathy*, and 11.17, *Neovascular or Exudative (Wet) Age-Related Macular Degeneration,* for a discussion on anti-VEGF agents.)

6. Goniophotocoagulation (laser photocoagulation of new vessels in the angle) in the very early stages may be used in addition to the previously described treatments in patients with significant angle NV but minimal angle closure. This procedure may reduce the risk of angle closure during the interval required for the PRP to take effect (often several weeks), but this has not been established and is rarely used.

7. In eyes without useful vision, topical steroids and cycloplegics may be adequate therapy for pain control. The pain in chronic neovascular glaucoma is not primarily a function of the IOP, and reducing IOP may not be needed if the goal is pain control only. In the acute stages, after a rapid rise in IOP, a paracentesis may be helpful. Beta-blockers, retrobulbar chlorpromazine or alcohol injection, or enucleation may be required to reduce pain. See 13.12, *Blind, Painful Eye.*

8. Treat the underlying disorder.

Follow-Up

The presence of NVI, especially with high IOP, requires urgent therapeutic intervention, usually within 1 to 2 days. Angle closure can proceed rapidly (days to weeks).

NOTE: NVI without glaucoma is managed similarly, but there is no need for pressure-reducing agents unless IOP increases.

9.15 IRIDOCORNEAL ENDOTHELIAL SYNDROME

Definition

Three overlapping syndromes—essential iris atrophy, Chandler, and iris nevus (Cogan–Reese)—that share an abnormal corneal endothelial cell layer, which can grow across the anterior chamber angle. Secondary angle closure can result from contraction of this membrane.

Symptoms

Asymptomatic early. Later, the patient may note an irregular pupil or iris appearance, blurred vision, monocular diplopia, or pain if IOP increases or corneal edema develops. Usually unilateral and most common in patients 20 to 50 years of age. More common in women. Familial cases are rare.

Signs

(See Figure 9.15.1.)

Critical. Corneal endothelial changes (fine, beaten-bronze appearance); microcystic corneal edema; localized, irregular, high PAS that often extend anterior to Schwalbe line; deep central anterior chamber; iris alterations as follows:

—Essential iris atrophy: Marked iris thinning leading to iris holes with displacement and distortion of the pupil (corectopia). Usually good prognosis.

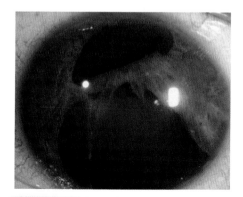

FIGURE 9.15.1. Essential iris atrophy.

—Chandler syndrome: Mild iris thinning and corectopia. The corneal and angle changes are most marked in this variant. However, findings are extremely variable with some cases having minimal changes and others marked. Patients often have corneal edema even at normal IOP. Accounts for about 50% of ICE syndrome cases. Variable prognosis.

—Iris nevus/Cogan–Reese syndrome: Pigmented nodules (not true nevi) on the iris surface, variable iris atrophy. Similar changes may be seen in Chandler syndrome and essential iris atrophy, resulting from contraction of the membrane over the iris, constricting around small islands of iris tissue. Usually poor prognosis.

Other. Corneal edema, elevated IOP, optic nerve cupping, or visual field loss. Unilateral but with occasional mild corneal changes in the fellow eye. However, the glaucoma is nearly always unilateral.

Differential Diagnosis

- Axenfeld–Rieger spectrum: Prominent, anteriorly displaced Schwalbe line (posterior embryotoxon); peripheral iris strands extending to (but not anterior to) Schwalbe line; iris thinning with atrophic holes. Bilateral. See 8.12, *Developmental Anterior Segment and Lens Anomalies/Dysgenesis.*

- Posterior polymorphous corneal dystrophy (PPCD): Bilateral. Endothelial vesicles or bandlike lesions, occasionally associated with iridocorneal adhesions, corneal edema, and glaucoma. No PAS. Autosomal dominant. See 4.26, *Corneal Dystrophies.*

- Fuchs endothelial dystrophy: Bilateral corneal edema and endothelial guttata. Normal iris and angle. See 4.27, *Fuchs Endothelial Dystrophy.*

- Prior uveitis with pigmented keratic precipitates and posterior synechiae.

- Iridoschisis: Usually bilateral separation of iris into an anterior and posterior layer.

9

Work-Up

1. Family history: ICE syndrome is not inherited, Axenfeld–Rieger spectrum and PPCD are often autosomal dominant.

2. Perform baseline glaucoma evaluation. See 9.1, *Primary Open-Angle Glaucoma*. Careful attention should be given to cornea and iris evaluation.

3. Consider slit-lamp photos and corneal endothelial specular microscopy.

Treatment

No treatment is needed unless glaucoma or corneal edema is present, at which point one or more of the following treatments may be used:

1. IOP-reducing medications. See 9.1, *Primary Open-Angle Glaucoma*. The IOP may need to be reduced dramatically to eliminate corneal edema. This critical level may become lower as the patient ages.

2. Hypertonic saline solutions (e.g., sodium chloride 5% drops q.i.d. and ointment q.h.s.) may reduce corneal edema.

3. Consider filtering procedure (trabeculectomy) when medical therapy fails because of persistent corneal edema or progression of glaucoma. Laser trabeculoplasty and laser PI are ineffective. If trabeculectomy fails, the procedure can often be salvaged with ab interno YAG sclerostomy in area of previous sclerostomy. If tube-shunt procedure is performed, place tube far into the anterior chamber to lessen the likelihood of occlusion with the endothelial membrane.

4. Consider a corneal transplant in cases of advanced chronic corneal edema in the presence of good IOP control.

Follow-Up

Varies according to the IOP and optic nerve damage. If asymptomatic with healthy optic nerve, may see every 6 to 12 months. If glaucoma is present, then every 1 to 3 months, depending on the severity.

9.16 POSTOPERATIVE GLAUCOMA

9.16.1. EARLY POSTOPERATIVE GLAUCOMA

IOP tends to start to increase approximately 1 hour after cataract extraction and usually returns to normal within 1 week. Etiologies include retained viscoelastic material or lens particles, pupillary block, hyphema, pigment dispersion, and generalized inflammation. Most normal eyes can tolerate an IOP up to 30 mm Hg for many months. However, eyes with preexisting optic nerve damage require IOP-lowering medications for any significant pressure increase. Prostaglandin agonists are generally avoided postoperatively because of their proinflammatory characteristics. Most eyes with an IOP >30 mm Hg should be treated. If inflammation is excessive, increase the topical steroid dose to every 30 to 60 minutes while awake and consider a topical NSAID (e.g., ketorolac or diclofenac q.i.d.). See 9.7, *Inflammatory Open-Angle Glaucoma*.

9.16.2. POSTOPERATIVE PUPILLARY BLOCK

Differential Diagnosis

Early Postoperative Period (within 2 weeks)

- Inflammation secondary to prostaglandin release, blood, fibrin, etc.

- Hyphema.

- Failure to filter after filtration surgery due to tight scleral flap, blocked sclerostomy (e.g., iris, vitreous, blood, fibrin).

- Aqueous misdirection syndrome (malignant glaucoma). See 9.17, *Aqueous Misdirection Syndrome/Malignant Glaucoma*.

- Suprachoroidal hemorrhage.

- Anterior chamber lens with vitreous loss: Vitreous plugs the pupil if iridectomy is not performed. Can also occur if patient is aphakic.

Late Postoperative Period (after 2 weeks)

- Pupillary block glaucoma. See 9.4, *Acute Angle-Closure Glaucoma.*

- Failing bleb (after filtering surgery).

- Suprachoroidal hemorrhage.

- UGH syndrome. See 9.16.3, *Uveitis, Glaucoma, Hyphema Syndrome.*

- Aqueous misdirection syndrome (malignant glaucoma): When cycloplegics are stopped. See 9.17, *Aqueous Misdirection Syndrome/Malignant Glaucoma.*

- Steroid-induced glaucoma. See 9.9, *Steroid-Response Glaucoma.*

Signs

Increased IOP, shallow or partially flat anterior chamber with anterior iris bowing (iris bombé), absence of a patent PI. Evidence of iris adhesions to lens, anterior capsule, or intraocular lens.

Treatment

1. If the cornea is clear and the eye is not significantly inflamed, a PI is performed, usually by YAG laser. Because the PI tends to close, it is often necessary to perform two or more iridotomies. They need to be larger than in the eye with primary angle-closure glaucoma. See Appendix 15, *YAG Laser Peripheral Iridotomy.*

2. If the cornea is hazy, the eye is inflamed, or a PI cannot be performed immediately, then:

   —Mydriatic agent (e.g., cyclopentolate 2% and phenylephrine 2.5%, every 15 minutes for four doses).

   —Topical therapy with β-blockers [(e.g., timolol 0.5%) caution with asthma or COPD], α-2 agonist (e.g., brimonidine 0.15%), and CAIs (dorzolamide 2%) should be initiated immediately. In urgent cases, three rounds of these medications may be given, with each round being separated by 15 minutes.

   —Systemic CAI (e.g., acetazolamide, 250 to 500 mg i.v., or two 250-mg tablets p.o. in one dose if unable to give i.v.) if IOP

decrease is urgent or if IOP is refractory to topical therapy.

—Topical steroid (e.g., prednisolone acetate 1%) every 15 to 30 minutes for four doses.

—PI, preferably YAG laser, when the eye is less inflamed. If the cornea is not clear, topical glycerin may help clear it temporarily.

—A surgical PI may be needed.

—A guarded filtration procedure or tube shunt may be needed, if the angle has become closed.

9.16.3. UVEITIS, GLAUCOMA, HYPHEMA SYNDROME

Signs

Anterior chamber cells and flare, increased IOP, and hyphema. Usually secondary to irritation from a malpositioned anterior or posterior chamber intraocular lens; often with a vitreous wick.

Treatment

1. Atropine 1% t.i.d.

2. Topical steroid (e.g., prednisolone acetate 1% four to eight times per day) and consider topical NSAID (e.g., ketorolac or diclofenac q.i.d.).

3. Systemic CAI (e.g., acetazolamide 500 mg sequel p.o. b.i.d.) or may consider topical CAI (e.g., dorzolamide 2% t.i.d.).

4. Topical β-blocker (e.g., timolol 0.5% b.i.d.) and α-2 agonist (e.g., brimonidine 0.1% to 0.2% b.i.d. to t.i.d.).

5. Consider laser ablation if a bleeding site can be identified.

6. Consider surgical repositioning, replacement, or removal of the intraocular lens, especially if patient experiences recurrent episodes, PAS are forming, or CME persists.

7. Consider YAG vitreolysis if vitreous strands can be seen.

9

9.16.4. GHOST CELL GLAUCOMA

Degenerated red blood cells pass from the vitreous into the anterior chamber and obstruct the TM. These cells are khaki colored. Often occurs after a large vitreous hemorrhage with a posterior capsular opening, but may also be seen in the absence of prior intraocular surgery. Usually occurs 1 to 3 months after the vitreous hemorrhage.

Treatment

1. Medical treatment: See 9.1, *Primary Open-Angle Glaucoma*.

2. Anterior chamber irrigation and posterior vitrectomy to clear the blood, if medical management fails.

9.17 AQUEOUS MISDIRECTION SYNDROME/ MALIGNANT GLAUCOMA

Symptoms

May be very mild early. Moderate pain, red eye, photophobia may develop. Classically follows surgery in eyes with small anterior segments (e.g., hyperopia, nanophthalmos) or surgery for primary angle-closure glaucoma; also may develop after trabeculectomy, tubeshunt operations, cataract surgery, various laser procedures, and many retinal surgeries. May occur spontaneously or be induced by miotics (even without surgery).

Signs

Critical. Diffusely shallow or flat anterior chamber and increased IOP in the presence of a patent PI and in the absence of both a choroidal detachment and iris bombé.

Differential Diagnosis

- Pupillary block glaucoma: Iris bombé, adhesions of iris to other anterior chamber structures. See 9.16.2, *Postoperative Pupillary Block*.

- Acute angle-closure glaucoma: See 9.4, *Acute Angle-Closure Glaucoma*.

- Choroidal detachment: Shallow or flat anterior chamber, but the IOP is typically low. See 11.27, *Choroidal Effusion/Detachment*.

- Postoperative wound leak: Shallow or flat anterior chamber often with positive Seidel test. IOP is typically low. See 13.11, *Hypotony Syndrome*. See Appendix 5, *Seidel Test to Detect a Wound Leak*.

- Suprachoroidal hemorrhage: Shallow or flat anterior chamber. IOP typically high. See 11.27, *Choroidal Effusion/Detachment*.

Etiology

Believed to result from anterior rotation of the ciliary body with posterior misdirection of the aqueous; aqueous accumulates in the vitreous resulting in forward displacement of the ciliary processes, the crystalline lens, the intraocular implant, or the anterior vitreous face, causing secondary angle closure.

Work-Up

1. History: Previous eye surgery?

2. Slit-lamp examination: Determine if a patent PI or iris bombé is present. Pupillary block is unlikely in the presence of a patent PI unless it is plugged, bound down, or plateau iris syndrome is present.

3. Gonioscopy.

4. Dilated retinal examination unless phakic angle closure is likely.

5. Consider B-scan US to rule out choroidal detachment and suprachoroidal hemorrhage.

6. Seidel test to detect postoperative wound leak if clinically indicated.

Treatment

1. If an iridectomy is not present or an existing PI is not clearly patent, pupillary block cannot be ruled out, and a PI should be performed. See 9.4, *Acute Angle-Closure Glaucoma*. If signs of malignant glaucoma are still present with a patent PI, attempt medical therapy to control IOP and return aqueous flow to the normal pathway.

2. Atropine 1% and phenylephrine 2.5% q.i.d. topically.

3. CAI (e.g., acetazolamide 500 mg i.v. or two 250-mg tablets p.o.).

4. Topical β-blocker (e.g., timolol 0.5% b.i.d.).

5. Topical α-2 agonist (e.g., apraclonidine 1.0% or brimonidine 0.1% to 0.2% b.i.d).

6. If needed, hyperosmotic agent (e.g., mannitol 20% 1 to 2 g/kg i.v. over 45 minutes).

If the attack is broken (the anterior chamber deepens and the IOP normalizes), continue atropine 1% q.d., indefinitely. At a later date, perform PI in the contralateral eye if the angle is occludable.

If steps 1 through 6 are unsuccessful, consider one or more of the following surgical interventions to disrupt the anterior hyaloid face in an attempt to restore the normal anatomic flow of aqueous:

—YAG laser disruption of the anterior hyaloid face and posterior capsule if aphakic or pseudophakic. If phakic, may attempt through a preexisting large PI.

—Vitrectomy and reformation of the anterior chamber with rupture of the anterior hyaloid face. Passing an activated vitrector from the posterior segment through a peripheral iridectomy is often helpful.

—Lensectomy with disruption of the anterior hyaloid or vitrectomy.

—Argon laser of the ciliary processes.

NOTE: An undetected anterior choroidal detachment may be present. Therefore, a sclerotomy to drain a choroidal detachment may be considered before vitrectomy.

Follow-Up

Variable, depending on the therapeutic modality used. PI is usually performed in an occludable contralateral eye within a week after treatment of the involved eye.

9

POSTOPERATIVE COMPLICATIONS OF GLAUCOMA SURGERY
9.18

BLEB INFECTION (BLEBITIS)

See 9.19, *Blebitis*.

INCREASED POSTOPERATIVE IOP AFTER FILTERING PROCEDURE

Grade of Shallowing of Anterior Chamber

I. Peripheral iris–cornea contact.

II. Entire iris in contact with cornea.

III. Lens (or lens implant or vitreous face)–corneal contact.

Differential Diagnosis

(See Table 9.18.1.)

If the Anterior Chamber is Flat or Shallow and IOP is Increased, Consider the Following:

■ Suprachoroidal hemorrhage: Sudden onset of excruciating pain (commonly 1 to 5 days after surgery), variable IOP, hazy cornea, shallow

TABLE 9.18.1	Postoperative Complications of Glaucoma Surgery				
Diagnosis	**IOP**	**Anterior Chamber**	**Iris Bombe**	**Pain**	**Bleb**
Inflammation	Variable	Deep	No	Possible	Varies
Hyphema	Mild to moderately elevated	Varies	Not early	Possible	Varies
Failure to filter	Moderately elevated	Deep	No	Moderate	Falling
Aqueous misdirection malignant glaucoma	Early: moderately elevated Late: moderately to markedly elevated	Diffusely shallow, Grade 2 or 3	No	Moderate	Falling or absent
Suprachoroidal hemorrhage	Early: markedly elevated Late: falling to mild to moderately elevated	Grade 1 and 2	No	Excruciating	Flat
Pupillary block	Early: moderately elevated, may become markedly elevated	Grade 1 to 3	Yes	None or mild	None
Serous choroidal detachment	Low	Grade 1 to 3	No	Ache frequently present	Usually excessive; may flatten with time

chamber. See 11.27, *Choroidal Effusion/ Detachment.*

■ Aqueous misdirection/malignant glaucoma: See 9.17, *Aqueous Misdirection Syndrome/ Malignant Glaucoma.*

■ Postoperative pupillary block: See 9.16.2, *Postoperative Pupillary Block.*

If the Anterior Chamber is Deep, Consider the Following:

■ Internal filtration occlusion by an iris plug, hemorrhage, fibrin, vitreous or viscoelastic material.

■ External filtration occlusion by a tight trabeculectomy flap (sutured tightly or scarred).

Treatment

Initial gonioscopy to assist in diagnosis is essential before starting any treatment.

1. If the bleb is not formed and the anterior chamber is deep, point pressure with an applicator on the anterior bleb edge should be used to determine if the sclerostomy will drain. In fornix-based procedures, take great care to not disrupt the limbal wound.

2. If the trabeculectomy flap is too tight, suture lysis may be indicated.

3. If the sclerostomy is blocked with iris, any pressure on the globe is contraindicated. Topical pilocarpine or slow intracameral injection of acetylcholine can pull the iris out of the sclerostomy if iris incarceration developed within the past 2 to 3 days. If this fails, and the sclerostomy is completely blocked by iris, transcorneal mechanical retraction of the iris may work. In rare cases, argon laser iridoplasty may be useful to pull the iris enough to restore filtration. If the sclerostomy is blocked with vitreous, photodisruption of the sclerostomy with a YAG laser may be attempted. Blood or fibrin at the sclerostomy may clear with time or tissue plasminogen activator (10 μg) injected intracamerally may reestablish aqueous flow through the sclerostomy.

4. For suprachoroidal hemorrhage, if the IOP is mildly increased and the chamber is formed, observation with medical management is indicated. Surgical drainage is indicated for persistent chamber flattening or IOP elevation, corneal–lenticular touch, chronic retinal fold apposition, intolerable pain. If possible, delay drainage for at least 4 days.

5. Medical therapy may be necessary if these measures are not successful. See 9.1, *Primary Open-Angle Glaucoma.*

6. If the above measures fail, reoperation may be necessary.

LOW POSTOPERATIVE IOP AFTER FILTERING PROCEDURE

Low pressures (5 to 9 mm Hg) are associated with complications such as flat anterior chamber, choroidal detachment, and suprachoroidal hemorrhage. An IOP <4 mm Hg is more likely associated with complications including macular hypotony and corneal edema.

Differential Diagnosis and Treatment

1. Large bleb with a deep chamber (overfiltration): It is often beneficial to have a large bleb in the first few weeks after trabeculec-tomy. However, treatment is appropriate if it is still present 6 to 8 weeks after surgery, the patient is symptomatic, IOP is decreasing, or the anterior chamber is shallowing. Treatment includes topical atropine 1% b.i.d., intracameral viscoelastic, and possibly autologous blood injection into the bleb. If IOP is stable and anterior chamber is deep, observe.

2. Large bleb with a flat chamber (Grade I or II): Treatment includes cycloplegics (atropine 1% t.i.d.) and careful observation. If the anterior chamber becomes more shallow (e.g., Grade I becoming Grade II), the IOP decreases as the bleb flattens, or choroidal detachment develops, the anterior chamber may be reformed with a viscoelastic material.

3. No bleb with flat chamber: Check carefully for a wound leak by Seidel testing (see Appendix 5, *Seidel Test to Detect a Wound Leak*). If positive, aqueous suppressants, patching, or surgical closure may be necessary. If negative, look for a cyclodialysis cleft (by gonioscopy) or serous choroidal detachments. Cyclodialysis clefts are managed by cycloplegics, laser or cryotherapy (to close the cleft), or surgical closure. Serous choroidal detachments are often observed, as they resolve when the IOP normalizes, in most cases. See 11.27, *Choroidal Effusion/Detachment.*

4. Grade III flat chamber: This is a surgical emergency and demands prompt correction. Methods include drainage of a choroidal detachment and reformation of the anterior chamber with or without revision of the scleral flap or tube, reformation of the anterior chamber with viscoelastic, and cataract extraction with or without other procedures.

COMPLICATIONS OF ANTIMETABOLITES (5-FLUOROURACIL, MITOMYCIN C)

Corneal epithelial defects, corneal edema, conjunctival wound leaks, bleb overfiltration, bleb rupture, scleral thinning, and perforation.

9

COMPLICATIONS OF CYCLODESTRUCTIVE PROCEDURES

Pain, uveitis, decreased vision, cataract, hypotony, scleral thinning, suprachoroidal effusion, suprachoroidal hemorrhage, sympathetic ophthalmia.

MISCELLANEOUS COMPLICATIONS OF FILTERING PROCEDURES

Cataracts, corneal edema, corneal dellen, endophthalmitis, uveitis, hyphema, bleb discomfort.

9.19 BLEBITIS

Definition

Infection of a filtering bleb. May occur any time after glaucoma filtering procedures (days to years).

- Grade 1 (mild): Bleb infection but no anterior chamber or vitreous involvement.

- Grade 2 (moderate): Bleb infection with anterior chamber inflammation but no vitreous involvement.

- Grade 3 (severe): Bleb infection with anterior chamber and vitreous involvement. See 12.13, *Postoperative Endophthalmitis*.

Symptoms

Red eye and discharge early. Later, aching pain, photophobia, decreased vision, mucous discharge.

Signs

(See Figure 9.19.1.)

- Grade 1: Bleb appears milky with loss of translucency, microhypopyon in loculations of the bleb, may have frank purulent material in or leaking from the bleb, intense conjunctival injection, IOP is usually unaffected.

- Grade 2: Grade 1 plus anterior chamber cell and flare, possibly an anterior chamber hypopyon, with no vitreous inflammation.

- Grade 3: Grade 2 plus vitreous involvement. Same appearance as endophthalmitis except with bleb involvement.

Differential Diagnosis

- Episcleritis: Sectoral inflammation, rarely superior. No bleb involvement. See 5.6, *Episcleritis*.

- Conjunctivitis: Minimal decrease in vision, no pain or photophobia. Bacterial conjunctivitis can progress to blebitis if not promptly treated. See 5.1, *Acute Conjunctivitis*.

- Anterior uveitis: Anterior chamber inflammation without bleb involvement. Photophobia. See 12.1, *Anterior Uveitis (Iritis/Iridocyclitis)*.

- Endophthalmitis: Similar findings as severe blebitis without bleb involvement. May have more intense pain, eyelid edema, chemosis, greater decrease in vision, hypopyon compared to blebitis. See 12.13, *Postoperative Endophthalmitis*.

- Ischemic bleb: Seen after the use of antimetabolites in immediate postoperative

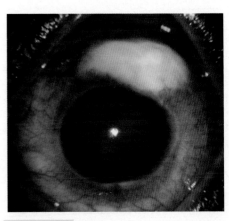

FIGURE 9.19.1. Blebitis.

period. Conjunctiva is opaque with sectoral conjunctival injection.

Work-Up

1. Slit-lamp examination with careful evaluation of the bleb, anterior chamber, and vitreous. Search for a hole in the bleb; perform Seidel test (see Appendix 5, *Seidel Test to Detect a Wound Leak*). Look for microhypopyon with gonioscopy.

2. Culture bleb or perform anterior chamber tap for moderate blebitis. If severe, see 12.13, *Postoperative Endophthalmitis*.

NOTE: The most frequent organisms in the early postoperative period include *Staphylococcus epidermidis*, *Staphylococcus aureus*, and other Gram-positive organisms. If blebitis occurs months to years later, Streptococcus, *Haemophilus influenzae*, *Staphylococcus aureus*, Moraxella, Pseudomonas, and Serratia are more common.

---

3. B-scan US may help identify vitritis if visualization is difficult.

Treatment

1. Grade 1: Intensive topical antibiotics with either of two regimens:

—Fortified cefazolin or vancomycin *and* fortified gentamicin, amikacin, or tobramycin alternating every half-hour for the first 24 hours. A loading dose of one drop of each every 5 minutes, repeated four times, is often given.

or

—Fluoroquinolones q1h after a loading dose.

—Reevaluate in 6 to 12 hours and again at 12 to 24 hours. Must not be getting worse.

—Start steroids 24 hours after antibiotics started and blebitis resolving.

2. Grade 2: Same approach as mild blebitis, plus cycloplegics and more careful monitoring. May consider use of oral fluoroquinolones as well (e.g., ciprofloxacin 500 mg p.o. b.i.d. or moxifloxacin 400 mg q.d.).

3. Grade 3: Treat as endophthalmitis. See 12.13, *Postoperative Endophthalmitis*.

Follow-Up

Daily until infection is resolving. Admission to the hospital is often indicated.

9

10 Neuro-Ophthalmology

ANISOCORIA

Eyelid position and extraocular motility MUST be evaluated when anisocoria is present (see Figure 10.1.1).

Classification

1. The abnormal pupil is constricted.

—Unilateral exposure to a miotic agent (e.g., pilocarpine).

—Iritis: Eye pain, redness, and anterior chamber cells and flare.

—Horner syndrome: Mild ptosis on the side of the small pupil. See 10.2, *Horner Syndrome.*

—Argyll Robertson (syphilitic) pupil: Always bilateral, irregularly round miotic pupils, but a mild degree of anisocoria is often present. See 10.3, *Argyll Robertson Pupils.*

—Long-standing Adie pupil: The pupil is initially dilated, but over time may constrict. Hypersensitive to pilocarpine 0.125%. See 10.4, *Adie (Tonic) Pupil.*

2. The abnormal pupil is dilated.

—Iris sphincter muscle damage from trauma: Torn pupillary margin or iris transillumination defects seen on slit-lamp examination.

—Adie (tonic) pupil: The pupil may be irregular, reacts minimally to light, and slowly and tonically to convergence. Hypersensitive to pilocarpine 0.125%. See 10.4, *Adie (Tonic) Pupil.*

—Third cranial nerve palsy: Always associated ptosis and/or extraocular muscle palsies. See 10.5, *Isolated Third Nerve Palsy.*

—Unilateral exposure to a mydriatic agent: Cycloplegic drops (e.g., atropine), scopolamine patch for motion sickness, ill-fitting mask in patients on nebulizers (using ipratropium bromide), possible use of sympathetic medications (e.g., pseudoephedrine). If the mydriatic exposure is recent, pupil will not react to pilocarpine 1%.

3. Physiologic anisocoria: Pupil size disparity is the same in light as in dark, and the pupils react normally to light. The size difference is usually, but not always, <2 mm in diameter.

Work-Up

1. History: When was the anisocoria first noted? Associated symptoms or signs? Ocular trauma? Eye drops or ointments? Syphilis? Old photographs?

2. Ocular examination: Try to determine which pupil is abnormal by comparing pupil sizes in light and in dark. Anisocoria greater in light suggests the abnormal pupil is the larger pupil; anisocoria greater in dark suggests the abnormal pupil is the smaller pupil. Test the pupillary reaction to both light and near. Evaluate for the presence of a relative afferent pupillary defect. Look for ptosis, evaluate ocular motility, and examine the pupillary margin with a slit lamp.

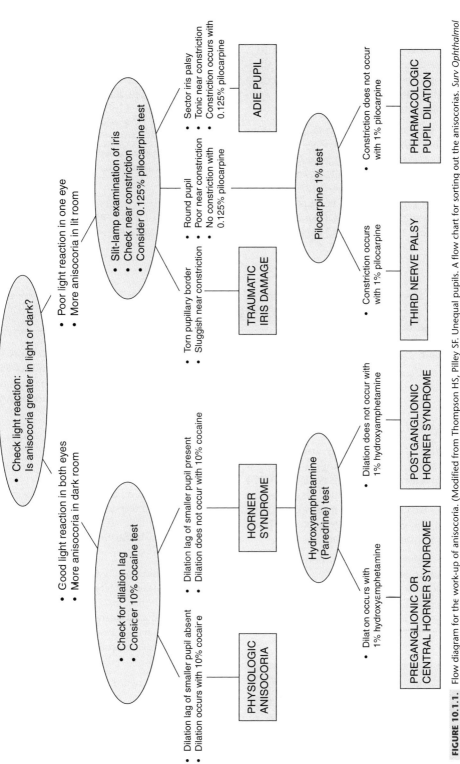

FIGURE 10.1.1. Flow diagram for the work-up of anisocoria. (Modified from Thompson HS, Pilley SF. Unequal pupils. A flow chart for sorting out the anisocorias. *Surv Ophthalmol* 1976;21:45–48, with permission.)

—If the abnormal pupil is small, a diagnosis of Horner syndrome may be confirmed by a cocaine or apraclonidine test (see 10.2, *Horner Syndrome*). In the presence of ptosis and an unequivocal increase in anisocoria in dim illumination, cocaine and apraclonidine testing may be unnecessary.

—If the abnormal pupil is large and there is no sphincter muscle damage or signs of third nerve palsy (e.g., extraocular motility deficit, ptosis), the pupils are tested with one drop of pilocarpine 0.125%. Within 10 to 15 minutes, an Adie pupil will constrict significantly more than the fellow pupil [see 10.4, *Adie (Tonic) Pupil*].

> **NOTE:** For an acute Adie pupil, the pupil may not react to a weak cholinergic agent.

—If the pupil does not constrict with pilocarpine 0.125%, or pharmacologic dilatation is suspected, pilocarpine 1% is instilled in both eyes. A normal pupil constricts sooner and to a greater extent than the pharmacologically dilated pupil. An eye that recently received a strong mydriatic agent such as atropine usually will not constrict at all.

See 10.2, *Horner Syndrome,* 10.3, *Argyll Robertson Pupils,* 10.4, *Adie (Tonic) Pupil,* and 10.5, *Isolated Third Nerve Palsy.*

10.2   HORNER SYNDROME

Symptoms

Ptosis and anisocoria. May have anhydrosis. Often asymptomatic.

Signs

(See Figure 10.2.1.)

Critical. Anisocoria that is greater in dim illumination (especially during the first few seconds after the room light is dimmed). The abnormal small pupil dilates less than the normal, larger pupil. Mild ptosis (2 mm) and lower eyelid elevation ("reverse ptosis") occur on the side of the small pupil.

Other. Lower intraocular pressure, lighter iris color in congenital cases (iris heterochromia), loss of sweating (anhydrosis, distribution depends on the site of lesion), transient increase in accommodation (older patients hold their reading card closer in the Horner eye). Involved eye may have conjunctival hyperemia due to decreased episcleral vascular tone. Light and near reactions are intact.

Differential Diagnosis

See 10.1, *Anisocoria.*

Etiology

■ First-order neuron disorder: Stroke (e.g., vertebrobasilar artery insufficiency or infarct), tumor, multiple sclerosis (MS). Rarely, severe osteoarthritis of the neck with bony spurs.

■ Second-order neuron disorder: Tumor (e.g., lung carcinoma, metastasis, thyroid adenoma, neurofibroma). Patients with pain in the arm or scapular region should be suspected of having a Pancoast tumor. In children, consider neuroblastoma, lymphoma, or metastasis.

■ Third-order neuron disorder: Headache syndrome (e.g., cluster, migraine, Raeder paratrigeminal syndrome), internal carotid dissection, varicella zoster virus, otitis media, Tolosa–Hunt syndrome, neck trauma/tumor/inflammation, cavernous sinus pathology.

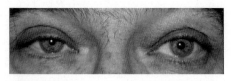

FIGURE 10.2.1. Right Horner syndrome with ptosis and miosis.

■ Congenital Horner syndrome: May also be caused by birth trauma.

■ Other rare causes: Cervical paraganglioma, ectopic cervical thymus.

Work-Up

1. Diagnosis confirmed with a positive cocaine test. Place one drop of 10% cocaine in both eyes. Check in 15 minutes. If no change in pupillary size is noted, repeat drops and recheck the pupils in 15 minutes (repeat until normal pupil dilates). A Horner pupil dilates less than the normal pupil. Alternatively, either 1% or 0.5% apraclonidine may be used. Apraclonidine causes relative reversal of anisocoria. The miotic pupil with Horner syndrome will appear larger than the normal pupil.

NOTE: There may be a high false-negative rate to pharmacologic testing in an acute Horner syndrome.

---

2. A third-order neuron disorder may be distinguished from a first- and second-order neuron disorder with hydroxyamphetamine. Place one drop of 1% hydroxyamphetamine in both eyes. Check in 15 minutes and repeat if no change in pupillary size is noted. Failure of the Horner pupil to dilate to an equivalent degree as the fellow eye indicates a third-order neuron lesion, which may help guide the work-up. However, most experts feel the entire sympathetic pathway should be imaged in Horner syndrome regardless of the results of pharmacologic testing.

NOTE: The hydroxyamphetamine test has a sensitivity of up to 93% and a specificity of 83% for identifying a third-order neuron lesion. Hydroxyamphetamine should not be used within 24 hours of cocaine or apraclonidine to avoid possible interference with each other. Both drops require an intact corneal epithelium and preferably no prior eye drops (including anesthetic drops) for accurate results.

---

3. Determine the duration of the Horner syndrome from the patient's history and an examination of old photographs. New-onset Horner syndrome requires a more urgent diagnostic work-up to exclude life-threatening etiologies [(e.g., internal carotid artery dissection, which can present with transient visual loss, head/neck/face pain, or dysgeusia (foul taste in the mouth)]. An old Horner syndrome is more likely to be benign.

4. History: Headaches? Arm pain? Previous stroke? Previous surgery that may have damaged the sympathetic chain, including cardiac, thoracic, thyroid, or neck surgery? History of head or neck trauma? Ipsilateral neck pain?

5. Physical examination (especially check for supraclavicular nodes, thyroid enlargement, or a neck mass).

6. Complete blood count (CBC) with differential.

7. Computed tomography (CT) of the chest to evaluate lung apex for possible mass (e.g., Pancoast tumor).

8. Magnetic resonance imaging (MRI) of the brain and neck.

9. Magnetic resonance angiography (MRA) or CT angiography (CTA) of head/neck or carotid Doppler ultrasonography (US) to evaluate for carotid artery dissection (especially with neck pain). MRA and CTA appear to be superior to Doppler US for evaluation of carotid artery dissection and allow for evaluation of the distal internal carotid artery. Additionally, imaging of the brain can be accomplished during the same examination which streamlines the work-up process. Obtain carotid angiography if MRA, CTA, or Doppler yield equivocal results.

10. Lymph node biopsy when lymphadenopathy is present.

Treatment

1. Treat the underlying disorder if possible.

NOTE: Carotid dissection usually requires anticoagulation or antiplatelet therapy to prevent carotid occlusion and hemispheric stroke in

---

10

consultation with Neurology and Neurosurgery. Rarely, ischemic symptoms in the distribution of the dissection persist despite anticoagulation. In these cases, surgical intervention may be considered.

2. Ptosis surgery may be performed electively.

Follow-Up

1. Work-up acute Horner syndromes as soon as possible to rule out life-threatening causes. MRA should be performed the same day for dissection (it is convenient to perform an MRI simultaneously). The other tests should be performed within 1 to 2 days.

2. Chronic Horner syndrome can be evaluated with less urgency. There are no ocular complications that necessitate close follow-up.

10.3 ARGYLL ROBERTSON PUPILS

Symptoms

Usually asymptomatic.

Signs

Critical. Small, irregular pupils that exhibit "light-near" dissociation (react poorly or not at all to light but constrict normally during convergence). By definition, vision must be intact.

Other. The pupils dilate poorly in darkness. Always bilateral, although may be asymmetric.

Differential Diagnosis of "Light-Near" Dissociation

- Bilateral optic neuropathy or severe retinopathy: Reduced visual acuity with normal pupil size.

- Adie (tonic) pupil: Unilateral or bilateral irregularly dilated pupil that constricts slowly and unevenly to light. Normal vision. See 10.4, *Adie (Tonic) Pupil.*

- Dorsal midbrain (Parinaud) syndrome: Bilateral, normal-to-large pupils. May be accompanied by convergence retraction nystagmus, lid retraction, and supranuclear upgaze palsy. See 10.4, *Adie (Tonic) Pupil* and "Convergence-retraction" in 10.21, *Nystagmus.*

- Rarely caused by third nerve palsy with aberrant regeneration. See 10.6, *Aberrant Regeneration of the Third Nerve.*

- Others: Diabetes, alcoholism, etc.

Etiology

- Tertiary syphilis.

Work-Up

1. Test the pupillary reaction to light and convergence: To test the reaction to convergence, patients are asked to look first at a distant target and then at their own finger, which the examiner holds in front of them and slowly brings in toward their face.

2. Slit-lamp examination: Look for interstitial keratitis (see 4.18, *Interstitial Keratitis*).

3. Dilated fundus examination: Search for chorioretinitis, papillitis, and uveitis.

4. Fluorescent treponemal antibody absorption (FTA-ABS) or microhemagglutination-*Treponema pallidum* (MHA-TP), rapid plasma reagin (RPR) or Venereal Disease Research Laboratories (VDRL) test.

5. If the diagnosis of syphilis is established, lumbar puncture (LP) may be indicated. See 12.12, *Syphilis,* for specific indications.

Treatment

1. Treatment based on the presence of active disease and previous appropriate treatment.

2. See 12.12, *Syphilis,* for treatment indications and specific antibiotic therapy.

Follow-Up

This is not an emergency. Diagnostic work-up and determination of syphilitic activity should be undertaken within a few days.

10.4   ADIE (TONIC) PUPIL

Symptoms

Difference in size of pupils, blurred near vision, photophobia. May be asymptomatic.

Signs

Critical. An irregularly dilated pupil that has minimal or no reactivity to light. Slow, tonic constriction with convergence, and slow redilation.

NOTE: It is typically unilateral initially and more common in young women.

Other. May have an acute onset and become bilateral. The involved pupil may become smaller than the normal pupil over time.

Differential Diagnosis

See 10.1, *Anisocoria.*

- Parinaud syndrome/dorsal midbrain lesion: Bilateral mid-dilated pupils that react poorly to light but constrict normally with convergence (not tonic). Associated with eyelid retraction (Collier Sign), supranuclear upgaze paralysis, and convergence retraction nystagmus. An MRI should be performed to rule out pinealoma and other midbrain pathology.

- Holmes–Adie syndrome: Tonic pupil and tendon areflexia. May be associated with autonomic and peripheral neuropathy.

Etiology

Idiopathic most commonly. Orbital trauma, surgery, and varicella zoster infection are seen frequently. Early syphilis, parvovirus B19, herpes simplex virus, botulism, paraneoplastic syndrome, giant cell arteritis (GCA), panretinal photocoagulation, and neurological Lyme disease less commonly. Rare associations reported with endometriosis, seminomas, and Sjogren syndrome.

Work-Up

See 10.1, *Anisocoria,* for a general work-up when the diagnosis is uncertain.

1. Evaluate pupils at slit lamp or with a muscle light for irregular and slow constriction.

2. Test for cholinergic hypersensitivity. Instill 0.125% pilocarpine in both eyes and recheck pupils in 10 to 15 minutes. An Adie pupil constricts while the normal pupil does not.

3. If bilateral simultaneous Adie pupils, consider further laboratory investigations including testing for the aforementioned etiologies. For unilateral involvement, no further laboratory investigations are necessary.

NOTE: The dilute pilocarpine test may occasionally be positive in familial dysautonomia. Hypersensitivity may not be present with an acute Adie pupil and may need to be retested a few weeks later.

---

4. If Adie pupil is present in a patient younger than 1 year, consult a pediatric neurologist to rule out familial dysautonomia (Riley–Day syndrome).

Treatment

Pilocarpine 0.125% b.i.d. to q.i.d. for cosmesis and to aid in accommodation, if desired.

Follow-Up

If the diagnosis is certain, follow-up is routine.

10

| **10.5** | **ISOLATED THIRD NERVE PALSY** |

Symptoms

Binocular diplopia and ptosis; with or without pain.

NOTE: Pain does not distinguish between microvascular infarction and compression.

Signs

(See Figures 10.5.1 through 10.5.4.)

Critical.

1. External ophthalmoplegia.

   —Complete palsy: Limitation of ocular movement in all fields of gaze except temporally.

   —Incomplete palsy: Partial limitation of ocular movement.

   —Superior division palsy: Ptosis and an inability to look up.

   —Inferior division palsy: Inability to look nasally or inferiorly.

2. Internal ophthalmoplegia.

   —Pupil-involving: A fixed, dilated, poorly reactive pupil.

   —Pupil-sparing: Pupil not dilated and normally reactive to light.

   —Relative pupil-sparing: Pupil partially dilated and sluggishly reactive to light.

Other.   An exotropia or hypotropia. Aberrant regeneration. See 10.6, *Aberrant Regeneration of the Third Nerve.*

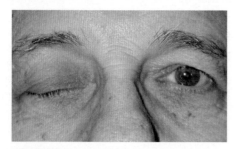

FIGURE 10.5.1. Isolated right third cranial nerve palsy with complete ptosis.

Differential Diagnosis

■ Myasthenia gravis: Diurnal variation of symptoms and signs, pupil never involved, increased eyelid droop after sustained upgaze. See 10.11, *Myasthenia Gravis.*

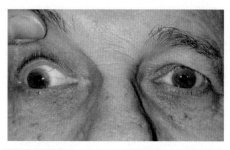

FIGURE 10.5.2. Isolated right third cranial nerve palsy: Primary gaze showing right exotropia and dilated pupil.

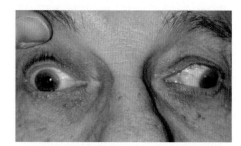

FIGURE 10.5.3. Isolated right third cranial nerve palsy: Left gaze showing inability to adduct right eye.

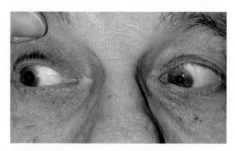

FIGURE 10.5.4. Isolated right third cranial nerve palsy: Right gaze showing normal abduction of right eye.

- Thyroid eye disease: Eyelid lag, lid retraction, injection over the rectus muscles, proptosis, positive forced-duction testing. See 7.2.1, *Thyroid Eye Disease*.

- Chronic progressive external ophthalmoplegia (CPEO): Bilateral, slowly progressive ptosis and motility limitation. Pupil spared, often no diplopia. See 10.12, *Chronic Progressive External Ophthalmoplegia*.

- Idiopathic orbital inflammatory syndrome: Pain and proptosis common. See 7.2.2, *Idiopathic Orbital Inflammatory Syndrome*.

- Internuclear ophthalmoplegia (INO): Unilateral or bilateral adduction deficit with horizontal nystagmus of opposite abducting eye. No ptosis. See 10.13, *Internuclear Ophthalmoplegia*.

- Skew deviation: Supranuclear brainstem lesion producing asymmetric, mainly vertical ocular deviation not consistent with single cranial nerve defect. See *Differential Diagnosis* in 10.7, *Isolated Fourth Nerve Palsy*.

- Parinaud syndrome/dorsal midbrain lesion: Bilateral mid-dilated pupils that react poorly to light but constrict normally with convergence (not tonic). Associated with eyelid retraction (Collier Sign), supranuclear upgaze paralysis, and convergence retraction nystagmus. No ptosis.

- GCA: Extraocular muscle ischemia due to involvement of the long posterior ciliary arteries. Any extraocular muscle may be affected, resulting in potentially complex horizontal and vertical motility deficits. Pupil typically not involved. Age ≥55 years. See 10.17, *Arteritic Ischemic Optic Neuropathy (Giant Cell Arteritis)*.

Etiology

- Pupil involving:

  —More common: Aneurysm, particularly posterior communicating artery aneurysm.

  —Less common: Tumor, trauma, congenital, uncal herniation, cavernous sinus mass lesion, pituitary apoplexy, orbital disease, varicella zoster virus, and leukemia. In children, ophthalmoplegic migraine.

- Pupil sparing: Ischemic microvascular disease; rarely cavernous sinus syndrome or GCA.

- Relative pupil sparing: Ischemic microvascular disease; less likely compressive.

- Aberrant regeneration present: Trauma, aneurysm, tumor, congenital. Not microvascular. See 10.6, *Aberrant Regeneration of the Third Nerve*.

Work-Up

1. History: Onset and duration of diplopia? Recent trauma? Pertinent medical history [e.g., diabetes, hypertension, known cancer or central nervous system (CNS) mass, recent infections]. If ≥55 years old, specifically ask about GCA symptoms.

2. Complete ocular examination: Check for pupillary involvement, the directions of motility restriction (in both eyes), ptosis, a visual field defect (visual fields by confrontation), proptosis, resistance to retropulsion, orbicularis muscle weakness, and eyelid fatigue with sustained upgaze. Look carefully for signs of aberrant regeneration. See 10.6, *Aberrant Regeneration of the Third Nerve*.

3. Full neurologic examination: Carefully assess the other cranial nerves on both sides.

NOTE: The ipsilateral fourth nerve can be assessed by focusing on a superior conjunctival blood vessel and asking the patient to look down and nasally. The eye should intort, and the blood vessel should turn down and toward the nose even if the eye cannot be adducted.

---

4. Immediate CNS imaging to rule out mass/aneurysm is indicated for:

   a. Pupil-involving (relatively or completely involved) third nerve palsies.

   b. Pupil-sparing third nerve palsies in the following groups of patients:

      —Patients ≤50 years of age (unless there is known long-standing diabetes or hypertension).

10

—Patients with incomplete third nerve palsies (with sparing of some muscle function) because this condition may be evolving into a pupil-involving third nerve palsy. If imaging not obtained, closely monitor patients for pupil involvement daily for at least 7 days.

—Patients with additional cranial nerve or neurologic abnormalities.

c. Children <10 years of age, regardless of the state of the pupil.

NOTE: Most sensitive modality is contrast-enhanced CT and CTA, though gadolinium-enhanced MRI and MRA are also very sensitive and can be done if CT and CTA are contraindicated or unavailable. Choice of imaging should be made in conjunction with neuroradiology. If initial imaging studies are negative but clinical suspicion remains high, catheter angiography may be indicated.

---

5. Prompt CNS imaging is required for:

a. All patients in whom aberrant regeneration develops, with the exception of regeneration after traumatic third nerve palsies.

b. Pupil-sparing third nerve palsy for >3 months in duration without improvement.

6. Imaging is usually not required in complete pupil-sparing third nerve palsies that do not fit these criteria, especially in patients >50 years of age with known vasculopathic risk factors such as diabetes or hypertension.

7. Cerebral angiography is indicated for all patients >10 years of age with pupil-involving third nerve palsies and whose imaging study is negative or shows a mass consistent with an aneurysm.

8. CBC with differential in children.

9. Edrophonium chloride test or ice-pack test when myasthenia gravis is suspected. See 10.11, *Myasthenia Gravis.*

10. For suspected ischemic disease: Check blood pressure, fasting blood sugar, glycosylated hemoglobin.

11. Immediate erythrocyte sedimentation rate (ESR), C-reactive protein (CRP), and platelets if GCA is suspected. See 10.17, *Arteritic Ischemic Optic Neuropathy (Giant Cell Arteritis).*

Treatment

1. Treat the underlying abnormality.

2. If the third nerve palsy is causing symptomatic diplopia, an occlusion patch or prism may be placed over the involved eye. Patching is usually not performed in children <11 years of age because of the risk of amblyopia. Children should be monitored closely for the development of amblyopia in the deviated eye.

3. Strabismus surgery may be considered for persistent significant misalignment.

Follow-Up

1. Pupil sparing: Observe daily for 7 days from onset of symptoms for delayed pupil involvement, and then recheck every 4 to 6 weeks. If secondary to ischemia, function should return within 3 months. If the palsy does not reverse or is not improving by 3 months, the pupil dilates, additional neurologic abnormalities develop, aberrant regeneration appears, or an incomplete third nerve palsy progresses, then urgent imaging is obtained. Refer to internist for management of vasculopathic disease risk factors.

2. Pupil involving: If imaging and angiography are negative, an LP should be considered and the patient should be followed as described above.

ABERRANT REGENERATION OF THE THIRD NERVE

Symptoms

See 10.5, *Isolated Third Nerve Palsy.*

Signs

(See Figures 10.6.1 and 10.6.2.)

The most common signs of aberrant third nerve regeneration include:

- Eyelid-gaze dyskinesis: Elevation of involved eyelid on downgaze (Pseudo-von Graefe sign) or adduction.

- Pupil-gaze dyskinesis: Pupil constricts on downgaze or adduction.

- Other signs may include limitation of elevation and depression of eye, adduction of involved eye on attempted elevation or depression, absent optokinetic response, or pupillary light-near dissociation.

Etiology

Thought to result from misdirection of the third nerve fibers from their original destination to alternate third nerve controlled muscles (e.g., inferior rectus to the pupil).

- Aberrancy from congenital third nerve palsies: Can be seen in up to two-thirds of these patients.

- Aberrancy from prior acquired third nerve palsies: Seen most often in patients recovering from third nerve damage by trauma or compression by a posterior communicating artery aneurysm.

- Primary aberrant regeneration: A term used to describe the presence of aberrant regeneration in a patient who has no history of a third nerve palsy. Usually indicates the presence of a progressively enlarging parasellar lesion such as a carotid aneurysm within the cavernous sinus or tumor such as meningioma.

Work-Up

1. Aberrancy from congenital: None. Document work-up of prior congenital third nerve palsy.

2. Aberrancy from acquired: See 10.5, *Isolated Third Nerve Palsy.* Document work-up of prior acquired third nerve palsy if previously obtained.

3. Primary aberrancy: All patients must undergo neuroimaging to rule out slowly compressive lesion or aneurysm.

NOTE: Ischemic third nerve palsies DO NOT produce aberrancy. If aberrant regeneration develops in a presumed ischemic palsy, neuroimaging should be performed.

Treatment

1. Treat the underlying disorder.

2. Consider strabismus surgery if significant symptoms are present.

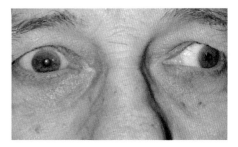

FIGURE 10.6.1. Aberrant regeneration of right third cranial nerve showing right-sided ptosis in primary gaze.

FIGURE 10.6.2. Aberrant regeneration of right third cranial nerve showing right upper eyelid retraction on attempted left gaze.

10

Follow-Up

1. Aberrancy from congenital: Routine.

2. Aberrancy from acquired: As per the underlying disorder identified in the work-up.

3. Primary aberrancy: As per neuroimaging findings. Patients are instructed to return immediately for any changes (e.g., ptosis, diplopia, sensory abnormality).

10.7   ISOLATED FOURTH NERVE PALSY

Symptoms

Binocular vertical (or oblique) diplopia, difficulty reading, sensation that objects appear tilted; may be asymptomatic.

Signs

(See Figures 10.7.1 and 10.7.2.)

Critical. Deficient inferior movement of an eye when attempting to look down and in. The three-step test isolates a palsy of the superior oblique muscle (see below).

Other. The involved eye is higher (hypertropic) in primary gaze. The hypertropia increases when looking in the direction of the uninvolved eye or tilting the head toward the ipsilateral shoulder. The patient often maintains a head tilt toward the contralateral shoulder to eliminate diplopia.

Differential Diagnosis

All of the following may produce binocular vertical diplopia, hypertropia, or both.

- Myasthenia gravis: Variable symptoms with fatigability. Ptosis common. Orbicularis oculi weakness often present. See 10.11, *Myasthenia Gravis.*

- Thyroid eye disease: May have proptosis, eyelid lag, lid retraction, or injection over the involved rectus muscles. Positive forced-duction test. See 7.2.1, *Thyroid Eye Disease.* See Appendix 6, *Forced-Duction Test and Active Force Generation Test.*

- Idiopathic orbital inflammatory syndrome: Pain and proptosis are common. See 7.2.2, *Idiopathic Orbital Inflammatory Syndrome.*

- Orbital fracture: History of trauma. Positive forced-duction test. See 3.9, *Orbital Blow-out Fracture.*

- Skew deviation: The three-step test does not isolate a particular muscle. Rule out a posterior fossa or brainstem lesion by MRI of the brain. See 10.13, *Internuclear Ophthalmoplegia.*

- Incomplete third nerve palsy: Inability to look down and in, usually with adduction weakness. Intorsion on attempted downgaze. Three-step test does not isolate the

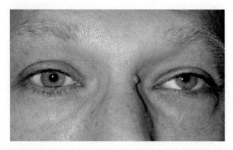

FIGURE 10.7.1. Isolated left fourth cranial nerve palsy: Primary gaze showing left hypertropia.

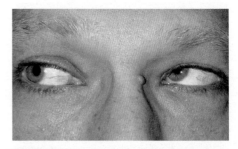

FIGURE 10.7.2. Isolated left fourth cranial nerve palsy: Right gaze with left inferior oblique overaction.

superior oblique. See 10.5, *Isolated Third Nerve Palsy*.

- Brown syndrome: Limitation of elevation in adduction due to restriction of superior oblique tendon. May be congenital or acquired (e.g., trauma, inflammation). Positive forced-duction test. See 8.6, *Strabismus Syndromes*.

- GCA: Extraocular muscle ischemia causing nonspecific motility deficits or neural ischemia mimicking a cranial nerve palsy. Age ≥55 years, usually associated systemic symptoms. See 10.17, *Arteritic Ischemic Optic Neuropathy (Giant Cell Arteritis)*.

Etiology

More common: Trauma, vascular infarct (often the result of underlying diabetes or hypertension), congenital, idiopathic, or demyelinating disease.

Rare: Tumor, hydrocephalus, aneurysm, GCA.

Work-Up

1. History: Onset and duration of the diplopia? Misaligned eyes or head tilt since early childhood? Trauma? Stroke?

2. Examine old photographs to determine whether the head tilt is long standing, indicating an old or congenital fourth nerve palsy.

3. Perform the three-step test:

   Step 1: Determine which eye is deviated upward in primary gaze. This is best seen with the cover–uncover test (see Appendix 3, *Cover/Uncover and Alternate Cover Tests*). The higher eye comes down after being uncovered.

   Step 2: Determine whether the upward deviation is greater when the patient looks to the left or to the right.

   Step 3: Determine whether the upward deviation is greater when tilting the head to the left shoulder or right shoulder.

   Patients with a superior oblique muscle paresis have a hyperdeviation that is worse when turning the elevated eye nasally and when tilting the head toward the shoulder ipsilateral to the elevated eye.

Patients with bilateral fourth nerve palsies demonstrate hypertropia of the right eye when looking left, hypertropia of the left eye when looking right, and a "V"-pattern esotropia (the eyes cross more when looking down).

In addition to the findings on the three-step test, the hypertropia should be greater in downgaze than in upgaze.

4. Perform the double Maddox rod test if bilateral fourth nerve palsies are suspected to measure total excyclotorsion.

   —A white Maddox rod is placed before one eye and a red Maddox rod is placed before the other eye in a trial frame or phoropter, aligning the axes of each rod along the 90-degrees vertical mark. While looking at a white light in the distance, the patient is asked if both the white and red lines seen through the Maddox rods are horizontal and parallel to each other. If not, the patient is asked to rotate the Maddox rod(s) until they are parallel. If he or she rotates the top of this vertical axis outward (away from the nose) for more than 10 degrees total for the two eyes, then a bilateral superior oblique muscle paresis is likely present.

5. Measure vertical fusional amplitudes with a vertical prism bar to distinguish a congenital from an acquired palsy.

   —A patient with an acquired fourth nerve palsy has a normal vertical fusional amplitude of 1 to 3 prism diopters. A patient with a congenital fourth nerve palsy has >3 prism diopters (sometimes up to 10 to 15 prism diopters) of fusional amplitude.

6. Edrophonium chloride test, ice test, or rest test if myasthenia gravis is suspected (see 10.11, *Myasthenia Gravis*).

7. CT scan of head and orbits (axial and coronal views) for suspected orbital disease.

8. Blood pressure measurement, fasting blood sugar, and glycosylated hemoglobin. Immediate ESR, CRP, and platelets if GCA is suspected.

9. MRI of the brain for:

   —A fourth nerve palsy accompanied by other cranial nerve or neurologic abnormalities.

10

—All patients <45 years of age with no history of significant head trauma, and patients aged 45 to 55 years with no vasculopathic risk factors or trauma.

Treatment

1. Treat the underlying disorder.

2. An occlusion patch may be placed over one eye or fogging plastic tape can be applied to one lens of patient's spectacles to relieve symptomatic double vision. Patching is usually not performed in children <11 years of age because of the risk of amblyopia.

3. Prisms in spectacles may be prescribed for small, stable hyperdeviations.

4. Strabismus surgery may be indicated for bothersome double vision in primary or reading position or for a cosmetically significant head tilt. Defer surgery at least 6 months after the onset of the palsy for the deviation to stabilize and because many palsies resolve spontaneously.

Follow-Up

1. Congenital fourth nerve palsy: Routine.

2. Acquired fourth nerve palsy: As per the underlying disorder. If the work-up is negative, the lesion is presumed vascular or idiopathic and the patient is reexamined in 1 to 3 months. If the palsy does not resolve in 3 months or if an additional neurologic abnormality develops, appropriate imaging studies of the brain are indicated. Patients are instructed to return immediately for any changes (e.g., ptosis, worsening diplopia, sensory abnormality, pupil abnormality).

10.8   ISOLATED SIXTH NERVE PALSY

Symptoms

Binocular horizontal diplopia, worse for distance than near, most pronounced in the direction of the paretic lateral rectus muscle.

Signs

(See Figures 10.8.1 and 10.8.2.)

Critical. Deficient lateral movement of an eye with negative forced-duction testing (see Appendix 6, *Forced-Duction Test and Active Force Generation Test*).

Other.   No proptosis.

Differential Diagnosis of Limited Abduction

■ Thyroid eye disease: May have proptosis, eyelid lag, lid retraction, injection over the involved rectus muscles, and positive forced-duction testing. See 7.2.1, *Thyroid Eye Disease.*

■ Myasthenia gravis: Variable symptoms with fatigability. Ptosis common. Positive edrophonium chloride test, ice test, and rest test. See 10.11, *Myasthenia Gravis.*

■ Idiopathic orbital inflammatory syndrome: Pain and proptosis are common. See 7.2.2, *Idiopathic Orbital Inflammatory Syndrome.*

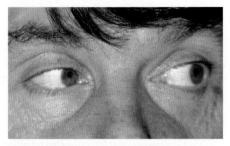

FIGURE 10.8.1. Isolated right sixth cranial nerve palsy: Left gaze showing full adduction.

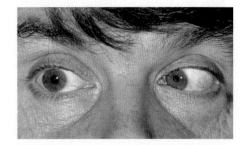

FIGURE 10.8.2. Isolated right sixth cranial nerve palsy: Right gaze showing limited abduction.

■ Orbital trauma: Fracture causing medial rectus entrapment, positive forced-duction testing. See 3.9, *Orbital Blow-out Fracture*.

■ Duane syndrome, type 1: Congenital; narrowing of the palpebral fissure and retraction of the globe on adduction. See 8.6, *Strabismus Syndromes*.

■ Möbius syndrome: Congenital; bilateral facial paralysis present. See 8.6, *Strabismus Syndromes*.

■ Convergence spasm: The pupils constrict on attempted abduction.

■ Primary divergence insufficiency: Usually acquired and benign; esotropia and diplopia only at distance and single binocular vision at near. Symptoms may improve spontaneously without treatment or may be corrected with base-out prisms or surgery. If the history reveals sudden onset, trauma, infection (e.g., meningitis, encephalitis), multiple sclerosis (MS), or malignancy, divergence paralysis should be considered and a neurologic work-up with MRI of the brain and brainstem obtained.

■ GCA: Extraocular muscle ischemia, age ≥55 years may be associated with systemic symptoms. See 10.17, *Arteritic Ischemic Optic Neuropathy (Giant Cell Arteritis)*.

Etiology

Adults

More common: Vasculopathic (e.g., diabetes, hypertension, other atherosclerotic risk factors), trauma, idiopathic.

Less common: Increased intracranial pressure, cavernous sinus mass (e.g., meningioma, aneurysm, metastasis), MS, sarcoidosis, vasculitis, after myelography or LP, stroke (usually with other neurologic deficits), meningeal inflammation/infection (e.g., Lyme disease, neurosyphilis), GCA.

Children

Benign and usually self-limited after viral infection or vaccination, trauma, increased intracranial pressure (e.g., obstructive hydrocephalus), pontine glioma, Gradenigo syndrome (petrositis causing sixth and often seventh nerve involvement, with or without eighth and fifth nerve involvement on the same side; associated with complicated otitis media).

Work-Up

Adults

1. History: Do the symptoms fluctuate during the day? Cancer, diabetes, or thyroid disease? Symptoms of GCA (in the appropriate age group)?

2. Complete neurologic and ophthalmic examinations; pay careful attention to the function of the other cranial nerves and the appearance of the optic disc. Because of the risk of corneal damage, it is especially important to evaluate the fifth cranial nerve. Corneal sensation (supplied by the first division) can be tested by touching a wisp of cotton or a tissue to the corneas before applying topical anesthetic. Ophthalmoscopy looking for papilledema is required because increased intracranial pressure from any cause can result in unilateral or bilateral sixth nerve palsies.

3. Check blood pressure, fasting blood sugar, and glycosylated hemoglobin.

4. MRI of the brain is indicated for the following patients:

   —Younger than 45 years of age (if MRI is negative, consider LP).

   —Consider MRI for patients aged 45 to 55 years with no vasculopathic risk factors.

   —Sixth nerve palsy accompanied by severe pain or any other neurologic or neuroophthalmic signs.

   —Any history of cancer.

   —Bilateral sixth nerve palsies.

   —Papilledema is present.

5. Immediate ESR, CRP, and platelet count if GCA is suspected. See 10.17, *Arteritic Ischemic Optic Neuropathy (Giant Cell Arteritis)*.

6. Consider RPR, FTA-ABS, Lyme titer.

Children

1. History: Recent illness or trauma? Neurologic symptoms, lethargy, or behavioral changes? Chronic ear infections?

10

2. Complete neurologic and ophthalmic examinations as described for adults.

3. Otoscopic examination to rule out complicated otitis media.

4. MRI of the brain in all children.

Treatment

1. Treat any underlying problem revealed by the work-up.

2. An occlusion patch may be placed over one eye or fogging plastic tape applied to one spectacle lens to relieve symptomatic diplopia. In patients <11 years, patching is avoided, and these patients are monitored closely for the development of amblyopia. See 8.7, *Amblyopia*.

3. Prisms in glasses may be fit acutely for temporary relief or for chronic stable deviations (e.g., after stroke). Consider strabismus surgery for a stable deviation that persists >6 months.

Follow-Up

Reexamine every 6 weeks after the onset of the palsy until it resolves. MRI of the head is indicated if any new neurologic signs or symptoms develop, the abduction deficit increases, or the isolated sixth nerve palsy does not resolve in 3 to 6 months.

10.9　ISOLATED SEVENTH NERVE PALSY

Symptoms

Weakness or paralysis of one side of the face, inability to close one eye, excessive drooling.

Signs

(See Figures 10.9.1 and 10.9.2.)

Critical. Unilateral weakness or paralysis of the facial musculature.

—Central lesion: Weakness or paralysis of lower facial musculature only. Upper eyelid closure and forehead wrinkling intact.

—Peripheral lesion: Weakness or paralysis of upper and lower facial musculature.

Other. Flattened nasolabial fold, droop of corner of the mouth, ectropion, and lagophthalmos. May have ipsilateral decreased taste on anterior two-thirds of tongue, decreased basic tear production, or hyperacusis. May have an injected eye with a corneal epithelial defect. Synkinesis, a simultaneous movement of muscles supplied by different branches of the facial nerve or simultaneous stimulation of visceral efferent fibers of facial nerve [e.g., corner of mouth contracts when eye closes, excessive lacrimation when eating ("crocodile" tears)], secondary to aberrant regeneration implying chronicity.

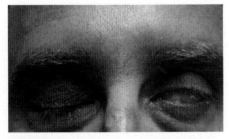

FIGURE 10.9.1. Isolated left seventh cranial nerve palsy: Lagophthalmos.

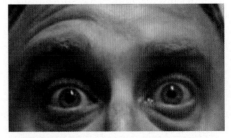

FIGURE 10.9.2. Isolated peripheral left seventh cranial nerve palsy.

Etiology

Central Lesions

- Cortical: Lesion of contralateral motor cortex or internal capsule (e.g., stroke, tumor). Loss of voluntary facial movement; emotional facial movement sometimes intact. May also have ipsilateral hemiparesis.

- Extrapyramidal: Lesion of basal ganglia (e.g., parkinsonism, tumor, vascular lesion of basal ganglia). Loss of emotional facial movement; volitional facial movement intact. Not a true facial paralysis.

- Brainstem: Lesion of ipsilateral pons (e.g., MS, stroke, tumor). Often with ipsilateral sixth nerve palsy, contralateral hemiparesis. Occasionally with cerebellar signs.

Peripheral Lesions

- Cerebellopontine angle (CPA) masses (e.g., acoustic neuroma, facial neuroma, meningioma, cholesteatoma, metastasis): Gradual progressive onset, although sometimes acute. May have facial pain, twitching, or a characteristic nystagmus. This is small-amplitude rapid jerk nystagmus in which the fast phase is directed away from the side of the lesion (peripheral vestibular) in conjunction with a slow, gaze-evoked nystagmus directed toward the side of the lesion (from brainstem compression). May have eighth nerve dysfunction, including hearing loss, tinnitus, vertigo, or dysequilibrium.

- Temporal bone fracture: History of head trauma. May have Battle sign (ecchymoses over mastoid region), cerebrospinal fluid otorrhea, hearing loss, vertigo, or vestibular nystagmus.

- Other trauma: Accidental or iatrogenic (e.g., facial laceration, local anesthetic block, parotid or mastoid surgery).

- Acute or chronic suppurative otitis media.

- Malignant otitis externa: Pseudomonas infection in diabetic or elderly patients. Begins in external auditory canal but may progress to osteomyelitis, meningitis, or abscess.

- Ramsay–Hunt syndrome (varicella zoster oticus): Viral prodrome followed by ear pain; vesicles on pinna, external auditory canal, tongue, face, or neck. Progresses over 10 days. May have sensorineural hearing loss, tinnitus, or vertigo.

- Guillain–Barré syndrome: Viral syndrome followed by progressive motor weakness or paralysis or cranial nerve palsies, or both. Loss of deep tendon reflexes. May have bilateral facial palsies.

- Lyme disease: May have rash, fever, fatigue, arthralgias, myalgias, or nausea. There may or may not be a history of tick bite. See 13.3, *Lyme Disease.*

- Sarcoidosis: May have uveitis, parotitis, skin lesions, or lymphadenopathy. May have bilateral facial palsies. See 12.6, *Sarcoidosis.*

- Parotid neoplasm: Slowly progressive paralysis of all or portion of facial musculature. Parotid mass with facial pain.

- Metastasis: History of primary tumor (e.g., breast, lung, prostate). Multiple cranial nerve palsies in rapid succession may be seen. Can be the result of basilar skull metastasis or carcinomatous meningitis.

- Bell palsy: Idiopathic seventh nerve palsy. Most common, but other etiologies must be ruled out. May have viral prodrome followed by ear pain, facial numbness, decreased tearing or taste. Facial palsy may be complete or incomplete and progress over 10 days. May be recurrent, rarely bilateral. Possible familial predisposition.

- Others: Diabetes mellitus, botulism, human immunodeficiency virus (HIV), syphilis, Epstein–Barr virus, acute porphyrias, nasopharyngeal carcinoma, collagen–vascular disease, and others.

Work-Up

1. History: Onset and duration of facial weakness? First episode or recurrence? Facial or ear pain? Trauma? Stroke? Recent infection? Hearing loss, tinnitus, dizziness, or vertigo? History of sarcoidosis or cancer?

2. Examine old photographs to determine chronicity of facial droop.

3. Complete neurologic examination: Determine if facial palsy is central or peripheral,

10

complete or incomplete. Assess taste with bitter or sweet solution on anterior two-thirds of tongue on affected side. Carefully assess other cranial nerves, especially the fifth, sixth, and seventh. Look for motor weakness and cerebellar signs.

4. Complete ocular examination: Check ocular motility and look for nystagmus. Assess orbicularis strength bilaterally, degree of ectropion, and Bell phenomenon. Examine cornea carefully for signs of exposure (superficial punctate keratopathy, epithelial defect, or ulcer). Perform Schirmer test (see 4.3, *Dry-Eye Syndrome*) to assess basic tear production. Check for signs of uveitis.

5. Otolaryngologic examination: Examine ear and oropharynx for vesicles, masses, or other lesions. Palpate parotid for mass or lymphadenopathy. Check hearing.

6. CT scan if history of trauma to rule out basilar skull fracture: Axial and coronal cuts with attention to temporal bone.

7. MRI or CT scan of brain if any other associated neurologic signs, history of cancer, or duration >3 months. Sixth nerve involvement warrants attention to the brainstem. Eighth nerve involvement warrants attention to the CPA. Multiple cranial nerve involvement warrants attention to the skull base.

8. Chest radiograph and angiotensin-converting enzyme (ACE) level if sarcoidosis suspected.

9. Consider Lyme titer, Epstein–Barr virus titer, RPR, HIV test, and CBC with differential, depending on suspected etiology.

10. Rheumatoid factor, ESR, antinuclear antibody (ANA), and antineutrophil cytoplasmic antibody if collagen–vascular disease suspected.

11. Echocardiogram, Holter monitor, carotid noninvasive studies in patients with a history of stroke.

12. LP in patients with history of primary neoplasm to rule out carcinomatous meningitis (repeat up to three times if negative to increase sensitivity).

Treatment

1. Treat the underlying disease as follows:

   —Stroke: Refer to neurologist.

   —CPA masses, temporal bone fracture, nerve laceration: Refer to neurosurgeon.

   —Otitis: Refer to otolaryngologist.

   —Ramsay–Hunt syndrome: If seen within 72 hours of onset, start acyclovir 800 mg five times per day for 7 to 10 days (contraindicated in pregnancy and renal failure). Refer to otolaryngologist.

   —Guillain–Barré syndrome: Refer to neurologist. May require urgent hospitalization for rapidly progressive motor weakness or respiratory distress.

   —Lyme disease: Refer to infectious disease specialist. May need LP. Treat with oral doxycycline, penicillin, or intravenous (i.v.) ceftriaxone. See 13.3, *Lyme Disease.*

   —Sarcoidosis: Treat uveitis if present. Consider brain MRI, LP, or both to rule out CNS involvement; if present, refer to neurologist. Refer to internist for systemic evaluation. May require systemic prednisone for extraocular or CNS disease. See 12.6, *Sarcoidosis.*

   —Metastatic disease: Refer to oncologist. Systemic chemotherapy, radiation, or both may be required.

2. Bell palsy: 86% of patients recover completely with observation alone within 2 months. Options for treatment include:

   —Facial massage or electrical stimulation of facial musculature.

   —Consider steroids (e.g., prednisone 60 mg p.o. q.d. for 4 days, tapering to 5 mg q.d. over 10 days). A short course of acyclovir or famciclovir, in combination with prednisone, may improve facial nerve function outcomes.

   —Consider referral to otorhinolaryngology for surgical decompression of the facial nerve.

3. The primary ocular complication of facial palsy is corneal exposure, which is

managed as follows (also see 4.5, *Exposure Keratopathy*):

—Mild exposure keratitis: Artificial tears q.i.d. with lubricating ointment q.h.s.

—Moderate exposure keratitis: Preservative-free artificial tears q1–2h, moisture chamber during the day with lubricating ointment, or tape tarsorrhaphy q.h.s. Consider a temporary tarsorrhaphy.

—Severe exposure keratitis: Temporary or permanent tarsorrhaphy. For expected chronic facial palsy, consider eyelid gold weight to facilitate eyelid closure.

Follow-Up

1. Recheck all patients at 1 and 3 months and more frequently if corneal complications arise.

2. If not resolved after 3 months, order MRI of brain to rule out mass lesion.

3. In nonresolving facial palsy with repeatedly negative work-up, consider referral to neurosurgeon or plastic surgeon for facial nerve graft, cranial nerve reanastomosis, or temporalis muscle transposition for patients who strongly desire facial reanimation.

CAVERNOUS SINUS AND ASSOCIATED SYNDROMES (MULTIPLE OCULAR MOTOR NERVE PALSIES)

10.10

Symptoms

Double vision, eyelid droop, facial pain, or numbness.

Signs

Critical. Limitation of eye movement corresponding to any combination of a third, fourth, or sixth nerve palsy on one side; facial pain or numbness or both corresponding to one or more branches of the fifth cranial nerve; ptosis and a small pupil (Horner syndrome); the pupil also may be dilated if the third cranial nerve is involved. Any combination of the above may be present simultaneously because of the anatomy of the cavernous sinus. All signs involve the same side of the face when one cavernous sinus/superior orbital fissure is involved. The circular sinus connects the cavernous sinuses, and its involvement can cause contralateral signs. Consider orbital apex syndrome when proptosis and optic neuropathy are present.

Other. Proptosis may be present when the superior orbital fissure is involved.

Differential Diagnosis

- Myasthenia gravis: Fatigable ptosis, orbicularis weakness, and limited motility. Pupils uninvolved. No proptosis. See 10.11, *Myasthenia Gravis.*

- CPEO: Progressive, painless, bilateral motility limitation with ptosis. Normal pupils. Orbicularis always weak. See 10.12, *Chronic Progressive External Ophthalmoplegia.*

- Orbital lesions (e.g., tumor, thyroid disease, inflammation). Proptosis and increased resistance to retropulsion are usually present, in addition to motility restriction. Results of forced-duction tests are abnormal (see Appendix 6, *Forced-Duction Test and Active Force Generation Test*). May have an afferent pupillary defect if the optic nerve is involved.

NOTE: Orbital apex syndrome combines the superior orbital fissure syndrome with optic nerve dysfunction, and most commonly results from an orbital lesion.

10

- Brainstem disease: Tumors and vascular lesions of the brainstem can produce ocular motor nerve palsies, particularly the sixth cranial nerve. MRI of the brain is best for making this diagnosis.

- Carcinomatous meningitis: Diffuse seeding of the leptomeninges by metastatic tumor cells can produce a rapidly sequential bilateral cranial nerve disorder. Diagnosis is made by serial LPs.

- Skull base tumors, especially nasopharyngeal carcinoma or clivus lesions: Most commonly affects the sixth cranial nerve, but the second, third, fourth, and fifth cranial nerves may be involved as well. Typically, one cranial nerve after another is affected by invasion of the base of the skull. The patient may have cervical lymphadenopathy, nasal obstruction, ear pain, or popping caused by serous otitis media or blockage of the Eustachian tube, weight loss, or proptosis.

- Progressive supranuclear palsy (PSP): Vertical limitation of eye movements, typically beginning with downward gaze. Postural instability, dementia, and rigidity of the neck and trunk may be present. All eye movements are eventually lost. See 10.12, *Chronic Progressive External Ophthalmoplegia.*

- Rare: Myotonic dystrophy, bulbar variant of the Guillain–Barré syndrome (Miller–Fisher variant), intracranial sarcoidosis, others.

Etiology

- Arteriovenous fistula [carotid–cavernous ("high-flow") or dural–cavernous ("low-flow")]: Proptosis, chemosis, dilated and tortuous ("corkscrew") episcleral and conjunctival blood vessels (see Figure 10.10.1). Intraocular pressure is often increased. Enhanced ocular pulsation ("pulsatile proptosis") may be present, usually only discernible on slit-lamp examination during applanation. A bruit may be heard by the patient, and sometimes by the physician if the globe or temple region is auscultated. Reversed, arterialized flow in the superior ophthalmic vein is detectable with orbital color Doppler US. Orbital CT scan or MRI may show an enlarged superior ophthalmic vein. High-flow fistulas have an abrupt onset and are most commonly caused by trauma or rupture of an intracavernous aneurysm, whereas low-flow fistulas have a more insidious presentation, most commonly in hypertensive women >50 years of age and are due to dural arteriovenous malformations. The Barrow classification is used for preoperative planning and further subdivides carotid–cavernous fistulas as follows:

A. Direct fistula.

B. Indirect with branches solely from internal carotid artery (rare).

C. Indirect with branches solely from external carotid artery.

D. Indirect with branches from both internal and external carotid arteries (most common).

- Tumors within the cavernous sinus: May be primary intracranial neoplasms with local invasion of the cavernous sinus (e.g., meningioma, pituitary adenoma, craniopharyngioma); or metastatic tumors to the cavernous sinus, either local (e.g., nasopharyngeal carcinoma, perineural spread of a periocular squamous cell carcinoma) or distant metastasis (e.g., breast, lung, lymphoma).

NOTE: Previously resected tumors may invade the cavernous sinus years after resection.

- Intracavernous aneurysm: Usually not ruptured. If aneurysm does rupture, the signs of a carotid–cavernous fistula develop.

- Mucormycosis/zygomycosis: Must be suspected in all diabetic patients, particularly those in ketoacidosis, and any debilitated or immunocompromised individual with multiple cranial nerve palsies, with or without proptosis. Onset is typically acute. Bloody nasal discharge may be present, and nasal examination may reveal a black, crusty material. This condition is life-threatening.

- Pituitary apoplexy: Acute onset of the critical signs listed previously; often bilateral with severe headache, decreased vision,

10

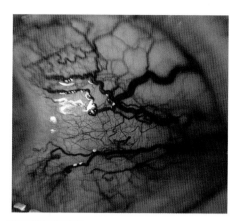

FIGURE 10.10.1. Carotid–cavernous fistula with dilated and tortuous episcleral and conjunctival vessels.

and possibly bitemporal hemianopsia or blindness. A preexisting pituitary adenoma may enlarge during pregnancy, owing to apoplexy. Peripartum hemorrhage or shock can cause an infarction of the pituitary gland, leading to apoplexy of a nontumorous pituitary gland (Sheehan syndrome). An enlarged sella turcica or an intrasellar mass, usually with acute hemorrhage, is seen on CT scan or MRI of the brain.

▪ Varicella zoster: Patients with the typical zoster rash may develop ocular motor nerve palsies as well as a mid-dilated pupil that reacts better to convergence than to light.

▪ Cavernous sinus thrombosis: Proptosis, chemosis, and eyelid edema. Usually bilateral. Fever, nausea, vomiting, and an altered level of consciousness often develop. May result from spread of infection from the face, mouth, throat, sinus, or orbit. Less commonly noninfectious, resulting from trauma or surgery.

▪ Tolosa–Hunt syndrome: Acute idiopathic inflammation of the superior orbital fissure or anterior cavernous sinus. Orbital pain often precedes restriction of eye movements. Recurrent episodes are common. This is a diagnosis of exclusion.

▪ Others: Sarcoidosis, Wegener granulomatosis, mucocele, tuberculosis, and other infections and inflammatory conditions.

Work-Up

1. History: Diabetes? Hypertension? Recent trauma? Prior cancer (including skin cancer)? Weight loss? Ocular bruit? Recent infection? Severe headache? Diurnal variation of symptoms?

2. Ophthalmic examination: Careful attention to pupils, extraocular motility, Hertel exophthalmometry, and resistance to retropulsion.

3. Examine the periocular skin for malignant or locally invasive lesions.

4. CT scan (axial and coronal views) or MRI of the sinuses, orbit, and brain, or both.

5. Consider orbital color Doppler imaging if arteriovenous fistula is suspected.

If the CT scan and MRI are negative, consider any or all of the following:

6. LP to rule out carcinomatous meningitis in patients with a history of primary carcinoma. More than one LP might be required in some cases.

7. Nasopharyngeal examination with or without a biopsy to rule out nasopharyngeal carcinoma.

8. Lymph node biopsy when lymphadenopathy is present.

9. CBC with differential, ESR, ANA, rheumatoid factor to rule out infection, malignancy, and systemic vasculitis. Antineutrophilic cytoplasmic antibody if Wegener granulomatosis is suspected.

10. Cerebral arteriography is rarely required to rule out an aneurysm or arteriovenous fistula because most of these are seen by noninvasive imaging studies.

NOTE: Patients suspected of having dural arteriovenous fistulas are recommended to undergo arteriography to look for cortical venous drainage. If present, this puts the patient at greater risk for intracranial hemorrhage.

---

11. If cavernous sinus thrombosis is being considered, obtain two to three sets of peripheral blood cultures and also

10

culture the presumed primary source of the infection.

Treatment and Follow-Up

Arteriovenous Fistula

1. Many dural fistulas close spontaneously, with intermittent ipsilateral carotid massage, or after arteriography. Others may require treatment via interventional neuroradiologic techniques.

2. Resolution of the fistula usually results in normalization of the intraocular pressure. However, medical treatment with aqueous suppressants for secondary glaucoma may be necessary. Drugs that increase outflow facility (e.g., latanoprost and pilocarpine) are usually not as effective because the intraocular pressure is increased as a result of increased episcleral venous pressure. See 9.1, *Primary Open-Angle Glaucoma.*

Metastatic Disease to the Cavernous Sinus

Often requires systemic chemotherapy (if a primary is found) with or without radiation therapy to the metastasis. Refer to an oncologist.

Intracavernous Aneurysm

Refer to a neurosurgeon for work-up and possible treatment.

Mucormycosis/Zygomycosis

1. Immediate hospitalization because this is a rapidly progressive, life-threatening disease.

2. Emergent CT scan of the sinuses, orbit, and brain.

3. Consult Infectious Disease, Neurosurgery, Otolaryngology, and Endocrinology as indicated.

4. Begin amphotericin B 0.25 to 0.30 mg/kg i.v. in D5W slowly over 3 to 6 hours on the first day, 0.5 mg/kg i.v. on the second day, and then up to 0.8 to 1.0 mg/kg i.v. q.d. The duration of treatment is determined by the clinical condition.

NOTE: Renal status and electrolytes must be checked before initiating therapy with amphotericin B and then monitored closely during treatment. Liposomal amphotericin has significantly less renal toxicity.

---

5. A biopsy should be obtained from any necrotic tissue (e.g., nasopharynx, paranasal sinuses) if mucormycosis/zygomycosis is suspected.

6. Early surgical debridement of all necrotic tissue (possibly including orbital exenteration), plus irrigation of the involved areas with amphotericin B, is often necessary to eradicate the infection.

7. Treat the underlying medical condition (e.g., diabetic ketoacidosis), with appropriate consultation as required.

Pituitary Apoplexy

Refer immediately to neurosurgeon for surgical consideration. These patients are often quite ill and require immediate steroid therapy.

Varicella Zoster

See 4.16, *Herpes Zoster Ophthalmicus/Varicella Zoster Virus.*

Cavernous Sinus Thrombosis

1. For possible infectious cases (usually caused by *Staphylococcus aureus*), hospitalize the patient for treatment with intravenous antibiotics for several weeks. Consult Infectious Disease for antibiotic management.

2. Intravenous fluid replacement is usually required.

3. For aseptic cavernous sinus thrombosis, consider systemic anticoagulation (heparin followed by warfarin) or aspirin 325 mg p.o. q.d. in collaboration with a medical internist.

4. Exposure keratopathy is treated with preservative-free lubricating ointment or drops (see 4.5, *Exposure Keratopathy*).

5. Treat secondary glaucoma. See 9.1, *Primary Open-Angle Glaucoma.*

Tolosa–Hunt Syndrome

Prednisone 60 to 100 mg p.o. q.d. for 2 to 3 days, and then a gradual taper over at least 4 to 6 weeks as the pain subsides. If pain persists after 72 hours, stop steroids and initiate reinvestigation to rule out other disorders.

NOTE: Other infectious or inflammatory disorders may also respond to steroids initially, so these patients need to be monitored closely.

MYASTHENIA GRAVIS

10.11

Symptoms

Droopy eyelid or double vision that is variable throughout the day or worse when the individual is fatigued; may have weakness of facial muscles, proximal limb muscles, and difficulty swallowing or breathing.

Signs

Critical. Worsening of ptosis with sustained upgaze or diplopia with continued eye movements, weakness of the orbicularis muscle (cannot close the eyelids forcefully to resist examiner's opening them). No pupillary abnormalities or pain.

Other. Upward twitch of ptotic eyelid when shifting gaze from inferior to primary position (Cogan eyelid twitch). Can have complete limitation of all ocular movements.

Differential Diagnosis

- Eaton–Lambert syndrome: A myasthenia-like paraneoplastic condition associated with carcinoma, especially lung cancer. Isolated eye signs do not occur, although eye signs may accompany systemic signs of weakness. Unlike myasthenia, muscle strength increases after exercise. Electromyography (EMG) distinguishes between the two conditions.

- Myasthenia-like syndrome due to medication (e.g., penicillamine, aminoglycosides).

- CPEO: No diurnal variation of symptoms or relation to fatigue; usually a negative intravenous edrophonium chloride test. Typically no diplopia. See 10.12, *Chronic Progressive External Ophthalmoplegia.*

- Kearns–Sayre syndrome: CPEO and retinal pigmentary degeneration in a young person; heart block develops. See 10.12, *Chronic Progressive External Ophthalmoplegia.*

- Third nerve palsy: Pupil may be involved, no orbicularis weakness, no fatigability, no diurnal variation. See 10.5, *Isolated Third Nerve Palsy.*

NOTE: Myasthenia may mimic specific cranial nerve palsies, but the pupil is never involved.

- Horner syndrome: Miosis accompanies the ptosis. Pupil does not dilate well in darkness. See 10.2, *Horner Syndrome.*

- Levator muscle dehiscence or disinsertion: High eyelid crease on the side of the droopy eyelid, no variability of eyelid droop, no orbicularis weakness.

- Thyroid eye disease: No ptosis. May have eyelid retraction or eyelid lag, may or may not have exophthalmos, no diurnal variation of diplopia. Graves disease occurs in 5% of patients with myasthenia gravis. See 7.2.1, *Thyroid Eye Disease.*

- Idiopathic orbital inflammatory syndrome: Proptosis, pain, ocular injection. See 7.2.2, *Idiopathic Orbital Inflammatory Syndrome.*

- Myotonic dystrophy: May have ptosis and rarely, gaze restriction. After a handshake, these patients are often unable to release their grip (myotonia). Polychromatic lenticular deposits, "Christmas tree" cataract and pigmentary retinopathy present.

Etiology

Autoimmune disease; sometimes associated with underlying thyroid dysfunction. May be associated with occult thymoma. Increased incidence of other autoimmune disease (e.g., lupus, MS, rheumatoid arthritis). All age groups may be affected.

Work-Up

1. History: Do the signs fluctuate throughout the day and worsen with fatigue? Any systemic weakness? Difficulty swallowing, chewing, or breathing? Medications?

2. Assess for presence of fatigability: Measure the degree of ptosis in primary gaze. Have the patient focus on your finger in upgaze for 1 minute. Observe whether the ptosis worsens.

10

3. Assess orbicularis strength by asking the patient to squeeze the eyelids shut while you attempt to force them open.

4. Test pupillary function.

5. Blood test for acetylcholine receptor antibodies. An elevated antibody titer establishes the diagnosis of myasthenia. However, values may be positive in only 60% to 88% of patients with myasthenia and are less likely to be positive in purely ocular myasthenia gravis.

6. In adults, edrophonium chloride or prostigmine tests, ice-pack test (see later), or rest test (see later) may confirm the diagnosis. Edrophonium chloride test is performed as follows:

   —Identify one prominent feature (e.g., ptosis, diplopia) to observe during test. Have a cardiac monitor (not portable) and injectable atropine readily available.

   —Inject edrophonium chloride 0.2 mL (2 mg) i.v. Observe for 1 minute. If an improvement in the selected feature is noted, the test is positive and may be stopped at this point. If no improvement with the medication develops, continue. Stop immediately if untoward reaction occurs.

   —Inject edrophonium chloride 0.4 mL (4 mg) i.v. Observe for 30 seconds for a response or side effect. If neither develops, proceed.

   —Inject edrophonium chloride 0.4 mL (4 mg) i.v. If no improvement is noted within two additional minutes, the test is negative.

—Improvement within the stated time period is diagnostic of myasthenia gravis (rarely a patient with CPEO, an intracavernous tumor, or some other rare disorder will have a false-positive result). A negative test does not exclude myasthenia.

NOTE: Cholinergic crisis, syncopal episode, and respiratory arrest, although rare, may be precipitated by the edrophonium chloride test. Treatment includes atropine 0.4 mg i.v., while monitoring vital signs. Consider pretreating with atropine to prevent problems.

Intramuscular prostigmine may be used instead of edrophonium chloride in children or in patients where injecting intravenous medication is problematic. The effect has a longer onset and lasts for approximately 30 minutes.

---

7. For the ice-pack test, an ice pack is placed over closed eyes for 2 minutes. Improvement of ptosis by at least 2 mm is a positive test (see Figures 10.11.1 and 10.11.2).

8. In children, observation for improvement immediately after a 1- to 2-hour nap (sleep test) is a safe alternative. A similar rest test (keeping eyes closed) for 30 minutes in adults may be similarly diagnostic.

9. Check swallowing and breathing function and proximal limb muscle strength to rule out systemic involvement.

10. Thyroid function tests [including thyroid-stimulating hormone (TSH)].

11. CT scan of the chest to rule out thymoma.

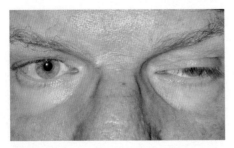

FIGURE 10.11.1. Myasthenia gravis with left ptosis.

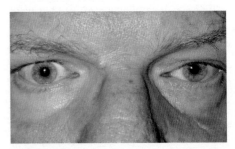

FIGURE 10.11.2. Myasthenia gravis after ice-pack test showing resolution of left ptosis.

12. Consider ANA, rheumatoid factor, and other tests to rule out other autoimmune disease.

13. A single-fiber EMG including the orbicularis muscle may be performed if other testing is negative and the diagnosis is still suspected. May be the most sensitive test for involvement of the ocular muscles.

Treatment

Refer to a neurologist familiar with this disease.

1. If the patient is having difficulty swallowing or breathing, urgent hospitalization for plasmapheresis, intravenous immunoglobulin (IVIG), and ventilatory support may be indicated.

2. If the condition is mild, purely ocular, and is not disturbing to the patient, therapy need not be instituted (the patient may patch one eye as needed).

3. If the condition is disturbing or more severe, an oral anticholinesterase agent such as pyridostigmine (gradually increasing to a dose of 60 mg p.o. q.i.d. for an adult) should be given. The dosage must be adjusted according to the response. Patients rarely benefit from >120 mg p.o. q3h of pyridostigmine. Overdosage may produce cholinergic crisis.

4. If symptoms persist, consider systemic steroids. There is no uniform agreement concerning the dosage. One option is to start with prednisone 20 mg p.o. q.d., increasing the dose slowly until the patient is receiving 100 mg/day. These patients may require hospitalization for several days when a high-dose regimen of steroids is employed.

NOTE: Steroid use in myasthenia may precipitate respiratory crisis in the first 2 weeks of treatment. Therefore, in patients with systemic symptoms, hospitalization to begin steroids is required.

---

5. Azathioprine (1 to 2 mg/kg/day) may be helpful in older patients. Other medications include mycophenolate mofetil and cyclosporine. Some patients with systemic myasthenia are treated with regularly scheduled IVIG or plasmapheresis.

6. Treat any underlying thyroid disease or infection.

7. Surgical removal of the thymus can be performed. This is indicated for anyone with thymoma. It may also improve symptoms in patients with generalized myasthenia without thymoma.

Follow-Up

1. If systemic muscular weakness is present, patients need to be monitored every 1 to 4 days by an appropriate medical specialist until improvement is demonstrated.

2. Patients who have had their isolated ocular abnormality for an extended time (e.g., months) should be seen every 4 to 6 months and if proven to be stable, every 6 to 12 months.

3. Patients should always be warned to return immediately if swallowing or breathing difficulties arise. After isolated ocular myasthenia has been present for 2 years, progression to systemic involvement is unlikely.

NOTE: Newborn infants of myasthenic mothers should be observed carefully for signs of myasthenia because acetylcholine receptor antibodies may cross the placenta. Poor sucking reflex, ptosis or decreased muscle tone may be seen.

10

Symptoms

Slowly progressive, symmetric ophthalmoplegia and droopy eyelids. Almost never have diplopia. Usually bilateral; there is no diurnal variation; there may be a family history.

Signs

Critical. Ptosis, limitation of ocular motility (sometimes complete limitation), normal pupils, orthophoric.

Other. Weak orbicularis oculi muscles, weakness of limb and facial muscles, exposure keratopathy.

Differential Diagnosis

See 10.11, *Myasthenia Gravis,* for a complete list. The following syndromes must be ruled out when CPEO is diagnosed:

- Kearns–Sayre syndrome: Onset of CPEO before age 20 years, retinal pigmentary degeneration with a salt-and-pepper appearance, heart block that usually occurs years after the ocular signs and may cause sudden death. Other signs may include hearing loss, mental retardation, cerebellar signs, short stature, delayed puberty, nephropathy, vestibular abnormalities, increased cerebrospinal fluid protein, and characteristic "ragged red fiber" findings on muscle biopsy. Although some are inherited maternally, the vast majority are due to spontaneous mitochondrial deletions.

- Abetalipoproteinemia (Bassen–Kornzweig syndrome): Retinal pigmentary degeneration similar to retinitis pigmentosa, diarrhea, ataxia, and other neurologic signs. Acanthocytosis of red blood cells are seen on peripheral blood smear and LP demonstrates increased cerebrospinal fluid protein. See 11.28, *Retinitis Pigmentosa and Inherited Chorioretinal Dystrophies.*

- Refsum disease: Retinitis pigmentosa and increased blood phytanic acid level. May have polyneuropathy, ataxia, hearing loss, anosmia, others. See 11.28, *Retinitis Pigmentosa and Inherited Chorioretinal Dystrophies.*

- Oculopharyngeal dystrophy: Difficulty swallowing, sometimes leading to aspiration of food; may have autosomal dominant inheritance.

- Mitochondrial myopathy and encephalopathy, lactic acidosis, and stroke-like episodes (MELAS): Occurs in children and young adults. May have headache, transient hemianopia, hemiparesis, nausea, vomiting. Elevated serum and cerebrospinal fluid lactate levels and may have abnormalities on MRI.

- Progressive supranuclear palsy (PSP; Steele-Richardson-Olszewski syndrome): Rare progressive neurodegenerative disorder affecting the brainstem that causes early gait instability and ophthalmoplegia. Often downgaze affected first followed by other gaze limitations; vertical more than horizontal. Other eye movement problems include abnormalities in the saccadic and pursuit subsystems of horizontal gaze. Often the eyelids are held wide open resulting in a "staring" type of facial expression. Neck and axial rigidity is an important sign.

Work-Up

1. Careful history: Determine the rate of onset (gradual versus sudden, as in cranial nerve disease).

2. Family history.

3. Carefully examine the pupils and ocular motility.

4. Test orbicularis oculi strength.

5. Fundus examination: Look for diffuse pigmentary changes.

6. Check swallowing function.

7. Edrophonium chloride test, ice-pack test, or rest test to check for myasthenia gravis. See 10.11, *Myasthenia Gravis.*

NOTE: Some patients with CPEO are super-sensitive to edrophonium chloride which may precipitate heart block and arrhythmias.

8. Prompt referral to a cardiologist for full cardiac work-up (including yearly electro-cardiograms) if Kearns–Sayre syndrome is suspected.

9. If neurologic signs and symptoms develop, consult a neurologist for work-up (including possible LP).

10. Lipoprotein electrophoresis and periph-eral blood smear if abetalipoproteinemia suspected.

11. Serum phytanic acid level if Refsum dis-ease suspected.

Treatment

There is no cure for CPEO, but associated abnormalities are managed as follows:

1. Treat exposure keratopathy with lubricants at night and artificial tears during the day. See 4.5, *Exposure Keratopathy.*

2. Single vision reading glasses or base-down prisms within reading glasses may help reading when downward gaze is restricted.

3. In Kearns–Sayre syndrome, a pacemaker may be required.

4. In oculopharyngeal dystrophy, dysphagia and aspirations may require cricopharyn-geal surgery.

5. In severe ptosis, consider ptosis crutches or surgical repair, but watch for worsening exposure keratopathy.

6. Genetic counseling.

Follow-Up

Depends on ocular and systemic findings.

10.13 INTERNUCLEAR OPHTHALMOPLEGIA

Definition

Ophthalmoplegia secondary to lesion in the medial longitudinal fasciculus (MLF).

Symptoms

Double vision, blurry vision, or vague visual complaints.

Signs

(See Figures 10.13.1 and 10.13.2.)

Critical. Weakness or paralysis of adduction, with horizontal jerk nystagmus of the abduct-ing eye.

NOTE: Internuclear ophthalmoplegia (INO) is local-ized to the side with the weak adduction.

Other. A skew deviation (a relatively comitant vertical deviation not caused by neuromuscular junction disease or intraorbital pathology). The

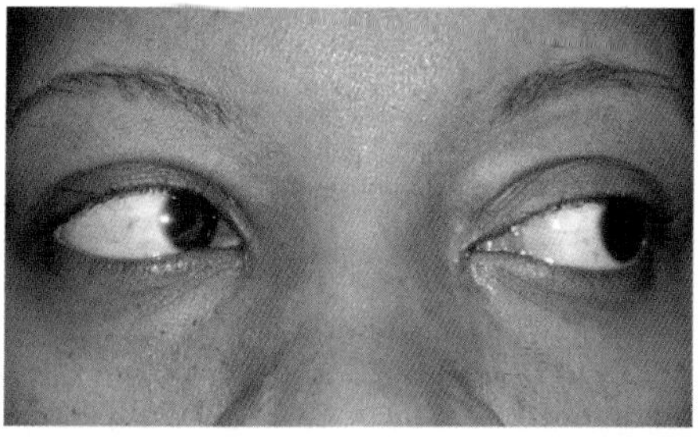

10

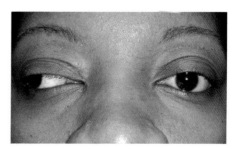

FIGURE 10.13.1. Left internuclear ophthalmoplegia: Left gaze showing full abduction.

FIGURE 10.13.2. Left internuclear ophthalmoplegia: Right gaze with severe adduction deficit.

three-step test cannot isolate a specific muscle. Localizes to the posterior fossa. See 10.7, *Isolated Fourth Nerve Palsy*. Upbeat nystagmus on upgaze when INO is bilateral. The involved eye can sometimes turn in when attempting to read (intact convergence). Unilateral or bilateral (WEBINO: "wall-eyed," bilateral INO).

Differential Diagnosis of Attenuated Adduction

■ Myasthenia gravis: May closely mimic INO; however, ptosis and orbicularis oculi weakness are common. Nystagmus of INO is faster; myasthenia gravis is more gaze paretic. Symptoms vary throughout the day. See 10.11, *Myasthenia Gravis*.

■ Orbital disease (e.g., tumor, thyroid disease, idiopathic orbital inflammatory syndrome): Proptosis, globe displacement, or pain may also be present. Nystagmus is usually not present. See 7.1, *Orbital Disease*.

■ One-and-a-half syndrome: Pontine lesion that includes the ipsilateral MLF and horizontal gaze center (sixth nerve nucleus). The only preserved horizontal movement is abduction of the eye contralateral to the lesion. This is because of an ipsilateral adduction deficit (from the MLF lesion) and a horizontal gaze paresis in the direction of the lesion (from the horizontal gaze center lesion). Causes include stroke and pontine neoplasia.

Etiology

■ MS: More common in young patients, usually bilateral.

■ Brainstem stroke: More common in elderly patients, usually unilateral.

■ Brainstem mass lesion.

■ Rare causes: CNS cryptococcosis, tuberculosis granuloma, pyoderma gangrenosum (all shown to cause WEBINO).

Work-Up

1. History: Age? Are symptoms constant or only toward the end of the day with fatigue? Prior optic neuritis, urinary incontinence, numbness or paralysis of an extremity, or another unexplained neurologic event (MS)?

2. Complete evaluation of eye movement to rule out other eye movement disorders (e.g., sixth nerve palsy, skew deviation).

NOTE: Ocular motility can appear to be full, but a muscular weakness can be detected by observing slower saccadic eye movement in the involved eye compared with the contralateral eye. The adducting saccade is assessed by having the patient fix on the examiner's finger held laterally and then asking the patient to make a rapid eye movement from lateral to primary gaze. If an INO is present, the involved eye will show a slower adducting saccade than the uninvolved eye. The contralateral eye may be tested in a similar fashion.

---

3. Edrophonium chloride test, ice-pack test, or rest test when the diagnosis of myasthenia gravis cannot be ruled out (see 10.11, *Myasthenia Gravis*).

4. MRI of the brainstem and midbrain.

Treatment/Follow-Up

1. If an acute stroke is diagnosed, admit to the hospital for neurologic evaluation and observation.

2. Otherwise, patients are managed by physicians familiar with the underlying disease.

10.14   OPTIC NEURITIS

Symptoms

Loss of vision over hours (rarely) to days (most commonly), with the nadir approximately 1 week after onset. Visual loss may be subtle or profound. Usually unilateral, but may be bilateral. Age typically 18 to 45 years. Orbital pain, especially with eye movement. Acquired loss of color vision. Reduced perception of light intensity. May have other focal neurologic symptoms (e.g., weakness, numbness, tingling in extremities). May have antecedent flulike viral syndrome. Occasionally altered perception of moving objects (Pulfrich phenomenon), or a worsening of symptoms with exercise or increase in body temperature (Uhthoff sign).

Signs

Critical. Relative afferent pupillary defect in unilateral or asymmetric cases; decreased color vision; central, cecocentral, arcuate, or altitudinal visual field defects.

Other. Swollen disc (in one-third of patients) with or without peripapillary flame-shaped hemorrhages (papillitis most commonly seen in children and young adults) or a normal disc (in two-thirds of patients, retrobulbar optic neuritis more common in adults). Posterior vitreous cells possible.

Differential Diagnosis

- Ischemic optic neuropathy: Visual loss is sudden but in up to 35% of patients may progress over 4 weeks. Typically, no pain with ocular motility, though pain may be present in 10% of cases (compared to 90% of patients with optic neuritis). Optic nerve swelling due to nonarteritic ischemic optic neuropathy (NAION) is initially hyperemic and then becomes pale. Optic nerve swelling in GCA is diffuse and chalk white. Patients tend to be older [40 to 60 for NAION and ≥55 in arteritic ischemic optic neuropathy (AION)]. See 10.17, *Arteritic Ischemic Optic Neuropathy (Giant Cell Arteritis)*, and 10.18, *Nonarteritic Ischemic Optic Neuropathy*.

- Acute papilledema: Bilateral disc edema, no decreased color vision, minimal to no decreased visual acuity, no pain with ocular motility, no vitreous cells. See 10.15, *Papilledema*.

- Severe systemic hypertension: Bilateral disc edema, increased blood pressure, flame-shaped retinal hemorrhages, and cotton-wool spots. See 11.10, *Hypertensive Retinopathy*.

- Orbital tumor compressing the optic nerve: Unilateral, often proptosis or restriction of extraocular motility is evident. See 7.4, *Orbital Tumors*.

- Intracranial mass compressing the afferent visual pathway: Normal or pale disc, afferent pupillary defect, decreased color vision, mass evident on CT scan or MRI of the brain.

- Leber hereditary optic neuropathy: Usually occurs in men in the second or third decade of life. Patients may have a family history and present with rapid visual loss of one and then the other eye within days to months. Early examination of the disc may reveal peripapillary telangiectases followed by optic atrophy. See 10.20, *Miscellaneous Optic Neuropathies*.

- Toxic or metabolic optic neuropathy: Progressive painless bilateral visual loss, may be secondary to alcohol, malnutrition, various toxins (e.g., ethambutol, chloroquine, isoniazid, chlorpropamide, heavy metals), anemia, and others. See 10.20, *Miscellaneous Optic Neuropathies*.

Etiology

- Idiopathic.

- MS: Frequently optic neuritis is the initial manifestation of MS. In the absence of demyelinating lesions on MRI, certain clinical features make MS unlikely including NLP vision, lack of pain, optic disc edema (particularly if severe), peripapillary hemorrhage, and retinal exudates.

- Childhood infections or vaccinations: Measles, mumps, chickenpox, and others.

- Other viral infections: Mononucleosis, varicella zoster, encephalitis, and others.

- Contiguous inflammation of the meninges, orbit, or sinuses.

- Granulomatous inflammations: Tuberculosis, syphilis, sarcoidosis, cryptococcus, and others.

Work-Up

1. For all cases, MRI of the brain and orbits with gadolinium and fat suppression (see Figure 10.14.1).

2. History: Determine the patient's age and rapidity of onset of the visual loss. Previous episode? Pain with eye movement?

10

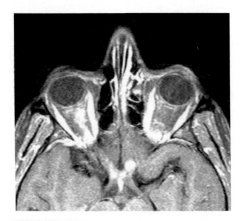

FIGURE 10.14.1. MRI of optic neuritis showing enhancement of the right optic nerve.

3. Complete ophthalmic and neurologic examinations, including pupillary assessment, color vision evaluation, evaluation for vitreous cells, and dilated retinal examination with optic nerve assessment.

4. Check blood pressure.

5. Visual field test, preferably automated (e.g., Humphrey).

6. Consider the following: CBC, RPR, FTA-ABS, Lyme titer, ESR ACE level, and chest X-ray.

Treatment

If patient seen acutely with no prior history of MS or optic neuritis:

1. If MRI reveals at least one typical area of demyelination, offer pulsed intravenous steroid in the following regimen within 14 days of decreased vision:

—Methylprednisolone 1 g/day i.v. for 3 days, then

—Prednisone 1 mg/kg/day p.o. for 11 days, then

—Taper prednisone over 4 days (20 mg on day 1, 10 mg on days 2 and 4).

—Antiulcer medication (e.g., ranitidine 150 mg p.o. b.i.d.) for gastric prophylaxis.

NOTE: The Optic Neuritis Treatment Trial (ONTT) found steroid treatment reduced initial progression to clinically definite multiple sclerosis (CDMS)

for 3 years. Steroid therapy only increases the rapidity of visual return but does not improve final visual outcome.

2. If MRI shows two or more characteristic demyelinating lesions, treat with the aforementioned steroid regimen. Refer to neurologist or neuroophthalmologist for possible treatment with interferon-β-1α, glatiramer acetate, or fingolimod within 28 days. Patients with one or more typical signal changes on MRI have a 72% chance of developing CDMS over 15 years.

NOTE: NEVER use oral prednisone as a primary treatment because of increased risk of recurrence. Interferon β-1α, interferon β-1b, and glatiramer acetate have been shown to reduce probability of progression to CDMS in high-risk patients.

3. With a negative MRI, the risk of MS is low, 25% at 15 years. Pulsed intravenous steroid may still be used to hasten visual recovery, though may be withheld unless the contralateral eye has preexisting visual compromise or the patient requests treatment and understands the risks, benefits, and alternatives. Repeat MRI in 3, 6, 9, and 12 months and then yearly after that.

In a patient with a diagnosis of prior MS or optic neuritis:

1. Observation.

Follow-Up

1. Reexamine the patient approximately 4 to 6 weeks after presentation and then every 3 to 6 months.

2. Patients at high risk for CDMS, including patients with CNS demyelination on MRI or a positive neurologic examination, should be referred to a neurologist or neuroophthalmologist for evaluation and management of possible MS.

Bibliography

Beck RW, Cleary PA, Anderson MM Jr, et al. A randomized, controlled trial of corticosteroids in the treatment of acute optic neuritis. *The Optic Neuritis Study Group. N Engl J Med* 1992;326:581–588.

Beck RW, Cleary PA, Trobe JD, et al. The effect of corticosteroids for acute optic neuritis on the subsequent development of multiple sclerosis. *The Optic Neuritis Study Group. N Engl J Med* 1993;329:1764–1769.

Jacobs LD, Beck RW, Simon JH, et al. Intramuscular interferon beta-1a therapy initiated during a first demyelinating event in multiple sclerosis. *CHAMPS Study Group. N Engl J Med* 2000;343:898–904.

Optic Neuritis Study Group. Multiple sclerosis risk after optic neuritis: final follow-up from the *Optic Neuritis Treatment Trial. Arch Neurol* 2008;65:727–732.

10.15   PAPILLEDEMA

Definition

Optic disc swelling produced by increased intracranial pressure.

Symptoms

Episodes of transient, often bilateral visual loss (lasting seconds), often precipitated after rising from a lying or sitting position (altering intracranial pressure); headache; double vision; nausea; vomiting; and, rarely, a decrease in visual acuity (a mild decrease in visual acuity can occur in the acute setting if associated with a macular disturbance). Visual field defects and severe loss of central visual acuity occur more often with chronic papilledema.

Signs

(See Figure 10.15.1.)

Critical.   Bilaterally swollen, hyperemic discs (in early papilledema, disc swelling may be asymmetric) with nerve fiber layer edema causing blurring of the disc margin, often obscuring the blood vessels.

Other.   Papillary or peripapillary retinal hemorrhages (often flame shaped); loss of venous pulsations (20% of the normal population do not have venous pulsations); dilated, tortuous retinal veins; normal pupillary response and color vision; an enlarged physiologic blind spot or other visual field defects by formal visual field testing.

In chronic papilledema, the hemorrhages and cotton-wool spots resolve, disc hyperemia disappears and the disc becomes gray in color, peripapillary gliosis and narrowing of the peripapillary retinal vessels occur, and optociliary shunt vessels may develop on the disc. Loss of color vision, central visual acuity, and visual field defects, especially inferonasally, also occur.

NOTE: Unilateral or bilateral sixth nerve palsy also may result from increased intracranial pressure.

Differential Diagnosis of Disc Edema or Elevation

■ Pseudopapilledema (e.g., optic disc drusen or congenitally anomalous disc): Not true disc swelling. Vessels overlying the disc are not obscured, the disc is not hyperemic, and the surrounding nerve fiber layer is normal. Spontaneous venous pulsations are often present. Buried drusen may be present and can be identified with B-scan US.

■ Papillitis: An afferent pupillary defect and decreased color vision are present, decreased visual acuity occurs in most

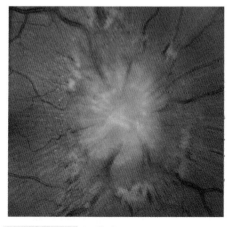

FIGURE 10.15.1. Papilledema.

10

cases, usually unilateral. See 10.14, *Optic Neuritis*.

- Hypertensive optic neuropathy: Extremely high blood pressure, narrowed arterioles, arteriovenous crossing changes, hemorrhages with or without cotton-wool spots extending into the peripheral retina. See 11.10, *Hypertensive Retinopathy*.

- Central retinal vein occlusion: Hemorrhages extend far beyond the peripapillary area, dilated and tortuous veins, generally unilateral, acute loss of vision in most cases. See 11.8, *Central Retinal Vein Occlusion*.

- Ischemic optic neuropathy: Disc swelling is pale but may be hyperemic; initially unilateral unless due to GCA, with sudden visual loss. See 10.17, *Arteritic Ischemic Optic Neuropathy (Giant Cell Arteritis)* and 10.18, *Nonarteritic Ischemic Optic Neuropathy*.

- Infiltration of the optic disc (e.g., sarcoid or tuberculous granuloma, leukemia, metastasis, other inflammatory disease or tumor): Other ocular or systemic abnormalities may be present. Usually unilateral.

- Leber hereditary optic neuropathy: Usually occurs in men in the second or third decade of life. Patients may have a family history and present with rapid visual loss of one and then the other eye within days to months. Early examination of the disc may reveal peripapillary telangiectases followed by optic atrophy. See 10.20, *Miscellaneous Optic Neuropathies*.

- Orbital optic nerve tumors: Unilateral disc swelling, may have proptosis. See 10.20, *Miscellaneous Optic Neuropathies*.

- Diabetic papillopathy: Benign disc edema in one or both eyes of a diabetic patient, most commonly with mild visual loss. No correlation with diabetic retinopathy. In addition to disc edema, disc hyperemia due to telangiectasis of the disc vessels may occur, simulating neovascularization. More common in patients with juvenile-onset diabetes. No treatment is indicated. Spontaneous resolution usually occurs after 3 to 4 months.

- Thyroid-related optic neuropathy: May have eyelid lag or retraction, ocular misalignment, resistance to retropulsion. See 7.2.1, *Thyroid Eye Disease*.

- Uveitis (e.g., syphilis or sarcoidosis): Pain or photophobia, anterior chamber, and vitreous cells. See 12.3, *Posterior Uveitis*.

- Amiodarone toxicity: May present with subacute visual loss and disc edema.

NOTE: Optic disc swelling in a patient with leukemia is often a sign of leukemic optic nerve infiltration. Immediate radiation therapy is usually required to preserve vision.

Etiology

- Primary and metastatic intracranial tumors.

- Hydrocephalus.

- Idiopathic intracranial hypertension: Often occurs in young, overweight females. See 10.16, *Idiopathic Intracranial Hypertension/Pseudotumor Cerebri*.

- Subdural and epidural hematomas.

- Subarachnoid hemorrhage: Severe headache, may have preretinal hemorrhages (Terson syndrome).

- Arteriovenous malformation.

- Brain abscess: Often produces high fever and mental status changes.

- Meningitis: Fever, stiff neck, headache (e.g., syphilis, tuberculosis, Lyme disease, bacterial, inflammatory, neoplastic).

- Encephalitis: Often produces mental status abnormalities.

- Cerebral venous sinus thrombosis.

Work-Up

1. History and physical examination, including blood pressure measurement.

2. Ocular examination, including a pupillary and color vision (using color plates) assessment, posterior vitreous evaluation for white blood cells, and a dilated fundus examination. The optic disc is best examined with a

slit lamp and a Hruby, fundus contact, or 60-diopter lens.

3. Emergency MRI with gadolinium and magnetic resonance venography (MRV) of the head are preferred. CT scan (axial and coronal views) may be done if MRI not available emergently.

4. LP with CSF analysis and opening pressure measurement if the CT or MRI/MRV do not reveal a mass lesion or hydrocephalus.

Treatment

Treatment should be directed at the underlying cause of the increased intracranial pressure.

10.16 IDIOPATHIC INTRACRANIAL HYPERTENSION/PSEUDOTUMOR CEREBRI

Definition

A syndrome in which patients present with symptoms and signs of elevated intracranial pressure, the nature of which may be either idiopathic or due to various causative factors.

Symptoms

Headache, transient episodes of visual loss (typically lasting seconds) often precipitated by changes in posture, double vision, pulsatile tinnitus, nausea, or vomiting accompanying the headache. Occurs predominantly in obese women.

Signs

Critical. By definition, the following findings are present:

- Papilledema due to increased intracranial pressure.

- Negative MRI/MRV of the brain.

- Increased opening pressure on LP with normal CSF composition.

Other. See 10.15, *Papilledema.* Unilateral or bilateral sixth nerve palsy may be present. There are no signs on neurologic examination besides possible sixth nerve palsy.

Differential Diagnosis

See 10.15, *Papilledema.*

Associated Factors

Obesity, significant weight gain, and pregnancy are often associated with the idiopathic form. Possible causative factors include various medications, including oral contraceptives, tetracyclines (including semisynthetics, e.g., minocycline), nalidixic acid, cyclosporine, and vitamin A (>100,000 U/day). Systemic steroid withdrawal may also be causative.

Work-Up

1. History: Inquire specifically about medications.

2. Ocular examination, including pupillary examination, ocular motility, color vision testing (color plates), and optic nerve evaluation.

3. Systemic examination, including blood pressure and temperature.

4. MRI/MRV of the orbit and brain. Any patient with papilledema needs to be imaged immediately. If normal, the patient should have an LP, to rule out other causes of optic nerve edema and to determine the opening pressure (see 10.15, *Papilledema*).

5. Visual field test is the most important method for following these patients (e.g., Humphrey).

Treatment

Idiopathic intracranial hypertension may be a self-limited process. Treatment is indicated in the following situations:

- Severe, intractable headache.

- Evidence of progressive decrease in visual acuity or visual field loss.

- Some ophthalmologists suggest treating all patients with papilledema.

10

Methods of treatment include the following:

1. Weight loss if overweight.

2. Acetazolamide 250 mg p.o. q.i.d. initially, building up to 500 mg q.i.d. if tolerated. Use with caution in sulfa-allergic patients.

3. Discontinuation of any causative medication.

If treatment by these methods is unsuccessful, one of the following may be tried:

4. A short course of systemic steroids in preparation for surgery.

5. Optic nerve sheath decompression surgery is often effective if vision is threatened and has been reported to improve headache in approximately 50% of patients.

6. A neurosurgical shunt (ventriculoperitoneal or lumboperitoneal) should be performed if intractable headache is a prominent symptom.

Special Circumstances

1. Pregnancy: Incidence of idiopathic intracranial hypertension does not increase during pregnancy beyond what would be expected from the weight gain. No increased risk of fetal loss. Acetazolamide may be used after 20 weeks gestation (in consultation with OB/GYN). Intense weight loss is contraindicated during pregnancy. Without visual compromise, close observation with serial visual fields is recommended. With visual compromise, consider steroids, optic nerve sheath decompression, shunting, or repeat LPs.

2. Children/adolescents: A secondary cause is identifiable in 50%.

Follow-Up

1. If acute, patients can be monitored every 3 months in the absence of visual field loss. If chronic, initially follow patient every 3 to 4 weeks to monitor visual acuity and visual fields, and then every 3 months, depending on the response to treatment.

2. In general, the frequency of follow-up depends on the severity of visual loss. The more severe, the more frequent the follow-up.

10.17 ARTERITIC ISCHEMIC OPTIC NEUROPATHY (GIANT CELL ARTERITIS)

Symptoms

Sudden, painless visual loss; initially unilateral, but may rapidly become bilateral; occurs in patients ≥55 years of age; antecedent or simultaneous headache, jaw claudication (pain with chewing), scalp tenderness especially over the superficial temporal arteries (tenderness with hair combing), proximal muscle and joint aches (polymyalgia rheumatica), anorexia, weight loss, or fever may occur.

Signs

(See Figure 10.17.1.)

Critical. Afferent pupillary defect; visual loss (often counting fingers or worse); pale, swollen disc, at times with flame-shaped hemorrhages. Later, optic atrophy and cupping occurs as the edema resolves. The ESR, CRP, and platelets may be markedly increased.

Other. Visual field defect (commonly altitudinal or involving the central field); a palpable, tender, and often nonpulsatile temporal artery; a central retinal artery occlusion or a cranial nerve palsy (especially a sixth nerve palsy) may occur.

Differential Diagnosis

■ NAION: Patients may be younger. Visual loss often less severe, do not have the accompanying symptoms of GCA listed previously, and usually have a normal ESR. See 10.18, *Nonarteritic Ischemic Optic Neuropathy.*

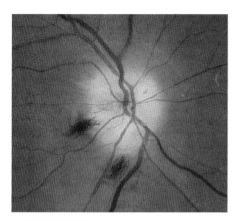

FIGURE 10.17.1. Giant cell arteritis.

- Inflammatory optic neuritis: Younger age group. Pain with eye movements. Optic disc swelling, if present, is more hyperemic. See 10.14, *Optic Neuritis*.

- Compressive optic nerve tumor: Slowly progressive visual loss, few to no symptoms in common with GCA. See 10.20, *Miscellaneous Optic Neuropathies*.

- Central retinal vein occlusion: Severe visual loss may be accompanied by an afferent pupillary defect and disc swelling, but the retina shows diffuse retinal hemorrhages extending out to the periphery. See 11.8, *Central Retinal Vein Occlusion*.

- Central retinal artery occlusion: Sudden, painless, severe visual loss with an afferent pupillary defect. No disc swelling. Retinal edema with a cherry-red spot frequently observed. See 11.6, *Central Retinal Artery Occlusion*.

Work-Up

1. History: GCA symptoms present? Age is critical.

2. Complete ocular examination, particularly pupillary assessment, color plates, dilated retinal examination to rule out retinal causes of severe visual loss, and optic nerve evaluation.

3. Immediate ESR (Westergren is the most reliable method), CRP (does not rise with age), and platelets (may have thrombocytosis). A guideline for top-normal ESR: men, age/2; women, (age + 10)/2. ESR may not be increased. CRP and platelet upper limit values based on laboratory-specific standards.

4. Perform a temporal artery biopsy if GCA is suspected.

NOTE: The biopsy should be performed within 1 week after starting systemic steroids, but a positive result may be seen up to 1 month later. Biopsy is especially important in patients in whom steroids are relatively contraindicated (e.g., diabetics).

Treatment

1. Systemic steroids should be given immediately once GCA is suspected. Methylprednisolone 250 mg i.v., q6h for 12 doses, and then switch to prednisone 80 to 100 mg p.o. q.d. A temporal artery biopsy specimen is obtained while the patient is in the hospital.

2. If the temporal artery biopsy is positive for GCA, the patient must be maintained on prednisone, about 1 mg/kg initially.

3. If the biopsy is negative on an adequate (2-3 cm) section, the likelihood of GCA is small. However, in highly suggestive cases, biopsy of the contralateral artery is performed.

4. Steroids are usually discontinued if the disease is not found in adequate biopsy specimens, unless the clinical presentation is classic and a response to treatment has occurred.

NOTE:

1. Without steroids (and occasionally on adequate steroids), the contralateral eye can become involved within 1 to 7 days

2. A histamine type 2 receptor blocker (e.g., ranitidine 150 mg p.o. b.i.d.) or another anti-ulcer medication should be used for prophylaxis while on steroids.

3. A medication to help prevent osteoporosis should be used as directed by an internist, particularly given the long-term need for steroids.

10

Follow-Up

1. Patients suspected of having GCA must be evaluated and treated immediately.

2. After the diagnosis is confirmed by biopsy, the initial oral steroid dosage is maintained until the symptoms resolve and ESR normalizes. The dosage is then tapered slowly, repeating the ESR with each dosage change or monthly to ensure that the new steroid dosage is enough to suppress the disease.

3. If the ESR increases or symptoms return, the dosage must be increased.

4. Treatment should last at least 6 to 12 months or more. The smallest dose that suppresses the disease is used.

10.18 NONARTERITIC ISCHEMIC OPTIC NEUROPATHY

Symptoms

Sudden, painless visual loss of moderate degree, initially unilateral, but may become bilateral. Typically occurs in patients 40 to 60 years of age. But well-documented cases have been reported in patients in their teenage years. In younger patients, NAION should be suspected when painless visual loss develops with a contralateral anomalous disc and normal MRI scan. The visual deficit may improve. Hyperlipidemia, labile hypertension, and sleep apnea are the common risk factors for younger patients.

Signs

(See Figure 10.18.1.)

Critical. Afferent pupillary defect, pale disc swelling (often segmental), flame-shaped hemorrhages, normal ESR.

- Nonprogressive NAION: Sudden initial decrease in visual acuity and visual field, which stabilizes.

- Progressive NAION: Sudden initial decrease in visual acuity and visual field followed by worsening in vision up to 3 to 4 weeks in acuity or visual field days to weeks later. As many as 35% of NAION cases may be progressive.

Other. Reduced color vision, altitudinal or central visual field defect, optic atrophy without cupping (segmental or diffuse) after the edema resolves. Congenitally anomalous disc in fellow eye.

Differential Diagnosis

See 10.17, *Arteritic Ischemic Optic Neuropathy (Giant Cell Arteritis).*

Etiology

Idiopathic: Arteriosclerosis, diabetes, hypertension, hyperlipidemia, hyperhomocysteinemia, anemia, and sleep apnea are associated risk factors, but causation has never been proven. Relative nocturnal hypotension may play a role, especially in patients taking antihypertensive medication. Nocturnal hypotension may be related to sleep apnea.

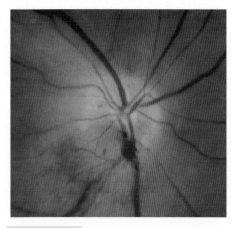

FIGURE 10.18.1. Nonarteritic ischemic optic neuropathy with segmental disc edema and hemorrhage.

10

NOTE: Erectile dysfunction medications have been implicated in a clinical picture that looks like NAION. Currently, there is no proven causation.

Work-Up

1. Same as 10.17, *Arteritic Ischemic Optic Neuropathy (Giant Cell Arteritis)*.

2. Consult internist to rule out cardiovascular disease, diabetes, and hypertension.

Treatment

1. Observation.

2. Cardiovascular risk factor modification.

3. Consider avoiding blood pressure medication at bedtime to help avoid nocturnal hypotension.

Follow-Up

1. One month.

2. Up to 40% of patients show mild improvement in vision over 3 to 6 months in some studies. Optic nerve edema resolves within 8 weeks.

10.19 POSTERIOR ISCHEMIC OPTIC NEUROPATHY

Symptoms

Painless visual loss. Most commonly occurs in the postoperative setting at any time from upon awakening from anesthesia to 4 to 7 days thereafter. May be unilateral or bilateral, with a partial or complete deficit.

Signs

See 10.18, *Nonarteritic Ischemic Optic Neuropathy*. Optic discs may appear normal initially in acute posterior ischemic optic neuropathy, but eventually pale disc edema, followed by pallor, develops.

Etiology

- Postoperative: May occur after head and neck surgery, spinal surgery, gastrointestinal surgery, open heart surgery, or any procedure in which hypotension, anemia, positioning of head in dependent, down-tilt position, increased surgical time, large amounts of blood loss, or increased central venous pressure occur. History of peripheral vascular disease, diabetes, and anemia may increase risk.

NOTE: Operative planning in high-risk patients should include: attention to head positioning and length of surgical time, balance of risk and benefits of hypotensive anesthesia, aggressive replacement of blood loss, monitoring vision early in the postoperative period, and prompt ophthalmic consultation if patient describes visual disturbances.

- Inflammatory/infectious: GCA, varicella zoster, systemic lupus erythematosus, and others.

Treatment

1. Although no controlled studies exist for postoperative posterior ischemic optic neuropathy, it has been suggested that prompt blood transfusion with correction of hypotension and anemia may be beneficial and should be considered.

2. Treat any inflammatory or infectious etiology as appropriate.

10

10.20   MISCELLANEOUS OPTIC NEUROPATHIES

TOXIC/METABOLIC OPTIC NEUROPATHY

Symptoms

Painless, progressive, bilateral loss of vision.

Signs

Critical.   Bilateral cecocentral or central visual field defects, signs of alcoholism, tobacco use, or poor nutrition.

Other.   Visual acuity of 20/50 to 20/200, reduced color vision, temporal disc pallor, optic atrophy, or normal-appearing disc initially.

Etiology

- Tobacco/alcohol abuse.

- Severe malnutrition with thiamine (vitamin B1) deficiency.

- Pernicious anemia: Usually due to vitamin B12 malabsorption.

- Toxic: Chloramphenicol, ethambutol, isoniazid, digitalis, streptomycin, chlorpropamide, ethchlorvynol, disulfiram, and lead.

Work-Up

1. History: Drug or substance abuse? Medications? Diet?

2. Complete ocular examination, including pupillary evaluation, color testing with color plates, and optic nerve examination.

3. Formal visual field test.

4. CBC.

5. Serum vitamin B1, B12, and folate levels.

6. Consider a heavy metal (e.g., lead, thallium) screen.

7. If disc is swollen, consider blood test for Leber hereditary optic neuropathy.

Treatment

1. Thiamine 100 mg p.o. b.i.d.

2. Folate 1.0 mg p.o. q.d.

3. Multivitamin tablet q.d.

4. Eliminate any causative agent (e.g., alcohol, medication).

5. Coordinated care with an internist, including vitamin B12 1,000 mg intramuscularly every month for pernicious anemia.

Follow-Up

Every month at first and then every 6 to 12 months.

COMPRESSIVE OPTIC NEUROPATHY

Symptoms

Slowly progressive visual loss, although occasionally acute or noticed acutely.

Signs

Critical.   Central visual field defect, relative afferent pupillary defect.

Other.   The optic nerve can be normal, pale, or, occasionally, swollen; proptosis; optociliary shunt vessels. Collateral vessels occur only with intrinsic lesions of the nerve (never with extrinsic lesions).

Etiology

- Optic nerve glioma: Age usually <20 years, often associated with neurofibromatosis.

- Optic nerve meningioma: Usually adult women. Orbital imaging may show an optic nerve mass, diffuse optic nerve thickening, or a railroad-track sign (increased contrast of the periphery of the nerve).

- Any intraorbital mass (e.g., hemangioma, schwannoma).

Work-Up

All patients with progressive visual loss and optic nerve dysfunction should have an MRI of the orbit and brain.

Treatment

1. Depends on the etiology.

2. Treatment for optic nerve glioma is controversial. These lesions are often monitored

unless there is evidence of intracranial involvement, at which point surgical excision may be indicated. Most of these patients are young children, who are very susceptible to cognitive complications of radiotherapy. Chemotherapy may be considered if there is progressive visual loss.

3. For optic nerve sheath meningiomas, conventional fractionated stereotactic radiotherapy treatment should be considered. Serial MRI and functional (111) In-octreotide single-photon emission CT scintigraphy may be used to monitor tumor control.

LEBER HEREDITARY OPTIC NEUROPATHY

Symptoms

Painless progressive visual loss in one and then the other eye within days to months of each other. Visual loss is bilateral at onset in approximately 25% of cases.

Signs

Critical. Mild swelling of optic disc progressing over weeks to optic atrophy; small, telangiectatic blood vessels near the disc that do not leak on intravenous fluorescein angiography (IVFA) are present acutely; usually occurs in young men aged 15 to 30 years, and less commonly in women in their second to third decade of life.

Other. Visual acuity 20/200 to counting fingers, cecocentral visual field defect.

Transmission

By mitochondrial DNA (transmitted by mothers to all offspring). However, 50% to 70% of sons and 10% to 15% of daughters manifest the disease. All daughters are carriers, and none of the sons can transmit the disease.

Work-Up

Genetic testing is available for the most frequent base-pair nucleotide substitutions at positions 11778, 3460, and 14484 in the mitochondrial gene for the NADH dehydrogenase protein.

Treatment

1. No effective treatment is available. Tobacco and alcohol avoidance are recommended.

2. Genetic counseling should be offered.

3. Consider cardiology consult because of increased incidence of cardiac conduction defects.

DOMINANT OPTIC ATROPHY

Mild-to-moderate bilateral visual loss (20/40 to 20/200) usually presenting at approximately age 4. Slow progression, temporal disc pallor, cecocentral visual field defect, tritanopic (blue-yellow) color defect on Farnsworth–Munsell 100-hue test, strong family history, no nystagmus.

COMPLICATED HEREDITARY OPTIC ATROPHY

Bilateral optic atrophy with spinocerebellar degenerations (e.g., Friedreich, Marie, Behr), polyneuropathy (e.g., Charcot–Marie–Tooth), or inborn errors of metabolism.

10

RADIATION OPTIC NEUROPATHY

Delayed effect (usually 1 to 5 years) after radiation therapy to the eye, orbit, sinus, nasopharynx, and occasionally brain with acute or gradual stepwise visual loss, often severe. Disc swelling, radiation retinopathy, or both may be present. Enhancement of optic nerve or chiasm on MRI.

10.21   NYSTAGMUS

Nystagmus is divided into congenital and acquired forms.

Symptoms

Congenital and acquired nystagmus may be symptomatic with decreased visual acuity. The environment may be noted to oscillate horizontally, vertically, or torsionally in cases of acquired nystagmus, but only rarely in congenital cases.

Signs

Critical. Repetitive oscillations of the eye horizontally, vertically, or torsionally.

- Jerk nystagmus: The eye repetitively slowly drifts in one direction (slow phase) and then rapidly returns to its original position (fast phase).

- Pendular nystagmus: Drift occurs in two phases of equal speed, giving a smooth back-and-forth movement of the eye.

CONGENITAL FORMS OF NYSTAGMUS

Infantile Nystagmus

Onset by age 2 to 3 months with wide, swinging eye movements. At age 4 to 6 months, small pendular eye movements are added. At age 6 to 12 months, jerk nystagmus and a null point (a position of gaze where the nystagmus is minimized) develop. Compensatory head positioning may develop at any point up to 20 years of age. Infantile nystagmus is usually horizontal and uniplanar (same direction in all gazes), and typically dampens with convergence. May have a latent component (worsens when one eye is occluded).

Differential Diagnosis

- Opsoclonus/saccadomania: Repetitive, conjugate, multidirectional eye movements associated with cerebellar or brainstem disease, postviral encephalitis, visceral carcinoma, or neuroblastoma.

- Spasmus nutans: Head nodding and head turn with vertical, horizontal, or torsional nystagmus appearing between 6 months and 3 years of age and resolving between 2 and 8 years of age. Unilateral, bilateral (but asymmetric), or alternating. Spasmus nutans is a benign condition; however, gliomas of the anterior visual pathway may produce an identical clinical picture and need to be ruled out with MRI.

- Latent nystagmus (see below).

- Nystagmus Blockage Syndrome (see below).

Etiology

- Idiopathic.

- Albinism: Iris transillumination defects and foveal hypoplasia. See 13.8, *Albinism.*

- Aniridia: Bilateral, near-total congenital iris absence. See 8.12, *Developmental Anterior Segment and Lens Anomalies/Dysgenesis.*

- Leber congenital amaurosis: Markedly abnormal or flat electroretinogram (ERG).

- Others: Bilateral optic nerve hypoplasia, bilateral congenital cataracts, rod monochromatism, or optic nerve or macular disease.

Work-Up

1. History: Age of onset? Head nodding or head positioning? Known ocular or systemic abnormalities? Medications? Family history?

2. Complete ocular examination: Observe the head position and eye movements, check iris transillumination, and carefully inspect the optic disc and macula.

3. Consider obtaining an eye movement recording if the diagnosis is uncertain.

4. If opsoclonus is present, obtain a urinary vanillylmandelic acid and an abdominal and chest CT scan to rule out neuroblastoma and visceral carcinoma.

5. In selected cases and in all cases of suspected spasmus nutans, obtain an MRI of the brain (axial and coronal views) to rule out an anterior optic pathway lesion.

Treatment

1. Maximize vision by refraction.

2. Treat amblyopia if indicated.

3. If small face turn: Prescribe prism in glasses with base in direction of face turn.

4. If large face turn: Consider muscle surgery.

Latent Nystagmus

Occurs only when one eye is viewing. Conjugate horizontal nystagmus with fast phase beating toward viewing eye.

Manifest latent nystagmus occurs in children with strabismus or decreased vision in one eye, in whom the nonfixating or poorly seeing eye behaves as an occluded eye.

NOTE: When testing visual acuity in one eye, fog (e.g., add plus lenses in front of) rather than occluding the opposite eye to minimize induction of latent nystagmus.

Treatment

1. Maximize vision by refraction.

2. Treat amblyopia if indicated.

3. Consider muscle surgery if symptomatic strabismus or cosmetically significant head turn exists.

Nystagmus Blockage Syndrome

Any nystagmus that decreases when the fixating eye is in adduction and demonstrates an esotropia to dampen the nystagmus.

Treatment

For large face turn, consider muscle surgery.

ACQUIRED FORMS OF NYSTAGMUS

Etiology

- Visual loss (e.g., dense cataract, trauma, cone dystrophy): Usually monocular and vertical nystagmus (Heimann–Bielschowsky phenomenon).

- Toxic/metabolic: Alcohol intoxication, lithium, barbiturates, phenytoin, salicylates, benzodiazepines, phencyclidine, other anticonvulsants or sedatives, Wernicke encephalopathy, thiamine deficiency.

- CNS disorders: Thalamic hemorrhage, tumor, stroke, trauma, MS, and others.

- Nonphysiologic: Voluntary, rapid, horizontal, small oscillatory movements of the eyes that usually cannot be sustained >30 seconds without fatigue.

Nystagmus with Localizing Neuroanatomic Significance

- See-saw: One eye rises and intorts while the other descends and extorts. Lesion typically involves the parasellar region and chiasm. Typically pendular when chiasmal region involved, and jerk if involving the midbrain. One proposal suggests a unilateral lesion of the interstitial nucleus of Cajal or its connections are responsible for this nystagmus subtype. May have a bitemporal hemianopia resulting from chiasmal compression. May be congenital or associated with septo-optic dysplasia.

- Convergence retraction: Convergence-like eye movements accompanied by globe retraction when the patient attempts an upward saccade. May be associated with limitation of upward gaze, eyelid retraction, and bilateral mid-dilated pupils that react poorly to light but constrict better with convergence. Papilledema may be present. Usually, a pineal region tumor or other dorsal midbrain abnormality is responsible. See 10.4, *Adie (Tonic) Pupil*.

- Upbeat: The fast phase of the nystagmus is up. If present in primary gaze, the lesion typically involves the brainstem or anterior vermis of the cerebellum. If present only in upgaze, the most likely etiology is drug effect.

- Gaze evoked: Absent in primary gaze, but appears as the eyes look to the side. Nystagmus increases when looking in the direction of fast phase. Slow frequency. Most commonly the result of alcohol intoxication, sedatives, cerebellar or brainstem disease.

10

- Downbeat: The fast phase of nystagmus is down and most prominent looking down and to the right and left. Most commonly, the lesion is at the cervicomedullary junction (e.g., Arnold–Chiari malformation) or a manifestation of cerebellar degeneration.

- Periodic alternating: In primary position, fast eye movements are in one direction for 60 to 90 seconds and then reverse direction for 60 to 90 seconds. The cycle repeats continuously. Patients may attempt to minimize nystagmus with periodic head turning. May be congenital. Acquired forms are most commonly the result of lesions of the cervicomedullary junction and posterior fossa. Other causes include MS, medication side effects, and rarely blindness.

- Peripheral vestibular: Horizontal or horizontal rotary nystagmus. May be accompanied by vertigo, tinnitus, or deafness. May be due to dysfunction of vestibular end organ (inner ear disease), eighth cranial nerve, or eighth nerve nucleus in brainstem. Destructive lesions produce fast phases opposite to lesion. Irritative lesions (e.g., Meniere disease) produce fast phase in the same direction as the lesion. Vestibular nystagmus associated with interstitial keratitis is called Cogan syndrome.

- Spasmus nutans: See above.

- Others: Rebound nystagmus (cerebellar lesions), Bruns nystagmus (cerebellopontine angle), oculomasticatory myorhythmia (Whipple disease), oculopalatal myoclonus (prior brainstem stroke).

Differential Diagnosis

- Superior oblique myokymia: Small, unilateral, vertical, and torsional movements of one eye can be seen with a slit lamp or ophthalmoscope. Patients complain of unilateral oscillopsia. Symptoms and signs are more pronounced when the involved eye looks inferonasally. Usually benign, resolving spontaneously, but rarely due to a mass lesion so consider neuroimaging. Consider carbamazepine 200 mg p.o. t.i.d. Consult internist for hematologic evaluation before carbamazepine use and periodic evaluation during therapy.

- Opsoclonus/saccadomania: Rapid, chaotic conjugate saccades. Etiology in children is a paraneoplastic effect of neuroblastoma or encephalitis. In adults, in addition to paraneoplastic or infectious, it can be seen with drug intoxication or following infarction.

Work-Up

1. History: Nystagmus, strabismus, or amblyopia in infancy? Oscillopsia? Drug or alcohol use? Vertigo? Episodes of weakness, numbness, or decreased vision in the past? MS?

2. Family history: Nystagmus? Albinism? Eye disorder?

3. Complete ocular examination: Careful motility examination. Slit-lamp or optic disc observation may be helpful in subtle cases. Iris transillumination should be performed to rule out albinism.

4. Obtain an eye movement recording if diagnosis unclear.

5. Visual field examination, particularly with see-saw nystagmus.

6. Consider a drug/toxin/nutritional screen of the urine, serum, or both.

7. CT scan or MRI as needed with careful attention to appropriate area of interest.

NOTE: The cervicomedullary junction and cerebellum are best evaluated with sagittal MRI.

Treatment

1. The underlying etiology must be treated.

2. The nystagmus of periodic alternating nystagmus may respond to baclofen. Baclofen is not recommended for pediatric use.

3. Although controversial, severe, disabling nystagmus can be treated with retrobulbar injections of botulinum toxin.

Follow-Up

Appropriate follow-up time is dictated by the condition responsible for the nystagmus.

10.22 TRANSIENT VISUAL LOSS/AMAUROSIS FUGAX

Symptoms

Monocular visual loss that usually lasts seconds to minutes, but may last up to 1 to 2 hours. Vision returns to normal.

Signs

Critical. May see an embolus within an arteriole or the ocular examination may be normal.

Other. Signs of ocular ischemic syndrome (see 11.11, *Ocular Ischemic Syndrome/Carotid Occlusive Disease*), an old branch retinal artery occlusion (sheathed arteriole), or neurologic signs caused by cerebral ischemia [transient ischemic attacks (TIAs); e.g., contralateral arm or leg weakness].

Differential Diagnosis of Transient Visual Loss

- Papilledema: Optic disc swelling is evident. Visual loss lasts seconds, is usually bilateral, and is often associated with postural change or Valsalva maneuver. See 10.15, *Papilledema.*

- GCA: ESR, CRP, and platelets typically elevated. GCA symptoms often present. Transient visual loss may precede an ischemic optic neuropathy or central retinal artery occlusion. See 10.17, *Arteritic Ischemic Optic Neuropathy (Giant Cell Arteritis).*

- Impending central retinal vein occlusion: Dilated, tortuous retinal veins are observed, though the fundus may be normal. See 11.8, *Central Retinal Vein Occlusion.*

- Migraine with aura: Visual loss/disturbance from 10 to 50 minutes, often with history of migraine headache or carsickness, or a family history of migraine. See 10.27, *Migraine.*

- Acephalgic migraine: Visual aura without migraine headache. Usually a diagnosis of exclusion. Typically occurs in patients <40 years of age. May have recurrent episodes. See 10.27, *Migraine.*

- Vertebrobasilar artery insufficiency: Transient (lasts seconds), bilateral blurred vision. Associated with vertigo, dysarthria or dysphasia, perioral numbness, and hemiparesis or hemisensory loss. History of drop attacks. See 10.23, *Vertebrobasilar Artery Insufficiency.*

- Basilar artery migraine: Mimics vertebrobasilar artery insufficiency. Bilateral blurring or blindness, vertigo, gait disturbances, formed hallucinations, and dysarthria in a patient with migraine. See 10.27, *Migraine,* and 10.23, *Vertebrobasilar Artery Insufficiency.*

- Vertebral artery dissection: After trauma or resulting from atherosclerotic disease.

- Intermittent intraocular hemorrhage (e.g., vitreous hemorrhage, UGH syndrome).

- Others: Optic nerve head drusen, intermittent angle closure, intermittent pigment dispersion.

Etiology

- Embolus from the carotid artery (most common), heart, or aorta.

- Vascular insufficiency as a result of arteriosclerotic disease of vessels anywhere along the path from the aorta to the globe causing hypoperfusion precipitated by a postural change or cardiac arrhythmia.

- Hypercoagulable/hyperviscosity state.

- Rarely, an intraorbital mass may compress the optic nerve or a nourishing vessel in certain gaze positions, causing gaze-evoked transient visual loss.

- Vasospasm.

Work-Up

1. Immediate ESR, CRP, and platelet count when GCA is suspected.

2. History: Monocular visual loss or homonymous hemianopsia (verified by covering each eye)? Duration of visual loss? Previous episodes of transient visual loss or TIA? Cardiovascular disease risk factors? Oral contraceptive use? Smoker? Vascular surgeries?

10

3. Ocular examination, including a confrontational visual field examination and a dilated retinal evaluation. Look for an embolus or signs of other aforementioned disorders.

4. Medical examination: cardiac and carotid auscultation.

5. Noninvasive carotid artery evaluation (e.g., duplex Doppler US). Consider orbital color Doppler US which may reveal a retrolaminar central retinal artery stenosis or embolus proximal to the lamina cribrosa. MRA or CTA may also be considered and may be superior to duplex Doppler US but cannot similarly evaluate flow.

6. CBC with differential, fasting blood sugar, glycosylated hemoglobin, and lipid profile (to rule out polycythemia, thrombocytosis, diabetes, and hyperlipidemia).

7. Cardiac evaluation including an echocardiogram.

Treatment

1. Carotid disease.

—Consider aspirin 81 mg or 325 mg p.o. q.d.

—Consult Vascular Surgery in select patients if a surgically accessible, high-grade carotid stenosis is present for consideration of carotid endarterectomy or endovascular stent.

—Control hypertension and diabetes (follow-up with a medical internist).

—Lifestyle modification (e.g., smoking cessation).

2. Cardiac disease.

—Consider aspirin 325 mg p.o. q.d.

—Consider hospitalization and anticoagulation (e.g., heparin therapy) in the presence of a mural thrombus.

—Consider referral to Cardiac Surgery as needed.

—Control arteriosclerotic risk factors (follow-up with medical internist).

3. If carotid and cardiac disease are ruled out, a vasospastic etiology can be considered (extremely rare). Treatment with a calcium channel blocker may be beneficial.

Follow-Up

Patients with recurrent episodes of amaurosis fugax (especially if accompanied by signs of cerebral TIA) require immediate diagnostic and sometimes therapeutic attention.

10

10.23 VERTEBROBASILAR ARTERY INSUFFICIENCY

Symptoms

Transient, bilateral blurred vision usually lasting a few seconds, sometimes accompanied by flashing lights. Ataxia, vertigo, dysarthria or dysphasia, perioral numbness, and hemiparesis or hemisensory loss may accompany the visual symptoms. History of drop attacks (the patient suddenly falls to the ground without warning or loss of consciousness). Recurrent attacks are common.

Signs

May have a hemianopsia, ocular motility deficits, or nystagmus, but often presents with a normal ocular examination.

Differential Diagnosis of Transient Visual Loss

See *Differential Diagnosis* in 10.22, *Transient Visual Loss/Amaurosis Fugax.*

Work-Up

1. History: Associated symptoms of vertebrobasilar insufficiency? History of carsickness or migraine? Symptoms of GCA? Smoker?

2. Dilated fundus examination to rule out retinal emboli or papilledema.

3. Blood pressure in each arm to rule out subclavian steal syndrome.

4. Cardiac auscultation to rule out arrhythmia.

5. Electrocardiography, echocardiography, and Holter monitor for 24 hours to rule out dysrhythmia.

6. Consider noninvasive carotid flow studies.

7. MRA or transcranial/vertebral artery Doppler US to evaluate posterior cerebral blood flow.

8. CBC to rule out anemia and polycythemia, with immediate ESR, CRP, and platelets if GCA is considered.

Treatment

1. Aspirin 81 mg p.o. q.d.

2. Consult internist for hypertension, diabetes, and hyperlipidemia control if present.

3. Lifestyle modification (e.g., smoking cessation).

4. Correct any underlying problem revealed by the work-up.

Follow-Up

One week to check test results.

10.24   CORTICAL BLINDNESS

Symptoms

Bilateral complete or severe loss of vision. Patients may deny they are blind (Anton syndrome) or may perceive moving targets but not stationary ones (Riddoch phenomenon).

Signs

Critical. Markedly decreased vision and visual field in both eyes (sometimes no light perception) with normal pupillary responses.

Etiology

- Most common: Bilateral occipital lobe infarctions.

- Other: Toxic, postpartum (amniotic embolus), posterior reversible encephalopathy syndromes (PRES).

- Rare: Neoplasm (e.g., metastasis, meningioma), incontinentia pigmenti.

Work-Up

1. Test vision at distance (patients with bilateral occipital lobe infarcts may appear completely blind, but actually have a very small residual visual field). Patients will do much worse with near card testing than distance if only a small island remains.

2. Complete ocular and neurologic examinations.

3. MRI of the brain.

4. Rule out nonphysiologic visual loss by appropriate testing (see 10.25, *Nonphysiologic Visual Loss*).

5. Cardiac auscultation and electrocardiography to rule out arrhythmia.

6. Check blood pressure.

7. Consult neurologist or internist for evaluation of stroke risk factors.

Treatment

1. Patients diagnosed with a stroke within 72 hours of symptom onset are admitted to the hospital for neurologic evaluation and observation.

2. If possible, treat the underlying condition.

3. Arrange for services to help the patient function at home and in the environment.

Follow-Up

As per the internist or neurologist.

10

Symptoms

Loss of vision. Malingerers frequently are involved with an insurance claim or are looking for other forms of financial gain. Those with psychogenic visual loss truly believe they have lost vision.

Signs

Critical. No ocular or neuroophthalmic findings that would account for the decreased vision. Normal pupillary light reaction.

Differential Diagnosis

- Amblyopia: Poor vision in one eye since childhood, rarely both eyes. Patient often has strabismus or anisometropia. Vision is no worse than counting fingers, especially in the temporal periphery of an amblyopic eye. See 8.7, *Amblyopia.*

- Cortical blindness: Bilateral complete or severe visual loss with normal pupils. See 10.24, *Cortical Blindness.*

- Retrobulbar optic neuritis: Afferent pupillary defect is present. See 10.14, *Optic Neuritis.*

- Cone–rod dystrophy: Positive family history, decreased color vision, abnormal results on dark adaptation studies and multifocal ERG. See 11.29, *Cone Dystrophies.*

- Chiasmal tumor: Visual loss may precede optic atrophy. Pupils usually react sluggishly to light, and an afferent pupillary defect is usually present. Visual fields are abnormal.

- Cancer- or melanoma-associated retinopathy (CAR or MAR): Immune-mediated attack of photoreceptors. Fundus often appears normal. Abnormal ERG.

Work-Up

The following tests may be used to diagnose a patient with nonphysiologic visual loss (to prove the malingerer or hysteric can see better than he or she admits to seeing).

Two codes are used in the list below:

U: This test may be used in patients feigning unilateral decreased vision;

B: This test may be used in patients feigning bilateral vision loss.

Patients Claiming No Light Perception

Determine whether each pupil reacts to light (U): When only one eye has no light perception, its pupil will not react to light. The pupil should not appear dilated unless the patient has bilateral lack of light perception or third nerve involvement.

Patients Claiming Hand Motion to No Light Perception

1. Test for an afferent pupillary defect (U): A defect should be present in unilateral or asymmetric visual loss to this degree. If not, the diagnosis of nonphysiologic visual loss is made.

2. Mirror test (U or B): If the patient claims unilateral visual loss, cover the better-seeing eye with a patch; with bilateral complaints leave both uncovered. Ask the patient to hold eyes still and slowly tilt a large mirror from side to side in front of the eyes, holding it beyond the patient's range of hand-motion vision. If the eyes move, the patient can see better than hand motion.

3. Optokinetic test (U or B): Patch the uninvolved eye when unilateral visual loss is claimed. Ask the patient to look straight ahead and slowly move an optokinetic tape in front of the eyes (or rotate an optokinetic drum). If nystagmus can be elicited, vision is better than counting fingers.

4. Worth four-dot test (U): Place red-green glasses on patient and quickly turn on four-dot pattern and ask patient how many dots are seen. If the patient closes one eye (cheating), try reversing the glasses and repeating test. If all four dots are seen, vision is better than hand motion.

Patients Claiming 20/40 to 20/400 Vision

1. Visual acuity testing (U or B): Start with the 20/10 line and ask the patient to read it. When the patient claims inability to read it, look amazed and then offer reassurance.

Inform the patient you will go to a larger line and show the 20/15 line. Again, force the patient to work to see this line. Slowly proceed up the chart, asking the patient to read each line as you pass it (including the three or four 20/20 lines). It may help to express disbelief that the patient cannot read such large letters. By the time the 20/30 or 20/40 lines are reached, the patient may in fact read one or two letters correctly. The visual acuity can then be recorded.

2. Fog test (U): Dial the patient's refractive correction into the phoropter. Add +4.00 to the normally seeing eye. Put the patient in the phoropter with both eyes open. Tell the patient to use both eyes to read each line, starting at the 20/15 line and working up the chart slowly, as described previously. Record visual acuity with both eyes open (this should be visual acuity of supposedly poorly seeing eye) and document the vision of the "good eye" through the +4.00 lens to prove the vision obtained was from the "bad eye."

3. Retest visual acuity in the supposedly poorly seeing eye at 10 feet from the chart (U or B): Vision should be twice as good (e.g., a patient with 20/100 vision at 20 feet should read 20/50 at 10 feet). If it is better than expected, record the better vision. If it worse, the patient has nonphysiologic visual loss.

4. Test near vision (U or B): If normal near vision can be documented, nonphysiologic visual loss or myopia has been documented.

5. Visual field testing (U or B): Goldmann visual field tests often reveal inconsistent responses and nonphysiologic field losses.

Children

1. Tell the child that there is an eye abnormality, but the strong drops about to be administered will cure it. Dilate the child's eyes (e.g., tropicamide 1%) and retest the visual acuity in 40 minutes. Children, as well as adults, sometimes need a "way out." Provide a reward (bribe them).

2. Test as described previously.

Treatment

1. Patients must be told the truth regarding the nature of their condition.

2. Patients are usually told that no ocular abnormality can be found that accounts for their decreased vision.

3. Hysterical patients often benefit from being told that their vision can be expected to return to normal by their next visit. Psychiatric referral is sometimes indicated.

Follow-Up

1. If nonphysiologic visual loss is highly suspected but cannot be proven, reexamine in 1 to 2 weeks.

2. Consider obtaining an ERG, visual-evoked response (VER), ocular coherence tomography (OCT), or an MRI of the brain.

3. If functional visual loss can be documented, have the patient return as needed.

NOTE: Always try to determine the patient's actual visual acuity if possible and carefully document your findings. Many patients with nonphysiologic visual loss have an underlying organic component that must be diagnosed and treated.

10

10.26 HEADACHE

Most headaches are not dangerous or ominous; however, they can be symptoms of a life- or vision-threatening problem. Accompanying signs and symptoms that may indicate a life- or vision-threatening headache and some of the specific signs and symptoms of various headaches are listed below.

Warning Symptoms and Signs of a Serious Disorder

■ Scalp tenderness, weight loss, pain with chewing, muscle pains, or malaise in patients at least 55 years of age (GCA).

■ Optic nerve swelling.

- Fever.

- Altered mentation or behavior.

- Stiff neck.

- Decreased vision.

- Neurologic signs.

- Subhyaloid (preretinal) hemorrhages on fundus examination.

Less Alarming but Suggestive Symptoms and Signs

- Onset in a previously headache-free individual.

- A different, more severe headache than the usual headache.

- A headache that is always in the same location.

- A headache that awakens the person from sleep.

- A headache that does not respond to pain medications that previously relieved it.

- Nausea and vomiting, particularly projectile vomiting.

- A headache followed by migraine-like visual symptoms (abnormal time course of events).

Etiology

Life or Vision Threatening

- GCA: Age ≥55 years. May have high ESR, CRP, and platelets. See 10.17, *Arteritic Ischemic Optic Neuropathy (Giant Cell Arteritis)*.

- Acute angle-closure glaucoma: Decreased vision, painful eye, fixed mid-dilated pupil, high intraocular pressure. See 9.4, *Acute Angle-Closure Glaucoma*.

- Ocular ischemic syndrome: Periorbital eye pain. See 11.11, *Ocular Ischemic Syndrome/ Carotid Occlusive Disease*.

- Malignant hypertension: Marked increase of blood pressure, often accompanied by retinal cotton-wool spots, hemorrhages, and, when severe, optic nerve swelling. Headaches typically are occipital in location. See 11.10, *Hypertensive Retinopathy*.

- Increased intracranial pressure: May have papilledema and/or a sixth cranial nerve palsy. Headaches usually worse in the morning and worsened with Valsalva. See 10.15, *Papilledema*.

- Infectious CNS disorder (meningitis or brain abscess): Fever, stiff neck, mental status changes, photophobia, neurologic signs.

- Structural abnormality of the brain (e.g., tumor, aneurysm, arteriovenous malformation): Mental status change, signs of increased intracranial pressure, or neurologic signs during, and often after, the headache episode.

- Subarachnoid hemorrhage: Extremely severe headache, stiff neck, mental status change; rarely, subhyaloid hemorrhages seen on fundus examination, usually from a ruptured aneurysm.

- Epidural or subdural hematoma: Follows head trauma; altered level of consciousness; may produce anisocoria.

Others

- Migraine (see 10.27, *Migraine*).

- Cluster headache (see 10.28, *Cluster Headache*).

- Tension headache.

- Varicella zoster virus: Headache or pain may precede the herpetic vesicles (see 4.16, *Herpes Zoster Ophthalmicus/Varicella Zoster Virus*).

- Sinus disease.

NOTE: A "sinus" headache may be a serious headache in diabetic patients and immunocompromised hosts given the possibility of mucormycosis/zygomycosis. See 10.10, *Cavernous Sinus and Associated Syndromes (Multiple Ocular Motor Nerve Palsies)*.

- Tolosa–Hunt syndrome: See 10.10, *Cavernous Sinus and Associated Syndromes (Multiple Ocular Motor Nerve Palsies)*.

- Cervical spine disease.

- Temporomandibular joint syndrome.

- Dental disease.

- Trigeminal neuralgia (tic douloureux).

- Anterior uveitis: See 12.1, *Anterior Uveitis (Iritis/Iridocyclitis)*.

- After lumbar puncture.

- Paget disease.

- Depression/psychogenic.

- Convergence insufficiency: See 13.4, *Convergence Insufficiency*.

- Accommodative spasm: See 13.5, *Accommodative Spasm*.

Work-Up

1. History: Location, intensity, frequency, possible precipitating factors, and time of day of the headaches? Determine the patient's age of onset, what relieves the headaches, and whether there are any associated signs or symptoms. Specifically ask about concerning symptoms and signs listed above. Also, trauma, medications and birth-control pills, family history of migraine, and motion sickness or cyclic vomiting as a child?

2. Complete ocular examination, including pupillary, motility, and visual field evaluation; intraocular pressure measurement, optic disc and venous pulsation assessment, and a dilated retinal examination. Manifest and cycloplegic refractions may be helpful.

NOTE: The presence of spontaneous venous pulsations indicates normal intracranial pressure at that moment; however, the absence of pulsations has little significance. About 20% of normal individuals do not have spontaneous venous pulsations. If there are spontaneous venous pulsations, at that moment, the intracranial pressure is <220 mm H_2O.

---

3. Neurologic examination (check neck flexibility and other meningeal signs).

4. Palpate the temporal arteries for tenderness, swelling, and hardness. Ask specifically about jaw claudication, scalp tenderness, temporal headaches, and unexpected weight loss. Immediate ESR, CRP, and platelet count when GCA is suspected [see 10.17, *Arteritic Ischemic Optic Neuropathy (Giant Cell Arteritis)*].

5. Temperature and blood pressure.

6. Refer the patient to a neurologist, otolaryngologist, or internist, as indicated.

Treatment/Follow-Up

See individual sections.

10.27   MIGRAINE

Symptoms

Typically unilateral (although it may occur behind both eyes or across the entire front of the head), throbbing or boring head pain accompanied at times by nausea, vomiting, mood changes, fatigue, or photophobia. An aura with visual disturbances, including flashing (zig-zagging) lights, blurred vision, or a visual field defect lasting 15 to 50 minutes, may precede the migraine. May experience temporary or permanent neurologic deficits, such as paralysis, numbness, tingling, or others. A family history is common. Motion sickness or cyclic vomiting as a child is also common. Migraine in children may be seen as recurrent abdominal pain and malaise. Of these patients, 60% to 70% are girls.

Migraine prevalence is highest between ages 30 and 39 years and progressively declines after age 40. Migraine attacks may be shorter and less typical with advancing age. New onset migraines are uncommon after the age of 50, and these patients should be worked up for secondary causes such as vascular lesions, intracranial hemorrhages, infarcts, masses, or GCA.

NOTE: Most unilateral migraine headaches at some point change sides of the head. Headaches always on the same side of the head may have another cause of headache (e.g., intracranial structural lesions).

Determine if headache precedes visual symptoms, which is more common with arteriovenous malformations, mass lesions with cerebral edema, or seizure foci.

Signs

Usually none. Complicated migraines may have a permanent neurologic or ocular deficit (see the following discussion).

Differential Diagnosis

See 10.26, *Headache.*

International Classification

Consult International Classification of Headache Disorders, 2nd edition, for further information.

1. Migraine without aura (common migraine; 80%): Lasts 4 to 72 hours. Unilateral location, pulsating quality, moderate-to-severe pain, and/or aggravation by physical activity. Nausea, vomiting, photophobia, and phonophobia.

2. Migraine with typical aura (classic migraine; 10%): Fully reversible binocular visual symptoms that may be perceived as monocular (e.g., flickering lights, spots, lines, loss of vision) or fully reversible unilateral sensory symptoms (e.g., numbness, "pins and needles"). Symptoms gradually develop over 5 minutes and last between 5 and 60 minutes. No motor symptoms are present.

3. Typical aura without headache (acephalgic migraine): Visual or sensory symptoms as above without accompanying or subsequent headache.

4. Familial hemiplegic and sporadic hemiplegic migraine: Migraine with aura as above with accompanying motor weakness with (familial) or without (sporadic) history in a first- or second-degree relative. Sporadic cases always require neuroimaging.

5. Retinal migraine: Fully reversible monocular visual phenomenon (e.g., scintillations, scotoma, blindness) accompanied by headache fulfilling migraine definition.

Appropriate investigations to exclude other causes of transient monocular blindness should be completed.

6. Basilar-type migraine: Aura symptoms mimic vertebrobasilar artery insufficiency in a patient with migraine. See 10.23, *Vertebrobasilar Artery Insufficiency.*

7. Ophthalmoplegic migraine: Onset in childhood. May develop a third cranial nerve palsy.

Associations or Precipitating Factors

Birth control or other hormonal pills, puberty, pregnancy, menopause, foods containing tyramine or phenylalanine (e.g., aged cheeses, wines, chocolate, cashew nuts), nitrates or nitrites, monosodium glutamate, alcohol, fatigue, emotional stress, or bright lights.

Work-Up

See 10.26, *Headache,* for a general headache work-up.

1. History: May establish the diagnosis.

2. Ocular and neurologic examinations, including refraction.

3. CT scan or MRI of the head is indicated for:

   —Atypical migraines: Migraines that are always on the same side of the head, those with an unusual sequence, such as visual disturbances persisting into or occurring after the headache phase.

   —Complicated migraines.

4. Consider checking for uncontrolled blood pressure or low blood sugar (hypoglycemic headaches are almost always precipitated by stress or fatigue).

Treatment

1. Avoid agents that precipitate the headaches (e.g., stop using birth control pills; avoid alcohol and any foods that may precipitate attacks; reduce stress).

2. Referral to neurologist or internist for pharmacologic management.

   a. Abortive therapy: Medications used at onset of the headache. Best for infrequent headaches.

i. Initial therapy: Aspirin or nonsteroidal antiinflammatory agents.
ii. More potent therapy (when initial therapy fails): ergotamines or selective serotonin receptor agonists (triptans). Check contraindications for specific agents.

NOTE: Opioid drugs should be avoided.

---

b. Prophylactic therapy: Used in patients with frequent or severe headache attacks (e.g., two or more headaches per month) or those with neurologic changes. Includes beta-blockers, calcium channel blockers, antidepressants, and others. Check contraindications for specific medications.

3. Antinausea medication as needed for an acute episode (e.g., prochlorperazine 25 mg rectally b.i.d.).

Follow-Up

Reevaluate in 4 to 6 weeks to assess the efficacy of the therapy.

10.28 CLUSTER HEADACHE

Symptoms

Typically unilateral, very painful (stabbing), periorbital, frontal, or temporal headache associated with ipsilateral tearing, rhinorrhea, sweating, nasal stuffiness, and/or a droopy eyelid. Usually lasts for minutes to hours. Typically recurs once or twice daily for several weeks, followed by a headache-free interval of months to years. The cycle may repeat. Predominantly affects men. Headache awakens patients, whereas migraine does not.

Signs

Ipsilateral conjunctival injection, facial flush, or Horner syndrome (third-order neuron etiology) may be present. Ptosis may become permanent.

Precipitating Factors

Alcohol, nitroglycerin.

Differential Diagnosis

- Migraine headache: Typically unilateral headache possibly associated with visual and neurologic symptoms. See 10.27, Migraine.

- Chronic paroxysmal hemicrania: Several attacks per day with a dramatic response to oral indomethacin.

- Others: See 10.26, Headache.

Work-Up

1. History and complete ocular examination.

2. Neurologic examination, particularly a cranial nerve evaluation.

3. If Horner syndrome present, consider imaging studies to eliminate other causes. See 10.2, Horner Syndrome.

4. Obtain an MRI of the brain when the history is atypical or a neurologic abnormality is present.

Treatment

1. No treatment is necessary if the headache is mild.

2. Avoid alcoholic beverages or cigarette smoking during a cluster cycle.

3. Refer patient to neurologist to help coordinate pharmacologic therapy.

4. Abortive therapy for acute attack:

—Oxygen, 5 to 8 L/min by face mask for 10 minutes at onset of attack. Relieves pain in 70% of adults.

—Sumatriptan used subcutaneously (6 mg) or intranasally (20 mg) is often effective in relieving pain.

—Zolmitriptan 5 or 10 mg intranasally also appears to be effective.

10

—Less frequent medications used include ergotamine inhalation, dihydroergotamine, or corticosteroids.

5. When headaches are moderate to severe and are unrelieved by nonprescription medication, one of the following drugs may be an effective prophylactic agent during cluster periods:

—Calcium channel blockers (e.g., verapamil 360 to 480 mg/day p.o. in divided doses).

—Lithium 600 to 900 mg p.o. q.d. is administered in conjunction with the patient's medical doctor. Baseline renal (blood urea nitrogen, creatinine, urine electrolytes) and thyroid function tests (triiodothyronine, thyroxine, TSH) are obtained. Lithium intoxication may occur in patients using indomethacin, tetracycline, or methyldopa.

—Ergotamine 1 to 2 mg p.o. q.d.

—Methysergide 2 mg p.o. b.i.d. with meals. Do not use for longer than 3 to 4 months because of the significant risk of retroperitoneal fibrosis. Methysergide is not recommended in patients with coronary artery or peripheral vascular disease, thrombophlebitis, hypertension, pregnancy, or hepatic or renal disease.

—Oral steroids (e.g., prednisone 40 to 80 mg p.o. for 1 week, tapering rapidly over an additional week if possible) and an antiulcer agent (e.g., ranitidine 150 mg p.o. b.i.d. or pantoprazole 40 mg p.o. q. d.).

6. If necessary, an acute, severe attack can be treated with intravenous diazepam.

Follow-Up

1. Patients started on systemic steroids are seen within a few days and then every several weeks to evaluate the effects of treatment and monitor intraocular pressure.

2. Patients taking methysergide or lithium are reevaluated in 7 to 10 days. Plasma lithium levels are monitored in patients taking this agent.

10

Retina

11

POSTERIOR VITREOUS DETACHMENT

Symptoms

Floaters ("cobwebs," "bugs," or "spots" that change position with eye movement), blurred vision, flashes of light, which are more common in dim illumination and the temporal visual field.

Signs

Critical. One or more discrete light gray to black vitreous opacities, one often in the shape of a ring ("Weiss ring") or broken ring, suspended over the optic disc (see Figure 11.1.1).

Other. Retinal break, retinal detachment (RD), or vitreous hemorrhage (VH) may occur with or without a posterior vitreous detachment (PVD), with similar symptoms. Peripheral retinal and disc margin hemorrhages,

released retinal pigment epithelial cells in the anterior vitreous ("tobacco dust" or Shafer sign).

NOTE: Approximately 8% to 10% of all patients with acute symptomatic PVD have a retinal break. The presence of pigmented cells in the anterior vitreous or VH in association with an acute PVD indicates a high probability (>70%) of a coexisting retinal break. See 11.2, *Retinal Break.*

Differential Diagnosis

- Vitritis: It may be difficult to distinguish PVD with anterior vitreous pigmented cells from inflammatory cells. In vitritis, vitreous cells may be found in both the posterior and anterior vitreous, the condition may be bilateral, and the cells are not typically pigmented. See 12.3, *Posterior Uveitis.*

- Migraine: Multicolored photopsias in a zig-zag pattern that obstructs vision, lasts approximately 20 minutes. A headache may or may not follow. Normal fundus examination. See 10.27, *Migraine.*

Work-Up

1. History: Distinguish retinal photopsias from the visual distortion of migraine, which may be accompanied by new floaters. Duration of the symptoms? Risk factors for retinal break (previous intraocular surgery, high myopia, family history of retinal tears, and/or detachments)?

2. Complete ocular examination, including examination of the anterior vitreous for pigmented cells and a dilated retinal examination

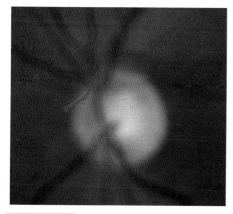

FIGURE 11.1.1. Posterior vitreous detachment.

293

with indirect ophthalmoscopy and scleral depression to rule out a retinal break and detachment.

3. Visualize the PVD at the slit lamp with a 60- or 90-diopter lens by identifying a gray-to-black strand suspended in the vitreous. If not visible, have the patient look up, down, and then straight to float the PVD into view.

4. If a VH obscures visualization of the retina, ultrasonography (US) is indicated to identify the PVD and rule out a RD, tumor, or hemorrhagic macular degeneration. Occasionally, the flap of a tear can be identified. See 11.13, *Vitreous Hemorrhage*.

Treatment

No treatment is indicated for PVD. If an acute retinal break is found, see 11.2, *Retinal Break*.

NOTE: A retinal break surrounded by pigment is old and usually does not require treatment.

Follow-Up

▪ The patient should be given a list of RD symptoms (an increase in floaters or flashing lights, worsening vision, or the appearance of a persistent curtain or shadow anywhere in the field of vision) and told to return immediately if these symptoms develop.

▪ If no retinal break or hemorrhage is found, the patient should be scheduled for repeated examination with scleral depression in 2 to 4 weeks, 2 to 3 months, and 6 months after the symptoms first develop.

▪ If no retinal break is found, but mild VH or peripheral punctate retinal hemorrhages are present, repeated examinations are performed 1 week, 2 to 4 weeks, 3 months, and 6 months after the event.

▪ If no retinal break is found but significant VH or anterior pigmented vitreous cells are present, repeat examination should be performed the next day by a retina specialist because of the high likelihood of a retinal break.

11.2   RETINAL BREAK

Symptoms

Acute retinal break: Flashes of light, floaters ("cobwebs" or "spots" that change position with eye movement), and sometimes blurred vision. Can be identical to symptoms associated with PVD.

Chronic retinal breaks or atrophic retinal holes: Usually asymptomatic.

Signs

(See Figure 11.2.1.)

Critical. A full-thickness retinal defect, usually seen in the periphery.

Other. Acute retinal break: Pigmented cells in the anterior vitreous, VH, PVD, retinal flap, subretinal fluid (SRF), or an operculum (a free-floating piece of retina) suspended in the vitreous cavity above the retinal hole.

Chronic retinal break: A surrounding ring of pigmentation, a demarcation line between attached and detached retina, and signs (but no symptoms) of an acute retinal break.

Predisposing Conditions

Lattice degeneration, high myopia, aphakia, pseudophakia, age-related retinoschisis, vitreoretinal tufts, meridional folds, history of previous retinal break or detachment in the fellow eye, family history of retinal break or detachment, and trauma.

Differential Diagnosis

▪ Meridional fold: Small radial fold of retina perpendicular to the ora serrata and overlying an oral tooth; may have small retinal hole at the base.

▪ Meridional complex: Meridional fold that extends to a ciliary process.

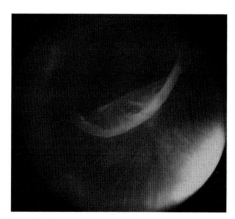

FIGURE 11.2.1. Giant retinal tear.

- Vitreoretinal tuft: Focal area of vitreous traction causing elevation of the retina.

- Paving stone degeneration.

- Lattice degeneration.

Work-Up

Complete ocular examination with a slit-lamp and indirect ophthalmoscopy of both eyes with scleral depression. Scleral depression is deferred until 2 to 4 weeks after a traumatic hyphema or microhyphema.

Treatment

In general, laser therapy or cryotherapy is required within 24 to 72 hours for acute retinal breaks, and only rarely for chronic breaks. Each case must be individualized; however, we follow these general guidelines:

1. Treatment recommended

    —Acute symptomatic break (e.g., a horseshoe or operculated tear).

    —Acute traumatic break (including a dialysis).

2. Treatment to be considered

    —Asymptomatic retinal break that is large (e.g., ≥1.5 mm), above the horizontal meridian, or both, particularly if there is no PVD.

    —Asymptomatic retinal break in an aphakic or pseudophakic eye, an eye in which the involved or the contralateral eye has had an RD, or in a highly myopic eye.

Follow-Up

1. Patients with predisposing conditions or retinal breaks that do not require treatment are followed every 6 to 12 months.

2. Patients treated for a retinal break are reexamined in 1 week, 1 month, 3 months, and then every 6 to 12 months.

3. RD symptoms (an increase in floaters or flashing lights, the appearance of a curtain, shadow, worsening vision, or a bubble anywhere in the field of vision) are explained and patients are told to return immediately if these symptoms develop.

11.3   RETINAL DETACHMENT

There are three distinct types of RD. All three forms show an elevation of the retina.

RHEGMATOGENOUS RETINAL DETACHMENT

Symptoms

Flashes of light, floaters, a curtain, or shadow moving over the field of vision, peripheral or central visual loss, or both.

Signs

(See Figures 11.3.1 to 11.3.3.)

Critical. Elevation of the retina from the retinal pigment epithelium (RPE) by fluid in the subretinal space due to an accompanying full-thickness retinal break or breaks. See 11.2, *Retinal Break.*

Other. Anterior vitreous pigmented cells, VH, PVD, usually lower intraocular pressure (IOP) in the affected eye, nonshifting clear SRF, sometimes fixed retinal folds. The detached retina is often corrugated and partially opaque in appearance. A mild relative afferent pupillary defect (RAPD) may be present.

11

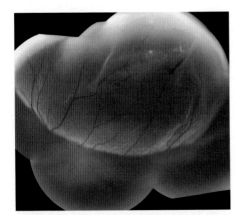

FIGURE 11.3.1. Rhegmatogenous retinal detachment.

NOTE: A chronic rhegmatogenous retinal detachment (RRD) often shows a pigmented demarcation line at the posterior extent of the RD, intraretinal cysts, fixed folds, white dots underneath the retina (subretinal precipitates), or a combination of these with a relative visual field defect. It should be differentiated from retinoschisis, which produces an absolute visual field defect.

Etiology

A retinal break allows fluid to move through the hole and separate the overlying retina from the RPE.

Work-Up

1. Indirect ophthalmoscopy with scleral depression. Slit-lamp examination with contact lens may help in finding small breaks.

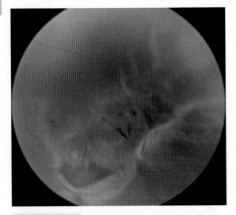

FIGURE 11.3.2. Retinal detachment with retinal break in lattice degeneration.

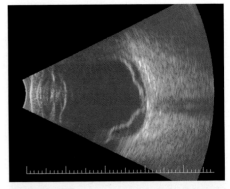

FIGURE 11.3.3. B-scan US of retinal detachment.

2. B-scan US may be helpful if media opacities are present.

EXUDATIVE RETINAL DETACHMENT

Symptoms

Minimal to severe visual loss or a visual field defect; visual changes may vary with changes in head position.

Signs

(See Figure 11.3.4.)
Critical. Serous elevation of the retina with shifting SRF. The area of detached retina changes when the patient changes position: While sitting, the SRF accumulates inferiorly, detaching the inferior retina; while in the supine position, the fluid accumulates in the posterior pole, detaching the macula. There is no retinal break; fluid accumulation is due to

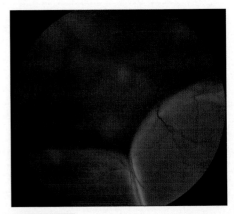

FIGURE 11.3.4. Exudative retinal detachment.

breakdown of the normal inner or outer blood-retinal barrier. The detachment does not extend to the ora serrata.

Other. The detached retina is smooth and may become quite bullous. A mild RAPD may be present if posterior pole involved.

Etiology

- Neoplastic: Choroidal malignant melanoma, metastasis, choroidal hemangioma, multiple myeloma, retinal capillary hemangioma (hemangioblastoma), etc.

- Inflammatory disease: Vogt–Koyanagi–Harada (VKH) syndrome, posterior scleritis, sympathetic ophthalmia, other chronic inflammatory processes.

- Congenital abnormalities: Optic pit, morning-glory syndrome, and choroidal coloboma (although these may have an associated retinal break).

- Vascular: Choroidal neovascularization (CNV), Coats disease, malignant hypertension (HTN), preeclampsia, and familial exudative vitreoretinopathy (FEVR). See specific sections.

- Nanophthalmos: Small eyes with a small cornea and a shallow anterior chamber but a large lens and a thick sclera.

- Idiopathic central serous chorioretinopathy (CSCR): May be seen with bullous RD from multiple, large RPE detachments. See 11.15, *Central Serous Chorioretinopathy.*

- Uveal effusion syndrome: Bilateral detachments of the peripheral choroid, ciliary body, and retina; leopard-spot RPE changes (when retina is reattached); cells in the vitreous; dilated episcleral vessels; more common in patients with high hyperopia, particularly nanophthalmic eyes.

Work-Up

1. Intravenous fluorescein angiography (IVFA) may show source of SRF.

2. Optical coherence tomography (OCT) may help identify SRF as well as the source (e.g., CNV).

3. B-scan US may help delineate the underlying cause.

4. Systemic work-up to rule out the above causes (e.g., HTN, multiple myeloma, etc.).

TRACTIONAL RETINAL DETACHMENT

Symptoms

Visual loss or visual field defect; may be asymptomatic.

Signs

(See Figure 11.3.5.)

Critical. The detached retina appears concave with a smooth surface; cellular and vitreous membranes exerting traction on the retina are present; retinal striae extending from these areas may also be seen. Detachment may become a convex RRD if a tractional retinal tear develops.

Other. The retina is immobile, and the detachment rarely extends to the ora serrata. A mild RAPD may be present.

Etiology

Fibrocellular bands in the vitreous (e.g., resulting from proliferative diabetic retinopathy (PDR), sickle cell retinopathy, retinopathy of prematurity, FEVR, toxocariasis, trauma, previous giant retinal tear) contract and detach the retina.

Work-Up

1. Indirect ophthalmoscopy with scleral depression. Slit-lamp examination with contact lens may help in finding small breaks.

2. B-scan US may be helpful if media opacities are present.

3. OCT is useful in identifying tractional membranes and can be useful in differentiating tractional membranes from detached retina.

11

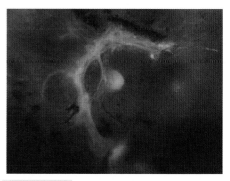

FIGURE 11.3.5. Traction retinal detachment.

Differential Diagnosis for All Three Types of Retinal Detachment

- Acquired/age-related degenerative retinoschisis: Commonly bilateral, usually inferotemporal, no pigmented cells or hemorrhage are present in the vitreous, the retinal vessels in the inner retinal layers are often sheathed peripherally, and white "snowflakes" are often seen on the inner retinal layers. See 11.4, *Retinoschisis.*

- X-linked retinoschisis: Petaloid foveal changes are present over 90% of the time. Dehiscences occur in the nerve fiber layer (NFL) 50% of the time. See 11.4, *Retinoschisis.*

- Choroidal detachment: Orange–brown, more solid in appearance than an RD, often extends 360 degrees. Hypotony is usually present. See 11.27, *Choroidal Effusion/Detachment.*

Treatment

1. Patients with an acute RRD that threatens the fovea should be placed on bed rest, with surgical repair performed urgently. The visual prognosis is significantly worse in detachments that progress to involve the fovea. Surgical options include laser photocoagulation, cryotherapy, pneumatic retinopexy, vitrectomy, and scleral buckle.

2. All RRDs that are macula-off, or tractional retinal detachments that involve the macula, are repaired preferably within a few days. Visual outcomes for macula-off detachments do not change if surgery is performed within 7–10 days of the onset.

3. Chronic RDs are treated within 1 week if possible.

4. For exudative RD, successful treatment of the underlying condition often leads to resolution of the detachment.

Follow-Up

Patients treated for RD are reexamined at 1 day, 1 week, 2 weeks, 1 month, 2 to 3 months, then every 6 to 12 months.

11.4   RETINOSCHISIS

Retinoschisis, a splitting of the retina, occurs in X-linked (juvenile) and age-related degenerative forms.

X-LINKED (JUVENILE) RETINOSCHISIS

Symptoms

Decreased vision due to VH (25%) and macular changes, or asymptomatic. The condition is congenital, but may not be detected at birth if an examination is not performed. A family history may or may not be elicited (X-linked recessive).

Signs

(See Figure 11.4.1.)

Critical.   Foveal schisis seen as stellate maculopathy: Cystoid foveal changes with retinal folds that radiate from the center of the fovea (petaloid pattern). Unlike the cysts of cystoid macular edema (CME), they do not stain or leak on IVFA, but can be seen with indocyanine green (ICG) and on OCT. The macular appearance changes in adulthood and the petaloid pattern may disappear.

Other.   Separation of the nerve fiber layer (NFL) from the outer retinal layers in the retinal periphery (bilaterally in the inferotemporal

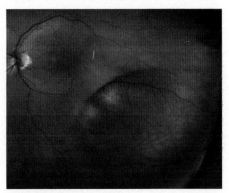

FIGURE 11.4.1.   Retinoschisis.

quadrant, most commonly) with the development of NFL breaks; this peripheral retinoschisis occurs in 50% of patients. However, schisis may occur between any two retinal layers. RD, VH, and pigmentary changes also may occur. Pigmented demarcation lines may be seen (indicating previous RD) even though the retina is not detached at the time, unlike acquired age-related degenerative retinoschisis.

Differential Diagnosis

- Age-related degenerative retinoschisis (see below).

- RRD: Usually unilateral, acquired, and associated with a retinal tear. Pigment in the anterior vitreous is seen. See 11.3, *Retinal Detachment*.

Work-Up

1. Family history.

2. Dilated retinal examination with scleral depression to rule out a retinal break or detachment.

3. OCT can help determine the layer of the schisis and help to differentiate schisis from an RD.

Treatment

1. No treatment for stellate maculopathy.

2. For non-clearing VH, consider vitrectomy.

3. Surgical repair of an RD should be performed.

4. Superimposed amblyopia may be present in children younger than 11 years of age when one eye is more severely affected and a trial of patching should be considered. See 8.7, *Amblyopia*.

Follow-Up

Every 6 months; sooner if treating amblyopia.

AGE-RELATED DEGENERATIVE RETINOSCHISIS

Symptoms

Usually asymptomatic; may have decreased vision.

Signs

Critical. The schisis cavity is dome-shaped with a smooth surface and is usually located temporally, especially inferotemporally. Usually bilateral and may show sheathing of retinal vessels and "snowflakes" or "frosting" (persistent Mueller fibers) on the elevated inner wall of the schisis cavity. Unlike X-linked juvenile retinoschisis, splitting usually occurs at the level of the outer plexiform layer. The area of schisis is not mobile, and there is no associated RPE pigmentation.

Other. Prominent cystoid degeneration near the ora serrata, an absolute scotoma corresponding to the area of schisis, hyperopia is common, no pigment cells or hemorrhage in the vitreous, and absence of a demarcation line. An RRD may occasionally develop.

Differential Diagnosis

- RRD: Surface is corrugated in appearance and moves more with eye movements. A long-standing RD may resemble retinoschisis, but intraretinal cysts, demarcation lines between attached and detached retina, and white sub-retinal dots may be seen. Only a relative scotoma is present. See 11.3, *Retinal Detachment*.

- X-linked juvenile retinoschisis (see above).

Work-Up

1. Slit-lamp evaluation for anterior chamber inflammation and pigmented anterior vitreous cells; neither should be present in isolated retinoschisis.

2. Dilated retinal examination with scleral depression to rule out a concomitant RD or an outer layer retinal hole, which may lead to an RD.

3. A fundus contact lens evaluation of the retina as needed to aid in recognizing outer layer retinal breaks.

4. OCT can help determine which layer of the retina is split.

5. Visual field testing will reveal an absolute scotoma in the area of schisis.

11

Treatment

1. Surgery is indicated when a clinically significant RD develops.

2. A small RD walled off by a demarcation line is usually not treated. This may take the form of pigmentation at the posterior border of outer layer breaks.

Follow-Up

Every 6 months. RD symptoms (an increase in floaters or flashing lights, blurry vision, or the appearance of a curtain or shadow anywhere in the field of vision) are explained to all patients, and patients are told to return immediately if these symptoms develop.

11.5 COTTON–WOOL SPOT

Symptoms

Visual acuity usually normal. Often asymptomatic.

Signs

(See Figure 11.5.1.)

Critical. Whitening in the superficial retinal NFL.

NOTE: The presence of even a single cotton–wool spot (CWS) is not normal. In a patient without diabetes mellitus, acute HTN, or a retinal vein occlusion, a work-up for an underlying systemic condition should be performed.

Differential Diagnosis

- Retinal whitening secondary to infectious retinitis, such as that seen in toxoplasmosis, herpes simplex virus, varicella zoster virus, and cytomegalovirus. These entities typically have vitritis and retinal hemorrhages associated with them. See 12.5, *Toxoplasmosis,* and 12.8, *Acute Retinal Necrosis.*

- Myelinated NFL: Develops postnatally. Usually peripapillary but may be in retinal areas remote from the disc (see Figure 11.5.2).

Etiology

Thought to be an acute obstruction of a precapillary retinal arteriole causing blockage of axoplasmic flow and buildup of axoplasmic debris in the NFL.

- Diabetes mellitus: Most common cause. Often associated with microaneurysms, dot-blot hemorrhages, and hard exudates. See 11.12, *Diabetic Retinopathy.*

- Chronic or acute HTN: May see retinal arteriolar narrowing and flame hemorrhages

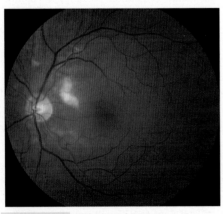

FIGURE 11.5.1. Cotton–wool spot.

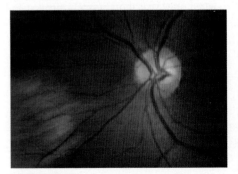

FIGURE 11.5.2. Myelinated nerve fiber layer.

in chronic HTN. Acute HTN may have hard exudates, optic nerve swelling, exudative RD. See 11.10, *Hypertensive Retinopathy.*

- Retinal vein occlusion: Unilateral, multiple hemorrhages, venous dilation, and tortuosity. Multiple CWS, usually ≥6, seen in ischemic varieties. See 11.8, *Central Retinal Vein Occlusion,* and 11.9, *Branch Retinal Vein Occlusion.*

- Retinal emboli: Often from carotid arteries or heart with resulting ischemia and subsequent CWS distal to arterial occlusion. Patients require carotid Doppler examination and echocardiography. See 10.22, *Transient Visual Loss/Amaurosis Fugax.*

- Collagen vascular disease: Systemic lupus erythematosus (most common), Wegener granulomatosis, polyarteritis nodosa, scleroderma, etc.

- Giant cell arteritis (GCA): Age ≥55 years. Symptoms include vision loss, scalp tenderness, jaw claudication, proximal muscle aches, etc. See 10.17, *Arteritic Ischemic Optic Neuropathy (Giant Cell Arteritis).*

- HIV retinopathy: Single or multiple cotton-wool spots in the posterior pole. See 12.10, *Noninfectious Retinal Microvasculopathy/HIV Retinopathy.*

- Other infections: Toxoplasmosis, orbital mucormycosis, Lyme, leptospirosis, Rocky Mountain spotted fever, onchocerciasis, subacute bacterial endocarditis.

- Hypercoagulable state: Polycythemia, multiple myeloma, cryoglobulinemia, Waldenström macroglobulinemia, antiphospholipid syndrome, factor V Leiden, activated protein C resistance, hyperhomocysteinemia, protein C and S deficiency, antithrombin III mutation, prothrombin mutation G20210A, etc.

- Radiation retinopathy: Follows radiation therapy to the eye or periocular structures when the eye is irradiated inadvertently. May occur any time after radiation, but occurs most commonly within a few years. Maintain a high suspicion even in patients in whom the eye was reportedly shielded. Usually, 3,000 cGy is necessary, but it has been noted to occur with 1,500 cGy. Resembles diabetic retinopathy.

- Interferon therapy.

- Purtscher and pseudo-Purtscher retinopathy: Multiple cotton-wool spots and/or superficial hemorrhages in a peripapillary configuration. Typically bilateral but can be unilateral and asymmetric. See 3.19, *Purtscher Retinopathy.*

- Cancer: Metastatic carcinoma, leukemia, lymphoma.

- Others: Migraine, hypotension, intravenous drug use, papilledema, papillitis, severe anemia, sickle cell, acute blood loss, etc.

Work-Up

1. History: Diabetes or HTN? Ocular or periocular radiation in past? GCA symptoms in appropriate age group? Symptoms of collagen vascular disease including joint pain, rashes, etc.? HIV risk factors?

2. Complete ocular examination, including dilated retinal examination with a slit lamp and a 60- or 90-diopter lens and indirect ophthalmoscopy. Look for concurrent hemorrhages, vascular occlusion, vasculitis, hard exudates.

3. Check a fasting blood sugar.

4. Check the blood pressure.

5. Consider erythrocyte sedimentation rate (ESR), c-reactive protein (CRP), and platelets if GCA is suspected.

6. Consider blood and urine cultures, chest x-ray, carotid Doppler examination, and echocardiography if emboli are suspected.

7. Consider HIV testing.

8. Fluorescein angiography is generally not helpful for an isolated CWS. IVFA reveals

areas of capillary nonperfusion adjacent to the location of the CWS.

Treatment

Treat underlying etiology.

Follow-Up

Depends on the underlying etiology. CWS typically fade in 5 to 7 weeks but can remain longer if associated with diabetic retinopathy.

11.6 CENTRAL RETINAL ARTERY OCCLUSION

Symptoms

Unilateral, painless, acute vision loss (counting fingers to light perception in 94% of eyes) occurring over seconds; may have a history of transient visual loss (amaurosis fugax).

Signs

(See Figure 11.6.1.)

Critical. Superficial opacification or whitening of the retina in the posterior pole, and a cherry-red spot in the center of the macula (may be subtle).

Other. Marked RAPD; narrowed retinal arterioles; boxcarring or segmentation of the blood column in the arterioles. Occasionally, retinal arteriolar emboli or cilioretinal artery sparing of the foveola is evident. If visual acuity is light perception or worse, strongly suspect ophthalmic artery occlusion.

Differential Diagnosis

- Acute ophthalmic artery occlusion: Usually no cherry-red spot; the entire retina appears whitened. The treatment is the same as for central retinal artery occlusion (CRAO).

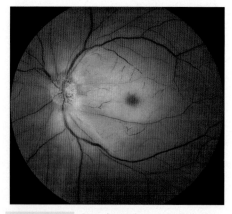

FIGURE 11.6.1. Central retinal artery occlusion.

- Commotio retinae: Retinal whitening from intracellular edema and fragmentation of the photoreceptor outer segments and RPE. Follows blunt trauma, resolves spontaneously. May mimic a cherry-red spot when the posterior pole is involved. See 3.16, *Commotio Retinae.*

- Other causes of a cherry-red spot: Tay–Sachs, Niemann–Pick disease type A, etc. These conditions present early in life with other, often severe, systemic manifestations. Ophthalmic findings are usually bilateral.

Etiology

- Embolus: Three main types include cholesterol, calcium, and platelet-fibrin emboli. All are seen within a vessel. Cholesterol emboli (Hollenhorst plaque) are typically refractile, orange, and seen at retinal vessel bifurcations. They arise from ulcerated atheromas, typically from the carotid arteries. Calcium emboli are white and frequently cause distal retinal infarction. They typically arise from cardiac valves. Platelet-fibrin emboli are a dull white and typically arise from atheromas in the carotid arteries.

- Thrombosis.

- GCA: May produce CRAO, ophthalmic artery occlusion, or an ischemic optic neuropathy. See 10.17, *Arteritic Ischemic Optic Neuropathy (Giant Cell Arteritis).*

- Other collagen–vascular disease: Systemic lupus erythematosus, polyarteritis nodosa, and others.

- Hypercoagulable state: Polycythemia, multiple myeloma, cryoglobulinemia, Waldenström macroglobulinemia, antiphospholipid syndrome, factor V Leiden, activated protein C resistance, hyperhomocysteinemia, protein

C and S deficiency, antithrombin III mutation, prothrombin mutation G20210A, etc.

- Rare causes: Migraine, Behçet disease, syphilis, sickle cell disease.
- Trauma.

Work-Up

1. Immediate ESR, CRP, and platelets to rule out GCA if the patient is 55 years of age or older. If the patient's history, laboratories, or both are consistent with GCA, start high-dose systemic steroids. See 10.17, *Arteritic Ischemic Optic Neuropathy (Giant Cell Arteritis)*.

2. Check the blood pressure.

3. Other blood tests: Fasting blood sugar, glycosylated hemoglobin, complete blood count (CBC) with differential, prothrombin time/activated partial thromboplastin time (PT/PTT). In patients younger than 50 years or with appropriate risk factors or positive review of systems, consider lipid profile, antinuclear antibody (ANA), rheumatoid factor, fluorescent treponemal antibody absorbed (FTA-ABS), serum protein electrophoresis, hemoglobin electrophoresis, and further evaluation for hypercoagulable state (see above).

4. Carotid artery evaluation by duplex Doppler US.

5. Cardiac evaluation with electrocardiography (ECG), echocardiography, and possibly Holter monitoring.

6. Consider IVFA, electroretinography (ERG), or both to confirm the diagnosis.

NOTE: It has been suggested that only patients with high-risk characteristics for cardioembolic disease merit echocardiography, including a history of subacute bacterial endocarditis, rheumatic heart disease, mitral valve prolapse, recent myocardial infarction, prosthetic valve, intravenous drug abuse, congenital heart disease, valvular heart disease, any detectable heart murmur, and ECG changes (atrial fibrillation, acute ST segment elevation, or Q waves).

Treatment

There are anecdotal reports of improvement after the following treatments, if instituted within 90 to 120 minutes of the occlusive event. None of these treatments have been proven effective in randomized, controlled clinical trials, and should not be considered the standard of care.

1. Immediate ocular massage with fundus contact lens or digital massage.

2. Anterior chamber paracentesis: See Appendix 13, *Anterior Chamber Paracentesis*.

3. IOP reduction with acetazolamide, 500 mg i.v., or two 250-mg tablets p.o. or a topical beta-blocker (e.g., timolol or levobunolol, 0.5% b.i.d.).

4. Hyperventilation into a paper bag to induce a respiratory acidosis and subsequent vasodilation.

Follow-Up

1. Refer to an internist for a complete work-up as above.

2. Repeat eye examination in 1 to 4 weeks, checking for neovascularization of the iris/disc/angle/retina (NVI/NVD/NVA/NVE), which develops in up to 20% of patients, at a mean of 4 weeks after onset. If neovascularization develops, perform panretinal photocoagulation (PRP) and/or administer an anti-vascular endothelial growth factor (anti-VEGF) agent.

11.7 BRANCH RETINAL ARTERY OCCLUSION

Symptoms

Unilateral, painless, abrupt loss of partial visual field; a history of transient visual loss (amaurosis fugax) may be elicited.

Signs

(See Figure 11.7.1.)

Critical. Superficial opacification or whitening along the distribution of a branch retinal

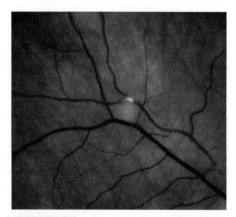

FIGURE 11.7.1. Branch retinal artery occlusion with Hollenhorst plaque.

artery. The affected retina becomes edematous.

Other. Narrowed branch retinal artery; boxcarring, segmentation of the blood column, or emboli are sometimes seen in the affected branch retinal artery. Cholesterol emboli appear as bright, reflective crystals, usually at a vessel bifurcation. Cotton-wool spots may appear in the involved area.

Etiology

See 11.6, *Central Retinal Artery Occlusion.*

Work-Up

See 11.6, *Central Retinal Artery Occlusion.* Unlike in CRAO, an ERG is not helpful.

NOTE: When a branch retinal artery occlusion (BRAO) is accompanied by optic nerve edema or retinitis, obtain appropriate serologic testing to rule out cat-scratch disease [Bartonella (Rochalimaea) henselae], syphilis, Lyme disease, and toxoplasmosis.

Treatment

1. No ocular therapy of proven value is available. See treatment in 11.6, *Central Retinal Artery Occlusion.*

2. Treat any underlying medical problem.

Follow-Up

1. Patients need immediate evaluation to treat any underlying disorders (especially GCA).

2. Reevaluate every 3 to 6 months initially to monitor progression. Ocular neovascularization after branch retinal artery occlusion is rare.

11.8 CENTRAL RETINAL VEIN OCCLUSION

Symptoms

Painless loss of vision, usually unilateral.

Signs

(See Figure 11.8.1.)

Critical. Diffuse retinal hemorrhages in all four quadrants of the retina; dilated, tortuous retinal veins.

Other. Cotton-wool spots; disc edema and hemorrhages; macular edema; optociliary collateral vessels on the disc; neovascularization of the optic disc (NVD), retina (NVE), iris (NVI), and angle (NVA).

Differential Diagnosis

- Ocular ischemic syndrome (OIS) or carotid occlusive disease: Dilated and irregular veins without tortuosity. Mid-peripheral retinal

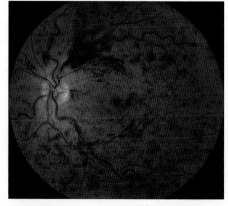

FIGURE 11.8.1. Central retinal vein occlusion.

hemorrhages are typically present, but disc edema and hemorrhages are not characteristic. Disc neovascularization is present in one-third of cases. Patients may have a history of transient visual loss (amaurosis fugax), transient ischemic attacks, or orbital pain. See 11.11, *Ocular Ischemic Syndrome/ Carotid Occlusive Disease*.

- Diabetic retinopathy: Hemorrhages and microaneurysms concentrated in the posterior pole. Typically bilateral. IVFA differentiates this condition from CRVO. See 11.12, *Diabetic Retinopathy*.

- Papilledema: Bilateral disc swelling with flame-shaped hemorrhages surrounding the disc. See 10.15, *Papilledema*.

- Radiation retinopathy: History of irradiation. Disc swelling with radiation papillopathy, and retinal neovascularization may be present. Generally, cotton-wool spots are a more prominent feature than hemorrhages.

Etiology

- Atherosclerosis of the adjacent central retinal artery: The artery compresses the central retinal vein in the region of the lamina cribrosa, secondarily inducing thrombosis in the lumen of the vein.

- HTN: Most common systemic disease associated with CRVO.

- Optic disc edema.

- Glaucoma: Most common ocular disease associated with CRVO.

- Optic disc drusen.

- Hypercoagulable state: Polycythemia, multiple myeloma, cryoglobulinemia, Waldenström macroglobulinemia, antiphospholipid syndrome, factor V Leiden, activated protein C resistance, hyperhomocysteinemia, protein C and S deficiency, antithrombin III mutation, prothrombin mutation G20210A, and others.

- Vasculitis: Sarcoidosis, syphilis, systemic lupus erythematosus, and others.

- Drugs: Oral contraceptives, diuretics, and others.

- Abnormal platelet function.

- Orbital disease: Thyroid eye disease, orbital tumors, arteriovenous fistula, and others.

- Migraine: Rare.

Types

- Ischemic CRVO: Multiple cotton-wool spots (usually ≥6), extensive retinal hemorrhage, and widespread capillary nonperfusion on IVFA. RAPD often present and visual acuity is typically 20/400 or worse with visual field constriction. ERG shows decreased b-wave amplitude.

- Nonischemic CRVO: Mild fundus changes. No RAPD is present and acuity is often better than 20/400.

Work-Up

Ocular

1. Complete ocular examination, including IOP measurement, careful slit-lamp examination and gonioscopy to rule out NVI and NVA (both of which are best observed before dilation), and dilated fundus examination.

2. IVFA: Risk of neovascularization proportional to degree of capillary nonperfusion.

3. Optical Coherence Tomography: Used to help detect presence and extent of macular edema as well as to monitor response to therapy.

4. If the diagnosis is uncertain, oculopneumoplethysmography or ophthalmodynamometry may help to distinguish CRVO from carotid disease. Ophthalmic artery pressure is low in carotid disease but is normal to increased in CRVO.

Systemic

1. History: Medical problems, medications, eye diseases?

2. Check blood pressure.

3. Blood tests: Fasting blood sugar, glycosylated hemoglobin, CBC with differential, platelets, PT/PTT, ESR, lipid profile.

4. If clinically indicated, particularly in younger patients, consider hemoglobin electrophoresis, VDRL or RPR, FTA-ABS, ANA, cryoglobulins, antiphospholipid antibodies, factor V Leiden mutation, protein C and S levels, antithrombin III mutation,

11

prothrombin G20210A mutation, homo-cysteine levels, serum protein electrophoresis, and chest radiograph.

5. Complete medical evaluation, with careful attention to cardiovascular disease or hypercoagulability.

Treatment

1. Discontinue oral contraceptives; change diuretics to other antihypertensive medications if possible.

2. Reduce IOP if increased in either eye. See 9.1, *Primary Open-Angle Glaucoma.*

3. Treat underlying medical disorders.

4. If NVI or NVA is present, perform PRP promptly. Consider PRP if NVD or retinal neovascularization is present. Prophylactic PRP is usually not recommended unless follow-up is in doubt. Intravitreal VEGF inhibitors are very effective in temporarily halting or reversing anterior and posterior segment neovascularization. They may be a useful adjunct to PRP, particularly when rapid reversal of neovascularization is needed.

5. Aspirin 81 to 325 mg p.o. q.d. is often recommended, but no clinical trials have demonstrated efficacy to date and it may increase the risk of hemorrhage.

CRVO-Related Macular Edema

1. Intravitreal ranibizumab 0.5 mg is U.S. Food and Drug Administration (FDA)-approved for treating RVO-related macular edema (ME). Phase III clinical trials have shown promise for the new intravitreal anti-VEGF agent, aflibercept, for the treatment of RVO-related ME. Intravitreal bevacizumab has been used off-label in a similar fashion. Risks of intravitreal injections are low, but include VH and endophthalmitis, among others.

2. Ozurdex, a biodegradable 0.7 mg dexamethasone implant, is FDA-approved for the treatment of ME associated with retinal vein occlusion. Complications include cataract formation and elevated IOP (typically manageable with medical therapy alone).

3. Intravitreal triamcinolone, in both 1 mg and 4 mg doses, is effective in both improving vision and reducing vision loss in patients with ME secondary to CRVO

NOTE: In a large, prospective, randomized trial (SCORE CRVO), a 1 mg dose of intravitreal triamcinolone was found to be equally as effective as a 4 mg dose, but with fewer side-effects (elevated IOP and cataract formation).

Follow-Up

1. Visual acuity 20/40 or better: Every 1 to 2 months for the first 6 months, with a gradual interval taper to annual follow-ups.

2. Visual acuity <20/200: Depends on the type of treatment employed, but in general, every month for the first 6 months, with a gradual taper based on the patient's condition.

3. Undilated gonioscopy looking for NVA, followed by careful dilated fundus examination looking for NVD or retinal neovascularization, should be performed at each follow-up visit. Evidence of early NVI or NVA should prompt immediate PRP and/or anti-VEGF therapy and monthly follow-up until stabilized or regressed.

4. Patients should be informed that there is an 8% to 10% risk for the development of a BRVO or CRVO in the fellow eye.

Bibliography

Brown DM, Campochiaro PA, Singh RP, et al. Ranibizumab for macular edema following central retinal vein occlusion: six-month primary end point results of a phase III study. *Ophthalmology* 2010;117(6):1124–1133.

Haller JA, Bandello F, Belfort R Jr, et al. Randomized sham-controlled trial of dexamethasone intravitreal implant in patients with macular edema due to retinal vein occlusion. *Ophthalmology* 2010;117(6):1134–1146.

Ip MS, Scott IU, VanVeldhuisen PC, et al. A randomized trial comparing the efficacy and safety of intravitreal triamcinolone with observation to treat vision loss associated with macular edema secondary to central retinal vein occlusion: the Standard Care vs Corticosteroid for Retinal Vein Occlusion (SCORE) study report 5. *Arch Ophthalmol* 2009;127(9):1101–1114.

11.9 BRANCH RETINAL VEIN OCCLUSION

Symptoms

Blind spot in the visual field or loss of vision, usually unilateral.

Signs

(See Figure 11.9.1.)

Critical. Superficial hemorrhages in a sector of the retina along a retinal vein. The hemorrhages usually do not cross the horizontal raphe (midline).

Other. Cotton-wool spots, retinal edema, a dilated and tortuous retinal vein, narrowing and sheathing of the adjacent artery, retinal neovascularization, VH.

Differential Diagnosis

- Diabetic retinopathy: Dot-blot hemorrhages and microaneurysms extend across the horizontal raphe. Nearly always bilateral. See 11.12, *Diabetic Retinopathy.*

- Hypertensive retinopathy: Narrowed retinal arterioles. Hemorrhages are not confined to a sector of the retina and usually cross the horizontal raphe. Bilateral in most. See 11.10, *Hypertensive Retinopathy.*

Etiology

Disease of the adjacent arterial wall (usually the result of HTN, arteriosclerosis, or diabetes) compresses the venous wall at a crossing point.

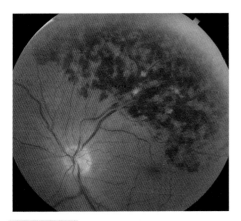

FIGURE 11.9.1. Branch retinal vein occlusion.

Work-Up

1. History: Systemic disease, particularly HTN or diabetes?

2. Complete ocular examination, including dilated retinal examination with indirect ophthalmoscopy to look for retinal neovascularization, and a macular examination with a slit lamp and a 60- or 90-diopter lens, or fundus contact lens to detect ME.

3. Optical Coherence Tomography: Used to help detect presence and extent of macular edema as well as monitor response to therapy.

4. Check blood pressure.

5. Blood tests: Fasting blood sugar, CBC with differential and platelets, PT/PTT, and ESR. If clinically indicated, consider a more comprehensive work-up. See 11.8, *Central Retinal Vein Occlusion.*

6. Medical examination: Performed by an internist to check for cardiovascular disease.

7. An IVFA is obtained after the hemorrhages clear or sooner if neovascularization is suspected.

Treatment

1. Retinal neovascularization: Sector PRP to the ischemic area, which corresponds to area of capillary nonperfusion on IVFA.

2. Prompt and appropriate treatment of underlying medical conditions (e.g., HTN).

BRVO-Related Macular Edema

1. Focal retinal laser photocoagulation is the traditional gold-standard treatment if edema is present for 3 to 6 months duration, and visual acuity is below 20/40 with macular capillary perfusion. Limitations of focal laser include length of time before effect (often several months) and the need to wait until retinal hemorrhages clear.

2. Intravitreal ranibizumab 0.5 mg is FDA approved for treating RVO-associated ME. Phase III clinical trials have shown promise for the new intravitreal anti-VEGF agent,

11

aflibercept, for the treatment of RVO-related ME. Intravitreal bevacizumab has been used off-label in a similar fashion. Risks of intravitreal injection are low, but include VH and endophthalmitis.

3. Ozurdex implant. See 11.8, *Central Retinal Vein Occlusion.*

NOTE: There is an evolving trend, particularly in cases of severe edema, to initiate treatment with pharmacologic agents for rapid visual recovery followed by focal laser for better durability of effect.

Follow-Up

In general, every 1 to 2 months for the first 4 months, and then every 3 to 12 months,

depending on the treatment employed. At each visit, the patient should be checked for neovascularization and ME.

Bibliography

Campochiaro PA, Heier JS, Feiner L, et al. Ranibizumab for macular edema following branch retinal vein occlusion: six-month primary end point results of a phase III study. *Ophthalmology* 2010;117(6):1102–1112.

Haller JA, Bandello F, Belfort R Jr, et al. Randomized sham-controlled trial of dexamethasone intravitreal implant in patients with macular edema due to retinal vein occlusion. *Ophthalmology* 2010;117(6):1134–1146.

11.10 — HYPERTENSIVE RETINOPATHY

Symptoms

Usually asymptomatic, although may have decreased vision.

Signs

(See Figure 11.10.1.)

Critical. Generalized or localized retinal arteriolar narrowing, almost always bilateral.

Other

- Chronic HTN: Arteriovenous crossing changes ("AV nicking"), retinal arteriolar sclerosis ("copper" or "silver" wiring), cotton-wool

spots, flame-shaped hemorrhages, arterial macroaneurysms, central or branch occlusion of an artery or vein. Rarely, neovascular complications can develop.

- Acute ("malignant") HTN: Hard exudates often in a "macular star" configuration, retinal edema, cotton-wool spots, flame-shaped hemorrhages, optic nerve head edema. Rarely serous RD or VH. Areas of focal chorioretinal atrophy [from previous choroidal infarcts (Elschnig spots)] are a sign of past episodes of acute HTN.

(See Figure 11.10.2.).

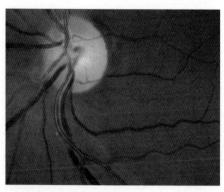

FIGURE 11.10.1. Chronic hypertensive retinopathy with arteriolar narrowing and arteriovenous nicking.

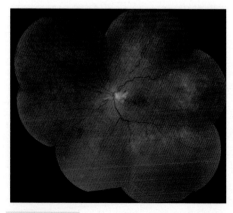

FIGURE 11.10.2. Acute ("malignant") hypertensive retinopathy.

NOTE: When unilateral, suspect carotid artery obstruction on the side of the normal-appearing eye, sparing the retina from the effects of the HTN.

Differential Diagnosis

- Diabetic retinopathy: Hemorrhages are usually dot-blot, microaneurysms are common, vessel attenuation is less common. See 11.12, *Diabetic Retinopathy.*

- Collagen–vascular disease: May show multiple cotton-wool spots, but few to no other fundus findings characteristic of HTN.

- Anemia: Mainly hemorrhage without marked arterial changes.

- Radiation retinopathy: History of irradiation. Most commonly occurs within a few years, but can develop at any time.

- CRVO or BRVO: Unilateral, multiple hemorrhages, venous dilation and tortuosity, no arteriolar narrowing. May be the result of HTN. See 11.8, *Central Retinal Vein Occlusion,* or 11.9, *Branch Retinal Vein Occlusion.*

Etiology

- Primary HTN: No known underlying cause.

- Secondary HTN: Typically the result of pre-eclampsia/eclampsia, pheochromocytoma, kidney disease, adrenal disease, or coarctation of the aorta.

Work-Up

1. History: Known HTN, diabetes, or adnexal radiation?

2. Check blood pressure.

3. Complete ocular examination, particularly dilated fundus examination.

4. Refer patient to a medical internist or an emergency department. The urgency depends on the blood pressure reading and whether the patient is symptomatic. As a general rule, a diastolic blood pressure of 110 to 120 mm Hg or the presence of chest pain, difficulty breathing, headache, change in mental status, or blurred vision with optic disc swelling requires immediate medical attention.

Treatment

Control the HTN, as per the internist.

Follow-Up

Every 2 to 3 months at first, and then every 6 to 12 months.

11.11 OCULAR ISCHEMIC SYNDROME/CAROTID OCCLUSIVE DISEASE

Symptoms

Decreased vision, ocular or periorbital pain, after images or prolonged recovery of vision after exposure to bright light, may have a history of transient monocular visual loss (amaurosis fugax). Usually unilateral. Typically occurs in patients who are aged 50 to 80 years. Men outnumber women by 2:1.

Signs

Critical. Although retinal veins are dilated and irregular in caliber, they are typically not tortuous. The retinal arterioles are narrowed. Associated findings include mid-peripheral retinal hemorrhages (80%), iris neovascularization (66%), and posterior segment neovascularization (37%).

Other. Episcleral injection, corneal edema, mild anterior uveitis, neovascular glaucoma, iris atrophy, cataract, retinal microaneurysms, cotton-wool spots, spontaneous pulsations of the central retinal artery, and cherry-red spot. CRAO may occur.

Differential Diagnosis

- CRVO: Similar signs. Decreased vision after exposure to light and orbital pain are not typically found. Ophthalmodynamometry may aid differentiating OIS from CRVO. See 11.8, *Central Retinal Vein Occlusion.*

- Diabetic retinopathy: Bilateral, usually symmetric. Hard exudates are often present. See 11.12, *Diabetic Retinopathy.*

- Aortic arch disease: Caused by atherosclerosis, syphilis, or Takayasu arteritis. Produces a clinical picture identical to OIS, but usually bilateral. Examination reveals absent arm and neck pulses, cold hands, and spasm of the arm muscles with exercise.

Etiology

- Carotid disease: Usually ≥90% stenosis.

- Ophthalmic artery disease: Less common.

Work-Up

1. History: Previous episodes of transient monocular visual loss? Cold hands or spasm of arm muscles with exercise?

2. Complete ocular examination: Search carefully for neovascularization of the iris, angle, disc, and retina.

3. Medical examination: Evaluate for HTN, diabetes, and atherosclerotic disease. Check pulses. Cardiac and carotid auscultation.

4. Consider IVFA for diagnostic or therapeutic purposes.

5. Noninvasive carotid artery evaluation: Duplex Doppler US, oculoplethysmography, magnetic resonance angiography, others.

6. Consider orbital color Doppler US.

7. Consider ophthalmodynamometry if the diagnosis of CRVO cannot be excluded.

8. Carotid arteriography is reserved for patients in whom surgery is to be performed.

9. Consider a cardiology consultation, given the high association with cardiac disease.

Treatment

Often unsuccessful.

1. Carotid endarterectomy for significant stenosis. Refer to neurovascular surgeon.

2. Consider PRP and anti-VEGF agents in the presence of neovascularization.

3. Manage glaucoma if present. See 9.14, *Neovascular Glaucoma.*

4. Control HTN, diabetes, and cholesterol. Refer to internist.

5. Lifestyle modification (e.g., smoking cessation).

Follow-Up

Depends on the age, general health of the patient, and the symptoms and signs of disease. Surgical candidates should be evaluated urgently.

11.12   DIABETIC RETINOPATHY

Diabetic Retinopathy Disease Severity Scale

- No apparent retinopathy.

- Mild nonproliferative diabetic retinopathy (NPDR): Microaneurysms only.

- Moderate NPDR: More than mild NPDR, but less than severe NPDR see Figure 11.12.1).

- Severe NPDR: Any of the following in the absence of proliferative diabetic retinopathy (PDR): diffuse (traditionally >20) intraretinal hemorrhages in all four quadrants, two quadrants of venous beading, or one quadrant of prominent intraretinal microvascular abnormalities (IRMA) (see Figure 11.12.2).

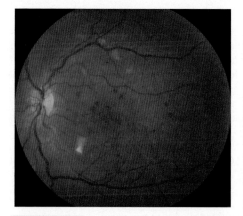

FIGURE 11.12.1. Moderate nonproliferative diabetic retinopathy with microaneurysms and cotton–wool spots.

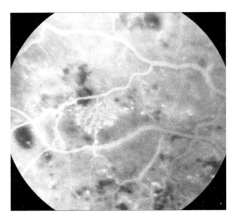

FIGURE 11.12.2. IVFA of intraretinal microvascular abnormality.

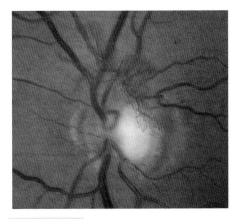

FIGURE 11.12.4. Proliferative diabetic retinopathy with neovascularization of the optic disc.

- PDR: Neovascularization of one or more of the following: iris, angle, optic disc, or elsewhere; or vitreous/preretinal hemorrhage (see Figures 11.12.3 and 11.12.4).

- Diabetic macular edema: May be present in any of the stages listed above. Clinically significant macular edema requires treatment and is defined as any one of the following (see Figures 11.12.5 and 11.12.6):

  1. Retinal thickening within 500 μm (one-third of disc diameter) of the foveal center.

  2. Hard exudates within 500 μm of the foveal center, if associated with thickening of the adjacent retina.

  3. Retinal thickening greater than one disc area in size, part of which is within one disc diameter of the center of the fovea.

Differential Diagnosis for Nonproliferative Diabetic Retinopathy

- CRVO: Optic disc swelling, veins are more dilated and tortuous, hard exudates usually not found, hemorrhages are nearly always in the NFL ("splinter hemorrhages"). CRVO

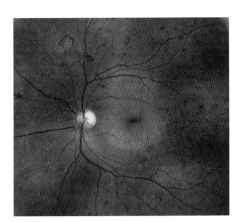

FIGURE 11.12.3. Proliferative diabetic retinopathy with neovascularization and scattered microaneurysms.

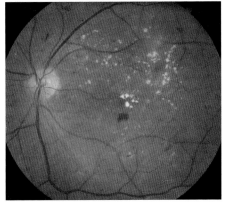

FIGURE 11.12.5. Nonproliferative diabetic retinopathy with clinically significant macular edema.

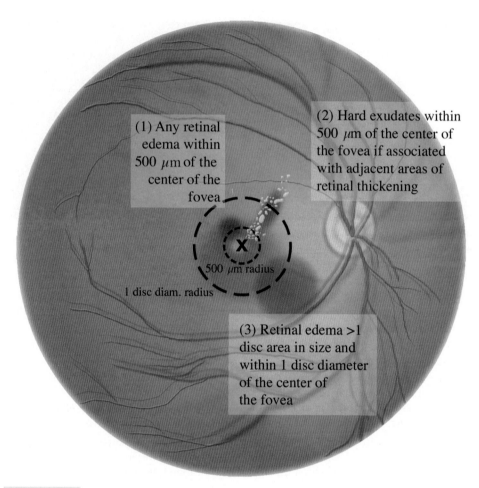

(1) Any retinal edema within 500 μm of the center of the fovea

(2) Hard exudates within 500 μm of the center of the fovea if associated with adjacent areas of retinal thickening

500 μm radius

x

1 disc diam. radius

(3) Retinal edema >1 disc area in size and within 1 disc diameter of the center of the fovea

FIGURE 11.12.6. Clinically significant macular edema.

is generally unilateral and of more sudden onset. See 11.8, *Central Retinal Vein Occlusion.*

- BRVO: Hemorrhages are distributed along a vein and do not cross the horizontal raphe (midline). See 11.9, *Branch Retinal Vein Occlusion.*

- Ocular ischemic syndrome: Hemorrhages mostly in the mid-periphery and larger; exudates are absent. Usually accompanied by pain; mild anterior chamber reaction; corneal edema; episcleral vascular congestion; a mid-dilated, poorly reactive pupil; iris neovascularization. See 11.11, *Ocular Ischemic Syndrome/ Carotid Occlusive Disease.*

- Hypertensive retinopathy: Hemorrhages fewer and typically flame-shaped, microaneurysms rare, and arteriolar narrowing present often with arteriovenous crossing changes ("AV nicking"). See 11.10, *Hypertensive Retinopathy.*

- Radiation retinopathy: Usually develops within a few years of radiation. Microaneurysms are rarely present. See 11.5, *Cotton–Wool Spot.*

Differential Diagnosis for Proliferative Diabetic Retinopathy

- Neovascular complications of CRAO, CRVO, or BRVO: See specific sections.

■ Sickle cell retinopathy: Peripheral retinal neovascularization. "Sea-fans" of neovascularization present. See 11.20, *Sickle Cell Disease (Including Sickle Cell Anemia, Sickle Trait).*

■ Embolization from intravenous drug abuse (talc retinopathy): History of intravenous drug abuse, peripheral retinal neovascularization, may see particles of talc in macular vessels. See 11.33, *Crystalline Retinopathy.*

■ Sarcoidosis: May have uveitis, exudates around veins ("candle-wax drippings"), NVE, or systemic findings. See 12.6, *Sarcoidosis.*

■ Other inflammatory syndromes (e.g., systemic lupus erythematosus).

■ Ocular ischemic syndrome: See 11.11, *Ocular Ischemic Syndrome/Carotid Occlusive Disease.*

■ Radiation retinopathy: See above.

■ Hypercoagulable states (e.g., antiphospholipid syndrome).

Work-Up

1. Slit-lamp examination with gonioscopy with careful attention for NVI and NVA, preferably before pharmacologic dilation.

2. Dilated fundus examination by using a 90- or 60-diopter or fundus contact lens with a slit lamp to rule out neovascularization and ME. Use indirect ophthalmoscopy to examine the retinal periphery.

3. Fasting blood sugar, glycosylated hemoglobin, and, if necessary, a glucose tolerance test if the diagnosis is not established.

4. Check the blood pressure.

5. Consider IVFA to determine areas of perfusion abnormalities, foveal ischemia, microaneurysms, and subclinical neovascularization, especially if considering focal macular laser therapy.

6. Consider OCT to evaluate for the presence and extent of ME.

7. Consider blood tests for hyperlipidemia if extensive exudate is present.

Treatment
Clinically Significant Macular Edema

1. Focal or grid laser treatment should be considered in patients with clinically significant macular edema. Patients with enlarged foveal avascular zones on IVFA are treated lightly, away from the regions of foveal ischemia, if they are treated at all. Patients with extensive foveal ischemia are poor laser candidates. Younger patients and diet-controlled diabetic patients tend to have a better response.

2. Patients with diffuse or extensive ME, isolated sub-foveal edema, ME in the presence of foveal ischemia, or those with poor response to prior focal/grid laser may benefit from intravitreal anti-VEGF or corticosteroid therapy, either alone or in combination with laser.

Proliferative Diabetic Retinopathy

Panretinal laser photocoagulation is indicated for any one of the following high-risk characteristics (see Figure 11.12.7):

1. NVD greater than one-fourth to one-third of the disc area in size.

2. Any degree of NVD when associated with preretinal hemorrhage or VH.

3. NVE greater than one-half of the disc area in size when associated with a preretinal hemorrhage or VH.

4. Any NVI or neovascularization of the angle.

NOTE: Some physicians treat NVE or any degree of NVD without preretinal hemorrhage or VH, especially in unreliable patients. If the ocular media is too hazy for an adequate fundus view, yet one of these criteria is met, anti-VEGF therapy and/or pars plana vitrectomy and endolaser therapy with or without lensectomy and posterior chamber intraocular lens implantation are other options. Anti-VEGF therapy alone must be used cautiously in the presence of retinal traction.

Indications for Vitrectomy

Vitrectomy may be indicated for any one of the following conditions:

11

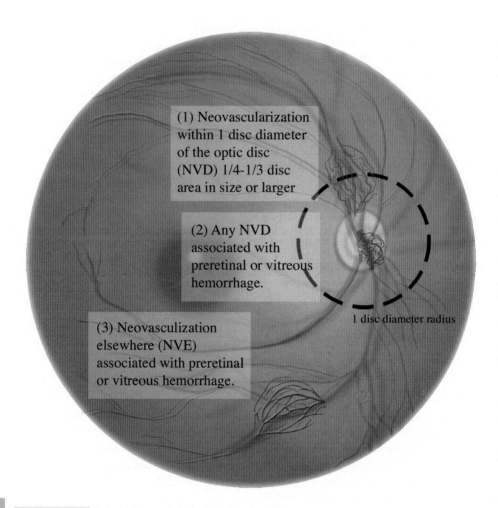

(1) Neovascularization within 1 disc diameter of the optic disc (NVD) 1/4-1/3 disc area in size or larger

(2) Any NVD associated with preretinal or vitreous hemorrhage.

(3) Neovasculization elsewhere (NVE) associated with preretinal or vitreous hemorrhage.

1 disc diameter radius

FIGURE 11.12.7.   High-risk characteristics for diabetic retinopathy.

11

1. Dense VH causing decreased vision, especially when present for several months.

2. Traction RD involving and progressing within the macula.

3. Macular epiretinal membranes or recent-onset displacement of the macula.

4. Severe retinal neovascularization and fibrous proliferation that is unresponsive to laser photocoagulation.

5. Dense premacular hemorrhage.

NOTE: Young patients with juvenile type 1 diabetes are known to have more aggressive PDR and therefore may benefit from earlier vitrectomy

and laser photocoagulation. B-scan US may be required to rule out tractional detachment of the macula in eyes with dense VH obscuring a fundus view.

Follow-Up

1. Diabetes without retinopathy. Annual dilated examination.

2. Mild NPDR. Dilated examination every 6 to 9 months.

3. Moderate to severe NPDR. Dilated examination every 4 to 6 months.

4. PDR (not meeting high-risk criteria). Dilated examination every 2 to 3 months.

TABLE 11.12.1 Recommendations Based on the Baseline Diabetic Retinopathy in Pregnancy					
Baseline Diabetic Retinopathy	Gestational Diabetes	None or Minimal NPDR	Mild to-Moderate NPDR	High-Risk NPDR	PDR
Gestational course	No risk of retinopathy.	No progression in vast majority. Of those who progress, only a few have visual impairment.	Progression in up to 50%. Postpartum regression in many.	Progression in up to 50%. Postpartum regression in some.	Tends to progress rapidly.
Eye exams	None.	First and third trimester.	Every trimester.	Monthly.	Monthly.
Treatment	None.	None	None, unless high-risk proliferative retinopathy develops.	None, unless high-risk proliferative retinopathy develops.	Treat PDR with PRP. Observe diabetic macular edema (high rate of spontaneous postpartum regression). Consider C-section to prevent VH due to Valsalva during labor. Not an indication to terminate pregnancy.

5. Diabetes and pregnancy. Changes that occur during pregnancy have a high likelihood of postpartum regression. See Table 11.12.1 for follow-up recommendations.

NOTE: The Diabetes Control and Complications Trial showed that strict control of blood sugar with insulin (in type 1 diabetes) decreases the progression of diabetic retinopathy, as well as nephropathy and neuropathy.

Bibliography

Diabetic Retinopathy Study Research Group. Photocoagulation treatment of proliferative diabetic retinopathy: Clinical application of Diabetic Retinopathy Study Research Group. *Arch Ophthalmol* 1979;97:654–655.

Early Treatment Diabetic Retinopathy Study Research Group. Treatment techniques and clinical guidelines for photocoagulation of diabetic macular edema. ETDRS report number 2. *Ophthalmology* 1987;94:761–774.

Early Treatment Diabetic Retinopathy Study Research Group. Early photocoagulation for diabetic retinopathy. ETDRS report number 9. *Ophthalmology* 1991;98:766–785.

Wilkinson CP, et al. Proposed international clinical diabetic retinopathy and diabetic macular edema disease severity scales. *Ophthalmology* 2003;110:1677–1682.

Nguyen QD, Shah SM, Khwaja AA, et al. Two-year outcomes of the ranibizumab for edema of the macula in diabetes (READ-2) study. *Ophthalmology* 2010;117:2146–51.

Elman MJ, Bressler NM, Qin H, et al. Expanded 2-Year Follow-up of Ranibizumab Plus Prompt or Deferred Laser or Triamcinolone Plus Prompt Laser for Diabetic Macular Edema. *Ophthalmology* 2011;118:609–14.

Mitchell P, Bandello F, Schmidt-Erfurth U, et al. The RESTORE Study Ranibizumab Monotherapy or Combined with Laser versus Laser Monotherapy for Diabetic Macular Edema. *Ophthalmology* 2011;118:615–25.

11

11.13   VITREOUS HEMORRHAGE

Symptoms

Sudden, painless loss of vision or sudden appearance of black spots, cobwebs, or haze in the vision.

Signs

(See Figure 11.13.1.)

Critical.   In a severe VH, the red fundus reflex may be absent, and there may be no view to the fundus. Red blood cells may be seen in the anterior vitreous. In a mild VH, there may be a partially obscured view to the fundus. Chronic VH has a yellow ochre appearance from hemoglobin breakdown.

Other.   A mild RAPD is possible in the setting of dense hemorrhage. Depending on the etiology, there may be other fundus abnormalities.

Differential Diagnosis

- Vitritis (white blood cells in the vitreous): Usually not sudden onset; anterior or posterior uveitis may also be present. No red blood cells are seen in the vitreous. See 12.3, *Posterior Uveitis.*

- Retinal detachment: May occur without a VH, but the symptoms may be identical. In VH due to RD, the peripheral retina is often obscured on indirect ophthalmoscopy. See 11.3, *Retinal Detachment.*

Etiology

- Diabetic retinopathy: Usually history of diabetes and usually diabetic retinopathy. Diabetic retinopathy is usually evident in the contralateral eye. In VH due to PDR, the peripheral retina is often visible on indirect ophthalmoscopy. See 11.12, *Diabetic Retinopathy.*

- PVD: Common in middle-aged or elderly patients. Usually patients note floaters and flashing lights. See 11.1, *Posterior Vitreous Detachment.*

- Retinal break: Commonly superior in cases of dense VH. This may be demonstrated by scleral depression and, if poor view, B-scan US. See 11.2, *Retinal Break.*

- Retinal detachment: May be diagnosed by B-scan US if the retina cannot be viewed on clinical examination. See 11.3, *Retinal Detachment.*

- Retinal vein occlusion (usually a BRVO): Commonly occurs in older patients with a history of high blood pressure. See 11.9, *Branch Retinal Vein Occlusion.*

- Exudative Age-Related Macular Degeneration (ARMD): Usually with a disciform scar or advanced choroidal neovascular membrane. Poor vision before the VH as a result of their underlying disease. Macular drusen and/or other findings of ARMD are found in the contralateral eye. B-scan US may aid in the diagnosis. See 11.17, *Neovascular or Exudative (Wet) Age-Related Macular Degeneration.*

- Sickle cell disease: May have peripheral retinal neovascularization in the contralateral eye, typically in a "sea-fan" configuration and salmon color. See 11.20, *Sickle Cell Disease (Including Sickle Cell Anemia, Sickle Trait).*

- Trauma: By history.

- Intraocular tumor: May be visible on ophthalmoscopy or B-scan US. See 5.13,

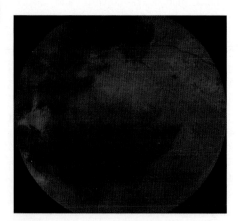

FIGURE 11.13.1.   Vitreous and preretinal hemorrhage due to proliferative diabetic retinopathy.

Malignant Melanoma of the Iris, and 11.36, *Choroidal Nevus and Malignant Melanoma of the Choroid.*

■ Subarachnoid or subdural hemorrhage (Terson syndrome): Frequently bilateral preretinal or VHs may occur. A severe headache usually precedes the fundus findings. Coma may occur.

■ Eales disease: Usually occurs in men aged 20 to 30 years with peripheral retinal ischemia and neovascularization of unknown etiology. Decreased vision as a result of VH is frequently the presenting sign. Typically bilateral. Diagnosis of exclusion.

■ Others: Ruptured arterial macroaneurysm, Coats disease, retinopathy of prematurity, retinal capillary angiomas of von Hippel–Lindau syndrome, congenital prepapillary vascular loop, retinal cavernous hemangioma, HTN, radiation retinopathy, anterior segment hemorrhage because of an intraocular lens, bleeding diathesis, hematologic malignancy, etc. See specific sections.

NOTE: In infancy and childhood, consider birth trauma, shaken baby syndrome, child abuse, congenital X-linked retinoschisis, pars planitis, bleeding dyscrasias, and hematologic malignancies.

Work-Up

1. History: Any ocular or systemic diseases, specifically the ones mentioned previously? Trauma?

2. Complete ocular examination, including slit-lamp examination with undilated pupils to check for iris neovascularization, IOP measurement, and dilated fundus examination of both eyes by using indirect ophthalmoscopy. In cases of spontaneous VH, scleral depression is performed if a retinal view can be obtained.

NOTE: We do not usually depress eyes until 2 weeks after traumatic hyphema/microhyphema.

---

3. When no retinal view can be obtained, B-scan US is performed to detect an associated RD or intraocular tumor. Flap retinal tears may be detected with scleral depression and sometimes can be seen on B-scan US (elevated flap).

4. IVFA may aid in defining the etiology, although the quality of the angiogram depends on the density of the hemorrhage. Additionally, it may be useful to highlight abnormalities in the contralateral eye.

Treatment

1. If the etiology of the VH is not known and a retinal break or an RD or both cannot be ruled out (i.e., there is no known history of one of the diseases mentioned previously, there are no changes in the contralateral eye, and the fundus is obscured by a total VH), the patient is monitored closely as an outpatient.

2. Bed rest with the head of the bed elevated for 2 to 3 days. This reduces the chance of recurrent bleeding and allows the blood to settle inferiorly, permitting a view of the superior peripheral fundus, a common site for responsible retinal breaks.

3. Eliminate aspirin, nonsteroidal anti-inflammatory drugs (NSAIDs), and other anticlotting agents unless they are medically necessary.

4. The underlying etiology is treated as soon as possible (e.g., retinal breaks are sealed with cryotherapy or laser photocoagulation, detached retinas are repaired, and proliferative retinal vascular diseases are treated with laser photocoagulation).

5. Surgical removal of the blood (vitrectomy) is usually performed for:

—VH accompanied by RD or RT on B-scan US.

—Nonclearing VH, usually persisting ≥3 to 6 months. However, two-thirds of patients with an idiopathic, fundus-obscuring hemorrhage will have retinal tears or an RD. Thus, early vitrectomy should be carefully considered.

—VH with neovascularization of the iris.

—Hemolytic or ghost cell glaucoma.

NOTE: Vitrectomy for isolated VH (e.g., without RD) may be considered earlier than 6 months for diabetic patients or those with bilateral VH, depending on their visual needs.

Follow-Up

The patient is evaluated daily for the first 2 to 3 days. If a total VH persists, and the etiology remains unknown, the patient is followed up with B-scan US every 1 to 3 weeks to rule out an RD.

11.14 CYSTOID MACULAR EDEMA

Symptoms

Decreased vision.

Signs

(See Figures 11.14.1 to 11.14.3.)

Critical. Irregularity and blunting of the foveal light reflex, thickening with or without small intraretinal cysts in the foveal region.

Other. Loss of the choroidal vascular pattern underlying the macula. Vitreous cells, optic nerve swelling, and dot hemorrhages can appear in severe cases. A lamellar macular hole causing permanent visual loss can develop.

Etiology

- Postoperative, following any ocular surgery, including laser photocoagulation and cryotherapy. The peak incidence of post-cataract extraction cystoid macular edema (CME), or Irvine–Gass, is approximately 6 to 10 weeks;

the incidence increases with surgical complications including vitreous loss, vitreous to the wound, and iris prolapse.

- Diabetic retinopathy: See 11.12, *Diabetic Retinopathy.*

- CRVO and BRVO: See 11.8, *Central Retinal Vein Occlusion,* and 11.9, *Branch Retinal Vein Occlusion.*

- Uveitis: Particularly pars planitis; see 12.2, *Intermediate Uveitis.*

- Retinitis pigmentosa (RP): See 11.28, *Retinitis Pigmentosa and Inherited Chorioretinal Dystrophies.*

- Topical drops: Epinephrine, dipivefrin, and prostaglandin analogs, especially in patients who have undergone cataract surgery.

- Retinal vasculitis: Eales disease, Behçet syndrome, sarcoidosis, necrotizing angiitis, multiple sclerosis, cytomegalovirus retinitis, others.

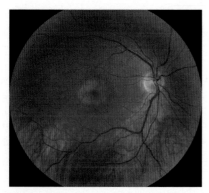

FIGURE 11.14.1. Cystoid macular edema.

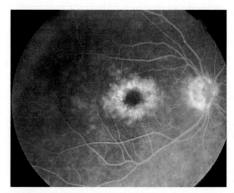

FIGURE 11.14.2. IVFA of cystoid macular edema.

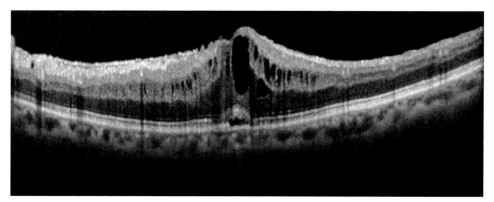

FIGURE 11.14.3. OCT of cystoid macular edema.

- Retinal telangiectasias: Coats disease, idiopathic macular telangiectasia, others.

- ARMD: See 11.16, *Nonexudative (Dry) Age-Related Macular Degeneration,* and 11.17, *Neovascular or Exudative (Wet) Age-Related Macular Degeneration.*

- Epiretinal membrane: See 11.26, *Epiretinal Membrane (Macular Pucker, Surface-Wrinkling Retinopathy, Cellophane Maculopathy).*

- Associated with other conditions: Occult inferior RRD, occult subfoveal CNV, others.

- Others: Intraocular tumors, systemic HTN, collagen–vascular disease, autosomal dominant CME, others.

- Pseudo-CME (no leakage on IVFA): Nicotinic acid maculopathy (typically seen only with relatively high doses of nicotinic acid), taxane drugs, X-linked retinoschisis (can see leakage with ICG), myopic foveal schisis, Goldmann–Favre disease (and other NR2E3-related retinopathies), pseudohole from an epiretinal membrane.

Work-Up

1. History: Recent intraocular surgery? Diabetes? Previous uveitis or ocular inflammation? Night blindness or family history of eye disease? Medications, including topical epinephrine, dipivefrin, or prostaglandin analogs?

2. Complete ocular examination, including a peripheral fundus evaluation (scleral depression inferiorly may be required to detect pars planitis). Macular examination is best performed with a slit lamp and a fundus contact lens, a Hruby lens, or a 60- or 90-diopter lens.

3. IVFA shows early leakage out of perifoveal capillaries and late macular staining, classically in a flower-petal or spoke-wheel pattern. Optic nerve head leakage is sometimes observed (Irvine–Gass syndrome). Fluorescein leakage does not occur in select cases of pseudo-CME (see above).

4. OCT can be utilized to document the presence of CME and demonstrate the efficacy of therapy. OCT outlines the loss of foveal contour resulting from cystic spaces within the retina.

5. Other diagnostic tests when indicated: Fasting blood sugar or glucose tolerance test, ERG, others.

NOTE: Subclinical CME commonly develops after cataract extraction and is noted on IVFA. These cases are not treated.

Treatment

Treat the underlying disorder if possible. For CME related to specific etiologies (e.g., diabetes, retinal vein occlusion, intermediate uveitis, etc.) see specific sections. Seventy percent of post-cataract CME cases resolve spontaneously within 6 months; treat if symptomatic with decreased vision.

1. Topical NSAID (e.g., ketorolac 0.5% q.i.d. for 3 months).

2. Discontinue topical epinephrine, dipivefrin, or prostaglandin analog drops and medications containing nicotinic acid.

3. Consider acetazolamide 500 mg p.o. q.d., especially for postoperative patients, but also for those with RP and uveitis.

4. Other forms of therapy that have unproven efficacy but are often used include:

   —Topical steroids (e.g., prednisolone acetate 1% q.i.d.); often used in combination with topical NSAID.

   —Subtenon steroid (e.g., triamcinolone 40 mg/mL, inject 0.5 to 1.0 mL).

   —Intravitreal steroid (e.g., triamcinolone 40 mg/mL, inject 0.05 to 0.1 mL).

—Intravitreal anti-VEGF therapy (e.g., bevacizumab 1.25 mg in 0.05 mL).

—Systemic steroids (e.g., prednisone 40 mg p.o. q.d. for 5 days and then taper over 2 weeks).

—Systemic NSAIDs (e.g., indomethacin 25 mg p.o. t.i.d. for 6 weeks).

—CME with or without vitreous incarceration in a surgical wound may be improved by vitrectomy or yttrium-aluminum garnet laser lysis of the vitreous strand.

Follow-Up

Postsurgical CME is not an emergency condition. Other forms of CME may require an etiologic work-up and may benefit from early treatment (e.g., elimination of nicotinic acid–containing medications).

11.15   CENTRAL SEROUS CHORIORETINOPATHY

Symptoms

Central scotoma, blurred or dim vision, objects appear distorted (metamorphopsia) and miniaturized (micropsia), colors appear washed out. Usually unilateral but 30% to 40% have evidence of bilateral disease (although may not be symptomatic at the same time). May be asymptomatic. Migraine-like headache may precede or accompany visual changes.

Signs

(See Figure 11.15.1.)

Critical. Localized serous detachment of the neurosensory retina in the region of the macula without subretinal blood or lipid exudates. The margins of the detachment are sloping and merge gradually into the attached retina.

Other. Visual acuity usually ranges from 20/20 to 20/80. Amsler grid testing reveals relative scotoma and distortion of straight lines. May see a small RAPD, a serous RPE detachment, deposition of subretinal fibrin. Focal

pigment epithelial irregularity may mark sites of previous episodes.

Differential Diagnosis

These entities may produce a serous detachment of the neurosensory retina in the macular area.

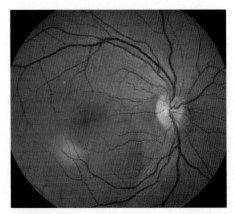

FIGURE 11.15.1. Central serous chorioretinopathy.

- ARMD: Patient usually ≥50 years old, drusen, pigment epithelial alterations, may have choroidal (subretinal) neovascularization, often bilateral. See 11.16, *Nonexudative (Dry) Age-Related Macular Degeneration,* and 11.17, *Neovascular or Exudative (Wet) Age-Related Macular Degeneration.*

- Optic pit: The optic disc has a small defect (a pit) in the nerve tissue. A serous RD may be present, contiguous with the optic disc. See 11.34, *Optic Pit.*

- Macular detachment as a result of an RRD or macular hole: In RRD, a hole in the retina can be found; see 11.3, *Retinal Detachment,* and 11.25, *Macular Hole.*

- Choroidal tumor: See 11.36, *Choroidal Nevus and Malignant Melanoma of the Choroid.*

- Hypertension: See 11.10, *Hypertensive Retinopathy.*

- Pigment epithelial detachment (PED): The margins of a PED are more distinct than those of CSCR, and the RPE is elevated. Occasionally, PED may accompany CSCR or ARMD.

- Others: Idiopathic choroidal effusion, inflammatory choroidal disorders, and chronic renal failure.

Etiology

- Idiopathic: Usually occurs in men aged 25 to 50 years. In women, CSCR typically occurs at a slightly older age and has an association with pregnancy. Increased incidence in patients with lupus.

- Increased endogenous cortisol: This helps explain a possible association with psychological or physiologic stress (type A personality). Rare cases exist with cortisol producing adrenal adenomas.

- Exogenous cortisol: Corticosteroid use, including nasal corticosteroid sprays and topical creams.

Work-Up

1. Amsler grid test to document the area of field involved. See Appendix 4, *Amsler Grid.*

2. Slit-lamp examination of the macula with a fundus contact, Hruby, or 60- or 90-diopter lens to rule out a concomitant CNV. In addition, search for an optic pit of the disc.

3. Dilated fundus examination with indirect ophthalmoscopy to rule out a choroidal tumor or RRD.

4. IVFA and ICG if the diagnosis is uncertain or presentation atypical, CNV is suspected, or laser treatment is to be considered. IVFA shows the nearly pathognomic "smokestack" pattern of dye leakage in 10% to 20% of cases. ICG shows choroidal artery and choriocapillaris filling delays and characteristic multifocal hyperfluorescent patches in the early phase. OCT can be helpful in demonstrating the subretinal or sub-RPE fluid and for monitoring purposes. Enhanced-depth imaging OCT often demonstrates choroidal thickening and may be a useful adjunct in diagnosis (see Figures 11.15.2 and 11.15.3).

5. In cases of chronic CSCR, a systemic work-up including cortisol levels and renal function should be considered.

Treatment

1. Observation: Prognosis for spontaneous recovery of visual acuity to at least 20/30 is excellent. Worse prognosis for patients with recurrent disease, multiple areas of detachment, or prolonged course.

2. Laser therapy: Accelerates visual recovery. Does not improve final visual outcome.

11

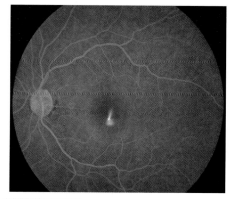

FIGURE 11.15.2. IVFA of CSCR showing "smokestack" pattern of dye leakage.

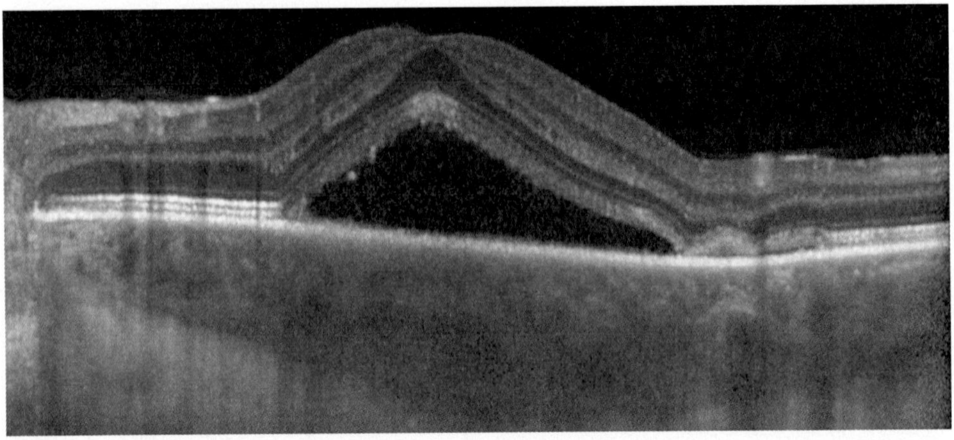

FIGURE 11.15.3. Enhanced-depth imaging OCT of CSCR showing subretinal fluid and choroidal thickening.

May increase risk of CNV formation. Given the CNV risk, use low laser intensity. Consider laser for:

—Persistence of a serous detachment for several months.

—Recurrence of the condition in an eye that sustained a permanent visual deficit from a previous episode.

—Occurrence in the contralateral eye after a permanent visual deficit resulted from a previous episode.

—Patient requires prompt restoration of vision (e.g., occupational necessity).

3. Stop steroids, if possible, including topical skin preparations and nasal sprays.

4. If CNV develops, consider anti-VEGF therapy.

5. Chronic CSCR may respond to treatment with photodynamic therapy (PDT).

Follow-Up

1. Examine patients every 6 to 8 weeks until resolution.

11.16 NONEXUDATIVE (DRY) AGE-RELATED MACULAR DEGENERATION

Symptoms

Gradual loss of central vision, Amsler grid changes; may be asymptomatic.

Signs

(See Figures 11.16.1 and 11.16.2.)

Critical. Macular drusen, clumps of pigment in the outer retina, and RPE atrophy, almost always in both eyes.

Other. Confluent retinal and choriocapillaris atrophy (e.g., geographic atrophy), dystrophic calcification.

Differential Diagnosis

■ Peripheral drusen: Drusen only located outside of the macular area.

■ Myopic degeneration: Characteristic peripapillary changes and macular changes without drusen. See 11.22, *High Myopia.*

■ CSCR: Parafoveal serous retinal elevation, RPE detachments, and mottled RPE atrophy, without drusen, usually in patients <50 years of age. See 11.15, *Central Serous Chorioretinopathy.*

■ Inherited central retinal dystrophies: Stargardt disease, pattern dystrophy, Best disease, others. Variable macular pigmentary changes, atrophy, or accumulation of lipofuscin or a combination of these. Usually <50 years, without drusen, familial occurrence. See specific entities.

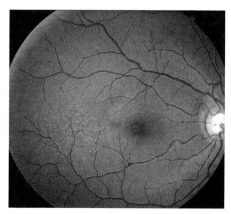

FIGURE 11.16.1. Dry ARMD with fine drusen.

■ Toxic retinopathies: e.g., chloroquine toxicity. Mottled hypopigmentation with ring of hyperpigmentation (bull's-eye maculopathy) without drusen. Possible history of drug ingestion or exposure.

■ Inflammatory maculopathies: Multifocal choroiditis, rubella, serpiginous choroidopathy, and others. Variable chorioretinal atrophy, often with vitreous cells and without drusen. See specific entities.

Work-Up

1. History: Presence of risk factors (e.g., family history, smoking, obesity, HTN, hypercholesterolemia)? See risk factors for loss of vision, 11.17, *Neovascular or Exudative (Wet) Age-Related Macular Degeneration.*

2. Amsler grid to document or detect a central or paracentral scotoma. See Appendix 4, *Amsler Grid.*

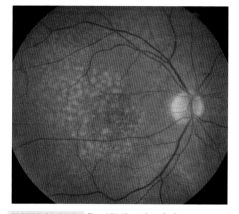

FIGURE 11.16.2. Dry ARMD with soft drusen.

3. Macular examination with a 60- or 90-diopter or a fundus contact lens: Look for risk factors for conversion to the exudative form, such as soft drusen or pigment clumping. Look for signs of the exudative form (disappearance of drusen may herald the development of CNV).

4. Baseline and periodic fundus autofluorecsence may be useful to monitor for progression.

5. IVFA or OCT when exudative ARMD cannot be ruled out clinically, when RPE detachment is present, or when visual acuity has declined rapidly to rule out CNV. Drusen and RPE atrophy are often more visible on IVFA.

Treatment

1. People with intermediate dry ARMD [one large druse (125 microns) and/or ≥20 medium drusen (63 to 125 microns)], or advanced dry or exudative ARMD in one eye but not the other eye, are at high risk for the development of advanced stages of ARMD. Per the Age-Related Eye Disease Study (AREDS) report, treatment with a high-dose combination of vitamin C (500 mg), vitamin E (400 IU), beta-carotene (15 mg), zinc (80 mg), and cupric oxide (5 mg) reduces the risk of progression to advanced ARMD by approximately 25% over 5 years and reduces the risk of vision loss caused by advanced ARMD by approximately 19% by 5 years.

NOTE: Beta-carotene should be withheld in past or present smokers because of increased risk of lung cancer. A formulation of the AREDS vitamins without beta-carotene for current or past smokers is available.

In addition, recommend consumption of green leafy vegetables if approved by primary care physician (intake of vitamin K decreases effectiveness of warfarin) and fish/fish oils containing high levels of omega-3 fatty acids..

2. Low-vision aids may benefit some patients with bilateral loss of macular function.

3. Refer to an internist for management of presumed risk factors: HTN, hypercholesterolemia, smoking cessation, etc.

4. Certain genetic mutations confer an increased risk for ARMD (e.g., Y402H mutation of the

11

complement factor H gene) and may influ-ence response to treatment. Genetic screening in ARMD patients is not routinely performed.

Follow-Up

Every 6 to 12 months, watching for signs of the exudative form. Daily use of Amsler grid with instructions to return promptly if a change is noted.

Bibliography

Age-Related Eye Disease Study Research Group. A randomized, placebo-controlled, clinical trial of high-dose supplementation with vitamins C and E, beta-carotene, and zinc for age-related macular degeneration and vision loss: AREDS report no. 8. *Arch Ophthalmol* 2001;119:1417–1436.

11.17 NEOVASCULAR OR EXUDATIVE (WET) AGE-RELATED MACULAR DEGENERATION

Symptoms

Variable onset of central visual loss, central or paracentral scotoma, metamorphopsia, photopsias in the central visual field.

Signs

(See Figures 11.17.1 and 11.17.2.)

Critical. Drusen and subretinal fluid or RPE detachment associated with CNV.

Other. Sub-, intra-, and/or pre-retinal blood. Retinal exudates, RPE loss, subretinal fibrosis (disciform scar). Retinal angiomatous prolifera-tion (RAP) may precede or follow the develop-ment of CNV and is characterized by focal telangiectatic retinal vessels with an adjacent superficial retinal hemorrhage and associated intraretinal edema and RPE detachment. Some neovascular ARMD patients may present with VH.

Risk Factors for Loss of Vision

Advanced age, hyperopia, blue eyes, family history, soft (large) drusen, focal subretinal pigment clumping, RPE detachments, sys-temic HTN, and smoking. Note that patients with wet ARMD in one eye have a 10% to 12% risk per year of developing a CNV in the fellow eye. The risk increases for eyes with multiple or confluent soft drusen with RPE clumping.

Differential Diagnosis

- Ocular histoplasmosis syndrome: Small white-yellow chorioretinal scars and

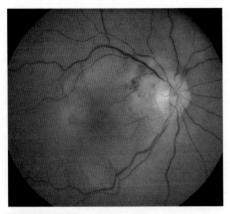

FIGURE 11.17.1. Exudative ARMD.

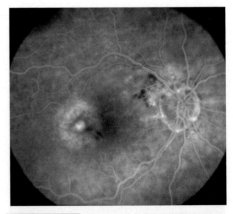

FIGURE 11.17.2. IVFA of exudative ARMD.

peripapillary atrophy. May also present with CNV. See 11.24, *Ocular Histoplasmosis.*

■ Angioid streaks: Bilateral subretinal red-brown or gray irregular bands often radiating from the optic disc. See 11.23, *Angioid Streaks.*

■ High myopia: Significant myopic refractive error, lacquer cracks, tilted disc. See 11.22, *High Myopia.*

■ Idiopathic polypoidal choroidal vasculopathy (IPCV): Multiple serosanguineous macular and RPE detachments. ICG angiography highlights characteristic polyplike aneurysmal dilations. Prognosis is more favorable than for exudative ARMD. See 11.18, *Idiopathic Polypoidal Choroidal Vasculopathy (Posterior Uveal Bleeding Syndrome).*

■ Other CNV-predisposing conditions include drusen of the optic nerve, choroidal rupture, choroidal tumors, photocoagulation scars, inflammatory focal chorioretinal spots, and idiopathic causes.

Types of Neovascular ARMD Lesions

■ Classic CNV: Early-phase IVFA demonstrates a well-delineated area of lacy hyperfluorescence with prominent leakage in later phases.

■ Occult CNV: Ill defined, stippled, flat, or elevated subtle late leakage.

■ RAP: Focal intraretinal hyperfluorescence on IVFA and ICGA. High-speed ICGA is particularly sensitive and may show characteristic "hair pin loop" with retinal feeder and draining vessels.

Work-Up

1. Slit-lamp biomicroscopy with a 60-, 78-, or 90-diopter, or fundus contact lens to detect CNV and associated exudation. Must examine both eyes.

2. Perform IVFA if CNV is suspected. IVFA is useful to confirm neovascular ARMD and specifically determine the size, type, and location of CNV, and monitor treatment response.

3. OCT is helpful in determining retinal thickness, CNV thickness, and extent of ME, SRF and RPE detachment. OCT is the primary modality for following response to treatment.

4. ICGA may help delineate the borders of certain obscured occult CNV, particularly with subretinal blood or exudation. It also shows RAP and IPCV lesions better than IVFA.

Treatment

Subfoveal CNV

—Ranibizumab: Anti-VEGF antibody fragment injected intravitreally that is FDA approved for all subfoveal CNV subtypes. The optimal dosing regimen has yet to be determined. In the original phase 3 efficacy trials (MARINA and ANCHOR), ranibizumab was given monthly to patients with close to 40% of patients in both studies gaining three or more lines of visual acuity at 1 year. While the best visual results may occur with monthly dosing, prn dosing using OCT guidance (PrONTO study) had similar 1 year visual results with half the number of injections.

—Aflibercept: Anti-VEGF fusion protein that binds all isoforms of VEGF-A and placental growth factor that is injected intravitreally and is FDA approved for the treatment of neovascular ARMD. The optimal dosing regimen has yet to be determined, but phase 3 studies showed similar efficacy at one year to monthly intravitreal ranibizumab with aflibercept dosed q8weeks after a 12 week monthly induction phase.

—Bevacizumab: Full-length anti-VEGF antibody. FDA approved for colon cancer. Off-label use as intravitreal injection at a dose of 1.25 mg is effective in treating all types of neovascular ARMD. It is cost-effective and commonly used in place of ranibizumab. The Comparison of Age-related macular degeneration Treatments Trial (CATT) study demonstrated the non-inferiority of bevacizumab as compared to ranibizumab at 1 year, when monthly or prn dosing was used.

—Pegaptanib: Anti-VEGF aptamer injected intravitreally every 6 weeks for 1 to 2 years. FDA approved for all subfoveal CNV subtypes. Pegaptanib reduces the risk of vision loss, but rarely improves visual acuity. Rarely used.

11

—PDT: FDA approved intravenous infusion of photosensitizing dye (verteporfin) followed by nondestructive (cold) laser application to activate the dye within the CNV. PDT can be performed as often as every 3 months for 1 to 2 years. Small, classic subfoveal CNV responds best, but small occult or minimally classic subfoveal CNV may also respond. PDT decreases vision loss, but does not improve vision as monotherapy. It is rarely used.

Nonsubfoveal CNV

—Anti-VEGF agents are the treatment of choice for nonsubfoveal CNV. See above for details.

—Thermal laser photocoagulation: Results are best for extrafoveal CNV (≥200 μm from fovea). Laser photocoagulation treatment is complicated by high CNV recurrence rates. Rarely used.

Follow-Up

Depends on the treatment algorithm used, but typically monthly follow up until the CNV lesion is inactive based on IVFA and/or OCT. Patients receiving anti-VEGF therapy need indefinite follow up, though the follow up frequency depends on treatment response and treatment algorithm.

Patients receiving intravitreal injections should be given warning symptoms for endophthalmitis and RD.

Bibliography

Rosenfeld PJ, Brown DM, Heier JS, et al. Ranibizumab for neovascular age-related macular degeneration. *N Engl J Med* 2006;355:1419–1431.

Brown DM, Kaiser PK, Michels M, et al. Ranibizumab versus verteporfin for neovascular age-related macular degeneration. *N Engl J Med* 2006;355:1432–1444.

Lalwani GA, Rosenfeld PJ, Fung AE, et al. A variable-dosing regimen with intravitreal ranibizumab for neovascular age-related macular degeneration: year 2 of the PrONTO Study. *Am J Ophthalmol* 2009;148(1):43–58.

The CATT Research Group, Martin DF, Maguire MG, Ying GS, Grunwald JE, Fine SL, Jaffe GJ. Ranibizumab and bevacizumab for neovascular age-related macular degeneration. *NEJM* 2011;364:1897–908.

Bayer and Regeneron Report Positive Top-Line Results of Two Phase 3 Studies with VEGF Trap-Eye in Wet Age-related Macular Degeneration. November 22, 2010. (Accessed December 1, 2010, at http://newsroom.regeneron.com/releasedetail.cfm?ReleaseID=532099.)

11.18 IDIOPATHIC POLYPOIDAL CHOROIDAL VASCULOPATHY (POSTERIOR UVEAL BLEEDING SYNDROME)

Symptoms

Decreased central vision; may be sudden or gradual.

Signs

Critical. Subretinal red-orange, polyp-like lesions of the choroidal vasculature. Can be macular (more symptomatic) or peripapillary.

Other. Subretinal and/or sub-RPE blood, VH, circinate subretinal exudates, subretinal fibrosis (disciform scar), subretinal fluid, atypical CNV, and multiple serous PEDs.

Risk Factors

More common in females, individuals of African or Asian descent, and in patients with HTN. Can occur at a younger age compared with neovascular ARMD without significant drusen or geographic atrophy.

Differential Diagnosis

- See 11.17, *Neovascular or Exudative (Wet) Age-Related Macular Degeneration.*

- See 11.19, *Retinal Arterial Macroaneurysm.*

- Peripheral exudative hemorrhagic chorio-retinopathy [PEHCR (extramacular degeneration)]: This is the peripheral form of ARMD and affects the ora serrata region with RPE atrophy, RPE detachment, subretinal blood, and exudation.

Work-Up

1. Slit-lamp biomicroscopy with a 60-, 90-diopter, or fundus contact lens to detect signs of exudation.

2. IVFA is performed to rule out other causes of CNV.

3. OCT is used to assess ME, subretinal fluid, and the presence of any PEDs.

4. ICG may confirm the presence of a branching network of vessels arising from the inner choroidal circulation with terminal aneurysmal dilations (popcorn lesions). Unlike occult CNV, the IPCV lesions do not stain late unless active leakage is present.

Treatment

Asymptomatic lesions may be observed. Many resolve spontaneously. IPCV with severe recurrent exudation and/or hemorrhagic complications has been treated with anti-VEGF agents, thermal laser photocoagulation, PDT, feeder vessel treatment, submacular surgery, macular translocation, steroid injection, and pneumatic displacement of large submacular hemorrhage.

Follow-Up

The prognosis of IPCV is generally better than for neovascular ARMD. Symptomatic or macular IPCV is followed every 1 to 2 months with repeat OCT, IVFA, and ICG as needed for new developments. Consider treatment or retreatment if symptomatic persistent or new leakage can be demonstrated.

11.19 RETINAL ARTERIAL MACROANEURYSM

Symptoms

Decreased vision; history of systemic HTN. Usually unilateral, but 10% bilateral.

Signs

(See Figures 11.19.1 and 11.19.2.)

Critical. Acute hemorrhages in multiple layers of the retina (subretinal, intraretinal, subinternal limiting membrane) and VH often with a white or yellow spot in the middle, which is probably fibrin. Chronic leakage may manifest as a ring of hard exudates and retinal edema

11

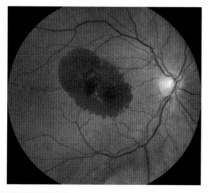

FIGURE 11.19.1. Retinal artery macroaneurysm on presentation.

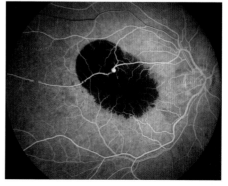

FIGURE 11.19.2. IVFA of a retinal artery macroaneurysm.

around the aneurysm resulting in decreased vision if the macula is involved.

Other. ME, arteriolar emboli, capillary telangiectasia, arterial or venous occlusions distal to macroaneurysm.

Differential Diagnosis

■ Coats disease: Unilateral retinal vascular telangiectasias. Extensive yellow intraretinal and subretinal exudates. Hemorrhages not typical. See 8.1, *Leukocoria.*

■ Idiopathic retinal vasculitis, aneurysms, and neuroretinitis (IRVAN): A syndrome characterized by retinal vasculitis, multiple arterial macroaneurysms, neuroretinitis, and peripheral capillary nonperfusion.

■ Diabetic retinopathy: Hemorrhages are not subretinal. See 11.12, *Diabetic Retinopathy.*

■ Valsalva retinopathy: No associated hard exudates. See 11.21, *Valsalva Retinopathy.*

■ Retinal telangiectasias: Juxtafoveal or parafoveal retinal telangiectasias cause hard exudates often in a circinate pattern usually temporal to macula. High association with diabetes.

■ Others: Retinal capillary hemangioma (hemangioblastoma), retinal cavernous hemangioma, choroidal melanoma, hemorrhagic RPE detachment seen in ARMD, IPCV, etc.

Etiology

Acquired vascular dilation of retinal artery or arteriole usually at site of arteriolar bifurcation or arteriovenous crossing. Usually related to systemic HTN and general arteriosclerotic disease.

Work-Up

1. History: Systemic disease, particularly HTN or diabetes?

2. Complete ocular examination with dilated retinal examination with a 60- or 90-diopter lens and indirect ophthalmoscopy. Look for concurrent retinal venous obstruction, present in one-third of cases and signs of hypertensive retinopathy (visible in fellow eye as well).

3. Check the blood pressure.

4. Consider checking fasting or random blood sugar and lipid panel.

5. IVFA may demonstrate early hyperfluorescence if there is no blockage from hemorrhage. Late frames may show leakage or staining of vessel wall.

6. OCT is helpful in demonstrating and following any ME that may be present.

Treatment

Bleeding is typically not treated since it usually only occurs once secondary to thrombosis and spontaneous involution. Consider laser treatment if edema and/or exudate threatens central vision. Caution must be taken when treating arterioles that supply the central macula since distal thrombosis and obstruction can occur. Laser can also cause aneurysmal rupture resulting in retinal and vitreous hemorrhage.

Follow-Up

Frequency based on the amount and location of exudate and hemorrhage.

11.20 SICKLE CELL DISEASE (INCLUDING SICKLE CELL ANEMIA, SICKLE TRAIT)

Symptoms

Usually without ocular symptoms. Floaters, flashing lights, or loss of vision with advanced disease. Systemically, patients often have painful crises with severe abdominal or musculoskeletal discomfort. Patients are of African or Mediterranean descent in most cases.

Signs

(See Figure 11.20.1.)

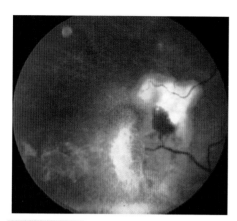

FIGURE 11.20.1. Sickle cell retinopathy neovascular sea-fan with associated vitreous hemorrhage.

Critical. Peripheral retinal neovascularization in the shape of a fan ("sea-fan sign"), sclerosed peripheral retinal vessels, or a dull gray peripheral fundus background color as a result of peripheral arteriolar occlusions and ischemia.

Other. Venous tortuosity, mid-peripheral fundus pigmented lesions with spiculated borders (black sunbursts), superficial intra-retinal hemorrhages (salmon patch), refractile (iridescent) intraretinal deposits following hemorrhage resorption, angioid streaks, comma-shaped capillaries of the conjunctiva (especially along the inferior fornix). VH and traction bands, RD, CRAO, macular arteriolar occlusions, and enlargement of the foveal avascular zone occasionally develop.

Staging

- Stage 1: Peripheral arteriolar occlusions.
- Stage 2: Peripheral arteriovenous anastomoses.
- Stage 3: Neovascular proliferation.
- Stage 4: Vitreous hemorrhage.
- Stage 5: Retinal detachment.

Differential Diagnosis of Peripheral Retinal Neovascularization

- Sarcoidosis: Peripheral sea-fan neovascularization often associated with uveitis.

Increased frequency in young patients of African descent. See 12.6, *Sarcoidosis.*

- Diabetic retinopathy: Posterior pathology more prominent. Associated dot-blot hemorrhages. See 11.12, *Diabetic Retinopathy.*

- Embolic (e.g., talc) retinopathy: History of intravenous drug abuse. May see refractile talc particles in the macular arterioles. See 11.33, *Crystalline Retinopathy.*

- Eales disease: Peripheral retinal vascular occlusion of unknown etiology; a diagnosis of exclusion.

- Others: Retinopathy of prematurity, FEVR, chronic myelogenous leukemia, radiation retinopathy, pars planitis, carotid–cavernous fistula, ocular ischemic syndrome OLS, collagen–vascular disease, hypercoagulable state. See specific sections.

Work-Up

1. Medical history and family history: Sickle cell disease, diabetes, or known medical problems? intravenous drug abuse?

2. Dilated fundus examination using indirect ophthalmoscopy.

3. Sickledex, sickle cell preparation, and hemoglobin electrophoresis.

NOTE: Patients with sickle cell trait, as well as hemoglobin C disease, may have a negative Sickledex preparation.

---

4. Consider IVFA to aid in diagnostic and therapeutic considerations. Rarely necessary.

Treatment

There are no well-established indications or guidelines for treatment. Isolated retinal neovascularization is not an indication. Neovascularization with associated VH is an indication for PRP to the avascular area anterior to the neovascularization. Retinal detachment and VH may be best treated with vitrectomy. Anti-VEGF agents may be beneficial, but caution should be used in cases of significant traction.

11

Follow-Up

1. No retinopathy: Annual dilated fundus examinations.

2. Retinopathy present: Repeat dilated fundus examination every 3 to 6 months, depending on severity.

11.21   VALSALVA RETINOPATHY

Symptoms

Decreased vision or asymptomatic. History of Valsalva maneuver (forceful exhalation against a closed glottis), which may occur during heavy lifting, coughing, vomiting, constipation, straining. Sometimes no history of Valsalva can be elicited.

Signs

(See Figure 11.21.1.)

Critical. Single or multiple hemorrhage(s) under the internal limiting membrane (ILM) in the area of the macula. Can be unilateral or bilateral. Blood may turn yellow after a few days.

Other. Vitreous and subretinal hemorrhage can occur, as well as subconjunctival hemorrhage.

Differential Diagnosis

- PVD: Can cause VH acutely as well as peripheral retinal and disc margin hemorrhages.

However, typically no sub-ILM hemorrhage. See 11.1, *Posterior Vitreous Detachment.*

- Retinal arterial macroaneurysm: Hemorrhages in multiple layers of the retina and vitreous. Can also have a circinate ring of hard exudates around a macroaneurysm. See 11.19, *Retinal Arterial Macroaneurysm.*

- Diabetic retinopathy: Microaneurysms, dot-blot hemorrhages, and hard exudates bilaterally, not isolated sub-ILM hemorrhage. Both can cause VH. See 11.12, *Diabetic Retinopathy.*

- CRVO or BRVO: Unilateral, multiple intraretinal hemorrhages, venous dilation, and tortuosity. See 11.8, *Central Retinal Vein Occlusion,* and 11.9, *Branch Retinal Vein Occlusion.*

- Anemia or leukemia: May have multiple, bilateral flame and dot-blot hemorrhages as well as cotton-wool spots. Can also present with sub-ILM hemorrhage.

- Retinal tear: Can be surrounded by hemorrhage obscuring the tear. Tears rarely occur in the macula.

Etiology

Valsalva causes sudden increase in intraocular venous pressure leading to rupture of superficial capillaries in macula. May be associated with anticoagulant therapy.

Work-Up

1. History: History of Valsalva including any recent heavy lifting, straining while constipated, coughing, sneezing, vomiting, etc.? The patient may not remember the incident.

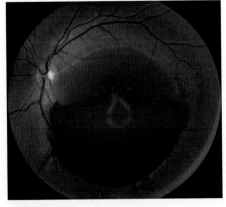

FIGURE 11.21.1. Valsalva retinopathy.

2. Complete ocular examination, including dilated retinal examination with a slit lamp and a 60- or 90-diopter lens, and indirect ophthalmoscopy. Look for findings suggestive of a different etiology including microaneurysms, dot-blot hemorrhages, cotton-wool spots, retinal tear, PVD.

3. If dense VH is present, then obtain B-scan US to rule out a retinal tear or detachment.

4. IVFA may be helpful to rule out other causes including retinal arterial macroaneurysm or diabetic retinopathy.

Treatment

Prognosis is excellent. Most patients are observed as sub-ILM hemorrhage usually resolves after a few days to weeks. Occasionally laser is used to permit the blood to drain into the vitreous cavity thereby uncovering the macula. Vitrectomy rarely considered, typically only for non-clearing VH.

Follow-Up

May follow-up every 2 weeks for the initial visits to monitor for resolution, then follow-up routinely.

11.22   HIGH MYOPIA

Symptoms

Decreased vision, usually does not progress until the fifth decade of life.

Signs

(See Figure 11.22.1.)

Critical. Myopic crescent (a crescent-shaped area of white sclera or choroidal vessels adjacent to the disc, separated from the normal-appearing fundus by a hyperpigmented line); an oblique (tilted) insertion of the optic disc, with or without vertical elongation; macular pigmentary abnormalities; a hyperpigmented spot in the macula (Fuchs spot); typically, a refractive correction of more than −6.00 to −8.00 diopters, axial length ≥26 mm.

Other. Temporal optic disc pallor, posterior staphyloma, entrance of the retinal vessels into the nasal part of the optic cup, the retina and choroid may be seen to extend over the nasal border of the optic disc, well-circumscribed areas of atrophy, spots of subretinal hemorrhage, choroidal sclerosis, yellow subretinal streaks (lacquer cracks), peripheral retinal thinning, lattice degeneration. Risk for CNV or RRD. Visual field defects may be present.

Differential Diagnosis

- ARMD: May develop CNV and a similar macular appearance, but typically drusen are present, and the myopic disc features are absent. See 11.16, *Nonexudative (Dry) Age-Related Macular Degeneration,* and 11.17, *Neovascular or Exudative (Wet) Age-Related Macular Degeneration.*

- Ocular histoplasmosis: Peripapillary atrophy with risk for CNV. A pigmented ring may separate the disc from the peripapillary atrophy, as opposed to pigmented ring separating the atrophic area from the adjacent retina. Round choroidal scars (punched-out lesions) are scattered throughout the fundus. See 11.24, *Ocular Histoplasmosis.*

- Tilted discs: Anomalous discs with a scleral crescent, most often inferonasally, an

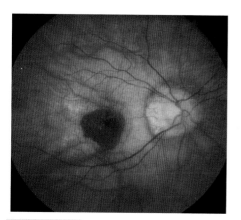

FIGURE 11.22.1. High myopia with macular hemorrhage.

11

irregular vascular pattern as the vessels emerge from the disc (situs inversus), and an area of fundus ectasia in the direction of the tilt (inferonasally). Many patients have myopia and astigmatism but no chorioretinal degeneration or lacquer cracks. Visual field defects corresponding to the areas of fundus ectasia are often seen. Most cases are bilateral.

▪ Gyrate atrophy: Rare. Multiple, well-demarcated areas of chorioretinal atrophy beginning in the mid-periphery in childhood and then coalescing to involve a large portion of the fundus. Increased blood levels of ornithine. Patients are often highly myopic. See 11.28, *Retinitis Pigmentosa and Inherited Chorioretinal Dystrophies.*

▪ Toxoplasmosis: Well-circumscribed chorioretinal scar that does not typically develop CNV; active disease shows retinitis and vitritis. See 12.5, *Toxoplasmosis.*

Work-Up

1. Manifest and/or cycloplegic refraction.

2. IOP measurement by applanation tonometry (Schiøtz tonometry may underestimate IOP in highly myopic eyes).

3. Dilated retinal examination with indirect ophthalmoscopy to search for retinal breaks or detachment. Scleral depression may be helpful but should be performed with care over a staphyloma.

4. Slit-lamp and fundus contact, or 60- or 90-diopter lens examination of the macula, searching for CNV (gray or green lesion beneath the retina, subretinal blood or exudate, or SRF).

5. IVFA for suspected CNV.

6. OCT can reveal macular detachment over a staphyloma. Additionally, OCT can be useful in identifying foveal schisis, a possible cause of vision loss in patients with high myopia.

Treatment

1. Symptomatic retinal breaks are treated with laser photocoagulation, cryotherapy, or scleral buckling surgery. Treatment of asymptomatic retinal breaks may be considered when there is no surrounding pigmentation or demarcation line.

2. Anti-VEGF agents are used for all CNV subtypes associated with high myopia. Laser photocoagulation therapy may be considered for extrafoveal or juxtafoveal CNV within several days of obtaining an IVFA. PDT may also be considered, but, like laser photocoagulation, is rarely used. See 11.17, *Neovascular or Exudative (Wet) Age-Related Macular Degeneration.*

3. For glaucoma suspects, a single visual field often cannot distinguish myopic visual field loss from early glaucoma. Progression of visual field loss in the absence of progressive myopia, however, suggests the presence of glaucoma and the need for therapy. See 9.1, *Primary Open-Angle Glaucoma.*

4. Recommend one-piece polycarbonate safety goggles for sports because of increased risk of choroidal rupture from minor trauma.

Follow-Up

In the absence of complications, reexamine every 6 to 12 months, watching for the related disorders discussed earlier.

11.23 ANGIOID STREAKS

Symptoms

Usually asymptomatic; decreased vision may result from CNV.

Signs

(See Figure 11.23.1.)

Critical. Bilateral reddish-brown or gray bands located deep to the retina, usually radiating in an irregular or spokelike pattern from the optic disc. CNV may occur.

Other. Mottled fundus appearance (peau d'orange), most common in the temporal

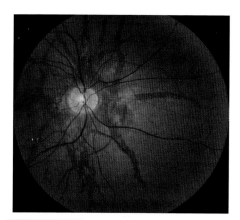

FIGURE 11.23.1. Angioid streaks.

mid-periphery; subretinal hemorrhages after mild blunt trauma; reticular pigmentary changes in the macula; small, white, pinpoint chorioretinal scars (histo-like spots) in the mid-periphery; drusen of the optic disc [especially with pseudoxanthoma elasticum (PXE)]; granular pattern of hyperfluorescent lines on IVFA.

Differential Diagnosis

- Lacquer cracks of myopic chorioretinal degeneration: High myopia present. See 11.22, *High Myopia*.

- Choroidal rupture: Subretinal streaks are usually concentric to the optic disc, yellow-white in color. See 3.17, *Traumatic Choroidal Rupture*.

Etiology

Fifty percent of cases are associated with systemic diseases; the remainder are idiopathic.

- PXE: Most common. Loose skin folds in the neck, axillae, and on flexor aspects of joints, cardiovascular complications, increased risk of gastrointestinal bleeds.

- Ehlers–Danlos syndrome: Hyperelasticity of skin, loose joints.

- Paget disease of bone: Enlarged skull, bone pain, history of bone fractures, hearing loss, possible cardiovascular complications. May be asymptomatic. Increased serum alkaline phosphatase and urine calcium.

Ten percent develop angioid streaks late; may develop visual loss due to optic nerve compression by enlarging bone.

- Sickle cell disease: May be asymptomatic or have decreased vision from fundus abnormalities. May have a history of recurrent infections and painless or painful crises. See 11.20, *Sickle Cell Disease (Including Sickle Cell Anemia, Sickle Trait)*.

- Less common: Acromegaly, senile elastosis, lead poisoning, Marfan syndrome, and others.

Work-Up

1. History: Any known systemic disorders? Previous ocular trauma?

2. Complete ocular examination: Look carefully at the macula with a slit lamp and a 60- or 90-diopter, or a fundus contact lens to detect CNV.

3. IVFA if diagnosis uncertain or CNV suspected.

4. Physical examination: Look for clinical signs of etiologic diseases.

5. Serum alkaline phosphatase and urine calcium levels if Paget disease of bone is suspected.

6. Sickle cell preparation and hemoglobin electrophoresis in patients of African descent.

7. Skin or scar biopsy if PXE is suspected.

Treatment

1. Anti-VEGF therapy is now used for angioid streak-associated CNV, as focal laser photocoagulation and PDT have disappointing outcomes. See 11.17, *Neovascular or Exudative (Wet) Age-Related Macular Degeneration*.

2. Management of any underlying systemic disease, if present, by an internist.

3. Recommend wearing one-piece polycarbonate safety glasses for sports because there is an increased risk of subretinal hemorrhage and choroidal rupture from minor trauma.

11

Follow-Up

1. Fundus examination every 6 months, monitoring for CNV.

2. Instruct patient to check Amsler grid daily and return immediately if changes are noted. See Appendix 4, *Amsler Grid*.

11.24   OCULAR HISTOPLASMOSIS

Symptoms

Most often asymptomatic; can present with decreased or distorted vision, especially when CNV develops. Patients often have lived in or visited the Ohio–Mississippi River Valley or areas where histoplasmosis is endemic. Usually in the 20- to 50-year age range.

Signs

(See Figure 11.24.1.)

Critical.   Classic triad. Need two of the three to make the diagnosis:

1. Yellow-white, punched-out round spots usually <1 mm in diameter, deep to the retina in any fundus location (histo-spots). Pigment clumps in or at the margin of the spots may be seen.

2. A macular CNV appearing as a gray–green patch beneath the retina, associated with detachment of the sensory retina, subretinal blood or exudate, or a pigment ring evolving into a disciform scar.

3. Peripapillary atrophy or scarring, sometimes with nodules or hemorrhage. There may be a rim of pigment separating the disc from the area of atrophy or scarring.

Other.   Linear rows of small histo-spots in the peripheral fundus. No vitreous or aqueous cells.

Differential Diagnosis

- High myopia: May have atrophic spots in the posterior pole and a myopic crescent on the temporal side of the disc with a rim of pigment on the outer (not inner) edge, separating the crescent from the retina. Atrophic spots are whiter than histo-spots and are not seen beyond the posterior pole. See 11.22, *High Myopia*.

- ARMD: Macular changes may appear similar, but typically there are macular drusen and patients are ≥50 years of age. There are no atrophic round spots similar to histoplasmosis and no scarring or atrophy around the disc. See 11.16, *Nonexudative (Dry)*

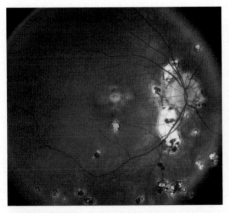 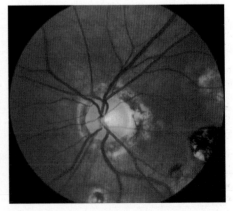

FIGURE 11.24.1. Ocular histoplasmosis.

Age-Related Macular Degeneration, and 11.17, *Neovascular or Exudative (Wet) Age-Related Macular Degeneration.*

■ Old toxoplasmosis: White chorioretinal lesion with vitreous and sometimes aqueous cells. See 12.5, *Toxoplasmosis.*

■ Angioid streaks: Histo-like spots in the mid-periphery and macular degeneration may occur. Jagged red, brown, or gray lines deep to the retinal vessels and radiating from the optic disc. See 11.23, *Angioid Streaks.*

■ Multifocal choroiditis with panuveitis: Similar clinical findings, except anterior or vitreous inflammatory cells or both are also present. See 12.3, *Posterior Uveitis.*

■ Multiple evanescent white dot syndrome (MEWDS): Multiple, creamy white lesions at the level of the outer retina or the RPE with an orange, granular appearance to the fovea, and occasional peripheral scintillation. Few vitreous cells and occasional sheathing of vessels. Enlarged blind spot. Vision typically returns to normal within weeks without treatment.

Etiology

Fungal infection caused by *Histoplasma capsulatum.* Once acquired by inhalation, the organisms can pass to the choroid through the bloodstream.

Work-Up

1. History: Time spent in the Ohio–Mississippi River Valley or endemic area? Prior exposure to fowl?

2. Amsler grid test (see Appendix 4, *Amsler Grid*) to evaluate the central visual field of each eye.

3. Slit-lamp examination: Anterior chamber or vitreous cells and flare should not be present.

4. Dilated fundus examination: Concentrate on the macular area with a slit lamp and fundus contact, or 60- or 90-diopter lens. Look for signs of CNV and vitreous cells.

5. IVFA and OCT to help detect CNV and monitor response to treatment.

Treatment

1. Antifungal treatment is not helpful.

2. Intravitreal anti-VEGF therapy for CNV. PDT (for subfoveal CNV) and focal laser photocoagulation (for extrafoveal CNV) may be used as initial treatments as well. Submacular surgery may be considered in the setting of medically unresponsive subfoveal CNV if vision is <20/100.

Follow-Up

1. Treatment should be instituted within 72 hours of confirming the presence of CNV by IVFA.

2. Instruct all patients to use an Amsler grid daily and return immediately if any sudden visual change is noted.

3. Patients treated with anti-VEGF injections are generally seen every 4 to 6 weeks, depending on the clinical response to therapy. Patients treated with PDT or focal laser are typically seen at 2 to 3 weeks, 4 to 6 weeks, 3 months, and 6 months after treatment and then every 6 months thereafter.

4. A careful macular examination and OCT is performed at each visit. IVFA may be repeated whenever renewed neovascular activity is suspected.

5. Patients without CNV are seen every 6 months when macular changes are present in one or both eyes and yearly when no macular disease is present in either eye.

11

11.25 MACULAR HOLE

Symptoms

Decreased vision, typically around the 20/200 level for a full-thickness hole, better for a partial-thickness hole; sometimes distortion of vision or central scotoma. Three times more likely in women; usually occurs in sixth to eighth decade. 10% bilateral.

Signs

(See Figures 11.25.1 and 11.25.2.)

Critical. A round, red spot in the center of the macula, usually from one-third to two-thirds of a disc diameter in size, surrounded by a gray halo [(cuff of subretinal fluid (SRF)]. A stage 1 idiopathic macular hole demonstrates loss of the normal foveolar depression and often a yellow spot or ring in the center of the macula.

Other. Small, yellow precipitates deep to the retina in the hole or surrounding retina; retinal cysts at the margin of the hole or a small operculum above the hole, anterior to the retina (stage 4); or both.

NOTE: A partial-thickness (lamellar) hole is not as red as a full-thickness hole, and the surrounding gray halo is usually not present. A sheen from ILM changes or epiretinal membrane can be seen.

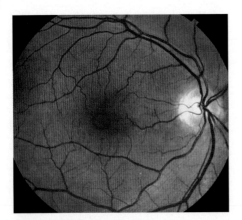

FIGURE 11.25.1. Macular hole.

Staging

- Stage 1: An impending hole, yellow spot, or ring in fovea.

- Stage 2: Small full-thickness hole.

- Stage 3: Full-thickness hole with cuff of SRF, no PVD.

- Stage 4: Full-thickness hole with cuff of SRF, with complete PVD.

Differential Diagnosis

- Macular pucker with a pseudohole: An epiretinal membrane (surface wrinkling) on the surface of the retina may simulate a macular hole. See 11.26, *Epiretinal Membrane (Macular Pucker, Surface-Wrinkling Retinopathy, Cellophane Maculopathy).*

- Solar retinopathy: Small, round, red or yellow lesion at the center of the fovea, with surrounding fine gray pigment in a sungazer or eclipse watcher. See 11.35, *Solar Retinopathy.*

- Intraretinal cysts: e.g., chronic CME with prominent central cyst.

Etiology

May be caused by vitreous or epiretinal membrane traction on the macula, trauma, or CME.

Work-Up

1. History: Previous trauma? Previous eye surgery? Sun-gazer?

2. Complete ocular examination, including a macular examination with a slit lamp and 60- or 90-diopter lens, or fundus contact lens. If a PVD is present, careful examination of the peripheral fundus to rule out peripheral breaks is important.

3. A true macular hole can be differentiated from a pseudohole by directing a thin, vertical slit beam across the area in question by using a 60- or 90-diopter lens with the slit-lamp biomicroscope. The patient with a true hole will report a break in the line (Watzke–

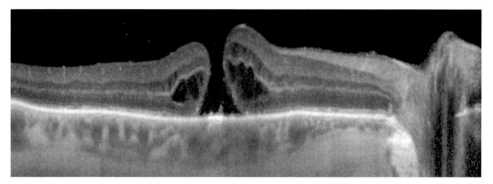

FIGURE 11.25.2. OCT of macular hole.

Allen test). A pseudohole may cause distortion of the line, but it should not be broken.

4. IVFA in stage 2 to 4 macular holes shows early foveal hyperfluorescence without evidence of leakage in the late phase.

5. OCT is helpful for staging, evaluating progression, and determining the degree of traction from vitreous or epiretinal membranes (see Figure 11.25.3).

Treatment

1. Fifty percent of stage 1 premacular holes resolve spontaneously.

2. In selected cases of more advanced macular holes, vitrectomy with membrane peel may be beneficial. It is preferable to operate within the first 6 months of onset with the possibility of regaining half of the visual angle. The risk of RD is very small. However, symptoms of an RD (e.g., sudden increase in flashes and floaters, abundant "cobwebs" in the vision, or a curtain coming across the field of vision) are explained to patients, particularly those with high myopia. It is in the latter group that the macular hole sometimes leads to an RD, which requires surgical repair.

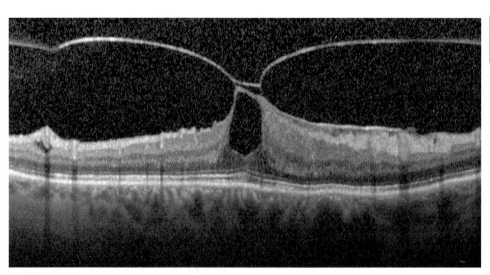

FIGURE 11.25.3. OCT of vitreomacular traction.

Follow-Up

1. Patients with high myopia are seen every 6 months.

2. Other patients may be seen yearly.

3. All patients are seen sooner if RD symptoms develop.

4. Because there is a small risk that the condition may develop in the contralateral eye, patients are given an Amsler grid for periodic home monitoring.

11.26 EPIRETINAL MEMBRANE (MACULAR PUCKER, SURFACE-WRINKLING RETINOPATHY, CELLOPHANE MACULOPATHY)

Symptoms

Most are asymptomatic; can have decreased or distorted vision or both. Typically occurs in middle-aged or elderly patients. Twenty percent bilateral.

Signs

(See Figure 11.26.1.)

Critical. Spectrum ranges from a fine, glistening membrane (cellophane maculopathy) to a thick, gray–white membrane (macular pucker) present on the surface of the retina in the macular area.

Other. Retinal folds radiating out from the membrane, displacement, straightening or tortuosity of the macular retinal vessels, ME, or detachment. A round, dark condensation of the epiretinal membrane in the macula may simulate a macular hole (pseudohole).

Differential Diagnosis

- Diabetic retinopathy: May produce preretinal fibrovascular tissue, which may displace retinal vessels or detach the macula. ME may be present. See 11.12, *Diabetic Retinopathy.*

- CME. See 11.14, *Cystoid Macular Edema.*

Etiology

- Idiopathic.

- Retinal break, RRD. See 11.2, *Retinal break,* and 11.3, *Retinal Detachment.*

- PVD. See 11.1, *Posterior Vitreous Detachment.*

- After retinal cryotherapy or photocoagulation.

- After intraocular surgery, trauma, or vitreous hemorrhage.

- Uveitis. See Chapter 12, *Uveitis.*

- Other retinal vascular disease.

Work-Up

1. History: Previous eye surgery or eye disease? Diabetes?

2. Complete ocular examination, particularly a thorough dilated fundus evaluation and careful macula evaluation with a slit lamp

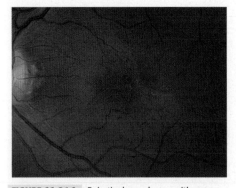

FIGURE 11.26.1. Epiretinal membrane with pseudohole.

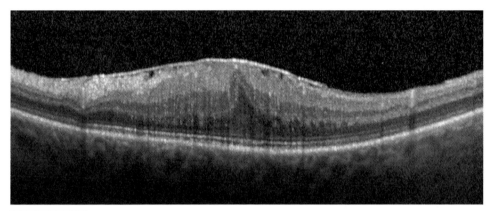

FIGURE 11.26.2. OCT of epiretinal membrane.

and a 60- or 90-diopter, Hruby, or fundus contact lens. A careful peripheral examination should be performed to rule out a retinal break.

3. OCT is helpful in evaluating epiretinal membranes (see Figure 11.26.2).

Treatment

1. Treat the underlying disorder.

2. Surgical peeling of the membrane can be considered when it significantly reduces the vision.

Follow-Up

This is not an emergent condition, and treatment may be instituted at any time. Rarely, membranes separate from the retina, resulting in spontaneously improved vision. A small percentage of epiretinal membranes recur after surgical removal.

11.27 CHOROIDAL EFFUSION/DETACHMENT

Symptoms

Decreased vision or asymptomatic in a serous choroidal detachment. Decreased vision may occur if the choroidal detachments extend through the macula. Moderate-to-severe pain and red eye may also occur with a hemorrhagic choroidal detachment.

Signs

(See Figure 11.27.1.)

Critical. Smooth, bullous, orange-brown elevation of the retina and choroid that usually extends 360 degrees around the periphery in a lobular configuration. The ora serrata can be seen without scleral depression.

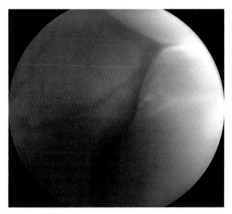

FIGURE 11.27.1. Choroidal detachment.

Other.

Serous choroidal *detachment:* Low IOP (often <6 mm Hg), shallow anterior chamber with mild cell and flare, positive transillumination.

Hemorrhagic choroidal *detachment:* High IOP (if detachment is large), shallow anterior chamber with mild cell and flare, no transillumination.

Differential Diagnosis

- Melanoma of the ciliary body: Not typically multilobular or symmetric in each quadrant of the globe. Pigmented melanomas do not transilluminate. B-scan US may help to differentiate between the two. See 11.36, *Choroidal Nevus and Malignant Melanoma of the Choroid.*

- Rhegmatogenous retinal detachment: Appears white and undulates with eye movements. A break is usually seen in the retina, and pigment cells are often present in the vitreous. See 11.3, *Retinal Detachment.*

Etiology

Serous

- Intraoperative or postoperative: Wound leak, perforation of the sclera from a superior rectus bridle suture, iritis, cyclodialysis cleft, leakage or excess filtration from a filtering bleb, or after laser photocoagulation or cryotherapy. May occur days to weeks after the surgery.

- Traumatic: Often associated with a ruptured globe.

- After retinal detachment repair by scleral buckling or vitrectomy.

- Other: Nanophthalmos, uveal effusion syndrome, carotid–cavernous fistula, primary or metastatic tumor, scleritis, VKH syndrome, etc. See specific sections.

Hemorrhagic

- Intraoperative or postoperative: From anterior displacement of the ocular contents and rupture of the short posterior ciliary arteries.

- Spontaneous: e.g., after perforation of a corneal ulcer.

Work-Up

1. History: Recent ocular surgery or trauma? Known eye or medical problem?

2. Slit-lamp examination: Check for the presence of a filtering bleb and perform Seidel test to rule out a wound leak. See Appendix 5, *Seidel Test to Detect a Wound Leak.*

3. Gonioscopy of the anterior chamber angle: Look for a cyclodialysis cleft.

4. Dilated retinal examination: Determine whether there is subretinal fluid, indicating a concomitant RD, and whether an underlying choroidal disease or tumor is present. Examination of the contralateral eye may be helpful in diagnosis.

5. In cases suggestive of melanoma, B-scan US and transillumination of the globe are helpful in making a diagnosis. B-scan US is also useful to distinguish between serous and hemorrhagic choroidal detachment and in determining if hemorrhage is mobile or coagulated.

6. Check the skin for vitiligo and the head for alopecia (e.g., VKH syndrome).

Treatment

General Treatment

1. Cycloplegic (e.g., atropine 1% t.i.d.).

2. Topical steroid (e.g., prednisolone acetate 1% four to six times per day).

3. Consider oral steroids.

4. Surgical drainage of the suprachoroidal fluid may be indicated for a flat or progressively shallow anterior chamber, particularly in the presence of inflammation (because of the risk of peripheral anterior synechiae), corneal decompensation resulting from lens–cornea touch, or "kissing" choroidals (apposition of two lobules of detached choroid).

Specific Treatment: Repair the Underlying Problem

1. Serous

　—Wound or filtering bleb leak: Patch for 24 hours, decrease steroids and add aqueous suppressants, suture the site, use cyanoacrylate glue, place a bandage contact lens on the eye, or a combination of these.

—Cyclodialysis cleft: Laser therapy, diathermy, cryotherapy, or suture the cleft to close it.

—Uveitis: Topical cycloplegic and steroid as discussed previously.

—Inflammatory disease: See the specific entity.

—RD: Surgical repair. Proliferative vitreoretinopathy after repair is common.

2. Hemorrhagic: Drainage of the choroidal detachment with or without vitrectomy is performed for severe cases with retina or vitreous to the wound. More successful if hemorrhage is liquefied, which occurs 7 to 10 days after the initial event. Otherwise use general treatment.

Follow-Up

In accordance with the underlying problem.

11.28 RETINITIS PIGMENTOSA AND INHERITED CHORIORETINAL DYSTROPHIES

RETINITIS PIGMENTOSA

Symptoms

Decreased night vision (often night blindness) and loss of peripheral vision. Decrease in central vision can occur early or late in the disease process. Color vision is intact until late.

Signs

(See Figure 11.28.1.)

Critical. Classically, vitreous cells (most consistent sign), clumps of pigment dispersed throughout the peripheral retina in a perivascular pattern, often assuming a "bone spicule" arrangement (though bone spicules may be absent), areas of depigmentation or atrophy of the RPE, narrowing of arterioles, and, later, waxy optic disc pallor. Progressive visual field loss, usually a ring scotoma, which progresses to a small central field. ERG usually moderately to markedly reduced.

Other. Focal or sectoral pigment clumping, CME, epiretinal membrane, posterior subcapsular cataract.

Inheritance Patterns

- Autosomal recessive (most common): Diminished vision (severe) and night blindness occur early in life.

- Autosomal dominant (least severe): More gradual onset of retinitis pigmentosa (RP), typically in adult life, variable penetrance, late onset of cataract. Visual loss less severe.

- X-linked recessive (rarest and most severe): Onset similar to autosomal recessive. Female carriers often have salt-and-pepper fundus. Visual loss is severe.

- Sporadic.

Treatment

Recently, epiretinal and subretinal microchip implants have been used with moderate

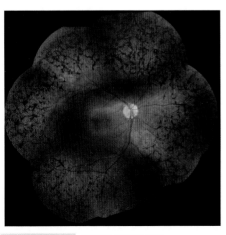

FIGURE 11.28.1. Retinitis pigmentosa.

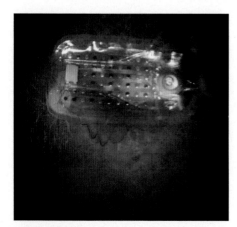

FIGURE 11.28.2. Epiretinal microchip implant in patient with advanced RP.

success to improve vision in patients with advanced RP (see Figure 11.28.2). Clinical trials are ongoing with a variety of designs to determine the safety and efficacy of retinal implant technology. In addition, research in gene therapy for specific types of RP is underway, though not yet clinically available.

SYSTEMIC DISEASES ASSOCIATED WITH HEREDITARY RETINAL DEGENERATION

Refsum Disease (Phytanoyl-CoA Hydroxylase Deficiency)

Autosomal recessive RP (often without bone spicules) with increased serum phytanic acid level. May have cerebellar ataxia, peripheral neuropathy, deafness, dry skin, anosmia, liver disease, and cardiac abnormalities. Treat with low-phytanic acid, low-phytol diet (minimize the amount of milk products, animal fats, and green leafy vegetables). Check serum phytanic acid levels every 6 months.

Hereditary Abetalipoproteinemia (Bassen–Kornzweig Syndrome)

Autosomal recessive RP (usually without bone spicules) with fat intolerance, diarrhea, crenated erythrocytes (acanthocytes), ataxia, progressive restriction of ocular motility, and other neurologic symptoms as a result of deficiency in lipoproteins and malabsorption of the fat-soluble vitamins (A, D, E, and K). Diagnosis based on serum apolipoprotein-B deficiency.

Treatment

1. Water-miscible vitamin A, 10,000 to 15,000 IU p.o. q.d.

2. Vitamin E, 200 to 300 IU/kg p.o. q.d.

3. Vitamin K, 5 mg p.o. weekly.

4. Restrict dietary fat to 15% of caloric intake.

5. Biannual serum levels of vitamins A and E; yearly ERG, and dark adaptometry.

6. Consider supplementing the patient's diet with zinc.

Leber Congenital Amaurosis

Group of autosomal recessive retinal dystrophies that represent the most common genetic cause of congenital blindness in children. Fundus appearance is variable, but typically shows a pigmentary retinopathy. Moderate-to-severe vision loss identified at or within a few months of birth, infantile nystagmus, poor and/or paradoxic papillary response, photophobia, oculodigital sign (eye poking), and markedly reduced or flat ERG. Associated with keratoconus. Gene therapy targeting the RPE65 gene has shown success in human trials.

Usher Syndrome

Multiple subtypes exist, all autosomal recessive. Associated with congenital sensorineural hearing loss which is usually stable throughout adult life. Genes involved code a protein complex present in inner ear hair cells and retinal photoreceptor cells. Molecular testing for certain subtypes is available.

Bardet–Biedl Complex

Mainly autosomal recessive group of different diseases with similar findings including pigmentary retinopathy, hypogonadism, obesity, polydactyly, mental retardation, and others. Lawrence–Moon syndrome is a related but separate entity associated with spastic paraplegia, but without the polydactyly and obesity.

Kearns–Sayre Syndrome

Salt-and-pepper pigmentary degeneration of the retina with normal arterioles, progressive limitation of ocular movement without diplopia, ptosis, short stature and, cardiac conduction defects. Ocular signs usually appear before age 20 years. Mitochondrial inheritance. Refer the patient to a cardiologist for yearly ECGs. Patients may need a pacemaker. See 10.12, *Chronic Progressive External Ophthalmoplegia.*

Other RP Syndromes

- Spielmeyer–Vogt–Batten–Mayou syndrome: Associated with seizures, dementia, and ataxia.

- Alström, Cockayne, and Alport syndromes: Associated with hearing loss.

- Zellweger syndrome: Associated with hypotonia, hypertelorism, and hepatomegaly.

- Others: Incontinentia pigmenti, Jansky–Bielschowsky, etc.

Differential Diagnosis

- Phenothiazine toxicity

    —Thioridazine

    Pigment clumps between the posterior pole and the equator, areas of retinal depigmentation, retinal edema, visual field abnormalities (central scotoma and general constriction), depressed or extinguished ERG. Symptoms and signs may occur within weeks of starting phenothiazine therapy, particularly if very large doses (≥2,000 mg/day) are taken. Usually, more than 800 mg/day chronically needed for toxicity. Discontinue if toxicity develops. Follow every 6 months.

    —Chlorpromazine

    Abnormal pigmentation of the eyelids, cornea, conjunctiva (especially within the palpebral fissure), and anterior lens capsule; anterior and posterior subcapsular cataract; rarely, a pigmentary retinopathy within the visual field and ERG changes described for thioridazine. Usually, 1,200 to 2,400 mg/day for longer than 12 months needed for toxicity. Discontinue if toxicity develops. Follow every 6 months.

- Syphilis: Positive FTA-ABS, asymmetric visual fields, abnormal fundus appearance, may have a history of recurrent uveitis, no family history of RP; the ERG is usually preserved to some degree.

- Congenital rubella: A salt-and-pepper fundus appearance may be accompanied by microphthalmos, cataract, deafness, a congenital heart abnormality, or another systemic abnormality. The ERG is usually normal.

- Bietti crystalline dystrophy: Autosomal recessive condition characterized by crystals of unknown composition in the peripheral corneal stroma and in the retina at different layers. Can cause choroidal atrophy, decreased night vision, decreased visual acuity, and a flat ERG.

- After resolution of a serous RD: e.g., toxemia of pregnancy or Harada disease. The history is diagnostic.

- Pigmented paravenous retinochoroidal atrophy: Paravenous localization of RPE degeneration and pigment deposition. No definite hereditary pattern. Variable visual fields and ERG (usually normal).

- After severe blunt trauma: Usually due to spontaneous resolution of RD.

- After ophthalmic artery occlusion.

- Carriers of ocular albinism: See 13.8, *Albinism.*

NOTE: The pigment abnormalities are at the level of the RPE with phenothiazine toxicity, syphilis, and congenital rubella. With resolved RD, the pigment is intraretinal.

11

Work-Up

1. Medical and ocular history pertaining to the diseases discussed previously.

2. Drug history.

3. Family history with pedigree and genetic testing for diagnostic and counseling purposes (see above).

4. Ophthalmoscopic examination.

5. Formal visual field testing (e.g., Humphrey).

6. ERG: May help distinguish stationary rod–cone dysfunction from RP (a progressive disease), and dark-adaptation studies.

7. Fundus photographs.

8. Consider FTA-ABS.

9. If the patient is male and the type of inheritance is unknown, examine his mother and perform an ERG on her. Women carriers of X-linked disease often have abnormal pigmentation in the mid-periphery and abnormal results on dark-adapted ERGs.

10. If neurologic abnormalities such as ataxia, polyneuropathy, deafness, or anosmia are present, obtain a fasting (at least 14 hours) serum phytanic acid level to rule out Refsum disease.

11. If hereditary abetalipoproteinemia is suspected, obtain serum cholesterol and triglyceride levels (levels are low), a serum protein and lipoprotein electrophoresis (lipoprotein deficiency is detected), and peripheral blood smears (acanthocytosis is seen).

12. If Kearns–Sayre syndrome is suspected, the patient must be examined by a cardiologist with sequential ECGs; patients can die of complete heart block. All family members should be evaluated.

Treatment

For syphilis, see 12.12, *Syphilis*. For vitamin A deficiency, see 13.7, *Vitamin A Deficiency*.

No definitive treatment for RP is currently known. However, vitamin A palmitate, 15,000 IU, has been shown to slow the reduction of ERG. This very controversial treatment (which showed no visual benefits) is considered only for nonpregnant patients ≥21 years of age. Monitor liver function test results and vitamin A levels.

Cataract surgery may improve central visual acuity. Topical or oral carbonic anhydrase inhibitors (e.g., acetazolamide 500 mg/day) may be effective for CME.

All patients benefit from genetic counseling and instruction on how to deal with their visual handicaps. Tinted lenses may provide comfort outdoors and may provide better contrast enhancement. In advanced cases, low-vision aids and vocational rehabilitation are helpful.

HEREDITARY CHORIORETINAL DYSTROPHIES AND OTHER CAUSES OF NYCTALOPIA (NIGHT BLINDNESS)

■ **Gyrate atrophy:** Nyctalopia and decreased peripheral vision usually presenting in the first decade of life, followed by progressive constriction of visual field. Scalloped RPE and choriocapillaris atrophy in the mid-periphery during childhood that coalesces to involve the entire fundus, posterior subcapsular cataract, high myopia with astigmatism. Constriction of visual fields and abnormal to nonrecordable ERG. Plasma ornithine level is 10 to 20 times normal; lysine is decreased. Consider ERG and IVFA if the ornithine level is not markedly increased. Autosomal recessive.

Treatment

1. Reduce dietary protein consumption and substitute artificially flavored solutions of essential amino acids without arginine (e.g., arginine-restricted diet). Monitor serum ammonia levels.

2. Supplemental vitamin B_6 (pyridoxine). The dose is not currently established; consider 20 mg/day p.o. initially and increase up to 500 mg/day p.o. if there is no response. Follow serum ornithine levels to determine the amount of supplemental vitamin B_6 and the degree to which dietary protein needs to be restricted. Serum ornithine levels between 0.15 and 0.2 mmol/L are optimal.

NOTE: Only a small percentage of patients are vitamin B_6 responders.

■ **Choroideremia:** Males present in the first to second decade of life with nyctalopia, followed by insidious loss of peripheral vision. Decreased central vision occurs late. In males, early findings include dispersed pigment granules in the periphery with focal areas of RPE atrophy. Late findings include total absence of RPE and choriocapillaris. No bone spicules. Retinal arteriolar narrowing and optic atrophy can

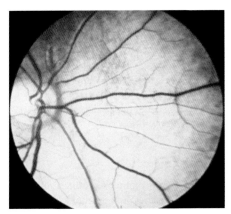

FIGURE 11.28.3. Oguchi disease with fundus exhibiting tapetum appearance in a light-adapted state.

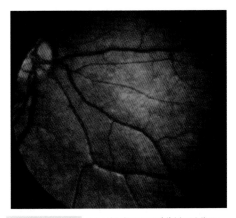

FIGURE 11.28.4. Oguchi disease exhibiting Mizuo phenomenon, with a normally colored fundus in dark-adapted state.

occur late in the process; constriction of visual fields, normal color vision, markedly reduced ERG. Female carriers have small, scattered, square intraretinal pigment granules overlying choroidal atrophy, most marked in the mid-periphery. No effective treatment for this condition is currently available. Darkly tinted sunglasses may ameliorate symptoms. X-linked recessive. Consider genetic counseling.

- **Vitamin A deficiency:** Marked night blindness; numerous small, yellow-white, well-demarcated spots deep in the retina seen peripherally; dry eye and/or Bitôt spots (white keratinized lesions) on the conjunctiva. See 13.7, *Vitamin A Deficiency.*

- **Zinc deficiency:** May cause abnormal dark adaptation (zinc is needed for vitamin A metabolism).

- **Congenital stationary night blindness:** Night blindness from birth, normal visual fields, may have a normal or abnormal fundus, not progressive. Paradoxic pupillary response. One variant is Oguchi disease, characterized by the Mizuo phenomenon—the fundus has a tapetum appearance in the light-adapted state, but appears normally colored when dark- adapted (takes about 12 hours) (see Figures 11.28.3 and 11.28.4).

- **Undercorrected myopia:** May be the most common cause of poor night vision.

11.29 CONE DYSTROPHIES

Symptoms

Slowly progressive visual loss, photophobia, and poor color vision, with onset during the first three decades of life. Vision is worse during the day than at night.

Signs

Critical.

- Early: Essentially normal fundus examination, even with poor visual acuity. Abnormal cone function on ERG (e.g., a reduced single-flash photopic response and a reduced flicker response).

- Late: Bull's-eye macular appearance or central geographic atrophy of the RPE and choriocapillaris.

Other. Nystagmus, temporal pallor of the optic disc, spotty pigment clumping in the macular area, tapetal-like retinal sheen. Rarely rod degeneration may ensue, leading to an RP-like picture (e.g., a cone–rod degeneration, which may have an autosomal dominant inheritance pattern).

Inheritance

Usually sporadic. Hereditary forms are usually autosomal dominant, or less often X- linked.

Differential Diagnosis

- Stargardt disease: Especially in an early stage when the fundus flavimaculatus is absent and ERG may be normal. See 11.30, *Stargardt Disease (Fundus Flavimaculatus).*

- Chloroquine/hydroxychloroquine maculopathy: May produce a bull's-eye macular appearance and poor color vision. History of medication use, no family history of cone degeneration, no nystagmus. See 11.32, *Chloroquine/Hydroxychloroquine Toxicity.*

- Central areolar choroidal dystrophy: Geographic atrophy of the RPE with normal photopic ERG.

- ARMD: Can have geographic atrophy of the RPE, but with normal color vision and photopic ERG. See 11.16, *Nonexudative (Dry) Age-Related Macular Degeneration,* and 11.17, *Neovascular or Exudative (Wet) Age-Related Macular Degeneration.*

- Congenital color blindness: Normal visual acuity, onset at birth, not progressive.

- RP: Night blindness and peripheral visual field loss. Often with peripheral retinal bone spicules. Can be distinguished by dark-adaptation testing and ERG. See 11.28, *Retinitis Pigmentosa and Inherited Chorioretinal Dystrophies.*

- Optic neuropathy or atrophy: Decreased acuity, impaired color vision, temporal or diffuse optic-disc pallor or both. See 10.17, *Arteritic*

Ischemic Optic Neuropathy (Giant Cell Arteritis), 10.18, *Nonarteritic Ischemic Optic Neuropathy,* and 10.20, *Miscellaneous Optic Neuropathies.*

- Nonphysiologic visual loss: Normal results on ophthalmoscopic examination, IVFA, OCT, ERG, and EOG. Patients can often be tricked into seeing better by special testing. See 10.25, *Nonphysiologic Visual Loss.*

Work-Up

1. Family history.

2. Complete ophthalmic examination, including color plates and formal color testing (e.g., Farnsworth–Munsell 100-hue test, red test object for chloroquine).

3. Formal visual field test.

4. ERG.

5. IVFA to help detect the bull's-eye macular pattern.

6. Fundus autofluorescence can be useful in the diagnosis (particularly sensitive to disturbances in the RPE), as well as for monitoring these diseases.

Treatment

There is no proven cure for this disease. The following measures may be palliative:

1. Heavily tinted glasses or contact lenses may help maximize vision.

2. Miotic drops (e.g., pilocarpine 0.5% to 1% q.i.d.) are occasionally tried to improve vision and reduce photophobia.

3. Genetic counseling.

4. Low-vision aids as needed.

Follow-Up

Yearly.

11.30　STARGARDT DISEASE (FUNDUS FLAVIMACULATUS)

Symptoms

Decreased vision in childhood or young adulthood. Early in the disease, the decrease in vision is often out of proportion to the clinical ophthalmoscopic appearance; there-

fore, care must be taken not to label the child a malingerer.

Signs

(See Figures 11.30.1 to 11.30.3.)

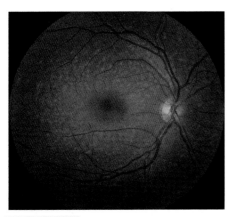

FIGURE 11.30.1. Stargardt disease.

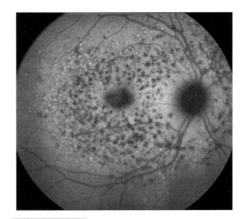

FIGURE 11.30.3. Fundus autofluorescence in Stargardt disease.

Critical. Any of the following may be present.

- A relatively normal-appearing fundus except for a heavily pigmented RPE.

- Yellow or yellow-white, flecklike deposits at the level of the RPE, usually in a pisciform (fish-tail) configuration.

- Atrophic macular degeneration: May have a bull's-eye appearance as a result of atrophy of the RPE around a normal central core of RPE, a "beaten-metal" appearance, pigment clumping, or marked geographic atrophy.

NOTE: In early stages, vision declines **before** visible macular changes develop.

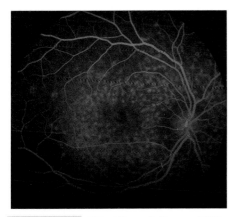

FIGURE 11.30.2. IVFA of Stargardt disease exhibiting silent choroid.

Other. Atrophy of the RPE just outside of the macula or in the mid-peripheral fundus, normal peripheral visual fields in most cases, and rarely an accompanying cone or rod dystrophy. The ERG is typically normal in the early stages, but may become abnormal late in the disease. The EOG can be subnormal.

Inheritance

Usually autosomal recessive, but occasionally autosomal dominant.

Differential Diagnosis

- Fundus albipunctatus: Diffuse, small, white, discrete dots, most prominent in the mid-peripheral fundus and rarely present in the fovea; congenital stationary night blindness variant; no atrophic macular degeneration or pigmentary changes. Visual acuity and visual fields remain normal. Prolonged dark-adaptation time with normal ERG.

- Retinitis punctata albescens: Similar clinical appearance to fundus albipunctatus, but visual acuity, visual field, and night blindness progressively worsen. A markedly abnormal ERG develops. Variant of RP.

- Drusen: Small, yellow-white spots deep to the retina, sometimes calcified, usually developing later in life. IVFA may be helpful (all drusen hyperfluoresce, whereas fundus flavimaculatus lesions show variable hyperfluorescence and some areas without flecks show hyperfluorescence).

11

■ Cone or cone-rod dystrophy: May have a bull's-eye macula, but have a significant color vision deficit and a characteristic ERG. See 11.29, *Cone Dystrophies.*

■ Batten disease and Spielmeyer–Vogt syndrome: May have bull's-eye maculopathy, autosomal recessive lysosomal storage disease, progressive dementia, seizures; may have variable degree of optic atrophy, attenuation of retinal vasculature, and peripheral RPE changes. Shows characteristic curvilinear or fingerprint inclusions on electron microscopy of peripheral blood or conjunctival biopsy. Variants of RP.

■ Chloroquine/hydroxychloroquine maculopathy: History of medication use. See 11.32, *Chloroquine/Hydroxychloroquine Toxicity.*

■ Nonphysiologic visual loss: Normal ophthalmoscopic examination, IVFA, OCT, ERG, and EOG. Patients can often be tricked into seeing better by special testing. See 10.25, *Nonphysiologic Visual Loss.*

Work-Up

Indicated when the diagnosis is uncertain or must be confirmed.

1. History: Age at onset, medications, family history?

2. Dilated fundus examination.

3. IVFA often shows blockage of choroidal fluorescence producing a "silent choroid" or "midnight fundus" as a result of increased lipofuscin in the RPE cells.

4. Fundus autofluorescence can be helpful in diagnosis and in monitoring disease progression.

5. ERG and EOG.

6. Formal visual field examination (e.g., Octopus, Humphrey).

7. Consider genetic testing: Sequencing of the ABCA4 gene (found to be abnormal in many cases of Stargardt disease and other related maculopathies).

Treatment

Ultraviolet light-blocking glasses when outdoors may be beneficial. Low-vision aids, services dedicated to helping the visually handicapped, and genetic counseling are helpful.

11.31 BEST DISEASE (VITELLIFORM MACULAR DYSTROPHY)

Symptoms

Decreased vision or asymptomatic.

Signs

(See Figure 11.31.1.)

Critical. Yellow, round, subretinal lesion(s) likened to an egg yolk (lipofuscin) or in some cases to a pseudohypopyon. Typically bilateral and located in the fovea, measuring approximately one to two disc areas in size. Likely present at birth, though may not be detected until examination is performed. Ten percent of lesions are multiple and extrafoveal. ERG is normal and EOG is abnormal, showing severe loss of the light response.

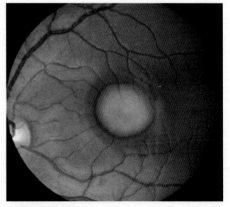

FIGURE 11.31.1. Best disease.

Other. The lesions may degenerate, and patients may develop macular CNV (20% of patients), hemorrhage, and scarring. In the scar stage, it may be indistinguishable from ARMD. May be hyperopic and have esophoria or esotropia.

Inheritance

Autosomal dominant with variable penetrance and expression. Carriers may have normal fundi but an abnormal EOG.

Differential Diagnosis

- Pattern dystrophy: A type of pattern dystrophy, adult-onset foveomacular dystrophy, can mimic Best disease. The egg-yolk lesions are usually smaller, appearing from ages 30 to 50 years. The condition is dominantly inherited, and the EOG may or may not be abnormal. Visual acuity is usually normal or slightly decreased until the sixth decade of life, when central vision may be compromised by geographic atrophy. There is no effective treatment for this entity.

- ARMD: See above and 11.16, *Nonexudative (Dry) Age-Related Macular Degeneration.*

Work-Up

1. Family history. It is often helpful to examine family members.

2. Complete ocular examination, including a dilated retinal examination, carefully inspecting the macula with a slit lamp and a fundus contact, or handheld (60-, 78-, 90-diopter) lens.

3. EOG is highly specific and can be used to confirm the diagnosis or to detect the carrier state of the disease.

4. Consider IVFA and OCT to detect the presence of or to delineate a CNV.

Treatment

There is no effective treatment for the underlying disease. Treatment for CNV is controversial because it may heal without devastating visual loss. Laser should be considered for well-defined CNV outside the foveal center. Subfoveal CNV treatment options include PDT and intravitreal anti-VEGF agents. See 11.17, *Neovascular or Exudative (Wet) Age-Related Macular Degeneration,* for detailed treatment options for CNV.

Follow-Up

Patients with CNV should be treated promptly. Otherwise, there is no urgency in seeing patients with this disease. Patients are given an Amsler grid (see Appendix 4, *Amsler Grid*), instructed on its use, and told to return immediately if a change is noted.

11.32   CHLOROQUINE/HYDROXYCHLOROQUINE TOXICITY

Symptoms

Decreased vision, abnormal color vision, difficulty adjusting to darkness.

Signs

Critical. Bull's-eye macula (a ring of depigmentation surrounded by a ring of increased pigmentation), loss of the foveal reflex.

Other. Increased pigmentation in the macula, arteriolar narrowing, vascular sheathing, peripheral pigmentation, decreased color vision, visual field abnormalities (central, paracentral, or peripheral scotoma), abnormal ERG and EOG, and normal dark adaptation. Whorl-like corneal changes also may be observed.

Dosage Usually Required to Produce Toxicity

Chloroquine: More than 300 g total cumulative dose.

Hydroxychloroquine: Toxicity much less common than with chloroquine. Typically more than 400 mg/day taken over months to years, with a cumulative dose of 1,000 g, though this is highly weight dependent.

Differential Diagnosis of Bull's-Eye Maculopathy

- Cone dystrophy: Family history, usually <30 years of age, severe photophobia, abnormal to nonrecordable photopic ERG. See 11.29, *Cone Dystrophies.*

- Stargardt disease: Family history, usually <25 years of age, may have white-yellow flecks in the posterior pole and mid-periphery. See 11.30, *Stargardt Disease (Fundus Flavimaculatus).*

- ARMD: Drusen; pigment clumping and atrophy and detachment of the RPE or sensory retina may or may not occur. See 11.16, *Nonexudative (Dry) Age-Related Macular Degeneration,* and 11.17, *Neovascular or Exudative (Wet) Age-Related Macular Degeneration.*

- Batten disease and Spielmeyer–Vogt syndrome: Pigmentary retinopathy, seizures, ataxia, and progressive dementia. See 11.30, *Stargardt Disease (Fundus Flavimaculatus).*

Treatment

Discontinue the medication if signs of toxicity develop.

Baseline Work-Up

Baseline evaluation should be performed within the 1st year of starting the medication.

1. Best corrected visual acuity.

2. Ophthalmoscopic examination, including dilated fundus exam with particular attention to any pigmentary alterations.

3. Consider posterior pole fundus photographs.

4. Visual field, preferably automated with a white target and 10-2 protocol.

5. Objective testing with multifocal ERG, fundus autofluorescence (FAF), or spectral

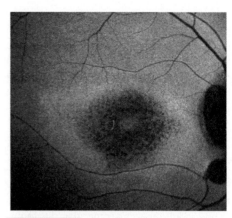

FIGURE 11.32.1. Fundus autofluorescence of hydroxychloroquine toxicity.

domain-OCT (SD-OCT) should be considered at baseline where available, but should be performed if any of the above screening tests are abnormal (see Figure 11.32.1).

Follow-Up

After the baseline examination, annual screening with multifocal ERG, FAF, or SD-OCT should begin after 5 years of medication use. These tests should be acquired sooner if any concern for toxicity exists or patients are at high risk.

NOTE: Once ocular toxicity develops, it usually does not regress even if the drug is withdrawn. In fact, new toxic effects may develop, and old ones may progress even after the chloroquine/hydroxychloroquine has been discontinued.

Bibliography

Marmor MF, Kellner U, Lai TY, et al. Revised recommendations on screening for chloroquine and hydroxychloroquine retinopathy. *Ophthalmology* 2011;118(2):415–422.

11.33 CRYSTALLINE RETINOPATHY

Symptoms

Decreased vision or asymptomatic.

Signs

Critical. Intraretinal refractile bodies.

Other. If crystals are intravascular and cause capillary nonperfusion, peripheral neovascularization as well as neovascularization of the optic nerve can develop (most commonly with talc). ME, macular pucker, and VH may also occur. Skin may reveal evidence of intravenous drug abuse.

Differential Diagnosis

- Hard exudates: Intraretinal lipid exudates as can be seen in multiple conditions (e.g., diabetic retinopathy, Coats, retinal telangiectasia, retinal arterial macroaneurysm). Hard exudates are not seen within retinal vessels.

- Calcific drusen: Seen in dry ARMD. Drusen are subretinal, not intravascular.

Etiology

- Canthaxanthin toxicity: Oral tanning agent causing ring-shaped deposits in the superficial retina. Generally asymptomatic and usually resolves over many years when the drug is stopped. Usually requires a total of 19 g over 2 years.

- Tamoxifen: Used in patients with hormone receptor-positive breast cancer. Toxicity usually requires 7.7 g total. Crystals appear in the inner retina usually around the macula and may cause ME. Vision may improve with discontinuation of drug, but crystals remain. Asymptomatic patients taking tamoxifen do not need to be screened. Consider medication change if evidence of toxicity in consultation with patient's oncologist.

- Retinal arterial emboli: Seen within vessel. See 11.6, *Central Retinal Artery Occlusion,* and 11.7, *Branch Retinal Artery Occlusion.*

- Talc: Red-yellow refractile particles seen intravascularly in intravenous drug users.

- Methoxyflurane: An anesthetic agent. Toxicity especially seen in patients with renal insufficiency.

- Bietti crystalline dystrophy: Crystals of unknown composition in the peripheral corneal stroma and in the retina at different layers. See 11.28, *Retinitis Pigmentosa and Inherited Chorioretinal Dystrophies.*

- Idiopathic juxtafoveal/parafoveal telangiectasis: Telangiectasis of juxtafoveal or parafoveal retinal capillaries leading to exudation and deposition of intraretinal crystals which may be Mueller foot plates or calcium or cholesterol deposits. Patients can develop ME and/or CNV. Vascular damage is very similar to that seen in diabetic retinopathy, and some patients with this condition are later found to have insulin resistance.

Work-Up

1. History: intravenous drug use? Cardiovascular risk factors such as HTN, elevated cholesterol? Breast cancer? Use of oral tanning agents? History of anesthesia in patient with renal failure?

2. Complete ocular examination, including dilated retinal examination with a slit lamp and a 60- or 90-diopter lens and indirect ophthalmoscopy carefully examining for the location, depth, color, and morphology of crystals as well as the presence of ME, neovascularization of the disc, or retinal infarction. Carefully examine retinal periphery for evidence of neovascularization. Carefully examine the cornea for crystals.

3. Consider carotid Doppler US and echocardiography in older patients and those with cardiovascular risk factors.

4. Examine patient for evidence of intravenous drug abuse.

5. Consider testing for diabetes if idiopathic juxtafoveal/parafoveal telangiectasis suspected.

6. IVFA may be helpful to demonstrate areas of nonperfusion distal to an intravascular crystal.

Treatment

1. Stop tamoxifen or canthaxanthin use if responsible for toxicity.

2. Stop intravenous drug use.

3. If cholesterol, calcium, or fibrin-platelet emboli, see 10.20, *Transient Visual Loss/ Amaurosis Fugax,* 11.6, *Central Retinal Artery Occlusion,* and 11.7, *Branch Retinal Artery Occlusion.*

11

4. If there is peripheral nonperfusion or neovascularization, consider PRP or anti-VEGF agents. Visual loss may be permanent if there has been vascular nonperfusion in the macula secondary to blockage from intraretinal crystals.

Follow-Up

Depends on the underlying etiology.

11.34 · OPTIC PIT

Symptoms

Asymptomatic if isolated. May notice distortion of straight lines or edges, blurred vision, a blind spot, or micropsia if a serous macular detachment develops.

Signs

(See Figure 11.34.1.)

Critical. Small, round depression (usually gray, yellow, or black in appearance) in the nerve tissue of the optic disc. Most are temporal, approximately one-third are central, but may be present anywhere on the nerve head.

Other. Peripapillary atrophy, white or gray membrane overlying pit, rarely RAPD, various visual field defects. May develop a localized detachment of the sensory retina or retinoschisis extending from the disc to the macula, often associated with subretinal precipitates, usually unilateral.

Differential Diagnosis

■ Acquired pit (pseudopit): Sometimes seen in patients with low-tension glaucoma or primary open-angle glaucoma. See 9.1, *Primary Open-Angle Glaucoma.*

■ Other causes of a serous macular detachment. See 11.15, *Central Serous Chorioretinopathy.*

Work-Up

1. Complete ophthalmologic examination including slit-lamp examination of the optic nerve and macula with a fundus contact lens or 60- or 90-diopter lens to evaluate for a serous macular detachment and CNV.

2. Measure IOP.

3. Obtain baseline automated visual field testing.

4. If a serous macular detachment is present, consider OCT or an IVFA to rule out a CNV.

Treatment

1. Isolated optic pit: No treatment required.

2. Optic pit with a serous macular detachment: Laser photocoagulation to the temporal margin of the optic disc is used in most cases. Vitrectomy with intravitreal gas may be used in refractory cases.

Follow-Up

1. Isolated optic pits: Yearly examination including IOP check, dilated fundus examination, and visual field testing if indicated; sooner if symptomatic. Patients should be given an Amsler grid. See Appendix 4, *Amsler Grid.*

2. Optic pits with serous macular detachment: Reexamine 3 to 4 weeks after treatment to check for resorption of subretinal fluid. Monitor for and treat amblyopia if present.

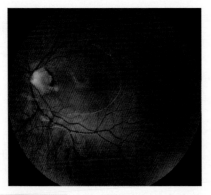

FIGURE 11.34.1. Optic pit with associated serous macular detachment.

11

11.35   SOLAR RETINOPATHY

Symptoms

Decreased visual acuity, central/paracentral scotomata, dyschromatopsia, metamorphopsia. Typically bilateral.

Signs

(See Figure 11.35.1.)

Critical. Acute findings include a yellow-white spot in the fovea with or without surrounding granular grey pigmentation. Classic late finding is a red, sharply demarcated, cyst-like lesion in the fovea.

Other. Visual acuity usually ranges from 20/25 to 20/100. Amsler grid testing may reveal central or paracentral scotoma. Resolution of acute findings within several weeks may leave a variable appearance to the fovea (e.g., pigmentary disturbance, lamellar hole, normal appearance, etc). Eyes with better initial visual acuities are more likely to have unremarkable fundoscopic examinations at follow-up.

Differential Diagnosis

- Macular hole or vitreomacular traction: See 11.25, *Macular Hole.*

- Idiopathic macular telangiectasia type 2: May have OCT findings similar to those seen in chronic solar retinopathy. This diagnosis is characaterized by bilateral juxtafoveal capillary telangiectasis with IVFA demonstrating leakage. May be complicated by CNV.

- Intraretinal cysts: e.g., chronic CME with prominent central cyst.

- Pattern dystrophy: Adult-onset foveomacular dystrophy. See 11.31, *Best Disease (Vitelliform Macular Dystrophy).*

Etiology

Unprotected solar eclipse viewing, sungazing (e.g., related to religious rituals, psychiatric illnesses, hallucinogenic drugs), sunbathing, vocational exposure (e.g., aviation, military service, astronomy).

Work-Up

1. History: Eclipse viewing or sungazing? Work exposure?

2. Complete ocular examination, including a dilated fundus examination and careful inspection of the macula with a slit lamp and a fundus contact, or handheld (60-, 78-, 90-diopter) lens.

3. Amsler grid testing may identify central or paracentral scotomata.

4. IVFA typically shows a window defect late in the disease course.

5. OCT findings in the acute setting include hyporeflectivity at the level of the RPE and occasional hyperreflectivity of the injured neurosensory retina. In the chronic stage, a central hyporeflective defect at the level of the photoreceptor inner segment–outer segment junction is seen (see Figure 11.35.2).

Treatment

1. Observation. Eyes with better visual acuities on initial examination tend to recover more vision. Long-term significant reduction in visual acuity is rare. However, central or paracentral scotomata may persist despite improvement in visual acuity.

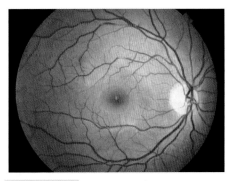

FIGURE 11.35.1. Solar retinopathy.

11

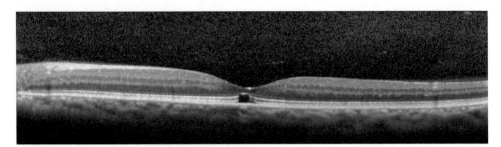

FIGURE 11.35.2.   OCT of solar retinopathy.

11.36   CHOROIDAL NEVUS AND MALIGNANT MELANOMA OF THE CHOROID

CHOROIDAL NEVUS

Symptoms

Usually asymptomatic. Rare symptoms include flashes of light (if subretinal fluid present) or decreased visual acuity (if directly subfoveal).

Signs

(See Figure 11.36.1.)

Critical. Flat or minimally elevated pigmented or nonpigmented choroidal lesion.

Other. Usually <2 mm thick with gradual elevation from the choroid. Overlying drusen become more prominent with age and can appear as hard cuticular drusen or soft drusen. RPE atrophy, hyperplasia, and detachment can occur. Rarely, overlying orange pigment (lipofuscin) or subretinal fluid is detected. Minimal growth of <1 mm over many years can be found. If >1 mm growth over shorter period (1 year), then transformation into melanoma should be considered.

Risk Factors for Malignant Transformation

These are remembered by mnemonic "To Find Small Ocular Melanoma" whereby the first letter of each word (TFSOM) represents a risk factor.

- ■ T: Thickness >2 mm.
- ■ F: Fluid (subretinal).
- ■ S: Symptoms (typically flashes or floaters).
- ■ O: Orange pigment over the lesion.
- ■ M: Margin of tumor ≤3 mm from the optic disc.

NOTE: If three or more factors are present, the lesion has a >50% chance to show growth and is likely to be a small choroidal melanoma.

Differential Diagnosis

See below for differential diagnosis of pigmented/nonpigmented choroidal lesions.

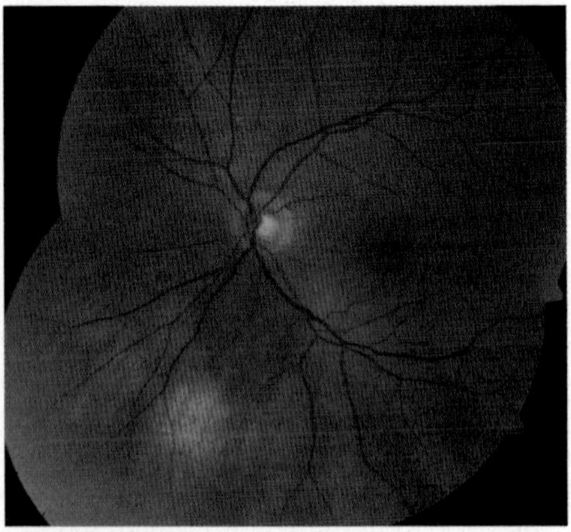

FIGURE 11.36.1.   Choroidal nevus.

Work-Up

1. Complete ophthalmologic examination including dilated fundus examination with evaluation of the lesion using a 20-diopter lens.

2. Detailed clinical drawing of the lesion with careful attention to location and size.

3. Baseline color photos of the lesion to assist in documenting growth.

4. OCT to document the overlying retinal features, subretinal fluid, and the lesion itself using enhanced-depth imaging.

5. Autofluorescence to document the presence of lipofuscin or retinal pigment epithelial disturbance.

6. US for tumor thickness measurement and internal acoustic qualities.

Treatment

Observation. First examination should be in 3 to 4 months to confirm stability, then one to two times yearly to document lack of change.

Follow-Up

Low-risk lesions can be followed with annual dilated fundus examination. High-risk lesions should be followed every 3 to 6 months.

MALIGNANT MELANOMA OF THE CHOROID

Symptoms

Decreased vision, visual field defect, floaters, light flashes, rarely pain; often asymptomatic.

Signs

(See Figure 11.36.2.)

Critical. Gray-green or brown (melanotic) or yellow (amelanotic) choroidal mass that exhibits one or more of the following:

- Presence of subretinal fluid.

- Thickness ≥2 mm, especially with an abrupt elevation from the choroid.

- Ill-defined, large areas of geographic orange pigment over the lesion.

- A dome, mushroom, or plateau shape with congested blood vessels in the apex of the tumor.

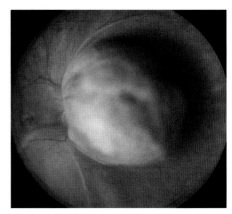

FIGURE 11.36.2. Choroidal melanoma.

- Break in Bruch membrane with subretinal hemorrhage.

- Growth.

NOTE: A diffuse choroidal melanoma can appear as a minimally thickened dark choroidal lesion without a prominently elevated mass and can simulate a nevus.

Other. Overlying cystoid retinal degeneration, VH or vitreous pigmented cells, drusen on the tumor surface, CNV, proptosis (from orbital invasion). Choroidal melanoma rarely occurs in blacks and more commonly occurs in light-skinned, blue- or green-eyed individuals.

Differential Diagnosis of Pigmented Lesions

- Choroidal nevus: See above.

- Congenital hypertrophy of the RPE: Flat black lesions that have crisp margins and often occur in the peripheral fundus. The margins are often well delineated with a surrounding depigmented and pigmented halo. Depigmented lacunae within the lesion appear as the lesion ages. Asymptomatic (see Figure 11.36.3).

- Reactive hyperplasia of the RPE: Related to previous trauma or inflammation. Lesions are black, flat, have irregular margins, and may have associated white gliosis. Often multifocal.

11

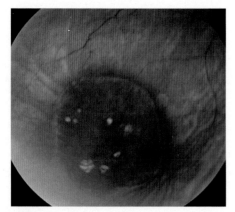

FIGURE 11.36.3. Congenital hypertrophy of the retinal pigment epithelium.

■ Subretinal blood: From any cause can simulate a melanoma, including ARMD, IPCV, PEHCR, others. IVFA and ICG may aid in differentiation. See specific sections.

■ Melanocytoma of the optic nerve: A black optic nerve lesion with fibrillated margins. It can grow slowly in approximately 15% cases. IVFA may allow differentiation.

■ Choroidal detachment: Follows ocular surgery, trauma, or hypotony of another etiology. Dark peripheral multilobular fundus mass. The ora serrata is often visible without scleral depression. Localized suprachoroidal hemorrhage can be very difficult to differentiate from melanoma based on appearance alone. Transillumination is helpful with serous detachment but is not helpful when there is a hemorrhagic component in distinguishing these entities from melanoma. In these situations, IVFA is the study of choice, usually allowing differentiation between the two entities. See 11.27, *Choroidal Effusion/Detachment.*

Differential Diagnosis of Nonpigmented Lesions

■ Choroidal hemangioma: Red-orange, may be elevated, not mushroom shaped.

■ Metastatic carcinoma: Cream or light brown, flat or slightly elevated, extensive subretinal fluid, may be multifocal or bilateral. Patient may have a history of cancer (especially breast or lung cancer).

■ Choroidal osteoma: Yellow-orange, usually close to the optic disc, pseudopod-like projections of the margin, often bilateral, typically occurs in young women in their teens or twenties. US may show a minimally elevated, calcified plaque-like lesion.

■ Posterior scleritis: Patients may have choroidal folds, pain, proptosis, uveitis, or anterior scleritis associated with an amelanotic mass. Look for the T-sign on US. See 5.7, *Scleritis.*

■ Lymphoma: Yellow-orange infiltration; can be unilateral or bilateral; often there is associated orbital or conjunctival lymphoma.

■ Sclerochoroidal calcification: Asymptomatic, yellow-white, sub-RPE and sub-choroidal plaques. Typically bilateral and commonly postequatorial and superotemporal. May be elevated. May be the result of calcification of the insertion of the oblique muscles. B scan US shows an elevated, calcified lesion. Typically idiopathic and seen in elderly patients. Can be associated with abnormalities of calcium-phosphorus metabolism and cases of renal tubular hypokalemic metabolic alkalosis (e.g., Gitelman and Bartter syndromes). Renal function, and serum electrolytes including calcium and magnesium should be checked.

Work-Up

1. History: Ocular surgery or trauma, cancer, anorexia, weight loss, or systemic illness?

2. Dilated fundus examination using indirect ophthalmoscopy.

3. IVFA: May rule out lesions that simulate melanoma, but may not differentiate melanoma from large nevus, metastases, or hemangioma.

4. A- and B-scan US: Documents thickness and confirms clinical impression. With choroidal melanoma, US usually shows low-to-moderate reflectivity with choroidal excavation. Thickness is often >2 mm. May show a mushroom appearance.

5. OCT: Often documents fresh subretinal fluid.

6. Autofluorescence: Often shows prominent overlying lipofuscin (orange pigment).

7. ICG angiography: Can show double circulation with prominent blood vessels within the melanoma.

8. Consider fine-needle aspiration biopsy in selected cases for cytologic confirmation and genetic analysis of the tumor for prognostication.

9. Consider CT scan or MRI of the orbit and brain (useful in patients with opaque media).

10. If melanoma is confirmed:

    —Blood work: lactate dehydrogenase, gamma-glutamyl transferase, aspartate and alanine aminotransferases, and alkaline phosphatase twice yearly. If liver enzymes are elevated, consider an MRI or liver scan to rule out a liver metastasis.

    —Annual chest radiograph or chest computed tomography.

    —Annual MRI of the liver.

    —Complete physical examination by a medical internist.

11. Referral to an internist or oncologist for breast examination, full skin examination, chest radiograph, and consider a carcinoembryonic antigen assay if a choroidal metastasis is suspected.

Treatment

Depending on the results of the metastatic work-up, the tumor characteristics, the status of the contralateral eye, and the age and general health of the patient, melanoma of the choroid may be managed by observation, photocoagulation, transpupillary thermotherapy, radiation therapy, local resection, enucleation, or exenteration. Most cases are managed with plaque radiotherapy followed by consolidation of the scar with thermotherapy. Methods to protect from ultimate vision loss from radiation retinopathy include anti-VEGF medications and sector photocoagulation.

11

12 Uveitis

12.1 ANTERIOR UVEITIS (IRITIS/IRIDOCYCLITIS)

Symptoms

- **Acute:** Pain, redness, photophobia, consensual photophobia (pain in the affected eye when a light is shone in the fellow eye), excessive tearing, decreased vision.

- **Chronic:** Decreased vision [from vitreous debris, cystoid macular edema (CME), or cataract]. May have periods of exacerbations and remissions with few acute symptoms [e.g., juvenile idiopathic (rheumatoid) arthritis (JIA/JRA)].

Signs

Critical. Cells and flare in the anterior chamber, ciliary flush, keratic precipitates (KP):

- Fine KP ("stellate"; typically covers entire corneal endothelium): Herpetic, Fuchs heterochromic iridocyclitis (FHIC), cytomegalovirus (CMV) retinitis, and others.

- Small, nongranulomatous KP: Human leukocyte antigen (HLA)-B27 associated, trauma, masquerade, JIA, Posner–Schlossman syndrome (glaucomatocyclitic crisis), and all the granulomatous entities.

- Granulomatous KP [large, greasy ("mutton-fat"); mostly on inferior cornea]: Sarcoidosis, syphilis, tuberculosis, sympathetic ophthalmia, lens-induced, Vogt–Koyanagi–Harada (VKH) syndrome, and others.

Other. Low intraocular pressure (IOP) more commonly seen (secondary to ciliary body hyposecretion), elevated IOP can occur (e.g., herpetic, lens-induced, FHIC, Posner–Schlossman syndrome), fibrin (HLA-B27 or endophthalmitis), hypopyon (HLA-B27, Behçet disease, infectious endophthalmitis, rifabutin, tumor), iris nodules (sarcoidosis, syphilis, tuberculosis), iris atrophy (herpetic), iris heterochromia (FHIC), iris synechiae (especially HLA-B27, sarcoidosis), band keratopathy (especially JIA in younger patients, any chronic uveitis in older), uveitis in a "quiet eye" (consider JIA, FHIC, masquerade syndromes), CME (see Figure 12.1.1).

Differential Diagnosis

- Posterior uveitis with spillover into the anterior chamber: Mainly floaters and decreased vision, positive fundoscopic findings (see 12.3, *Posterior Uveitis*).

- Traumatic iritis. See 3.5, *Traumatic Iritis.*

- Posner–Schlossman syndrome: Recurrent episodes of very high IOP and minimal inflammation. See 9.8, *Glaucomatocyclitic Crisis/Posner–Schlossman Syndrome.*

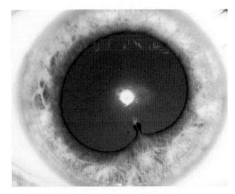

FIGURE 12.1.1. Anterior uveitis with posterior synechiae.

- Drug-induced uveitis (e.g., rifabutin, cidofovir, sulfonamides, pamidronate, systemic moxifloxacin).

- Sclerouveitis: Uveitis secondary to scleritis; typically presents with profound pain.

- CLARE (contact lens-associated red eye): Red eye, corneal edema, epithelial defects, iritis with or without hypopyon, and no stromal infiltrates.

- Infectious keratouveitis: Corneal infiltrate is present. See 4.11, *Bacterial Keratitis.*

- Infectious endophthalmitis: History of recent surgery or penetrating trauma, pain, hypopyon, fibrin, vitritis, decreased vision, red eye; may have endogenous source with fever, elevated white count. See 12.13 to 12.16, *Endophthalmitis* sections.

- Schwartz–Matsuo syndrome: Pigment released from a chronic retinal detachment clogs the trabecular meshwork resulting in elevated IOP.

- Tumor: Retinoblastoma in children, intraocular lymphoma in elderly, metastatic disease in all ages, and others.

- Pseudouveitis from pigment dispersion syndromes. Other findings include krukenburg spindle and iris transillumination defects.

Etiology

- Idiopathic.

- HLA-B27 associated uveitis: Systemic associations include ankylosing spondylitis, reactive arthritis (Reiter syndrome), psoriatic arthritis, inflammatory bowel disease.

NOTE: Bilateral recurrent alternating anterior uveitis is very characteristic of HLA-B27 uveitis.

- Lens-induced uveitis: Immune reaction to lens material, often secondary to incomplete cataract extraction, trauma with lens capsule damage, or hypermature cataract. See 9.12, *Lens-Induced (Phacogenic) Glaucoma.*

- Postoperative iritis: Anterior chamber inflammation following intraocular surgery. Endophthalmitis must be considered if severe inflammation and pain are present. See 12.14, *Chronic Postoperative Uveitis.*

- Uveitis–Glaucoma–Hyphema (UGH) syndrome: Usually secondary to irritation from an intraocular lens (particularly a closed-loop anterior chamber lens or single-piece lens in ciliary sulcus). See 9.16, *Postoperative Glaucoma.*

- Behçet disease: Young adults, acute hypopyon, iritis, aphthous ulcers, genital ulcerations, erythema nodosum, retinal vasculitis (arteries and/or veins) and hemorrhages, may have recurrent episodes.

- Lyme disease: May have history of a tick bite and rash. See 13.3, *Lyme Disease.*

- Anterior segment ischemia: Flare out of proportion to cellular reaction. Pain. Secondary to carotid insufficiency, tight scleral buckle, or previous muscle surgeries.

- Other rare etiologies of anterior uveitis: Mumps, influenza, adenovirus, measles, Chlamydia, Leptospirosis, Kawasaki disease, rickettsial disease, and others.

Chronic

- JIA: Usually young girls, may be painless and asymptomatic with minimal injection. Often bilateral. Iritis may precede the typical pauciarticular arthritis (four or fewer joints involved). Positive antinuclear antibody (ANA), negative rheumatoid factor, and increased erythrocyte sedimentation rate (ESR) most commonly seen. Associated with glaucoma, cataracts, band keratopathy, and CME. Uveitis may occur in polyarticular and less frequently in systemic JIA.

- Chronic iridocyclitis of children: Usually young girls, similar to JIA except no arthritis.

- FHIC: Few symptoms, diffuse iris stromal atrophy often causing a lighter-colored iris with transillumination defects and blunting of the iris architecture. Gonioscopy may reveal fine vessels that cross the trabecular meshwork, typically without posterior synechiae. Fine KP over the entire corneal endothelium, mild anterior chamber reaction. Vitreous opacities, glaucoma, and cataracts are common.

- Sarcoidosis: More common in African-Americans and Scandinavians. Usually bilateral; can have extensive posterior synechiae or conjunctival nodules. See 12.6, *Sarcoidosis.*

12

■ Herpes simplex/varicella zoster: Corneal scars, history of unilateral recurrent red eye, occasionally history of skin vesicles, associated with decreased corneal sensation, increased IOP and iris atrophy.

■ Syphilis: May have a maculopapular rash, iris roseola (vascular papules on the iris), and interstitial keratitis with ghost vessels in late stages. Inflammation of any ocular structure may occur. Neurosyphilis can have vitritis and meningismus. See 12.12, *Syphilis*.

■ Tuberculosis: Positive protein derivative of tuberculin (PPD), typical chest radiograph findings, occasionally phlyctenular or interstitial keratitis, sometimes signs of posterior uveitis. See 12.3, *Posterior Uveitis*.

■ Others: Leprosy, brucellosis, etc.

Work-Up

1. Obtain a thorough history and review of systems (Tables 12.1.1 and 12.1.2).

NOTE: Autoimmune diseases are less common in the very young and very old—consider masquerades.

Inflammatory arthritis typically presents with stiffness in the morning that improves after activity.

---

2. Complete ocular examination, including an IOP check, gonioscopy, and a dilated fundus examination. The vitreous should be evaluated for cells.

3. A laboratory work-up may be unnecessary in certain situations:

—First episode of a mild, unilateral, nongranulomatous uveitis with a history and examination that is not suggestive of systemic disease.

—Uveitis in the setting of known systemic disease such as sarcoidosis or the use of medicines known to cause uveitis (e.g., rifabutin).

—Clinical findings are classic for a particular diagnosis (e.g., herpetic keratouveitis, FHIC, toxoplasmosis).

4. If the uveitis is bilateral, granulomatous, or recurrent, and the history and examination are unremarkable, then a nonspecific initial work-up is conducted:

—Rapid plasma reagin (RPR) or venereal disease research laboratories test (VDRL).

—Fluorescent treponemal antibody absorption (FTA-ABS).

—PPD and anergy panel.

—Chest radiograph to rule out sarcoidosis and tuberculosis.

—Angiotensin-converting enzyme [(ACE); questionable utility].

—Lyme titer.

—ESR.

—HLA-B27.

TABLE 12.1.1	**Epidemiology of Anterior Uveitis**			
Age:	**Infants**	**Children**	**Young Adults**	**Elderly**
	TORCH infections, retinoblastoma	JIA, toxocariasis, toxoplasmosis	HLA-B27, Fuchs heterochromic iridocyclitis, pars planitis, idiopathic	Lymphoma, other masquerades, serpiginous, birdshot, ARN
Sex:	**Female**	**Male**		
	JIA, SLE	Ankylosing spondylitis, Reactive arthritis		
Race:	**Caucasian**	**African-American**	**Mediterranean, Middle Eastern**	**Asian**
	HLA-B27, white dot syndromes, MS	Sarcoidosis, SLE	Behçet disease	Behçet disease, VKH syndrome

TABLE **12.1.2** Review of Systems	
Musculoskeletal	
Arthritis	Behçet disease, Lyme disease, SLE, HLA-B27, relapsing polychondritis, JIA
Heel pain	Reactive arthritis, HLA-B27
Pulmonary	
Asthma	Sarcoidosis, TB, Wegener
Pneumonia	Cytomegalovirus, AIDS, aspergillosis, SLE, sarcoidosis, Wegener
Ear–Nose–Throat	
Auditory	VKH, sympathetic ophthalmia
Gastrointestinal	
Diet/hygiene	Poor handwashing-toxoplasmosis and toxocariasis; uncooked meat-toxoplasmosis and cysticercosis; unpasteurized milk-brucellosis and TB
Diarrhea	Whipple disease, ulcerative colitis, Crohn disease
Oral ulcers	Behçet disease, reactive arthritis, ulcerative colitis, herpes, sarcoidosis
Genitourinary	
Genital ulcers	Behçet disease, reactive arthritis, syphilis
Hematuria	Polyarteritis nodosum, SLE, Wegener, TINU
Urethral discharge	Reactive arthritis, syphilis, Chlamydia
Skin	
Erythema nodosum	Behçet disease, sarcoidosis
Rash on palms and soles	Syphilis
Erythema chronicum migrans	Lyme disease
Lupus pernio (purple malar rash)	Sarcoidosis
Psoriasis	Psoriatic arthritis
Vitiligo and poliosis	VKH
Shingles	Varicella-zoster virus, acute retinal necrosis
Pets	
Puppy	Toxocariasis
Cat	Toxoplasmosis
Social History	
Drug abuse	Candida, HIV/AIDS
Venereal disease	Syphilis, HIV/AIDS, reactive arthritis

12

TABLE 12.1.3	Suggested Diagnostic Workup for Anterior Uveitis
Ankylosing Spondylitis	HLA B27, SI joint films, rheumatology consult
Reactive arthritis	HLA B27, SI joint films (if symptomatic), swab for Chlamydia
Psoriatic arthritis	HLA B27, rheumatology and/or dermatology consult
Lyme disease	Lyme immunofluorescent assay or ELISA
Juvenile idiopathic arthritis or any suspect uveitis in children	Rheumatoid factor, antinuclear antibodies, rheumatology consult, radiographs of affected joints
Sarcoidosis	Chest radiograph, PPD and anergy panel, angiotensin-converting enzyme
Syphilis	RPR or VDRL, MHA-TP or FTA-ABS, consider HIV
Ocular ischemic syndrome	Intravenous fluorescein angiography, carotid Doppler studies

NOTE: In children with uveitis, it is recommended to perform ANA, RF, and HLA-B27. Lyme titer and ACE may also be considered. Evaluation for systemic disease by a pediatric rheumatologist may be warranted.

5. If a specific diagnosis is suspected, perform the appropriate work-up. If too many tests are ordered unnecessarily, a portion of them may come back false-positive and confuse the diagnosis. See Table 12.1.3.

Treatment

1. Cycloplegic (e.g., scopolamine 0.25% b.i.d. for mild to moderate inflammation; atropine 1% b.i.d. for severe inflammation).

2. Topical steroid (prednisolone acetate 1% one drop q1–6h, depending on the severity, brand name is better than generic and often necessary). Most cases of moderate to severe acute uveitis require q1–2h dosing initially. Difluprednate 0.05% may allow less frequent dosing than prednisolone acetate. Consider FML ophthalmic ointment at night. If the anterior uveitis is severe, unilateral, and is not responding to topical steroids, then consider periocular repository steroids (e.g., triamcinolone 20 to 40 mg subtenon injection). See Appendix 10, *Technique for Retrobulbar/Subtenon/Subconjunctival Injections*.

NOTE: This is an off-label use of medication and patients must be advised appropriately. A trial of topical steroids at full strength for several weeks may help identify patients at risk of a significant IOP increase from steroids. Additionally, periocular depot steroids are relatively contraindicated in patients with scleritis.

3. If there is no improvement on maximal topical and repository steroids, or if the uveitis is bilateral and severe, consider systemic steroids, or immunosuppressive therapy. Consider referral to a uveitis specialist and rheumatologist.

NOTE: Prior to initiating systemic steroids or periocular depot steroids, it is important to rule out infectious causes.

4. Treat secondary glaucoma with aqueous suppressants. Avoid pilocarpine. Glaucoma may result from:

—Cellular blockage of the trabecular meshwork. See 9.7, *Inflammatory Open-Angle Glaucoma*.

—Secondary angle closure from synechiae formation. See 9.4, *Acute Angle-Closure Glaucoma*.

—Neovascularization of the iris and angle. See 9.14, *Neovascular Glaucoma*.

—Steroid-response. See 9.9, *Steroid-Response Glaucoma*.

5. If an exact etiology for the anterior uveitis is determined, then systemic management is required.

—Ankylosing spondylitis: Often requires systemic antiinflammatory agents (e.g., NSAIDs such as naproxen). Consider cardiology consult (high incidence of cardiomegaly, conduction defects, and aortic insufficiency), rheumatology consult, and physical therapy consult.

—Inflammatory bowel disease: Often benefits from systemic steroids, sulfadiazine, or other immunosuppressive agents. Obtain a medical or gastrointestinal consult.

—Reactive arthritis (Reiter syndrome): If urethritis is present, then the patient and sexual partners are treated for chlamydia (e.g., azithromycin 1 g, single dose). Obtain medical and/or rheumatology consult.

—Psoriatic arthritis: Consider a rheumatology and/or dermatology consult.

—Glaucomatocyclitic crisis: See 9.8, *Glaucomatocyclitic Crisis/Posner–Schlossman Syndrome.*

—Lens-induced uveitis: Usually requires removal of lens material. See 9.12, *Lens-Induced (Phacogenic) Glaucoma.*

—Herpetic uveitis: Herpes simplex typically requires topical or oral antivirals and steroid drops for corneal disease. Herpetic iridocyclitis benefits from topical steroids and systemic antiviral medications (e.g., acyclovir/valacyclovir). See 4.15, *Herpes Simplex Virus* and 4.16, *Herpes Zoster Ophthalmicus/ Varicella Zoster Virus.*

—UGH syndrome: See 9.16, *Postoperative Glaucoma.*

—Behçet disease: See 12.7, *Behçet Disease.*

—Lyme disease: See 13.3, *Lyme Disease.*

—JIA: Steroid dosage is adjusted according to the degree of anterior chamber cells, not flare. Prolonged cycloplegic therapy may be required. Consult rheumatology or pediatrics as systemic steroid therapy or other systemic immunomdulatory therapy is often needed. Regular follow up is essential as flares may be asymptomatic but can cause extensive damage from synechiae, glaucoma, cystoid macular edema, and cataract formation.

NOTE: JIA has a high complication rate with cataract surgery. Avoid cataract surgery if possible until patient is free of inflammation for at least 3 months. An intraocular lens (IOL) may be placed in select circumstances.

—Chronic iridocyclitis of children: Same as JIA.

—FHIC: Usually does not respond to or require steroids (a trial of steroids may be attempted, but they should be tapered quickly if there is no response); cycloplegics are rarely necessary.

NOTE: Patients with FHIC usually do well with cataract surgery, however they may develop a hyphema.

—Sarcoidosis: See 12.6, *Sarcoidosis.*

—Syphilis: See 12.12, *Syphilis.*

—Tuberculosis: Avoid systemic steroids. Refer the patient to an internist or infectious disease specialist for consideration of systemic antituberculous treatment.

Follow-Up

1. Every 1 to 7 days in the acute phase, depending on the severity; every 1 to 6 months when stable.

2. At each visit, the anterior chamber reaction and IOP should be evaluated.

3. A vitreous and fundus examination should be performed for all flare-ups, when vision is affected, or every 3 to 6 months.

4. If the anterior chamber reaction has resolved, then the steroid drops can be slowly tapered [usually one drop per day every 3 to 7 days (e.g., q.i.d. for 1 week, then t.i.d. for 1 week, then b.i.d. for 1 week)]. Steroids are usually discontinued following the taper when the anterior chamber does not have any cellular reaction (flare may still be present). Rarely, long-term low-dose steroids every day or every other day are required to keep the inflammation from recurring. Punctal occlusion techniques may increase potency of drug and decrease systemic absorption.

12

The cycloplegic agents also can be tapered as the anterior chamber reaction improves. Cycloplegics should be used at least every evening until the anterior chamber is free of cells.

NOTE: As with most ocular and systemic diseases requiring steroid therapy, the steroid should be tapered. Sudden discontinuation of steroids can lead to severe rebound inflammation.

12.2　INTERMEDIATE UVEITIS

Symptoms

Painless floaters and decreased vision. Minimal photophobia or external inflammation. Usually, 15 to 40 years of age and bilateral.

Signs

(See Figure 12.2.1.)

Critical. Vitreous cells, white exudative material over the inferior ora serrata and pars plana (snowbank), cellular aggregates floating predominantly in the inferior vitreous (snowballs). Younger patients may present with vitreous hemorrhage.

NOTE: Snowbanking is typically in the inferior vitreous and can often be seen only with indirect ophthalmoscopy and scleral depression.

Other. Peripheral retinal vascular sheathing, peripheral neovascularization, mild anterior chamber inflammation, CME, posterior subcapsular cataract, band keratopathy, secondary glaucoma, epiretinal membrane, and exudative retinal detachment.

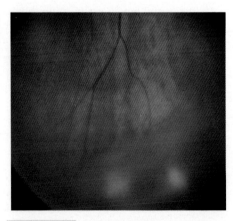

FIGURE 12.2.1. Pars planitis/intermediate uveitis with snowballs.

Etiology

- Idiopathic pars planitis (>70%).

- Sarcoidosis. See 12.6, *Sarcoidosis.*

- Multiple sclerosis. See 10.14, *Optic Neuritis.*

- Lyme disease. See 13.3, *Lyme Disease.*

- Syphilis. See 12.12, *Syphilis.*

- Toxocariasis. See 12.3, *Posterior Uveitis,* and 8.1, *Leukocoria.*

- Others: Inflammatory bowel disease, Bartonella, Whipple syndrome, primary Sjogrens syndrome, lymphoma, tubulointerstitial nephritis uveitis (TINU) syndrome, etc.

Work-Up

1. Chest radiograph, PPD, ACE level, RPR, FTA-ABS.

2. Consider intravenous fluorescein angiography (IVFA) and/or optical coherence tomography (OCT) to document CME or retinal vasculitis.

3. Consider lab testing for Lyme disease, toxoplasmosis, cat-scratch disease. In older individuals, consider work-up for malignancy/lymphoma.

4. Consider magnetic resonance imaging (MRI) of the brain with gadolinium to evaluate for demyelinating lesions if review of systems is positive for current or previous focal neurologic deficits. Refer to neurologist for multiple sclerosis work-up if necessary.

Treatment

Treat all vision-threatening complications in symptomatic patients with active disease. Mild vitreous cell in the absence of symptoms or vision loss may be observed.

1. Topical prednisolone acetate 1% or difluprednate 0.05% q1–2h, and consider simultaneous subtenon steroid (0.5 to 1.0 mL of triamcinolone 40 mg/mL). Repeat the injections every 6 to 8 weeks until the vision and CME have stabilized. Slowly taper the frequency of injections. Subtenon steroid injections must be used with extreme caution in patients with steroid-responsive glaucoma. See Appendix 10, *Technique for Retrobulbar/Subtenon/Subconjunctival Injections*.

2. If no improvement after three injections, consider systemic steroids (e.g., prednisone 40 to 60 mg p.o. q.d. for 4 to 6 weeks), tapering gradually according to the patient's response. Systemic steroid therapy should be no longer than 3 months, including taper. Other options include slow release steroid implants (dexamethasone 0.7 mg intravitreal implant, and fluocinolone acetonide 0.59 mg intravitreal implant), and immunomodulatory therapy, often in conjunction with Rheumatology.

NOTE: In bilateral cases, systemic steroid therapy is often preferred to periocular injections.

---

3. Transscleral cryotherapy to the area of snowbanking should be considered in patients who fail to respond to either oral or subtenon corticosteroids.

4. Pars plana vitrectomy may be useful in cases refractory to systemic steroids or to treat vitreous opacification, tractional retinal detachment, epiretinal membrane, and other complications. Additionally, vitreous biopsy through a pars plana vitrectomy may be indicated in cases of suspected masquerade syndromes, particularly, intraocular lymphoma.

NOTE:

1. Some physicians delay steroid injections for several weeks to observe whether the IOP increases on topical steroids (steroid response). If a steroid response is found, depot injections should be avoided.

2. Topical NSAIDs (e.g., ketorolac q.i.d.) may be added in patients with CME.

3. Cataracts are a frequent complication of intermediate uveitis. If cataract extraction is performed, the patient should ideally be free of inflammation for 3 months. Consider starting the patient on oral prednisone 60 mg daily 5 days prior to surgery and tapering the prednisone over the next month. Consider a combined pars plana vitrectomy at the time of cataract surgery if significant vitreous opacification is present.

Follow-Up

1. In the acute phase, patients are reevaluated every 1 to 4 weeks, depending on the severity of the condition.

2. In the chronic phase, reexamination is performed every 3 to 6 months.

12.3 POSTERIOR UVEITIS

12

Symptoms

Blurred vision and floaters. Pain, redness, and photophobia are typically absent unless anterior chamber inflammation is present.

NOTE: Posterior uveitis with significant pain suggests bacterial endophthalmitis or posterior scleritis.

Signs

Critical. Cells in the anterior and/or posterior vitreous, vitreous haze, retinal or choroidal inflammatory lesions, vasculitis (sheathing and exudates around vessels).

Other. Anterior segment inflammatory signs, CME.

Differential Diagnosis

Panuveitis

Describes a pattern of severe, diffuse inflammation of both anterior and posterior segments. Often bilateral. Possible etiologies are listed below:

- Sarcoidosis: See 12.6, *Sarcoidosis.*

- Syphilis: See 12.12, *Syphilis.*

- VKH syndrome: See 12.11, *Vogt–Koyanagi–Harada Syndrome.*

■ Behçet disease: See 12.1, *Anterior Uveitis (Iritis/Iridocyclitis)*, and 12.7, *Behçet Disease*.

■ Lens-induced uveitis: See 9.12, *Lens-Induced (Phacogenic) Glaucoma*.

■ Sympathetic ophthalmia: See 12.18, *Sympathetic Ophthalmia*.

■ Tuberculosis: Produces varied clinical manifestations. The diagnosis is usually made by ancillary laboratory tests. Miliary tuberculosis may produce multifocal, small, yellow-white choroidal lesions. Most patients have concomitant anterior granulomatous or nongranulomatous uveitis.

Postsurgical/Trauma

See 12.13, *Postoperative Endophthalmitis;* 12.14, *Chronic Postoperative Uveitis;* 12.15, *Traumatic Endophthalmitis;* and 12.18, *Sympathetic Ophthalmia*.

Choroiditis

■ Acute posterior multifocal placoid pigment epitheliopathy (APMPPE): Acute visual loss in young adults, often after a viral illness. Multiple, creamy yellow-white, plaque-like subretinal lesions in both eyes. Lesions block early and stain late on IVFA. Usually spontaneously improves. Rarely associated with a cerebral vasculitis.

■ Birdshot retinochoroidopathy: Usually middle-aged, with bilateral, multiple, creamy-yellow spots deep to the retina, approximately 1 mm in diameter, scattered throughout the fundus. A mild to moderate vitritis is present. Retinal or optic nerve edema or both may be present. Positive HLA-A29 in approximately 90% of patients. Consider systemic immunosuppression.

■ Multifocal choroiditis: Visual loss in young myopic women, typically bilateral. Multiple, small, round, pale inflammatory lesions (similar to histoplasmosis) are located at the level of the pigment epithelium and choriocapillaris. Unlike histoplasmosis, vitritis occurs in 98% of patients. The lesions are predominantly in the macula and frequently respond to oral or periocular steroids, but typically recur. Choroidal neovascularization (CNV) is common, and

so patients should return for urgent evaluation if they have decreased vision or metamorphopsia.

■ Punctate inner choroidopathy: Blurred vision, paracentral scotoma, and/or photopsias, usually in young myopic women. Multiple, small round yellow-white spots predominantly in posterior pole with minimal intraocular inflammation. Lesions become well-demarcated atrophic scars within weeks. CNV may develop in up to 40% of patients.

■ Serpiginous choroidopathy: Typically bilateral, recurrent chorioretinitis characterized by acute lesions (yellow-white subretinal patches with indistinct margins) bordering old atrophic scars. The chorioretinal changes usually extend from the optic disc outward; however, one-third may begin peripherally. Patients are typically aged 30 to 60 years. Strongly consider systemic immunosuppression. CNV may develop.

■ Toxocariasis: Typically unilateral. Usually occurs in children. The most common presentations are a macular granuloma (elevated white retinal/subretinal lesion) with poor vision, unilateral pars planitis with peripheral granuloma, or endophthalmitis. A peripheral lesion may be associated with a fibrous band extending to the optic disc, sometimes resulting in macular vessel dragging. A severe vitritis and anterior uveitis may be present. A negative undiluted Toxocara titer in an immunocompetent host usually rules out this disease. See 8.1, *Leukocoria*.

■ Presumed ocular histoplasmosis syndrome: Punched-out chorioretinal scars, peripapillary atrophy, and often CNV. Vitreous cells are absent. See 11.24, *Ocular Histoplasmosis*.

Retinitis

■ Multiple evanescent white-dot syndrome: Photopsias and acute unilateral visual loss, often after a viral illness, usually in young women. Uncommonly bilateral or sequential. Multiple, small, creamy white lesions deep in the retina or at the level of the retinal pigment epithelium with foveal granularity and occasionally vitreous cells. There is often an enlarged blind spot on formal visual field testing. May have a shimmering scotoma. Vision typically returns to normal within weeks without treatment.

- CMV: Whitish patches of necrotic retina are mixed with retinal hemorrhage. Seen in neonates and immunocompromised patients. See 12.9, *Cytomegalovirus Retinitis*.

- Acute retinal necrosis (ARN): Unilateral or bilateral peripheral white patches of thickened necrotic retina with vascular sheathing that progress rapidly. A significant vitritis is typically present. See 12.8, *Acute Retinal Necrosis*.

- Progressive outer retinal necrosis (PORN): Clinically similar to ARN, but may not have vitreous cells and involves the posterior pole early. Often in immunocompromised patients. See 12.8, *Acute Retinal Necrosis*.

- Toxoplasmosis: Retinal lesion associated with a pigmented chorioretinal scar. Focal dense vitritis. See 12.5, *Toxoplasmosis*.

- Candida: Early discrete drusen-like choroidal lesions progressing to yellow–white, fluffy retinal or preretinal lesions. See 12.17, *Candida Retinitis/Uveitis/Endophthalmitis*.

Vasculitis

Retinal sheathing around vessels. Branch retinal vein and branch retinal artery occlusions may occur.

- Periphlebitis (predominantly veins).

  —Sarcoidosis: Yellow "candlewax" exudates around veins.

  —Syphilis.

  —Pars planitis: Most prominent in the inferior periphery, NVE may be present.

  —Eales disease: Peripheral neovascularization and/or avascular retina.

  —Multiple sclerosis.

  —Birdshot retinochoroidopathy.

- Arteritis (predominantly arteries).

  —Giant cell arteritis.

  —Polyarteritis nodosum.

  —Frosted branch angiitis.

  —Churg-Strauss.

  —ARN.

  —IRVAN (idiopathic retinal vasculitis, aneurysms, and neuroretinitis).

- Both arteries and veins.

  —Systemic lupus erythematosus.

  —Wegener granulomatosis.

  —Behçet disease.

  —HLA-B27-associated.

Other Infectious Causes of Posterior Uveitis

- Cat-scratch disease: Stellate macular exudates, optic nerve swelling, vitreous cells, positive Bartonella serology. See 5.3, *Parinaud Oculoglandular Conjunctivitis*.

- Diffuse unilateral subacute neuroretinitis: Typically unilateral visual loss in children and young adults, caused by a nematode. Optic nerve swelling, vitreous cells, and deep gray–white retinal lesions are present initially, but may be subtle. Later, optic atrophy, narrowing of retinal vessels, and atrophic pigment epithelial changes develop. Vision, visual fields, and ERG deteriorate with time. Treatment is to laser nematode.

- Lyme disease: Produces varied forms of posterior uveitis. See 13.3, *Lyme Disease*.

- Nocardia, Coccidioides species, Aspergillus species, Cryptococcus species, meningococcus, ophthalmomyiasis, onchocerciasis, and cysticercosis (seen more commonly in Africa and Central and South America).

Other Causes of Vitreous Cells

- Ocular ischemia.

- Spillover from anterior uveitis.

- Masquerade syndromes: Always consider these in the very old or very young patient.

  —Large cell lymphoma (reticulum cell sarcoma): Persistent vitreous cells in patients >50 years, which usually do not respond completely to systemic steroids. Yellow–white subretinal infiltrates, retinal edema and hemorrhage, anterior chamber inflammation, or neurologic signs may be present.

12

—Malignant melanoma: A retinal detachment and associated vitritis may obscure the underlying tumor. See 11.36, *Choroidal Nevus and Malignant Melanoma of the Choroid.*

—Retinitis pigmentosa: Vitreous cells and macular edema may accompany waxy pallor of the optic disc, "bone-spicule" pigmentary changes, and attenuated retinal vessels. See 11.28, *Retinitis Pigmentosa and Inherited Chorioretinal Dystrophies.*

—Rhegmatogenous retinal detachment (RRD): A small number of pigmented anterior vitreous and anterior chamber cells frequently accompany an RRD. See 11.3, *Retinal Detachment.*

—Retained intraocular foreign body: Persistent inflammation after a penetrating ocular injury. May have iris heterochromia. Diagnosed by indirect ophthalmoscopy, gonioscopy, B-scan ultrasonography (US), US biomicroscopy, or computed tomography (CT) scan of the globe. See 3.15, *Intraocular Foreign Body.*

—Retinoblastoma: Almost always occurs in young children. May also present with a pseudohypopyon and vitreous cells. One or more elevated white retinal lesions are usually, but not always, present. See 8.1, *Leukocoria.*

—Leukemia: Unilateral retinitis and vitritis may occur in patients already known to have leukemia.

—Amyloidosis: Retrolenticular footplate-like deposits, vitreous globules, or membranes without any signs of anterior segment inflammation. Serum protein electrophoresis and diagnostic vitrectomy confirm the diagnosis. Rare.

—Asteroid hyalosis: Small, white, refractile particles (calcium soaps) adherent to collagen fibers and floating in the vitreous. Usually asymptomatic and of no clinical significance.

Work-Up

1. Complete history and review of systems: Systemic disease or infection, skin rash, intravenous (i.v.) drug abuse, indwelling catheter, risk factors for AIDS? Recent eye trauma or surgery? Travel to the Ohio–Mississippi River Valley, Southwestern United States, New England, or Middle Atlantic area? Tick bite?

2. Complete ocular examination, including IOP measurement and careful ophthalmoscopic examination. Indirect ophthalmoscopy with scleral depression of the ora serrata.

3. Consider IVFA to help in diagnosis or plan for therapy.

4. Blood tests (any of the following are obtained, depending on the suspected diagnosis): Toxoplasma titer, ACE level, serum lysozyme, FTA-ABS, RPR, ESR, ANA, HLA-B51 (Behçet disease), HLA-A29 (birdshot retinochoroidopathy), Toxocara titer, Lyme immunofluorescent assay or ELISA. In neonates or immunocompromised patients, consider checking titers for CMV, herpes simplex, varicella zoster, and rubella virus. Cultures of blood and i.v. sites may be helpful when infectious etiologies are suspected. Polymerase chain reaction (PCR) techniques are available for varicella zoster, herpes simplex, Toxoplasma, and other pathogens.

5. PPD with anergy panel.

6. Chest radiograph.

7. Urine for CMV in immunocompromised patients.

8. CT/MRI scan of the brain and lumbar puncture when reticulum cell sarcoma is suspected and when human immunodeficiency virus (HIV)-associated opportunistic infections indicate a potential for central nervous system (CNS) involvement.

9. Diagnostic vitrectomy when appropriate (see individual sections).

See the individual sections for more specific guidelines for work-up and treatment.

12.4 HUMAN LEUKOCYTE ANTIGEN–B27–ASSOCIATED UVEITIS

Symptoms

Acute pain, blurred vision, photophobia. Associated systemic complaints include back pain, arthritis, oral ulcers (typically not as painful as those seen in Behçet disease), pain with urination, gastrointestinal complaints, rashes.

Signs

Critical. Recurrent, unilateral (or bilateral) nongranulomatous anterior uveitis.

Other. Severe anterior chamber reaction with cell, flare, and fibrin. May have hypopyon. Tendency to form posterior synechiae early. Ciliary flush. More common in men than women.

Differential Diagnosis

- Other hypopyon uveitides: Behçet disease (posterior involvement more common than in HLA-B27), infectious endophthalmitis, retinoblastoma, metastatic tumors, rifabutin, sarcoidosis, masquerade syndromes.
- Idiopathic anterior uveitis.

Types of HLA-B27 Disease

- HLA-B27-associated uveitis without systemic disease.
- Ankylosing spondylitis: Young adult men, often with low back pain or stiffness, abnormalities on sacroiliac spine radiographs, increased ESR, positive HLA-B27.
- Inflammatory bowel disease: Crohn disease and ulcerative colitis. Chronic diarrhea.

- Reactive arthritis (Reiter syndrome): Young adult men, conjunctivitis, urethritis, polyarthritis, occasionally keratitis, increased ESR, positive HLA-B27, may have recurrent episodes. Arthritis tends to involve the lower extremities.
- Psoriatic arthritis: Characteristic skin findings with arthritis typically involving the upper extremities.

Work-Up

1. HLA-B27 to confirm diagnosis.
2. Ankylosing spondylitis: Sacroiliac spine radiographs show sclerosis and narrowing of the joint spaces, ESR.
3. Inflammatory bowel disease: Medicine or Gastroenterology consult.
4. Reactive arthritis: Conjunctival and urethral swabs for Chlamydia if indicated; a Medicine or Rheumatology consult.
5. Psoriatic arthritis: A Rheumatology or Dermatology consult.

Treatment

See 12.1, *Anterior Uveitis* (*Iritis/Iridocyclitis*). Patients with HLA-B27 uveitis often suffer multiple recurrences. For particularly relapsing cases, consider longer-term steroid sparing immunomodulatory therapy, often in conjunction with Rheumatology.

12

12.5 TOXOPLASMOSIS

Symptoms

Blurred vision and floaters. May have redness and photophobia. Pain is typically absent, except with iridocyclitis.

Signs

(See Figure 12.5.1.)

Critical. New, unilateral white–yellow retinal lesion often associated with an old pigmented chorioretinal scar. There is a moderate to severe focal vitreous inflammatory reaction directly over the lesion. Scar may be absent in cases of newly acquired toxoplasmosis.

Other.
- Anterior: Mild anterior chamber spillover may be present, increased IOP in 10% to 20%.

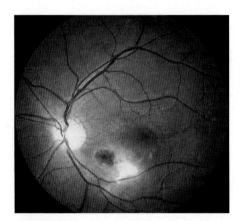

FIGURE 12.5.1. Toxoplasmosis.

■ Posterior: Vitreous debris, optic disc swelling often with edema extending into the retina, neuroretinitis with/without macular star, optic neuritis with significant vitritis, retinal vasculitis, rarely retinal artery or vein occlusion in the area of the inflammation. Kyrieleis arterialitis is periarterial exudate accumulation which may occur near the retinitis or elsewhere in the retina. Chorioretinal scars are occasionally found in the uninvolved eye. CME may be present.

NOTE: Toxoplasmosis is the most common cause of posterior uveitis and accounts for approximately 90% of focal necrotizing retinitis.

Toxoplasmosis can also develop in the deep retina (punctate outer retinal toxoplasmosis) with few to no vitreous cells present. More common in HIV-infected patients. See below.

Differential Diagnosis

See 12.3, *Posterior Uveitis,* for a complete list. The following rarely may closely simulate toxoplasmosis.

■ Syphilis (See 12.12, *Syphilis*) and tuberculosis.

■ Toxocariasis: Usually affects children. Chorioretinal scars are not typically seen. See 12.3, *Posterior Uveitis,* and 8.1, *Leukocoria.*

■ Acute retinal necrosis. See 12.8, *Acute Retinal Necrosis* (see Table 12.8.1).

Work-Up

See 12.3, *Posterior Uveitis,* for a nonspecific work-up when the diagnosis is in doubt.

1. History: Does the patient eat raw meat or has the patient been exposed to cats (sources of acquired infection)? Inquire about risk factors for HIV in atypical cases (e.g., several active lesions without old chorioretinal scars).

2. Complete ocular examination, including a dilated fundus evaluation.

3. Serum anti-toxoplasma antibody titer to indicate previous or current infection (usually not necessary). The high population seropositivity reduces the positive predictive value of a positive titer, but a negative titer should give strong consideration to an alternate diagnosis. Immunoglobulin M (IgM) is found approximately 2 weeks to 6 months after initial infection, after which only IgG remains.

NOTE: Request a 1:1 dilution because any titer of serum antibodies is significant in the setting of classic fundus findings.

---

4. Toxoplasmosis antibody titers and PCR may be performed on anterior chamber taps or through diagnostic vitrectomy in equivocal cases.

5. FTA-ABS, PPD, chest radiograph, and a Toxocara ELISA when the diagnosis is uncertain.

6. Consider HIV testing in atypical cases or high-risk patients. See below.

Treatment

1. Mild peripheral retinochoroiditis.

   a. Self-limited in immunocompetent patients. Consider observation only for extramacular lesions.

   b. Treat elevated IOP with antiglaucoma medications and if anterior chamber involved use topical cycloplegic (e.g., cyclopentolate 1% to 2% t.i.d.) with or without topical steroid (e.g., prednisolone acetate 1% q.i.d.).

2. Consider treatment for lesions in the macula, within 2 to 3 mm of the disc, threatening a large retinal vessel, vitritis severe enough to cause a two-line decrease in vision, or disease in an immunocompromised patient. Extended treatment may be required for patients who are immunocompromised.

a. Classic first-line therapy (for 4 to 6 weeks):

—Pyrimethamine, 200 mg p.o. load (or two 100-mg doses p.o. 12 hours apart), and then 25 to 50 mg p.o. daily. Do not give pyrimethamine to pregnant or breast-feeding women. (Spiramycin 1 g p.o. t.i.d. for women who seroconvert in pregnancy.)

—Folinic acid 10 mg p.o. every other day (to minimize bone marrow toxicity of pyrimethamine).

—Sulfadiazine 2 g p.o. load and then 1 g p.o. q.i.d.

—Prednisone may be added 20 to 60 mg p.o. q.d. beginning at least 24 hours after initiating antimicrobial therapy and tapered 10 days before stopping antibiotics. Periocular steroids should not be given.

NOTE: Due to potential bone marrow suppression, a complete blood count (CBC) must be obtained once per week while a patient is taking pyrimethamine. If the platelet count decreases below 100,000, then reduce the dosage of pyrimethamine and increase the folinic acid. Patients taking pyrimethamine should not take vitamins that contain folic acid. The medication should be given with meals to reduce anorexia.

Systemic steroids should only rarely be used in immunocompromised patients. Before systemic steroid use, evaluation of fasting blood sugar and studies to rule out tuberculosis are prudent.

---

b. Alternate regimens:

—Clindamycin 150 to 450 mg p.o. t.i.d. to q.i.d. (maximum 1.8 g/d) may be used alone, with pyrimethamine as alternative therapy (if the patient is sulfa allergic), or as an adjunct (quadruple therapy) to previously discussed therapy. Patients on clindamycin should be warned about pseudomembranous colitis, and the medication should be stopped if diarrhea develops. Intravitreal injection of clindamycin (0.1 mg/0.1 mL) can be effective for macular threatening cases, or when the patient is intolerant to systemic medication. May be combined with intravitreal steroid injection (i.e., dexamethasone 400 micrograms).

—Atovaquone 750 mg p.o. q.i.d., used as alternative similar to clindamycin.

—Trimethoprim/sulfamethoxazole (160 mg/800 mg) one tablet p.o. b.i.d., with or without clindamycin and prednisone.

—Azithromycin loading dose 1 g (day 1) then 250 to 500 mg daily. May be used alone or in combination with pyrimethamine (50 mg q.d.)

c. Anterior segment inflammation is treated as above.

3. Vitrectomy has been used for nonclearing dense vitritis or other complications.

4. Maintenance therapy (if patient is immunosuppressed)

—Trimethoprim/sulfamethoxazole 160 mg/800 mg one tablet p.o. b.i.d. Recurrences may be avoided with dosing as infrequently as one tablet every 3 days.

or

—Pyrimethamine 25 to 50 mg p.o. q.d. Sulfadiazine 500 to 1,000 mg p.o. q.i.d. Folinic acid 10 mg p.o. q.i.d.

—If sulfa-allergic, may use clindamycin 300 mg p.o. q.i.d.

5. Prophylaxis: Prior to cataract or refractive surgery in a patient with a history of toxoplasmosis consider using trimethoprim/sulfamethoxazole b.i.d. during the perioperative period.

Follow-Up

In 3 to 7 days for blood tests and/or ocular assessment, and then every 1 to 2 weeks on therapy.

SPECIAL CONSIDERATION IN IMMUNOCOMPROMISED PATIENTS

Vitritis is much less prominent. Adjacent retinochoroidal scars are usually not observed. The lesions may be single or multifocal, discrete or diffuse, and unilateral or bilateral. CNS imaging is essential because of high association with CNS disease (e.g., toxoplasmosis encephalitis in HIV patients). Diagnostic vitrectomy may be necessary because of the multiple simulating entities and the variability of laboratory diagnostic tests. Systemic steroids for ocular toxoplasmosis are contraindicated in AIDS.

12

12.6 ▸ SARCOIDOSIS

Symptoms

Bilateral ocular pain, photophobia, and decreased vision. May have insidious onset, especially in older patients with chronic disease. Systemic findings may include shortness of breath, parotid enlargement, fever, arthralgias, and rarely neurologic symptoms. Most common in 20- to 50-year age group. Most common in African Americans and Scandinavians.

Signs

Critical. Iris nodules, large mutton-fat KP (especially in a triangular distribution on the inferior corneal endothelium), sheathing along peripheral retinal veins (candle-wax drippings), peripheral retinal neovascularization.

Other. Conjunctival nodules, enlargement of lacrimal gland, dry eyes, posterior synechiae, glaucoma, cataract, intermediate uveitis, CME, vitritis, Dalen–Fuchs nodules (pale choroidal lesions that may simulate multifocal choroiditis or birdshot retinochoroidopathy), peripheral retinal neovascularization (see Figure 12.6.1).

Systemic. Tachypnea, facial nerve palsy, enlargement of salivary or lacrimal glands, bilateral symmetric hilar adenopathy on chest radiograph or CT, erythema nodosum (erythematous, tender nodules beneath the skin, often found on the shins), lupus pernio (a dusky purple rash on nose and cheeks), arthritis, lymphadenopathy, hepatosplenomegaly.

NOTE: Uveitis, secondary glaucoma, cataracts, and macular edema are the most common vision-threatening complications of ocular sarcoidosis.

Differential Diagnosis

■ Other causes of mutton-fat KP and iris nodules include syphilis, tuberculosis, sympathetic ophthalmia, and lens-induced uveitis. See 12.1, *Anterior Uveitis (Iritis/Iridocyclitis).*

■ Intermediate uveitis may be idiopathic or secondary to sarcoid, multiple sclerosis, Lyme disease, and others. See 12.2, *Intermediate Uveitis.*

■ Posterior uveitis with multiple chorioretinal lesions may be from birdshot retinochoroidopathy, intraocular lymphoma, syphilis, sympathetic ophthalmia, multifocal choroiditis, VKH syndrome, and others. See 12.3, *Posterior Uveitis.*

Work-Up

The following are the tests that are obtained when sarcoidosis is suspected clinically. See 12.1, *Anterior Uveitis (Iritis/Iridocyclitis),* and 12.3, *Posterior Uveitis,* for nonspecific uveitis work-up.
   Initial work-up:

1. Chest radiography is the single most useful test. Typically shows bilateral and symmetric hilar adenopathy and/or infiltrates indicative of pulmonary fibrosis. In cases of unilateral or atypical lung disease, consider malignancy. Consider chest CT scan if chest x-ray normal but clinical suspicion high.

2. Serum ACE is elevated in 60% to 90% of patients with active sarcoidosis. Normal level does not rule out sarcoidosis and elevation is not specific. Leprosy, histoplasmosis, and tuberculosis may also present with elevated ACE. Patients on oral steroids and ACE inhibitors (e.g., captopril for hypertension) may have falsely low ACE levels. ACE

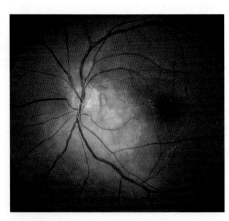

FIGURE 12.6.1. Sarcoid choroidal granuloma.

levels in children are variable and less helpful in diagnosis.

3. PPD with anergy panel: Useful for differentiating tuberculosis from sarcoidosis. Up to 50% of sarcoidosis patients are anergic and have no response to PPD or controls.

4. Obtain biopsy of accessible affected lesions to confirm noncaseating granulomatous inflammation. Sample at the edges of skin plaques or nodules. Sarcoid granulomas are not present in erythema nodosum and these lesions should not be sampled. An acid-fast stain and a methenamine–silver stain may be performed to rule out tuberculosis and fungal infection. A nondirected conjunctival biopsy in the absence of visible lesions has a low yield and is not recommended.

5. Some authors recommend serum and urine calcium levels, liver function tests, and a serum lysozyme. A positive result on one of these tests in the absence of chest radiographic or other findings is usually not helpful in diagnosis. A serum lysozyme may be useful in children, where ACE levels are unreliable.

If laboratory and chest radiographic studies suggest sarcoidosis or in the setting of a negative work-up but a high clinical suspicion of sarcoidosis, the following tests should be considered:

1. Chest CT scan may be more sensitive than plain films because of better visualization.

2. Whole-body gallium scan is sensitive for sarcoidosis. A "panda sign" indicates involvement of lacrimal, parotid, and submandibular glands. A "lambda sign" indicates involvement of perihilar and paratracheal lymph nodes. A positive gallium scan and an elevated ACE level is 73% sensitive and 100% specific for sarcoidosis.

3. Referral to pulmonologist for pulmonary function tests and transbronchial lung biopsy.

Treatment

Consider referring patients to an internist or pulmonologist for systemic evaluation and medical management. Consider early referral to a uveitis specialist in complicated cases. A poor visual outcome has been reported with posterior uveitis, glaucoma, delay in definitive treatment, or presence of macula-threatening conditions such as CME.

1. Anterior uveitis:

   • Cycloplegic (e.g., scopolamine 0.25% t.i.d.).

   • Topical steroid (e.g., prednisolone acetate 1% q1–6h).

2. Posterior uveitis:

   • Systemic steroids (e.g., prednisone 20 to 100 mg p.o. q.d.) and a histamine type 2 receptor (H2) blocker (e.g., ranitidine 150 mg p.o. b.i.d.) are often required in the presence of posterior uveitis (including optic neuritis) or bilateral severe anterior disease.

   • Periocular steroids (e.g., triamcinolone 40 mg/mL in 0.5 mL subtenon injection every 3 to 4 weeks) may be considered instead of systemic steroids, especially in unilateral or asymmetric cases. See Appendix 10, *Technique for Retrobulbar/Subtenon/Subconjunctival Injections*.

3. Immunosuppressives (e.g., methotrexate, azathioprine, mycophenolate mofetil, cyclosporine, cyclophosphamide, hydroxychloroquine, infliximab) have been used effectively as steroid-sparing agents.

NOTE: Topical steroids alone are inadequate for treatment of significant posterior uveitis.

---

4. Cystoid macular edema: See 11.14, *Cystoid Macular Edema*.

5. Glaucoma: See 9.7, *Inflammatory Open-Angle Glaucoma*; 9.9, *Steroid-Response Glaucoma*; 9.4, *Acute Angle-Closure Glaucoma*; or 9.14, *Neovascular Glaucoma*, depending on the etiology of the glaucoma.

6. Retinal neovascularization: May require panretinal photocoagulation.

7. Orbital disease is managed with systemic steroids as described previously.

8. Pulmonary disease, seventh nerve palsy, CNS disease, and renal disease require systemic steroids and management by an internist.

12

Follow-Up

1. Patients are reexamined in 1 to 7 days, depending on the severity of inflammation. The steroid dosages are adjusted in accordance with the treatment response. Slowly taper the steroids and cycloplegic agent as the inflammation subsides. Monitor IOP and reevaluate the fundus at each visit.

2. Patients with quiescent disease are seen every 3 to 6 months.

3. Patients being treated with steroids are monitored every 3 to 6 weeks.

4. Poor response to steroid treatment should prompt a work-up for other causes of uveitis or referral to a subspecialist.

12.7   BEHÇET DISEASE

Symptoms

Sudden onset of bilateral decreased vision, floaters, pain, photophobia.

Signs

Critical.   Painful oral aphthous ulcers (98% to 100% of patients) at least three times per year and two of the following: genital ulcers, skin lesions, positive Behçetine (pathergy) test (formation of a local pustule in response to skin puncture with needle), and eye lesions. May have other skin lesions including erythema nodosum and folliculitis. Systemic manifestations include arthritis and CNS disease.

Other.   Arthritis, bowel ulceration, epididymitis, vasculitis or vasculopathy, neuropyschiatric symptoms.

Ocular Signs

- Anterior: Hypopyon, anterior chamber reaction, and scleritis.

NOTE: Patients with Behçet disease almost never have fibrin even if anterior chamber reaction is severe, thus the hypopyon appears mobile, in contrast to HLA-B27-associated uveitis.

- Posterior: Vitritis, retinal vasculitis affecting both arteries and veins, venous obstruction, arterial attenuation, focal necrotizing retinitis, waxy optic nerve pallor, and retinal detachment.

Epidemiology

Age 20 to 40 years, especially Japanese, Turkish, or Middle Eastern descent.

Differential Diagnosis

- Sarcoidosis: May occasionally present with oral ulcers. See 12.6, *Sarcoidosis*.

- HLA-B27: Severe fibrinous uveitis. Oral ulcers are less painful and severe. See 12.4, *Human Leukocyte Antigen–B27–Associated Uveitis*.

- ARN: Confluent retinal whitening in periphery. More pain than Behçet disease. See 12.8, *Acute Retinal Necrosis*.

- Wegener granulomatosis: Nephritis, orbital inflammation, sinus, and pulmonary inflammation.

- Syphilis. See 12.12, *Syphilis*.

- Systemic lupus erythematosus and other collagen vascular diseases.

Work-Up

- Chest radiograph, ACE level, PPD, RPR, and FTA-ABS.

- Consider HLA-B27 in young men with positive review of systems.

- Granular-staining antineutrophil cytoplasmic antibody (c-ANCA) if Wegener granulomatosis suspected.

- Consider HLA-B51 and HLA-DR5 testing for Behçet disease.

- Consider Behçetine (pathergy) test.

Treatment

Untreated, bilateral blindness often develops within 3 to 4 years. Death may result from CNS involvement. Therefore, all patients with Behçet disease and posterior uveitis should be referred to a specialist for consideration of immunosuppressive therapy.

1. Systemic corticosteroids should be started (prednisone 1 to 2 mg/kg p.o. q.d. with ranitidine 150 mg p.o. b.i.d.). Steroids have been shown to delay the onset of blindness but not to alter the long-term outcome. Prior to starting steroids it is important to obtain a negative PPD and RPR/FTA-ABS.

2. All patients with Behçet disease and posterior uveitis should be referred to a specialist for immunosuppressive therapy.

Follow-Up

Daily during acute episode to monitor inflammation and IOP. Refer to uveitis specialist for further follow-up.

12.8 ACUTE RETINAL NECROSIS

Symptoms

Blurred vision, floaters, ocular pain, photophobia. Most patients are immunocompetent.

Signs

(See Figure 12.8.1.)

Critical. Focal, well-demarcated areas of retinal whitening (full-thickness necrosis) in the peripheral retina; rapid, circumferential progression of necrosis which may approach the posterior pole; occlusive vasculitis and prominent inflammatory reaction in the vitreous and anterior chamber. The macula is typically spared early in the disease course.

Other. Anterior chamber reaction; conjunctival injection; scleritis; increased IOP; sheathed retinal arterioles and sometimes venules, especially in the periphery; retinal hemorrhages (minor finding); optic disc edema; delayed RRD occurs in approximately 70% of patients secondary to large irregular posterior breaks. Usually begins unilaterally but may involve second eye in one-third of cases within weeks to months. An optic neuropathy with disc edema or pallor sometimes develops.

Etiology

ARN is a clinical syndrome caused by the herpesvirus family: varicella-zoster virus (older patients), herpes simplex virus (younger patients), or, rarely, CMV or EBV.

Differential Diagnosis

See 12.3, *Posterior Uveitis.*

- CMV retinitis (Table 12.8.1).

- PORN: Rapidly progressive retinitis characterized by clear vitreous and sheet-like opacification deep to normal-looking retinal vessels, and occasional spontaneous vitreous hemorrhage. PORN is usually found in immunocompromised individuals and frequently leads to rapid bilateral blindness due either to the infection itself or to secondary retinal detachment, making prompt diagnosis and treatment essential. Unlike ARN, pain and vitritis are minimal and macular involvement is early in PORN.

- Syphilis.

- Toxoplasmosis.

- Behçet disease.

- Fungal or bacterial endophthalmitis.

- Large cell lymphoma. Consider in patients >50 years of age with refractory unilateral vitritis, yellow–white subretinal infiltrates, and absence of pain.

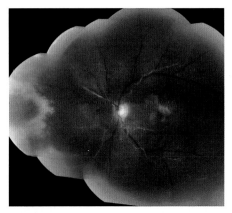

FIGURE 12.8.1. Acute retinal necrosis.

12

TABLE 12.8.1	Cytomegalovirus (CMV) Retinitis Versus Acute Retinal Necrosis (ARN) Versus Progressive Outer Retinal Necrosis (PORN) Versus Toxoplasmosis			
	CMV	**ARN**	**PORN**	**Toxoplasmosis**
Retinal hemorrhages	Significant	Uncommon	Uncommon	Absent
Vitritis	Minimal	Significant	Minimal	Significant
Pain	Absent	Significant	Absent	Moderate
Immune status	Immunocompromised	Usually healthy	Immunocompromised	Either
Appearance	"Brushfire" border with leading edge of active retinitis and necrotic retina and mottled retinal pigment epithelium in its wake	Sharply demarcated lesions with nearly homogeneous appearance and same age	Multifocal patches of deep retinal necrosis, rapid progression with involvement of macula	"Headlight in fog" with dense vitritis and smooth edges

Work-Up

See 12.3, *Posterior Uveitis,* for a nonspecific uveitis work-up.

1. History: Risk factors for AIDS? Immuno-compromised? If yes, the differential diagnosis includes CMV retinitis and PORN.

2. Complete ocular examination: Evaluate the anterior chamber and vitreous for cells, measure the IOP, and perform a dilated retinal examination using indirect ophthalmoscopy and scleral depression.

3. Consider a CBC with differential, FTA-ABS and RPR, ESR, toxoplasmosis titers, PPD, and chest radiograph to rule out other etiologies.

4. Consider HIV testing.

5. Consider anterior chamber paracentesis for herpes virus and toxoplasmosis PCR in atypical cases. See Appendix 13, *Anterior Chamber Paracentesis.*

6. Consider IVFA.

7. An orbital CT scan or B-scan US to look for an enlarged optic nerve in cases of suspected optic nerve dysfunction.

8. CT scan or MRI of the brain and lumbar puncture if large cell lymphoma, tertiary syphilis, or encephalitis is suspected.

Treatment

NOTE: All patients with ARN should be referred to a specialist.

1. Prompt inpatient or outpatient treatment. The goal is to decrease the incidence of the disease in the fellow eye. Treatment does not reduce the rate of retinal detachment in the first eye.

2. Acyclovir, 1,500 mg/m^2 of body surface area/day i.v., in three divided doses for 5 to 14 days (requires dose adjustment for renal insufficiency) with supplemental intravitreal injections with foscarnet (1200 micrograms/ 0.1 mL) or ganciclovir (2 mg/0.1 mL) given 1–2 times per week. This is then followed with oral valacyclovir 1 g t.i.d. or acyclovir (400 to 800 mg five times per day), for up to 14 weeks from the onset of infection. Involvement of the second eye typically starts within 6 weeks of initial infection. Recent reports suggest that primary treatment with oral antivirals (valacyclovir 1–2 grams t.i.d. to q.i.d., famciclovir 500 mg t.i.d., or acyclovir 800 mg five times per day) in conjunction with the above intravitreal injections, has similar efficacy as intravenous therapy. Stabilization and early regression of retinitis is usually seen within 4 days. The lesions may progress during the first 48 hours of treatment.

3. Topical cycloplegic (e.g., atropine 1% t.i.d.) and topical steroid (e.g., prednisolone acetate 1% q2–6h) in the presence of anterior segment inflammation.

4. Consider antiplatelet therapy (e.g., aspirin 81 to 650 mg daily).

5. Systemic steroids may be considered, particularly when the optic nerve is thought to be involved. Steroids are usually delayed at least 24 hours after the initiation of antiviral therapy. A typical oral corticosteroid regimen is prednisone 60 to 80 mg/day for 1 to 2 weeks followed by a taper over 2 to 6 weeks. Subtenon injection of triamcinolone (40 mg/ 1 mL) can be considered after adequate loading of antiviral therapy.

6. See 9.7, *Inflammatory Open-Angle Glaucoma,* for increased IOP.

7. Consider prophylactic barrier laser photocoagulation posterior to active retinitis to wall off or prevent subsequent RRD (controversial).

8. Pars plana vitrectomy, with long-acting gas or silicone oil, is the best way to repair the associated complex RRD. Proliferative vitreoretinopathy is common.

Follow-Up

1. Patients are seen daily and are examined every few weeks to months for the following year.

2. A careful fundus evaluation with scleral depression is performed at each visit to rule out retinal holes that may lead to a detachment. If the retinitis crosses the margin of laser demarcation, consider applying additional laser therapy.

3. Pupillary evaluation should be performed, and optic neuropathy should be considered if the retinopathy does not explain the amount of visual loss.

12.9   CYTOMEGALOVIRUS RETINITIS

CMV is the most frequent ocular opportunistic infection in patients with AIDS, but is becoming less common. CMV is almost never seen unless the CD4+ count is <50 cells/mm^3. Because active retinitis may be asymptomatic, patients with CD4+ counts <0 cells/mm^3 should be seen at least every 3 months. May also be seen in other immunocompromised states (e.g., leukemia and post-transplant).

Symptoms

Scotoma or decreased vision in one or both eyes and floaters. Pain and photophobia are uncommon. Often asymptomatic.

Signs

Critical.

- Indolent form: Peripheral granular opacities with occasional hemorrhage.

- Fulminant form: Confluent areas of necrosis with prominent hemorrhage, starting along the major retinal vascular arcades.

Progressive retinal atrophy may also indicate active CMV (see Figure 12.9.1).

Other. Minimal inflammation with few to no aqueous or vitreous cells. Retinal pigment epithelial (RPE) atrophy and pigment clumping result once the active process resolves.

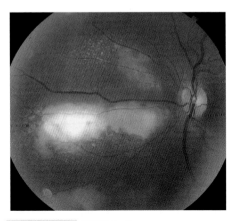

FIGURE 12.9.1. CMV Retinitis.

12

RRD occurs in approximately one-third of patients with CMV retinitis with increased risk when >25% of the retina is involved. Stellate keratic precipitates may signify concomitant CMV uveitis.

Work-Up

1. History and complete ocular examination.

2. Consider anterior chamber paracentesis with viral PCR in equivocal cases. See Appendix 13, *Anterior Chamber Paracentesis*.

3. Serial fundus photographs to document progression should be taken at each visit.

4. Refer patient to an internist or infectious disease specialist for systemic evaluation and treatment.

Treatment

See Table 12.9.1 for treatment details.

1. Intravenous ganciclovir, cidofovir, and foscarnet are used individually or in combi-

TABLE 12.9.1	Therapy for CMV Retinitis		
Drug	**Dosing**	**Toxicities**	**Contraindications**
Ganciclovir	Induction: 5 mg/kg i.v. b.i.d. 2 to 3 times/per wk Maintenance: 5 mg/kg i.v. q.d. or 6 mg/kg i.v. 5 d/wk	Neutropenia,[a] thrombocytopenia, anemia, renal toxicity Discontinue nursing	Absolute neutrophil count <500/mm³ Platelets <25,000/mm³; potentially embryotoxic
Valganciclovir	Induction: 900 mg p.o. b.i.d. Maintenance: 900 mg p.o. daily	Neutropenia,[a] thrombocytopenia, anemia, renal toxicity Discontinue nursing	Absolute neutrophil count <500/mm³ Platelets <25,000/mm³; potentially embryotoxic
Ganciclovir implant	4.5 mg sustained release	Well-tolerated[b] device implanted in the anterior vitreous Lasts 6 to 10 months	Surgical complications occur (e.g., retinal detachment, vitreous hemorrhage)
Foscarnet	Induction: 90 mg/kg i.v. b.i.d. twice/per wk Maintenance: 120 mg/kg i.v. q.d.[c] Monitor creatinine electrolytes and adjust dosing as needed	Renal impairment; neutropenia; anemia electrolyte imbalances	Use caution with renal impairment or electrolyte imbalances
Cidofovir, HPMPC	Induction: 5 mg/kg i.v. weekly for 3 weeks. Intravenous maintenance 3 to 5 mg/kg biweekly Intravitreal: 20 mg every 5 to 6 wk	Dose- and schedule-dependent nephrotoxicity; hypotony (necessitates discontinuation); iritis (steroid responsive)	Intravitreal injection in the fellow eye is contraindicated if permanent hypotony develops in the first (treated) eye

[a]Granulocyte colony-stimulating factor can reduce neutropenia incidence.
[b]Compared with i.v. ganciclovir, there is an increased risk of systemic disease (30%) and fellow eye involvement (50%) after 6 months. However, the relapse-free interval is greatly increased.
[c]During induction phase, 500 mL of normal saline is used for each dose. During maintenance, 1,000 mL of saline should be used.

nation. The goal of treatment is quiescent retinitis: nonprogressive areas of RPE atrophy with a stable opacified border. Patients who respond may be switched to oral therapy (e.g., ganciclovir 1,000 mg p.o. t.i.d. or valganciclovir 900 mg p.o. b.i.d. for 21 days then 900 mg p.o. q.d.). Oral therapy with valganciclovir [900 mg p.o. b.i.d. for induction (21 days), followed by 900 mg p.o. daily for maintenance] is an acceptable alternative to i.v. therapy. Patients with progression of retinitis despite induction or who have disease that threatens the macula may benefit from intravitreal antiviral injections. Patients who cannot tolerate systemic medications (e.g., myelosuppression) may benefit from insertion of a ganciclovir vitreal implant. Systemic therapy may still be necessary to prevent involvement of the fellow eye.

2. Under the direction of an internist or infectious disease specialist, highly active antiretroviral therapy (HAART) should be initiated or optimized

3. Macula-sparing RRDs may be treated with laser demarcation. Pars plana vitrectomy with silicone oil is indicated for detachments involving the macula.

4. The role of oral ganciclovir prophylaxis against CMV is controversial.

Follow-Up

1. Ganciclovir resistance (reflected by positive blood or urine CMV cultures) may occur at any point during treatment.

2. Almost all patients eventually relapse. Serial fundus photographs are quite useful. Relapse is defined as recurrent or new retinitis, movement of opacified border, or expansion of the atrophic zone.

3. Relapse does not necessarily indicate drug resistance. Reinduction with the same medication is the first line of treatment. Subtherapeutic intraocular drug levels may occur in patients on maintenance and allow for relapse.

4. Clinical resistance is defined as persistent or progressive retinitis despite induction-level medication for 6 weeks. Laboratory confirmation is possible for ganciclovir resistance (screen for UL97 mutation).

5. If resistance is recognized, a change in therapy is indicated. Cross-resistance may be a problem since the three common drugs are all DNA polymerase inhibitors. Cross-resistance between ganciclovir and cidofovir is especially common. Ganciclovir–foscarnet cross-resistance is uncommon.

6. Discontinuation of anti-CMV maintenance therapy may be considered in selected patients receiving HAART who have CD4+ counts >100 cells/mm^3 for greater than 6 months and completely quiescent CMV retinitis. In these patients, whose immune system can control CMV, stopping maintenance therapy may prevent drug toxicity and drug-resistant organisms.

7. Immune recovery uveitis (IRU): Occurs in previously immunocompromised patients (HIV/transplant) with CMV after the CD4+ count or immune system reconstitutes. In the presence of a functioning immune system, the CMV antigens elicit an inflammatory response that is predominantly posterior (i.e., vitritis, papillitis, cystoid macular edema). Treatment may require topical, periocular, or intraocular steroids. Antivirals should be continued to avoid reactivation of CMV in cases of borderline CD4+ counts.

12

12.10 NONINFECTIOUS RETINAL MICROVASCULOPATHY/HIV RETINOPATHY

Noninfectious retinopathy is the most common ocular manifestation of HIV/AIDS. About 50% to 70% of patients with AIDS have this condition.

Symptoms

Usually asymptomatic.

Signs

Cotton–wool spots, intraretinal hemorrhages, and microaneurysms. An ischemic maculopathy may occur with significant visual loss in 3% of patients.

Work-Up

HIV retinopathy is a marker of low CD4+ counts. Look for concomitant opportunistic infections (see 12.9, *Cytomegalovirus Retinitis*). Rule out the other causes for unexplained cotton–wool spots (see 11.5, *Cotton–Wool Spot*).

Treatment

No specific ocular treatment necessary, but often improves with HAART and increased CD4+ counts.

Follow-Up

Patients with CD4+ counts <50 should be examined every 4–6 months.

12.11 VOGT–KOYANAGI–HARADA SYNDROME

Symptoms

Decreased vision, photophobia, pain, and red eyes, accompanied or preceded by a headache, stiff neck, nausea, vomiting, fever, and malaise. Hearing loss, dysacusia, and tinnitus frequently occur. Typically bilateral.

NOTE: Harada disease refers to isolated ocular findings without associated systemic signs of VKH syndrome.

Signs

(See Figure 12.11.1.)

Critical.

- Anterior: Anterior chamber flare and cells, granulomatous (mutton-fat) keratic precipitates, perilimbal vitiligo (e.g., depigmentation around the limbus).

- Posterior: Bilateral serous retinal detachments with underlying choroidal thickening, vitreous cells and opacities, optic disc edema.

- Systemic:

　—Early: loss of high-frequency hearing, meningismus.

　—Late: alopecia, vitiligo, poliosis.

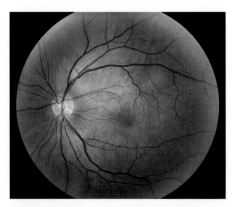

FIGURE 12.11.1. Vogt–Koyanagi–Harada (VKH) disease.

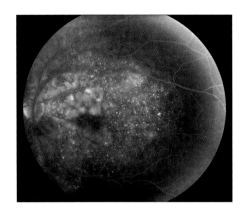

FIGURE 12.11.2. IVFA of VKH.

- IVFA: Multiple pinpoint leaking areas of hyperfluorescence at the level of the retinal pigment epithelium (see Figure 12.11.2).

Other.
- Anterior: Iris nodules, peripheral anterior or posterior synechiae, scleritis, hypotony or increased IOP from forward rotation of ciliary processes.

- Posterior: Mottling and atrophy of the retinal pigment epithelium after the serous retinal detachment resolves (sunset glow fundus), retinal vasculitis, choroidal neovascularization, Dalen–Fuchs nodules.

- Systemic: Neurologic signs, including loss of consciousness, paralysis, seizures.

Epidemiology

Typically, patients are aged 20 to 50 years, female (77%), and have pigmented skin, especially Asian, Hispanic, or Native American.

Differential Diagnosis

See Table 12.11.1 for the differential of serous retinal detachments and 12.3, *Posterior Uveitis.* In particular, consider the following:

- Sympathetic ophthalmia: History of trauma or surgery to the uninvolved eye. Usually no systemic signs. See 12.18, *Sympathetic Ophthalmia.*

- APMPPE: Ophthalmoscopic and IVFA features may be very similar, but there is less vitreous inflammation and no anterior

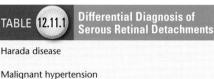

TABLE 12.11.1	Differential Diagnosis of Serous Retinal Detachments
Harada disease	
Malignant hypertension	
Toxemia of pregnancy	
Disseminated intravascular coagulopathy	
Idiopathic uveal effusion syndrome	
Sympathetic ophthalmia	
Posterior scleritis	
Central serous chorioretinopathy	
Choroidal tumors (including metastases)	
Choroidal neovascularization	
Congenital optic disc pit	
Nanophthalmos	

segment involvement. See 12.3, *Posterior Uveitis.*

- Other granulomatous panuveitides (e.g., syphilis, sarcoidosis, tuberculosis).

Work-Up

See 12.3, *Posterior Uveitis,* for a nonspecific uveitis work-up.

1. History: Neurologic symptoms, hearing loss, or hair loss? Previous eye surgery or trauma?

2. Complete ocular examination, including a dilated retinal evaluation.

3. CBC, RPR, FTA-ABS, ACE, PPD, and possibly chest radiograph to rule out similar-appearing disorders.

4. Consider a CT scan with or without contrast or MRI of the brain in the presence of neurologic signs to rule out a CNS disorder.

5. Lumbar puncture during attacks with meningeal symptoms for cell count and differential, protein, glucose, VDRL, Gram and

12

methenamine–silver stains, and culture. CSF pleocytosis is often seen in VKH and APMPPE.

6. Consider IVFA to evaluate for pinpoint leaking areas of hyperfluorescence at the level of the retinal pigment epithelium.

Treatment

Inflammation is initially controlled with steroids; the dose depends on the severity of the inflammation. In moderate to severe cases, the following regimen can be used. Steroids are tapered very slowly as the condition improves.

1. Topical steroids (e.g., prednisolone acetate 1% q1h).

2. Systemic steroids (e.g., prednisone 60 to 80 mg p.o. q.d.) and a histamine blocker (e.g., ranitidine 150 mg p.o. b.i.d.).

3. Topical cycloplegic (e.g., scopolamine 0.25% t.i.d.).

4. Treatment of any specific neurologic disorders (e.g., seizures or coma).

5. For patients who cannot tolerate or are unresponsive to systemic steroids, consider immunosuppressive agents (e.g., methotrexate, azathioprine, chlorambucil, cyclosporine, TNF-alpha inhibitors).

Follow-Up

1. Initial management may require hospitalization.

2. Weekly, then monthly reexamination is performed, watching for recurrent inflammation and increased IOP.

3. Steroids are tapered very slowly and most patients should be transitioned to steroid-sparing immunosuppressants for long-term management. Inflammation may recur up to 9 months after the steroids have been discontinued. If this occurs, steroids should be reinstituted.

12.12 — SYPHILIS

ACQUIRED SYPHILIS

Signs

Systemic

- Primary: Chancre (ulcerated, painless lesion), regional lymphadenopathy.

- Secondary: Skin or mucous membrane lesions, generalized lymphadenopathy, constitutional symptoms (e.g., sore throat, fever), symptomatic or asymptomatic meningitis, less common.

- Latent: No clinical manifestations.

- Tertiary: Cardiovascular disease (e.g., aortitis), CNS disease (e.g., meningovascular disease, general paresis, tabes dorsalis).

Ocular

- Primary: A chancre may occur on the eyelid or conjunctiva.

- Secondary: Uveitis, optic neuritis, active chorioretinitis, retinitis, retinal vasculitis, conjunctivitis, dacryoadenitis, dacryocystitis, episcleritis, scleritis, monocular interstitial keratitis, and others.

- Tertiary: Optic atrophy, old chorioretinitis, interstitial keratitis, chronic iritis, Argyll Robertson pupil (see 10.3, *Argyll Robertson Pupil*), in addition to the other signs seen in secondary disease.

NOTE: Patchy hyperemia of the iris with fleshy, pink nodules near the iris sphincter is pathognomonic of syphilis.

Differential Diagnosis

See 12.1, *Anterior Uveitis* (*Iritis/Iridocyclitis*), and 12.3, *Posterior Uveitis*.

Work-Up

See 12.1, *Anterior Uveitis* (*Iritis/Iridocyclitis*), and 12.3, *Posterior Uveitis,* for a nonspecific uveitis work-up.

1. Complete ophthalmic examination, including pupillary and dilated fundus examination.

2. VDRL and RPR reflect the activity of the disease and are important in monitoring the patient's response to treatment. Used for screening, but many false-negative results can occur in early primary, latent, or late syphilis. Not as specific.

3. FTA-ABS and treponema pallidum microhemagglutination assay (MHA-TP) are very sensitive and specific in all stages of syphilis. They are the tests of choice in suspected ocular syphilis. Once reactive, these tests do not normalize and cannot be used to assess the patient's response to treatment.

4. HIV testing is indicated in any patient with syphilis because of the relatively aggressive course in HIV-infected individuals as well as the frequency of co-infection.

5. Patients should be evaluated for concomitant sexually transmitted diseases, with notification sent to the local health department when indicated.

6. Lumbar puncture is controversial. We consider lumbar puncture in the following clinical situations:

—Positive FTA-ABS and neurological or neuro-ophthalmological signs, papillitis, active chorioretinitis, or anterior or posterior uveitis.

—HIV and FTA-ABS positive patients.

—Treatment failure.

—Treatment with a nonpenicillin regimen (as a baseline).

—Untreated syphilis of unknown duration or longer than 1 year's duration.

Treatment Indications

1. FTA-ABS negative: No treatment indicated. Likely not syphilis.

2. FTA-ABS positive and VDRL negative

   a. If appropriate past treatment cannot be documented, treatment is indicated.

   b. If appropriate past treatment can be documented, treatment is not indicated.

3. FTA-ABS positive and VDRL positive: A VDRL titer of 1:8 or greater (e.g., 1:64) is expected to decline at least fourfold within 1 year of appropriate treatment, and should revert to at least 1:4 or less within 1 year in primary syphilis, 2 years in secondary syphilis, and 5 years in tertiary syphilis. A VDRL titer of <1:8 (e.g., 1:4) often does not decrease fourfold. Therefore, the following recommendations are made:

   a. No documentation of appropriate past treatment, treatment is indicated.

   b. Documentation of appropriate past treatment, and:

      —If a previous VDRL titer greater than or equal to four times the current titer can be documented, no treatment is indicated (unless 5 years have passed and the titer is still >1:4).

      —If a previous VDRL titer was at least 1:8 and did not decrease fourfold, treatment is indicated.

      —If the previous VDRL titer was <1:8, treatment is not indicated, unless the current titer has increased fourfold.

      —If a previous VDRL is unavailable, treatment is not required unless treatment was >5 years earlier and the VDRL is still >1:4.

NOTE:

1. If active syphilitic signs (e.g., active chorioretinitis, papillitis) are present despite appropriate past treatment (regardless of the VDRL titer), lumbar puncture and treatment may be needed.

2. Patients with concurrent HIV and active syphilis may have negative serologies (FTA-ABS, RPR) because of their immunocompromised state. These patients manifest aggressive, recalcitrant syphilis and should be treated with neurosyphilis dosages over longer treatment periods. Consultation with infectious disease is recommended.

Treatment

1. Neurosyphilis (positive FTA-ABS in the serum and either cell count >5 white blood cells/mm^3, protein >45 mg/dL, or positive

12

CSF VDRL on lumbar puncture): Aqueous crystalline penicillin G 2 to 4 million U i.v. q4h for 10 to 14 days, followed by benzathine penicillin 2.4 million U intramuscularly (i.m.) weekly for 3 weeks (1.2 million U in each buttock).

2. Syphilis with abnormal ocular but normal CSF findings: Benzathine penicillin 2.4 million U i.m. weekly for 3 weeks. Some experts believe that any retinal or optic nerve involvement be considered as neurosyphilis and treated accordingly.

3. If anterior segment inflammation is present, treatment with a cycloplegic (e.g., cyclopentolate 2% t.i.d.) and topical steroid (e.g., prednisolone acetate 1% q.i.d.) may be beneficial.

NOTE:

1. Treatment for chlamydial infection with a single dose of azithromycin 1 g p.o. is typically indicated.

2. Therapy for penicillin-allergic patients is not well established and should be managed in consultation with an infectious disease specialist. Ceftriaxone 2 g i.v./i.m. for 10 to 14 days is usually the first-choice alternative, but is contraindicated with severe allergy. Tetracycline 500 mg p.o. q.i.d. for 30 days is used by some for both late syphilis and neurosyphilis. Some believe that using penicillin is critical in neurosyphilis and merits ICU admission and desensitization in penicillin-allergic patients.

Follow-Up

1. Neurosyphilis: Repeat lumbar puncture every 6 months for 2 years, less frequently if the cell count returns to normal sooner. The cell count should decrease to a normal level within this period, and the CSF VDRL titer should decrease fourfold within 6 to 12 months. An increased CSF protein decreases more slowly. If these indices do not decrease as expected, retreatment may be indicated.

2. Other forms of syphilis: Repeat the VDRL titer at 3 and 6 months after treatment. If a VDRL titer of 1:8 or more does not decline fourfold within 6 months, if the VDRL titer increases fourfold at any point, or if clinical symptoms or signs of syphilis persist or recur, lumbar puncture and retreatment are indicated. If a pretreatment VDRL titer is <1:8, retreatment is indicated only when the titer increases when signs of syphilis recur.

Congenital Syphilis

Ocular signs include bilateral interstitial keratitis, secondary cataracts, salt-and-pepper chorioretinitis, and iridocyclitis. Hutchinson triad of congenital syphilis includs peg-shaped widely spaced incisors, interstitial keratitis, and deafness. Serologic testing is similar to acquired syphilis above. Standard treatment is with penicillin G, but dosing should be managed by a pediatrician or infectious disease specialist.

---

12 | **12.13** POSTOPERATIVE ENDOPHTHALMITIS

ACUTE [DAY(S) AFTER SURGERY]

Symptoms

Sudden onset of decreased vision and increasing eye pain after surgical procedure.

Signs

(See Figure 12.13.1.)

Critical. Hypopyon, fibrin, severe anterior chamber reaction, vitreous cells and haze, decreased red reflex.

Other. Eyelid edema, corneal edema, intense conjunctival injection, chemosis (all are highly variable).

Organisms

■ Most common: *Staphylococcus epidermidis.*

■ Common: *Staphylococcus aureus,* Streptococcal species (except Pneumococcus).

■ Less common: Gram-negative bacteria (Pseudomonas, Aerobacter, Proteus species, *Haemophilus influenzae,* Klebsiella species,

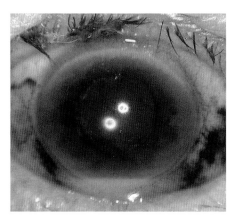

FIGURE 12.13.1. Postoperative endophthalmitis with hypopyon.

Escherichia coli, Bacillus species, Enterobacter species) and anaerobes.

- Bleb associated: Streptococcus or gram-negative infections.

Differential Diagnosis

See 12.14, *Chronic Postoperative Uveitis.*

Work-Up

1. Complete ocular history and examination. Look for wound/bleb leak, exposed suture, vitreous to wound, blepharitis, or other predisposing factors for endophthalmitis.

2. Consider B-scan US if limited view to posterior segment, which may confirm marked vitritis and establishes a baseline against which the success of therapy can be measured.

3. If vision is light perception or worse, a diagnostic (and therapeutic) vitrectomy is often indicated. Cultures (blood, chocolate, Sabouraud, thioglycolate) and smears (Gram and Giemsa stains) are obtained, and intravitreal antibiotics are given. Otherwise, an anterior chamber paracentesis and vitreous aspiration of 0.2 mL are usually performed, although some physicians consider them nonessential. See Appendix 13, *Anterior Chamber Paracentesis.*

Treatment

1. Prevention: Standard practice for prophylaxis of postoperative endophthalmitis includes preparation of eyelids and conjunctiva with 5% povidone-iodine prior to surgery. Perioperative use of topical broad-spectrum antibiotics may decrease bacterial load, but has not been proven to lower rates of endophthalmitis and may promote antibiotic resistance.

2. Anterior chamber and/or vitreous tap for Gram stain, culture, and sensitivities and timely intravitreal injections with broad-spectrum antibiotics (often vancomycin and ceftazidime). See Appendix 11, *Intravitreal Tap and Inject,* and Appendix 12, *Intravitreal Antibiotics.* Consider intravitreal steroids (e.g., triamcinolone acetate 4 mg/0.1 mL) in select cases with severe vitreous inflammation.

3. Consider admission to hospital for observation.

4. Consider intensive topical steroids (e.g., prednisolone acetate 1% q1h around the clock) and intensive topical fortified antibiotics (e.g., vancomycin and tobramycin, q1h around the clock for 24 to 48 hours). Intensive topical antibiotics are more important in the setting of filtering blebs, wound leaks, or exposed sutures. See Appendix 9, *Fortified Topical Antibiotics/Antifungals.*

5. Atropine 1% t.i.d. to q.i.d.

6. For postcataract endophthalmitis, immediate pars plana vitrectomy is beneficial if visual acuity on presentation is light perception. Vitrectomy for other causes of endophthalmitis (bleb-related, posttraumatic, or endogenous) may be beneficial in selected cases.

7. Systemic antibiotics may be considered. Intravenous antibiotics are not routinely used. Consider i.v. fluoroquinolones (e.g., moxifloxacin) in special circumstances (e.g., bleb-related endophthalmitis or trauma). Third- and fourth-generation fluoroquinolones may penetrate the vitreous enough to reach therapeutic levels, especially in inflamed eyes. Some oral antibiotics (e.g., moxifloxacin 400 mg p.o. q.d.) may reach therapeutic vitreous levels and could be considered as alternatives to intravenous antibiotics.

12

Follow-Up

1. Monitor the clinical course q12h.

2. Relief of pain is a useful early sign of response to therapy.

3. Consider starting oral steroids (prednisone 60 mg p.o. each morning with ranitidine 150 mg p.o. b.i.d.) in patients who can tolerate steroids.

4. After 48 hours, patients should show clinical improvement (e.g., relief of pain, decreased inflammation, decreased hypopyon). Consider reinjecting antibiotics if no improvement or if Gram stain shows an unusual organism. Consider vitrectomy if patient is deteriorating.

5. The antibiotic regimen is refined according to the treatment response and to the culture and sensitivity results.

6. If the patient is responding well, topical fortified antibiotics may be slowly tapered after 48 hours and then switched to regular strength antibiotics (e.g., fluoroquinolone). Close outpatient follow-up is warranted.

SUBACUTE (WEEKS TO MONTHS AFTER SURGERY)

Symptoms

Variable. Insidious decreased vision, increasing redness and pain.

Signs

Critical. Anterior chamber and vitreous inflammation, vitreous abscesses, hypopyon; clumps of exudate in the anterior chamber, on the iris surface, or along the pupillary border.

Other. Corneal infiltrate and edema; may have a surgical bleb.

Organisms

- *S. epidermidis* or other common bacteria (e.g., Streptococci with a filtering bleb).

- *Propionibacteriam acnes* or other rare, indolent bacteria: Recurrent, granulomatous anterior uveitis, often with a hypopyon and granulomatous keratic precipitates, but with minimal conjunctival injection and pain. A white plaque or opacities on the lens capsule may be evident. Only a transient response to steroids.

- Fungi (Aspergillus, Candida, Cephalosporium, Penicillium species; others).

Differential Diagnosis

See 12.14, *Chronic Postoperative Uveitis.*

Work-Up

1. Complete ocular history and examination.

2. Aspiration of vitreous for smears (Gram, Giemsa, and methenamine–silver) and cultures (blood, chocolate, Sabouraud, thioglycolate, and a solid medium for anaerobic culture; *P. acnes* will be missed unless proper anaerobic cultures are obtained). See Appendix 11, *Intravitreal Tap and Inject.* Intravitreal antibiotics are given as described previously. See Appendix 12, *Intravitreal Antibiotics.*

3. Consider CBC with differential, serum electrolytes, liver function tests.

Treatment

1. Initially treat as acute postoperative endophthalmitis, as described previously, but do not start steroids.

2. Immediate pars plana vitrectomy is beneficial if visual acuity on presentation is light perception or worse up to 6 weeks after surgery. Benefit beyond 6 weeks is not known.

3. If a fungal infection is suspected or vitreous smear is consistent with fungus, administer intravitreal amphotericin B, 5 to 10 µg or intravitreal voriconazole (50 to 100 µg/0.1 mL) at the time of vitrectomy. If fungus is identified on Gram stain, Giemsa stain, or calcofluor white, then consider topical antifungals (e.g., natamycin 5% or voriconazole 1% q1h), and/or systemic antifungal medications until specific organism is known (consider consulting an infectious disease specialist for recommendations). Antifungal therapy is modified in accordance with sensitivity testing, clinical course, and tolerance to antifungal agents.

   - A therapeutic vitrectomy should be performed if it was not done with the initial cultures.

4. Removal of the lens and capsular remnants may be required for diagnosis and treatment of *P. acnes*, which may be sensitive to intravitreal penicillin, cefoxitin, clindamycin, or vancomycin.

5. If *S. epidermidis* is isolated, intraocular vancomycin alone may be sufficient.

Follow-Up

1. Dependent on the organism.

2. In general, follow-up is as described previously for acute postoperative endophthalmitis.

3. Repeat CBC, serum electrolytes, and liver function tests two times per week during treatment for fungal endophthalmitis.

12.14 CHRONIC POSTOPERATIVE UVEITIS

Postoperative inflammation is typically mild, responds promptly to steroids, and usually resolves within 6 weeks. Consider the following etiologies when postoperative inflammation is atypical.

Etiology

■ Severe intraocular inflammation in the early postoperative course:

—Infectious endophthalmitis: Deteriorating vision, fibrin in the anterior chamber, vitritis. See 12.13, *Postoperative Endophthalmitis.*

—Retained lens material: A severe granulomatous inflammation with mutton-fat keratic precipitates, resulting from an autoimmune reaction to lens protein exposed during surgery. See 9.12, *Lens-Induced (Phacogenic) Glaucoma.*

—Aseptic endophthalmitis: A severe sterile postoperative uveitis caused by excess tissue manipulation, especially vitreous manipulation, during surgery. A hypopyon and a mild vitreous cellular reaction may develop. Usually not characterized by profound or progressive pain or visual loss. Eyelid swelling and chemosis are atypical. Usually resolves with topical steroid therapy.

—Toxic anterior segment syndrome: An acute, sterile inflammation following uneventful surgery that develops rapidly within 12 to 24 hours. Characterized by anterior chamber cell and flare, possibly with fibrin or hypopyon, and severe corneal edema in excess of what would be expected following surgery. Intraocular pressure may be increased. May be caused by any material placed in the eye during surgery including irrigating or injected solutions (e.g., due to presence of a preservative or incorrect pH or concentration of a solution) or improperly cleaned instruments.

■ Persistent postoperative inflammation (e.g., beyond 6 weeks):

—Poor compliance with topical steroids.

—Steroid drops tapered too rapidly.

—Retained lens material.

—Iris or vitreous incarceration in the wound.

—UGH syndrome: Irritation of the iris or ciliary body by an intraocular lens. Increased IOP and red blood cells in the anterior chamber accompany the anterior segment inflammation. See 9.16, *Postoperative Glaucoma.*

—Retinal detachment: Often produces a low-grade anterior chamber reaction. See 11.3, *Retinal Detachment.*

—Low-grade endophthalmitis (e.g., *P. acnes* and other indolent bacteria, fungal, or partially treated bacterial endophthalmitis).

—Epithelial downgrowth: Corneal or conjunctival epithelium grows into the eye through a corneal wound and may be seen on the posterior corneal surface. The iris may appear flattened because of the

12

spread of the membrane over the anterior chamber angle onto the iris. Large cells may be seen in the anterior chamber, and glaucoma may be present. The diagnosis of epithelial downgrowth can be confirmed by observing the immediate appearance of white spots after medium-power argon laser treatment to the areas of iris covered by the membrane.

—Preexisting uveitis: See 12.1, *Anterior Uveitis (Irtitis/Iridocyclitis)*.

—Sympathetic ophthalmia: Diffuse granulomatous inflammation in both eyes, after trauma or surgery to one eye. See 12.18, *Sympathetic Ophthalmia*.

Work-Up

1. History: Is the patient taking the steroid drops properly? Did the patient stop the steroid drops abruptly? Was there a postoperative wound leak allowing epithelial downgrowth or fibrous ingrowth? Previous history of uveitis?

2. Complete ocular examination of both eyes, including a slit-lamp assessment of the anterior chamber reaction, a determination of whether vitreous or residual lens material is present in the anterior chamber, and an inspection of the lens capsule looking for capsular opacities (e.g., *P. acnes* capsular plaque). Perform gonioscopy (to evaluate for iris or vitreous to the wound or small retained lens fragments), an IOP measurement, a dilated indirect ophthalmoscopic examination (to rule out retained lens material in the inferior pars plana, retinal detachment, or signs of chorioretinitis), and a posterior vitreous evaluation with a slit lamp and hand-held lens looking for inflammatory cells.

3. Obtain B-scan US when the fundus view is obscured. Consider ultrasound biomicroscopy if available to assess IOL position, irido-IOL contact for possible UGH syndrome, and to evaluate for retained lens material.

4. For postoperative endophthalmitis. Anaerobic cultures, using both solid media and broth, should be obtained to isolate *P. acnes* (routine cultures also are obtained; see 12.13, *Postoperative Endophthalmitis*). The anaerobic cultures should be incubated in an anaerobic environment as rapidly as possible and allowed to grow for at least 2 weeks.

5. Consider an anterior chamber paracentesis for diagnostic smears and cultures. See Appendix 13, *Anterior Chamber Paracentesis*.

6. Consider diagnostic medium-power argon laser treatment to the areas of iris thought to be covered by epithelial downgrowth.

If this work-up is negative and steroid trial reduces the inflammation only transiently, surgery may be required. Consider a limited surgical capsulectomy, vitrectomy, and injection of intravitreal antibiotics in an effort to isolate and treat *P. acnes*. Inflammation, however, often recurs due to persistent organisms in which case removal of the capsular bag and intraocular lens with reinjection of antibiotics may be required.

See 12.1, *Anterior Uveitis (Iritis/Iridocyclitis)*; 12.3, *Posterior Uveitis*; 12.13, *Postoperative Endophthalmitis*; and 12.18, *Sympathetic Ophthalmia* for more specific information on diagnosis and treatment.

12.15 TRAUMATIC ENDOPHTHALMITIS

This condition constitutes an emergency requiring prompt attention.

Symptoms and Signs

Similar to 12.13, *Postoperative Endophthalmitis*. An occult or missed intraocular foreign body (IOFB) must be ruled out. See 3.15, *Intraocular Foreign Body*.

NOTE: Patients with Bacillus endophthalmitis may have a high fever, leukocytosis, proptosis, a corneal abscess in the form of a ring, and rapid visual deterioration.

Organisms

Bacillus species, *Staphylococcus epidermidis,* Gram-negative species, fungi, Streptococcus species, and others. Mixed flora may be present. Understanding the mechanism of injury is helpful in predicting the type of infecting organism.

Differential Diagnosis

- Phacoanaphylactic inflammation: A sterile autoimmune inflammatory reaction as a result of exposed lens protein. See 9.12, *Lens-Induced (Phacogenic) Glaucoma.*

- Lens cortex: Fluffed up and hydrated cortical lens material, especially in younger patients with soft nuclei after violation of the lens capsule.

- Sterile inflammatory response from a retained IOFB, blood in the vitreous, or as a result of surgical manipulation.

Work-Up

Same as for 12.13, *Postoperative Endophthalmitis.* Orbital CT scan (axial and coronal views) with 1-mm cuts and/or B-scan US to evaluate for IOFB is essential.

Treatment

1. Consider hospitalization.

2. Management for a ruptured globe or penetrating ocular injury if present. See 3.14, *Ruptured Globe and Penetrating Ocular Injury.*

3. Topical antibiotics (e.g., fortified tobramycin q1h, and fortified cefazolin or fortified vancomycin q1h, alternating every half hour) in the absence of globe rupture. See Appendix 9, *Fortified Topical Antibiotics/Antifungals.*

4. Systemic antibiotics (e.g., ciprofloxacin 400 mg i.v. q12h or moxifloxacin 400 mg p.o. q.d.; and cefazolin 1 g i.v. q8h). Consider an infectious disease consult for guidance in specific cases. May need to adjust dose for renal insufficiency and for children.

5. Intravitreal antibiotics (e.g., amikacin 0.4 mg in 0.1 mL and vancomycin 1 mg in 0.1 mL, or clindamycin 1 mg in 0.1 mL). These may be repeated every 48 to 72 hours, as needed. See Appendix 12, *Intravitreal Antibiotics.*

6. The benefit of pars plana vitrectomy is unknown for traumatic endophthalmitis without IOFB. However, pars plana vitrectomy reduces infectious and inflammatory load and provides sufficient material for diagnostic culture and pathologic investigation.

7. If tetanus immunization is not up to date, give tetanus toxoid 0.5 mL intramuscularly. See Appendix 2, *Tetanus Prophylaxis.*

8. Steroids should not be used until fungal organisms are ruled out. If no fungi are isolated, may use prednisolone acetate 1% q4h. Oral prednisone use is at the discretion of the surgeon. If fungus is isolated, specific antifungal regimens may be used.

Follow-Up

Same as for 12.13, *Postoperative Endophthalmitis.*

12.16

ENDOGENOUS BACTERIAL ENDOPHTHALMITIS

12

Symptoms

Decreased vision in an acutely ill (e.g., septic) or recently hospitalized patient, an immunocompromised host, or an intravenous drug abuser. No history of recent intraocular surgery.

Signs

Critical. Vitreous cells and debris, anterior chamber cell and flare, or a hypopyon.

Other. Iris microabscess, absent red reflex, retinal inflammatory infiltrates, flame-shaped retinal hemorrhages with or without white centers, retinal or subretinal abscess, corneal edema, eyelid edema, chemosis, conjunctival injection, panophthalmitis with orbital involvement (proptosis, restricted ocular motility). May be bilateral.

Organisms

Bacillus cereus (especially in i.v. drug abusers), Streptococci, *Neisseria meningitidis, Staphylococcus aureus, Haemophilus influenzae,* and others.

Differential Diagnosis

- Endogenous fungal endophthalmitis: May see fluffy, white vitreous opacities. Organisms include Aspergillus and Candida. See 12.17, *Candida Retinitis/Uveitis/Endophthalmitis.*

- Retinochoroidal infection (e.g., toxoplasmosis and toxocariasis): Yellow or white retinochoroidal lesion present.

- Noninfectious posterior or intermediate uveitis (e.g., sarcoidosis, pars planitis). Unlikely to get the first episode coincidentally during sepsis.

- Neoplastic conditions (e.g., large cell lymphoma and retinoblastoma).

Work-Up

1. History: Duration of symptoms? Underlying disease or infections? Intravenous drug abuse? Immunocompromised?

2. Complete ocular examination, including a dilated fundus evaluation.

3. B-scan US if there is no view to the fundus.

4. Complete medical work-up by an Infectious Disease specialist.

5. Chest x-ray, cultures of blood, urine, all indwelling catheters, and i.v. lines, as well as Gram stain of any discharge. Consider transesophageal or transthoracic echocardiogram to rule out endocarditis. A lumbar puncture is indicated when meningeal signs are present.

Treatment

All treatment should be coordinated with a medical internist.

1. Hospitalize the patient.

2. Broad-spectrum (i.v. and/or oral) antibiotics are started after appropriate smears and cultures are obtained. Antibiotic choices vary according to the suspected source of septic infection (e.g., gastrointestinal tract, genitourinary tract, cardiac) and are determined in consultation with an infectious disease spe-

cialist. Dosages recommended for meningitis and severe infections are used. If oral antibiotics are used, confirm that the regimen includes antibiotics with good vitreous penetration.

NOTE: Intravenous drug abusers are given an aminoglycoside and clindamycin to eradicate Bacillus cereus.

---

3. Topical cycloplegic (e.g., atropine 1% t.i.d.).

4. Topical steroid (e.g., prednisolone acetate 1% q1–6h depending on the degree of anterior segment inflammation).

5. Consider intravitreal antibiotics (e.g., amikacin 0.4 mg in 0.1 mL and vancomycin 1 mg in 0.1 mL; clindamycin 1 mg in 0.1 mL may be used in place of vancomycin). The timing of this procedure is controversial. Some vitreoretinal surgeons perform it as soon as possible. Others initially perform aqueous and vitreous aspirations when the systemic cultures are negative and the organism remains unknown. Intravitreal antibiotics offer higher intraocular concentrations. Consider intravitreal antifungal agents, if clinically warranted. See Appendix 11, *Intravitreal Tap and Inject,* and Appendix 12, *Intravitreal Antibiotics.*

6. Consider pars plana vitrectomy. Vitrectomy offers the benefit of reducing infective and inflammatory load and providing sufficient material for diagnostic culture and pathologic study. Additionally, intravitreal antibiotics may be administered at the time of surgery.

7. Periocular antibiotics (e.g., subconjunctival or subtenon injections) are sometimes used. See Appendix 10, *Technique for Retrobulbar/Subtenon/Subconjunctival Injections.*

Follow-Up

1. Daily in the hospital.

2. Peak and trough levels for many antibiotic agents are obtained every few days. Blood urea nitrogen and creatinine levels are monitored during aminoglycoside therapy. The antibiotic regimen is guided by the culture and sensitivity results, as well as the patient's clinical response to treatment. Intravenous antibiotics are maintained for at least 2 weeks and until the condition has resolved.

12.17 CANDIDA RETINITIS/UVEITIS/ ENDOPHTHALMITIS

Symptoms

Decreased vision, floaters, pain, often bilateral. Patients are typically intravenous drug abusers, immunocompromised, or possess a long-term indwelling catheter (e.g., for hyperalimentation, hemodialysis, or antibiotics).

Signs

(See Figure 12.17.1.)

Critical. Discrete, multifocal, yellow–white, choroidal or deep retinal lesions progressing to fluffy lesions from one to several disc diameters in size. With time, the lesions increase in size, spread into the vitreous, and appear as "cotton balls."

Other. Vitreous cells and haze, vitreous abscesses, retinal hemorrhages with or without pale centers, anterior chamber cells, hypopyon. Retinal detachment may develop.

Differential Diagnosis

The following should be considered in immunocompromised patients.

- CMV retinitis: Minimal to mild vitreous reaction, more retinal hemorrhage. See 12.9, *Cytomegalovirus Retinitis.*

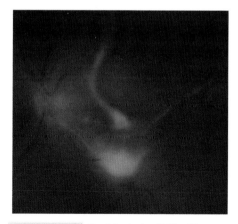

FIGURE 12.17.1. Candida chorioretinitis with vitreous involvement.

- Toxoplasmosis: Yellow–white retinal lesions often with adjacent chorioretinal scar. See 12.5, *Toxoplasmosis.*

- Pneumocystis choroidopathy: Rare manifestation of widely disseminated *Pneumocystis carinii* infection. Usually in AIDS patients. Often asymptomatic. History of *P. carinii* and treatment with aerosolized pentamidine. Multifocal, yellow, round, deep choroidal lesions approximately one-half to two disc diameters in size, located in the posterior pole. No vitritis. Patients are often very ill. Treatment is with i.v. trimethoprim/sulfamethoxazole or i.v. pentamidine in conjunction with an infectious disease specialist.

- Others: Herpes viruses; Mycobacterium avium-intracellulare; Nocardia, Aspergillus, and Cryptococcus species; coccidioidomycosis, and others.

Work-Up

1. History: History of bacteremia or fungemia? Underlying medical conditions? Medications? Intravenous drug abuse? Other risk factors for immunocompromisation?

2. Skin examination for signs of intravenous drug injection.

3. Complete ocular examination, including a dilated retinal evaluation. It is recommended that all patients with candidemia have a baseline fundoscopic examination (ideally within 72 hours), as ocular involvement may be asymptomatic. A repeat fundoscopic examination is recommended 2 weeks after initial examination.

4. Blood, urine, and catheter tip fungal cultures; these often need to be repeated several times and may be negative despite ocular candidiasis. Blood cultures may need to be held a full 7 days and may take 3 to 4 days to become positive for Candida species.

12

5. Consider vitrectomy to obtain a specimen and remove opacified vitreous. Cultures and smears can confirm the diagnosis. Amphotericin B 5 μg in 0.1 mL is injected into the vitreous cavity at the conclusion of the procedure. Intravitreal voriconazole (50 to 100 μg in 0.1 mL) may be considered as an alternative.

6. Baseline CBC, renal function tests, and liver function tests.

Treatment

1. Hospitalize all unreliable patients, systemically ill patients, or those with moderate to severe vitreous involvement.

2. An infectious disease specialist should be consulted. Systemic work-up for other sites of involvement as needed.

3. Typically, chorioretinitis can be successfully treated with systemic therapy alone with one of the following regimens: Fluconazole 400 to 600 mg i.v. or p.o. loading dose followed by 200 to 400 mg i.v. or p.o. daily. Voriconazole 200 mg i.v. or p.o. twice daily may also

be considered. Caspofungin 70 mg i.v. loading dose followed by 50 mg i.v. daily may also be considered. Other agents that may be used include liposomal amphotericin, itraconazole, and micafungin.

4. Intravitreal injection of antifungal agents as above (amphotericin B or voriconazole) if there is vitreous involvement.

5. Topical cycloplegic agent (e.g., atropine 1% t.i.d.).

6. See 9.7, *Inflammatory Open-Angle Glaucoma*, for IOP control. However, steroids are usually contraindicated in candidiasis.

Follow-Up

1. Patients are seen daily. Visual acuity, IOP, and the degree of anterior chamber and vitreous inflammation are assessed.

2. Patients receiving -azole antifungals require liver function tests at least once every other week and as clinically indicated. Patients receiving amphotericin require monitoring of electrolytes, creatinine, and CBC as directed by an infectious disease specialist.

12.18 SYMPATHETIC OPHTHALMIA

Symptoms

Bilateral eye pain, photophobia, decreased vision (near vision is often affected before distance vision), red eye. A history of penetrating trauma or intraocular surgery (most commonly vitreoretinal surgery) to one eye (usually 4 to 8 weeks before, but the range is from 5 days to 66 years, with 90% occurring within 1 year) may be elicited.

Signs

Critical. Suspect any inflammation in the uninvolved eye after unilateral ocular trauma. Bilateral severe anterior chamber reaction with large mutton-fat KP; may have asymmetric involvement with typically more reaction in sympathetic eye. Posterior segment findings include small depigmented nodules at the level of the retinal pigment epithelium

(Dalen–Fuchs nodules), and thickening of the uveal tract. Signs of previous injury or surgery in one eye are usually present.

Other. Nodular infiltration of the iris, peripheral anterior synechiae, neovascularization of the iris, occlusion and seclusion of the pupil, cataract, exudative retinal detachment, papillitis. The earliest sign may be loss of accommodation or a mild anterior or posterior uveitis in the uninjured eye.

Differential Diagnosis

- VKH syndrome: Similar signs, but no history of ocular trauma or surgery. Other systemic symptoms. See 12.11, *Vogt–Koyanagi–Harada Syndrome.*

- Phacoanaphylactic endophthalmitis: Severe anterior chamber reaction from injury to the lens capsule. Contralateral eye is uninvolved. See 9.12, *Lens-Induced (Phacogenic) Glaucoma.*

■ Sarcoidosis: Often elevated ACE level. May cause a bilateral granulomatous panuveitis. See 12.6, *Sarcoidosis.*

■ Syphilis: Positive FTA-ABS. May cause bilateral granulomatous panuveitis. See 12.12, *Syphilis.*

■ Tuberculosis: Positive PPD and CXR. May cause bilateral granulomatous panuveitis.

Work-Up

1. History: Any prior eye surgery or injury? Venereal disease? Difficulty breathing?

2. Complete ophthalmic examination, including a dilated retinal examination.

3. CBC, RPR, FTA-ABS, and ACE level.

4. Consider a chest radiograph to evaluate for tuberculosis or sarcoidosis.

5. IVFA or B-scan US, or both, to help confirm the diagnosis.

Treatment

1. Prevention: Enucleation of a blind, traumatized eye before a sympathetic reaction can develop (usually considered within 14 days of the trauma). If sympathetic ophthalmia develops, the role of enucleation is unclear.

2. Topical steroids (e.g., prednisolone acetate 1% q1–2h). Topical steroids are tapered slowly as condition improves.

3. Periocular or intravitreal steroids (e.g., subconjunctival triamcinolone acetate 40 mg in 1 mL). See Appendix 10, *Technique for Retrobulbar/Subtenon/Subconjunctival Injections.*

4. Systemic steroids [e.g., prednisone 60 to 80 mg p.o. q.d. and an antacid or histamine blocker (e.g., ranitidine 150 mg p.o. b.i.d.)].

5. Slow release intravitreal steroid implants (fluocinolone acetonide 0.59 mg intravitreal implant and dexamethasone 0.7 mg intravitreal implant) are alternatives to oral steroids.

6. Cycloplegic (e.g., scopolamine 0.25% t.i.d.).

7. Long-term systemic immunosuppression with corticosteroid sparing agents may be needed for chronic or relapsing cases.

Follow-Up

1. Every 1 to 7 days initially, to monitor the effectiveness of therapy and IOP.

2. As the condition improves, the follow-up interval may be extended to every 3 to 4 weeks.

3. Steroids should be maintained for 3 to 6 months after all signs of inflammation have resolved and should be tapered slowly. Because of the possibility of recurrence, periodic checkups are important.

12

General Ophthalmic Problems

ACQUIRED CATARACT

Symptoms

Slowly progressive visual loss or blurring, usually over months to years, affecting one or both eyes. Glare, particularly from oncoming headlights while driving at night, and reduced color perception may occur, but not to the same degree as in optic neuropathies. The characteristics of the cataract determine the particular symptoms.

Signs

(See Figure 13.1.1.)

Critical. Opacification of the normally clear crystalline lens.

Other. Blurred view of the retina with dimming of red reflex on retinoscopy. Myopic shift or the so-called "second sight." A cataract alone does not cause a relative afferent pupillary defect (RAPD).

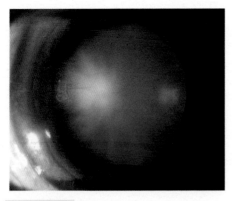

FIGURE 13.1.1. Cataract.

Etiology

- Age-related: Most common. Mature, hypermature, and morgagnian.

- Presenile: Diabetes, myotonic dystrophy, and atopic dermatitis.

- Trauma: Penetrating, concussion (vossius ring), and electric shock.

- Toxic: Steroids, miotics, antipsychotics (e.g., phenothiazines), and others.

- Secondary.

  —Chronic anterior uveitis. See 12.1, *Anterior Uveitis (Iritis/Iridocyclitis)*.

  —Ionizing radiation.

  —Tumor (ciliary body).

  —Acute angle-closure glaucoma: Glaucomflecken. See 9.4, *Acute Angle-Closure Glaucoma*.

  —Degenerative ocular disease: Retinitis pigmentosa, Leber congenital amaurosis, Gyrate atrophy, Wagner and Stickler syndromes associated with posterior subcapsular cataracts, and others.

- Endocrine/Metabolic.

  —Diabetes: Juvenile form characterized by rapidly progressing white "snowflake" opacities in the anterior and posterior subcapsular locations. Age-related cataracts form earlier than in nondiabetics.

  —Hypocalcemia: Small, white, iridescent cortical changes, usually seen in the presence of tetany.

—Wilson disease: Red–brown pigment deposition in the cortex beneath the anterior capsule (a "sunflower" cataract). See 13.9, *Wilson Disease*.

—Myotonic dystrophy: Multicolored opacities, "Christmas-tree cataract," behind the anterior capsule.

—Others: Down syndrome, Neurofibromatosis Type 2 (posterior subcapsular cataract), etc.

Types

1. Nuclear: Yellow or brown discoloration of the central lens. Typically blurs distance vision more than near (myopic shift).

2. Posterior subcapsular: Plaque-like opacity near the posterior aspect of the lens. Best seen in retroillumination against the red reflex. Glare and difficulty reading are common complaints. Associated with ocular inflammation, steroid use, diabetes, trauma, or radiation. Classically occurs in patients <50 years of age.

3. Cortical: Radial or spoke-like opacities in the periphery that expand to involve the anterior and posterior lens and can cause glare. Often asymptomatic until central changes develop.

NOTE: A mature cataract is defined as lenticular changes sufficiently dense to totally obscure the view of the posterior lens and posterior segment of the eye. No iris shadow is seen on oblique illumination at the pupillary margin. Rarely, the cortex may liquefy and the nucleus becomes free-floating within the capsule, this is known as a hypermature or Morgagnian cataract. If the liquefied cortex leaks through the intact capsule, wrinkling of the lens capsule may be seen and phacolytic glaucoma may develop. See 9.12.1, *Phacolytic Glaucoma*.

Work-Up

Determine the etiology, whether the cataract is responsible for the decreased vision, and whether surgical removal would improve vision.

1. History: Medications? [e.g., tamsulosin or any medications used for urinary retention (alpha-1 blockers) strongly associated with intraoperative floppy iris syndrome]

Systemic diseases? Trauma? Ocular disease or poor vision before the cataract?

2. Complete ocular examination, including distance and near vision, pupillary examination, and refraction. A dilated slit-lamp examination using both direct and retroillumination techniques is required to view the cataract properly. Fundus examination, concentrating on the macula, is essential in ruling out other causes of decreased vision.

3. For preoperative planning, note the degree of pupil dilation, density of the cataract, and presence or absence of pseudoexfoliation syndrome, phacodonesis (quivering of the lens indicating zonular damage or weakness), or cornea guttata.

4. B-scan ultrasonography (US) if the fundus is obscured to rule out detectable posterior segment disease.

5. The potential acuity meter (PAM) or laser interferometry can be used to estimate the visual potential when cataract extraction is considered in an eye with posterior segment disease.

NOTE: Laser interferometry and PAM often overestimate the eye's visual potential in the presence of macular holes or macular pigment epithelial detachments. Interferometry also overestimates results in cases of amblyopia. Near vision is often the most accurate manner of evaluating macular function if the cataract is not too dense. Nonetheless, both laser interferometry and PAM are useful clinical tools.

---

6. Keratometry readings and an A-scan US measurement of axial length are required for determining the power of the desired intraocular lens (IOL). Corneal pachymetry or endothelial cell count is occasionally helpful if cornea guttata are present.

13

Treatment

1. Cataract surgery may be performed for the following reasons:

—To improve visual function in patients with symptomatic visual disability.

—As surgical therapy for ocular disease (e.g., lens-related glaucoma or uveitis).

—To facilitate management of ocular disease (e.g., to allow a view of the fundus to monitor or treat diabetic retinopathy or glaucoma).

2. Correct any refractive error if the patient declines cataract surgery.

3. A trial of mydriasis (e.g., scopolamine 0.25% q.d.) may be used successfully in some patients who desire nonsurgical treatment. The benefits of this therapy are only temporary. Most useful for posterior subcapsular cataracts.

Follow-Up

Unless there is a secondary complication from the cataract (e.g., glaucoma), a cataract itself does not require urgent action. Patients who decline surgical removal are reexamined annually, sooner if symptoms worsen.

If congenital, see 8.8, *Congenital Cataract.*

13.2 — PREGNANCY

ANTERIOR SEGMENT CHANGES

Transient loss of accommodation and increased corneal thickness/edema and curvature. Refractive change likely results from a shift in fluid or hormonal status and will likely normalize after delivery. Defer prescribing new glasses until several weeks postpartum.

PREECLAMPSIA/ECLAMPSIA

A worldwide leading cause of maternal/fetal/neonatal morbidity and mortality. Occurs in 2% to 5% of pregnancies but may approach 10% in developing countries. Occurs after 20 weeks of gestation; most commonly in primigravids.

Symptoms

Headaches, blurred vision, photopsias, diplopia, and scotomas.

Signs

Systemic

■ Preeclampsia or pregnancy-induced hypertension: Hypertension and proteinuria in previously normotensive women. Other signs include peripheral edema, liver failure, renal failure, and HELLP syndrome (hemolysis, elevated liver enzymes, and low platelet counts).

■ Eclampsia: Preeclampsia with seizures.

Ocular. Focal retinal arteriolar spasm and narrowing, peripapillary or focal areas of retinal edema, retinal hemorrhages, exudates, nerve fiber layer infarcts, vitreous hemorrhage secondary to neovascularization, serous retinal detachments in 1% of preeclamptic and 10% of eclamptic patients, acute nonarteritic ischemic optic neuropathy, and bilateral occipital lobe infarcts (preeclampsia–eclampsia hypertensive posterior encephalopathy syndrome, or PEHPES). Differential diagnosis of PEHPES includes posterior circulation stroke, infectious cerebritis, coagulation disorder causing intracranial venous thrombosis, intracranial hemorrhage, occult tumor with secondary bleed, migraines, atypical seizure, or demyelination.

Natural History

1. Magnetic resonance imaging (MRI) abnormalities resolve 1 to 2 weeks after blood pressure control, at which time complete neurologic recovery can be expected.

2. Serous retinal detachments; often bilateral and bullous; resolve postpartum with residual pigment epithelial changes (see Figure 13.2.1).

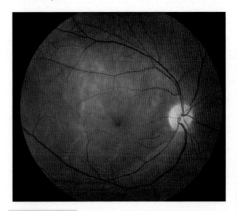

FIGURE 13.2.1. Serous macular detachment in a patient with preeclampsia.

3. Retinal vascular changes also normalize postpartum.

Work-Up

1. Complete neuro-ophthalmologic and fundus examinations. Poor vision with brisk pupils without an RAPD suggests occipital lesions.

2. MRI findings in PEHPES include bilateral occipital lobe lesions involving subcortical white matter with possible extension into the gray–white junction, cortical surface, external capsule, and basal ganglia. MRI abnormalities are identical in obstetric and nonobstetric hypertensive encephalopathy.

3. With typical presentation, further invasive studies are discouraged.

4. Systemic work-up, including blood pressure monitoring and urinalysis, in conjunction with an OB/GYN specialist.

Treatment

1. Control blood pressure and electrolyte imbalances.

2. Prompt delivery ideal.

OCCLUSIVE VASCULAR DISORDERS

Pregnancy represents a hypercoagulable state possibly resulting in the development of retinal artery and vein occlusions, disseminated intravascular coagulopathy (DIC), and thrombotic thrombocytopenia purpura. Ocular DIC is characterized by widespread small-vessel thrombosis, particularly in the choroid, associated with hemorrhage, tissue necrosis, and serous retinal detachments.

MENINGIOMA OF PREGNANCY

Meningiomas may have a very aggressive growth pattern during pregnancy that is difficult to manage. They may regress postpartum but may reoccur during subsequent pregnancies.

NOTE: All pregnant women complaining of a headache should have their blood pressure, visual fields, and fundus checked (particularly looking for papilledema). MRI/MRV or lumbar puncture is often required if a hemorrhage or cortical venous thrombosis is suspected.

OTHER CONDITIONS INFLUENCED BY PREGNANCY

Multiple conditions can be impacted by pregnancy. See 3.19, *Purtscher Retinopathy;* 10.10, *Cavernous Sinus and Associated Syndromes (Multiple Ocular Motor Nerve Palsies);* 10.16, *Idiopathic Intracranial Hypertension/Pseudotumor Cerebri;* 10.27, *Migraine;* 11.12, *Diabetic Retinopathy;* and 11.15, *Central Serous Chorioretinopathy.* Medications deserve special attention during pregnancy.

13.3   LYME DISEASE

13

Symptoms

Decreased vision, double vision, pain, photophobia, facial weakness. Also may have headache, malaise, fatigue, fever, chills, palpitations, or muscle or joint pains. A history of a tick bite within the previous few months may be elicited.

Signs

Ocular.   Optic neuritis; vitritis; iritis; stromal keratitis; choroiditis; exudative retinal detachment; third, fourth, or sixth cranial nerve palsy; bilateral optic nerve swelling; conjunctivitis; episcleritis; exposure keratopathy; other rare abnormalities, including idiopathic orbital inflammatory syndrome. See specific sections.

Critical Systemic.   One or more flat, erythematous or "bull's-eye" skin lesions, which enlarge in all directions (erythema migrans); unilateral or bilateral facial nerve palsies; polyarticular migratory arthritis. May not be present at the time the ocular signs develop. A high serum antibody titer against *Borrelia burgdorferi*, is often, but not always present.

Other Systemic.   Meningitis, peripheral radiculoneuropathy, synovitis, joint effusions, cardiac abnormalities, or a low false-positive FTA-ABS titer.

Differential Diagnosis

- Syphilis: High-positive FTA-ABS titer may produce a low false-positive antibody titer against *B. burgdorferi*. See 12.12, *Syphilis*.

- Others: Rickettsial infections, acute rheumatic fever, juvenile idiopathic arthritis, sarcoidosis, tuberculosis, herpes virus infections, etc.

Work-Up

1. History: Does patient live in endemic area? Prior tick bite, skin rash, facial nerve palsy, joint or muscle pains, flulike illness? Meningeal symptoms? Prior positive Lyme titer?

2. Complete systemic, neurologic, and ocular examinations.

3. Two-step diagnosis with a screening assay and confirmatory Western blot for *B. burgdorferi*.

4. Serum RPR and FTA-ABS. Consider serum ACE, chest x-ray, and PPD.

5. Consider lumbar puncture when meningitis is suspected or neurologic signs or symptoms are present.

Treatment

Early Lyme Disease (Including Lyme-Related Uveitis, Keratitis, or Facial Nerve Palsy):

1. Doxycycline 100 mg p.o. b.i.d. for 10 to 21 days.

2. In children, pregnant women, and those who cannot take doxycycline, substitute amoxicillin 500 mg p.o. t.i.d., cefuroxime axetil 500 mg p.o. b.i.d., clarithromycin 500 mg p.o. b.i.d., or azithromycin 500 mg p.o. q.d.

Patients with Neuro-ophthalmic Signs or Recurrent or Resistant Infection:

1. Ceftriaxone 2 g intravenously q.d. for 2 to 3 weeks.

2. Alternatively, penicillin G, 20 million units intravenously q.d. for 2 to 3 weeks.

Follow-Up

Every 1 to 3 days until improvement is demonstrated, and then weekly until resolved.

13.4   CONVERGENCE INSUFFICIENCY

Symptoms

Eye discomfort or blurred vision from reading or near work. Most common in young adults, but may be seen in older people.

Signs

Critical. An exophoria at near in the presence of poor near-fusional convergence amplitudes, a low accommodative convergence/accommodation (AC/A) ratio, and a remote near point of convergence.

Differential Diagnosis

- Uncorrected refractive error: Hyperopia or over-minused myopia.

- Accommodative insufficiency (AI): Often in prepresbyopia age range from uncorrected low hyperopia or over-minused myopia. While reading, a 4-diopter base-in prism placed in front of the eye blurs the print in AI, but improves clarity in CI. Rarely, adolescents may develop transient paresis of accommodation, requiring reading glasses or bifocals. This idiopathic condition resolves in several years. Patients with AI may benefit from reading glasses with base-in prism.

- Convergence paralysis: Acute onset of exotropia and diplopia on near fixation only; normal adduction and accommodation. Usually results from a lesion in the corpora quadrigemina or the third cranial nerve nucleus, and may be associated with Parinaud syndrome.

NOTE: A diagnosis of convergence paralysis should prompt neuroimaging to rule out an intracranial lesion.

Etiology

- Fatigue or illness.

- Drugs (parasympatholytics).

- Uveitis.

- Adie tonic pupil.

- Glasses inducing a base-out prism effect.

- Post-exanthematous encephalitis.

- Traumatic injury.

- Idiopathic.

Work-Up

1. Manifest (without cycloplegia) refraction.

2. Determine the near point of convergence: Ask patient to focus on an accommodative target (e.g., a pencil eraser) and to state when double vision develops as you bring the target toward them; a normal near point of convergence is <8 cm.

3. Check for exodeviations or esodeviations at distance and near using the cover tests (see Appendix 3, *Cover/Uncover and Alternate Cover Tests*) or the Maddox rod test.

4. Measure the patient's fusional ability at near. Have patient focus on an accommodative target at their reading distance. With a prism bar, slowly increase the amount of base-out prism in front of one eye until patient notes double vision (the break point), and then slowly reduce the amount of base-out prism until a single image is again noted (the recovery point). A low break point (10 to 15 prism diopters), a low recovery point, or both, are consistent with CI.

5. Place a 4-diopter base-in prism in front of one eye while patient is reading. Determine whether the print becomes clearer or more blurred to rule out AI.

6. Perform cycloplegic refraction after the previous tests.

NOTE: These tests are performed with the patient's spectacle correction in place (if glasses are worn for near work).

Treatment

1. Correct any refractive error. Slightly undercorrect hyperopia, and fully correct myopia.

2. Near-point exercises (e.g., pencil push-ups): The patient focuses on a pencil eraser while slowly moving it from arm's length toward the face. Concentrate on maintaining one image of the eraser, repeating the maneuver when diplopia manifests. Try to bring the pencil in closer each time while maintaining single vision. Repeat the exercise 15 times, 5 times per day.

3. Near-point exercises with base-out prisms (for patients whose near point of convergence is satisfactory or for those who have mastered pencil push-ups without a prism): The patient performs pencil push-ups as described previously, while holding a 6-diopter base-out prism in front of one eye.

4. Encourage good lighting and relaxation time between periods of close work.

5. For older patients, or those whose condition shows no improvement despite near-point exercises, reading glasses with base-in prism can be useful.

Follow-Up

Nonurgent. Patients are reexamined in 1 month.

13.5 ACCOMMODATIVE SPASM

13

Symptoms

Bilateral blurred distance vision, fluctuating vision, blurred vision when shifting gaze from near to far, headache, and eye strain while reading. Often seen in teenagers under stress. Symptoms may occur after prolonged and intense periods of near work.

Signs

Critical. Cycloplegic refraction reveals substantially less myopia (or more hyperopia) than was originally found when the refraction was performed without cycloplegia (manifest refraction). Manifest myopia may be as high as 10 diopters. Spasm of the near reflex is associated with excess accommodation, excess convergence, and miosis.

Other. Abnormally close near point of focus, miosis, and a normal amplitude of accommodation that may appear low.

Etiology

- Inability to relax the ciliary muscles. Involuntary and associated with stressful situations or functional neuroses.

- Fatigue.

- Prolonged reading may precipitate episodes.

Differential Diagnosis

- Uncorrected hyperopia: Increased plus accepted during manifest refraction.

- Other causes of pseudomyopia: Hyperglycemia, medication induced (e.g., sulfa drugs and anticholinesterase medications), anterior displacement of the lens-iris diaphragm.

- Manifestation of iridocyclitis.

Work-Up

1. Complete ophthalmic examination. The manifest refraction may be highly variable, but it is important to determine the least amount of minus power or the most amount of plus power that provides clear distance vision.

2. Cycloplegic refraction.

Treatment

1. True refractive errors should be corrected. If a significant amount of esophoria at near is present, additional plus power (e.g., +2.50 diopters) in reading glasses or bifocal form may be helpful.

2. Counseling patient and parents to provide a more relaxed atmosphere and avoid stressful situations.

3. Cycloplegics have been used to break the spasm, but are rarely needed except in resistant cases.

Follow-Up

Reevaluate in several weeks.

13.6 STEVENS–JOHNSON SYNDROME (ERYTHEMA MULTIFORME MAJOR)

Symptoms

Acute onset of fever, rash, red eyes, malaise, arthralgias, and respiratory tract symptoms.

Signs

Systemic. Classic "target" skin lesions (maculopapules with a red center and a white surrounding area on an erythematous base) concentrated on hands and feet; ulcerative stomatitis; and hemorrhagic lip crusting. Mortality rate is 10% to 33%.

Ocular

- Acute phase: Mucopurulent or pseudomembranous conjunctivitis, episcleritis, and iritis.

- Late complications: Conjunctival scarring and symblepharon; trichiasis; eyelid defor-

mities; tear deficiency; corneal neovascularization, ulcer, perforation, or scarring.

Etiology

Precipitated by many agents, including:

- Drugs: Sulfonamides, barbiturates, chlorpropamide, thiazide diuretics, phenytoin, salicylates, allopurinol, chlormezanone, corticosteroids, isoniazid, tetracycline, codeine, aminopenicillins, chemotherapeutic agents, and others.

- Infectious agents: Most commonly *Mycoplasma pneumoniae*, herpes simplex virus, and adenovirus.

- Allergy and autoimmune diseases.

- Genetics: HLA B-12 may confer increased risk.

13

- Radiation therapy.
- Malignancy.

Types

1. Erythema multiforme minor: Only skin involvement.

2. Erythema multiforme major (Stevens–Johnson syndrome): Immune complex deposition in dermis with subepithelial vesiculobullous reaction of skin and mucous membranes.

3. Toxic epidermal necrolysis: Most severe form with extensive vesiculobullous eruptions and epidermal sloughing. More common in children and immunosuppressed patients.

Work-Up

1. History: Attempt to determine the precipitating factor.

2. Slit-lamp examination, including eyelid eversion with examination of the fornices.

3. Conjunctival or corneal cultures if infection is suspected. See Appendix 8, *Corneal Culture Procedure.*

4. Consult Internal Medicine for a systemic work-up.

5. Skin biopsy may aid in the diagnosis.

Treatment

1. Hospitalization, often requiring burn unit if available.

2. Remove (e.g., drug) or treat (e.g., infection) the inciting factor.

3. Supportive care is the mainstay of therapy.

4. Co-management with Dermatology and Internal Medicine.

Ocular:

a. Tear deficiency: Aggressive lubrication with preservative-free artificial tears, gels, and ointments. Topical cyclosporine 0.05%, punctal occlusion, moisture chambers, or tarsorrhaphy.

b. Iritis: Topical steroid drops (e.g., prednisolone acetate 1% four to eight times per day) and cycloplegic (e.g., atropine 1% t.i.d.).

c. Infections: Treat as outlined in 4.11, *Bacterial Keratitis.*

d. Controversial treatments:

—Topical steroids for ocular surface inflammation.

—Daily pseudomembrane peel and symblepharon lysis with glass rod or moistened cotton swab.

—Systemic or topical vitamin A.

—Intravenous immunoglobulin.

Systemic: Manage by burn unit protocol, including hydration, wound care, and system antibiotics. Medical and dermatological consultation recommended.

Follow-Up

1. During hospitalization: Follow daily, with infection and IOP surveillance.

2. Outpatient: Weekly follow-ups initially, watching for long-term ocular complications.

—Topical steroids and antibiotics are maintained for 48 hours after resolution and are then tapered.

—If there is severe conjunctival scarring, artificial tears and lubricating ointment may need to be maintained indefinitely.

3. Possible late surgical interventions.

—Trichiasis: Repeated epilation, electrolysis, cryotherapy, or surgical repair.

—Entropion repair with buccal mucosal grafts.

—Penetrating keratoplasty: Poor prognosis even when combined with limbal stem cell or amniotic membrane transplantation because of underlying deficiencies, such as dry eyes and limbal stem cell abnormality.

—Permanent keratoprosthesis.

13

VITAMIN A DEFICIENCY

See Table 13.7.1.

Symptoms

Night blindness (earliest and most common manifestation), dry eyes, ocular pain, and severe vision loss.

Signs

Ocular: Bitôt spots (triangular, perilimbal, gray, foamy plaques of keratinized conjunctival debris); decreased tear breakup time; bilateral conjunctival and corneal dryness; corneal epithelial defects, sterile or infectious ulceration (often peripheral with a punched-out appearance), perforation, scarring; keratomalacia (often preceded by a gastrointestinal, respiratory, or measles infection); fundus abnormalities [yellow or white peripheral retinal dots representing focal retinal pigment epithelium (RPE) defects].

Systemic: Growth retardation in children; dry, hyperkeratotic skin; increased susceptibility to infections.

Differential Diagnosis

See 4.3, *Dry-Eye Syndrome,* and 11.28, *Retinitis Pigmentosa and Inherited Chorioretinal Dystrophies.*

Etiology

■ Primary: Dietary deficiency or chronic alcoholism (relatively uncommon in developed countries). Beyond 6 months postpartum, breast milk in vitamin A-deficient mothers is unlikely to sufficiently maintain vitamin A stores in nursing infants.

■ Secondary: Lipid malabsorption [e.g., cystic fibrosis, chronic pancreatitis, inflammatory bowel disease, celiac sprue, postgastrectomy or postintestinal bypass surgery, chronic liver disease, abetalipoproteinemia (Bassen–Kornzweig syndrome)].

Work-Up

1. History: Malnutrition? Poor or extreme diet? Gastrointestinal or liver disease? Previous surgery? Measles?

2. Complete ophthalmic examination, including careful inspection of eyelid margins and inferior fornices.

3. A positive response to treatment is a simple, cost-effective way to confirm the diagnosis.

4. Consider serum vitamin A level before treatment is initiated.

5. Consider impression cytology of the conjunctiva, looking for decreased goblet cell density.

6. Consider dark-adaptation studies and electroretinogram (may be more sensitive than the serum vitamin A level).

TABLE **13.7.1** World Health Organization Classification of Vitamin A Deficiency	
XN	Night blindness
X1A	Conjunctival xerosis
X1B	Bitôt spot
X2	Corneal xerosis
X3A	Corneal ulceration or keratomalacia with less than one-third corneal involvement
X3B	Corneal ulceration or keratomalacia with one-third or more corneal involvement
XS	Corneal scar
XF	Xerophthalmia fundus

7. Corneal cultures if an infection is suspected. See Appendix 8, *Corneal Culture Procedure.*

Treatment

1. Immediate vitamin A replacement therapy orally (preferred) or intramuscularly in the following WHO recommended dosages for clinical xerophthalmia:

—Children <12 months: 100,000 IU q.d. for 2 days, repeat in 2 weeks.

—Adults and children >12 months: 200,000 IU q.d. for 2 days, repeat in 2 weeks.

—Women of childbearing age (reduce dose due to possible teratogenic effects): night blindness or Bitôt spots only, 10,000 IU q.d. for 2 weeks or 25,000 IU weekly for 4 weeks; any corneal lesions, give full adult dose as above.

2. Intensive ocular lubrication with preservative-free artificial tears every 15 to 60 minutes and preservative-free artificial tear ointment q.h.s.

3. Treat malnutrition/underlying disease if present.

4. Consider supplementing the patient's diet with zinc and vitamin A.

5. Consider a penetrating keratoplasty or keratoprosthesis for corneal scars in eyes with potentially good vision.

6. Prophylaxis in endemic regions:

—Infants: consider 50,000 IU.

—6 to 12 months: 100,000 IU q 4 to 6 months.

—Children >12 months: 200,000 IU q 4 to 6 months.

—Retinyl palmitate has been used to fortify sugars in developing countries.

Follow-Up

Determined by the clinical presentation and response to treatment, ranges from hospitalization to daily or weekly follow-up. Vitamin A deficiency associated with measles may be especially severe.

13.8   ALBINISM

Symptoms

Decreased vision. Photosensitivity in some patients.

Signs

Best corrected visual acuity of 20/40 to 20/200; may have high refractive error; strabismus; reduced stereopsis; nystagmus starting at age 2 to 3 months; amblyopia secondary to strabismus or anisometropia; iris transillumination defects; retinal hypopigmentation with highly visible choroidal vasculature; failure of the retinal vessels to wreathe the fovea; in true albinism the fovea is hypoplastic, with no foveal pit or reflex (the only ocular finding consistently present).

NOTE: Patients with albinism show a wide range of visual acuities, refractive errors, nystagmus, and amblyopia.

Associated Disorders

- Hermansky–Pudlak syndrome: An autosomal recessive defect in platelet function leading to easy bruisability and bleeding. More common in patients of Puerto Rican descent. Most common gene involved is HPS-1 on chromosome 10q23.1.

- Chediak–Higashi syndrome: An autosomal recessive disorder affecting white blood cell function, resulting in an increased susceptibility to infections and a predisposition for a lymphoma-like condition. LYST gene on chromosome 1q42.1-q42.2.

Types

1. Oculocutaneous albinism: Autosomal recessive, hypopigmentation of hair, skin, and eye.

   - Tyrosinase positive (OCA2): Varying degree of pigmentation.

13

- Tyrosinase intermediate (OC1B): No pigmentation at birth. Varying degree of pigmentation with age.

- Tyrosinase negative (OCA1A): No pigmentation.

2. Ocular albinism: Only ocular hypopigmentation is clinically apparent. Usually inherited as X-linked recessive (Nettleship–Falls). Female carriers may have partial iris transillumination and mottled areas of hypopigmentation in peripheral retina. In the autosomal recessive form, females and males are affected with equal severity.

Work-Up

1. History: Easy bruisability? Frequent nosebleeds? Prolonged bleeding after dental work? Frequent infections? Family history? Puerto Rican heritage?

2. External (including hair and skin color) examination.

3. Complete ocular examination.

4. Before surgery, obtain bleeding time. Platelet aggregation studies and platelet electron microscopy are also indicated if Hermansky–Pudlak syndrome is suspected.

5. If Chediak–Higashi syndrome is suspected, check polymorphonuclear leukocyte function.

6. Flash visual evoked potential testing to demonstrate excessive decussation of retinal ganglion cell axons at the chiasm.

Treatment

There is currently no effective treatment for albinism, but the following may be helpful:

1. Treating amblyopia may reduce nystagmus, if present. See 8.7, *Amblyopia.*

2. Appropriate refraction and early use of bifocals may be necessary as amplitude of accommodation diminishes.

3. Eye muscle surgery may be considered for patients with significant strabismus or an abnormal head position due to nystagmus. However, patients with albinism and strabismus rarely achieve binocularity after surgical correction.

4. Genetic counseling.

5. Dermatologic consultation. Advise ultraviolet sun protection.

6. Hematology evaluation if either Chediak–Higashi syndrome or Hermansky–Pudlak syndrome is suspected. Patients with Hermansky–Pudlak syndrome may require platelet transfusions before surgery.

13.9   WILSON DISEASE

Symptoms

Ocular complaints are rare. Patients experience symptoms of cirrhosis, neurologic disorders, psychiatric problems, or renal disease. Onset typically between 5 and 40 years of age.

Signs

Critical. Kayser–Fleischer ring: a 1- to 3-mm, brown, green, or red band that represents copper deposition in the peripheral Descemet membrane (see Figure 13.9.1). Present in 50% to 60% of patients with isolated hepatic involvement and more than 90% of patients with neurologic manifestations. First appears superiorly (may only be visible on gonioscopy)

and eventually forms a ring involving the entire corneal periphery extending to the limbus. This autosomal recessive inborn error of metabolism results in low serum copper and ceruloplasmin levels with elevated urine copper.

Other. "Sunflower" cataract due to anterior and posterior subcapsular copper deposition.

Differential Diagnosis

- Kayser–Fleischer-like ring: Seen in primary biliary cirrhosis, chronic active hepatitis, progressive intrahepatic cholestasis, and multiple myeloma. These patients have a normal serum ceruloplasmin level and no neurologic symptoms.

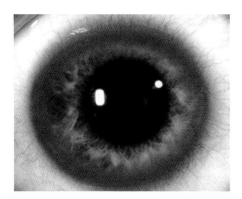

FIGURE 13.9.1. Kayser–Fleischer ring in Wilson disease.

- Arcus senilis: Corneal stromal lipid deposition, initially appears inferiorly and superiorly before extending. A clear zone of cornea separates the edge of the arcus from the limbus. Check a fasting lipid profile in patients <40 years.

- Chalcosis: Copper deposition in basement membranes, including Descemet membrane, secondary to copper-containing intraocular foreign body. Alloys containing more than 85% copper may induce severe inflammation, those with lower amounts may cause retinal toxicity.

Work-Up

1. Slit-lamp examination: Deposition at Descemet membrane is apparent with a narrow slit beam.

2. Gonioscopy if the Kayser–Fleischer ring is not evident on slit-lamp examination.

3. Serum copper and ceruloplasmin levels. Urine copper level.

4. Referral to an internist or neurologist.

Treatment

1. Lifelong systemic therapy (e.g., zinc, D-penicillamine, trientine) is instituted by an internist or neurologist. Liver transplantation may be required for fulminant hepatic failure or disease progression after medical therapy.

2. The ocular manifestations usually require no specific treatment.

Follow-Up

1. Systemic therapy and monitoring with an internist or neurologist.

2. Successful treatment should lead to resorption of the corneal copper deposition and clearing of the Kayser–Fleischer ring, although residual corneal changes may remain. This change can be used to monitor treatment response. Reappearance of ring may suggest noncompliance with treatment.

3. Consider referral of family members for genetic testing for early detection and prevention, specifically defects of the ATP7B gene on chromosome 13q14.3-q21.1.

13.10 SUBLUXED OR DISLOCATED CRYSTALLINE LENS

Definition

- Subluxation: Partial disruption of the zonular fibers. Lens is decentered but remains partially visible through the pupil.

- Dislocation: Complete disruption of the zonular fibers. Lens is fully displaced out of the pupillary aperture.

Symptoms

Decreased vision, double vision that persists when covering one eye (monocular diplopia).

Signs

(See Figure 13.10.1.)

Critical. Decentered or displaced lens, iridodonesis (quivering of the iris), phacodonesis (quivering of the lens).

Other. Change in refractive error, marked astigmatism, cataract, angle-closure glaucoma as a result of pupillary block, acquired high myopia, vitreous in the anterior chamber, asymmetry of the anterior chamber depth.

13

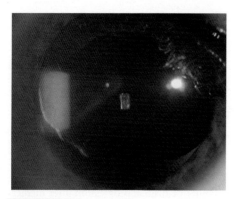

FIGURE 13.10.1. Ectopia lentis.

Etiology

■ Trauma: Most common. Results in sub-luxation if >25% of the zonular fibers are ruptured. Need to rule out a predisposing condition (see other etiologies).

■ Pseudoexfoliation: Flaky material seen as scrolls in a "target pattern" on anterior lens capsule; associated with glaucoma; poor pupillary dilation; patients at higher risk of complications during cataract surgery due to weak zonular fibers (see 9.11, *Pseudoexfoliation Syndrome/Exfoliative Glaucoma*).

■ Marfan syndrome: Bilateral lens sublux-ation, classically superiorly and temporally, with increased risk for retinal detachment. Autosomal dominant with cardiomyopa-thy, aortic aneurysm, tall stature with long extremities, and kyphoscoliosis.

■ Homocystinuria: Bilateral lens subluxation, classically inferiorly and nasally. Increased risk of retinal detachment. Autosomal recessive with frequent mental retarda-tion, skeletal deformities, high incidence of thromboembolic events (particularly with general anesthesia). Lens subluxation may be first manifestation in patients with mild disease.

■ Weill–Marchesani syndrome: Small lens can dislocate into the anterior chamber, caus-ing reverse pupillary block. Often autoso-mal recessive with short fingers and stature, seizures, microspherophakia (small, round lens), myopia, no mental retardation.

■ Others: Acquired syphilis, congenital ectopia lentis, simple ectopia lentis, aniridia, Ehlers–Danlos syndrome, Crouzon syndrome, hyperlysinemia, sulfite oxidase deficiency, high myopia, chronic inflammations, hyper-mature cataract, etc.

Work-Up

1. History: Family history of the disorders listed? Trauma? Systemic illness (e.g., syphilis)? Neurologic symptoms (e.g., sei-zures)?

2. Complete ocular examination: Determine whether the condition is unilateral or bilateral and direction of displacement. Check for pseudoexfoliation. Evaluation for subtle phacodonesis by observing the lens during back and forth eye move-ment. Evaluate for signs of ocular trauma including hyphema, angle recession, iri-dodialysis, cyclodialysis, retinal tears, and detachments.

3. Systemic examination: Evaluate stature, extremities, hands, and fingers; often in con-junction with an internist, including sodium nitroprusside test or urine chromatography to rule out homocystinuria and echocar-diography to rule out aortic aneurysms in patients with possible Marfan syndrome. Consider genetic testing when appropriate and available.

4. RPR and FTA-ABS.

Treatment

1. Lens dislocated into the anterior chamber.

—Dilate the pupil, place the patient on his or her back, and replace the lens into the posterior chamber by head manipu-lation. It may be necessary to indent the cornea after topical anesthesia with a Zeiss gonioprism or cotton swab to reposition the lens. After the lens is repo-sitioned in the posterior chamber, con-strict the pupil with pilocarpine 0.5% to 1% q.i.d. and perform a peripheral laser iridotomy.

or

—Surgically remove the lens (usually per-formed if a significant cataract is present, treatment described previously fails, recurrent dislocations occur, or there are compliance issues with pilocarpine) and consider placing an IOL.

2. Lens dislocated into the vitreous.

—Lens capsule intact, patient asymptomatic, no signs of inflammation: Observation versus pars plana lensectomy and consider IOL placement.

—Lens capsule broken with intraocular inflammation: Pars plana lensectomy with possible IOL placement.

3. Subluxation.

—Asymptomatic: Observe.

—Uncorrectable astigmatism or monocular diplopia: Surgical removal of the lens and possible IOL placement.

—Symptomatic cataract: Options include surgical removal of the lens, mydriasis (e.g., scopolamine 0.25% q.d.) and aphakic correction, pupillary constriction (e.g., pilocarpine 4% gel q.h.s.) and phakic correction, or a large optical iridectomy (away from the lens).

4. Pupillary block: Treatment is identical to that for aphakic pupillary block. See 9.16, *Postoperative Glaucoma.*

5. If Marfan syndrome suspected: Refer the patient to a cardiologist for an annual echocardiogram and management of any cardiac-related abnormalities. Prophylactic systemic antibiotics are required if the patient undergoes surgery (or a dental procedure) to prevent endocarditis.

6. If homocystinuria is suspected: Refer to an internist. The usual therapy consists of:

—Pyridoxine (Vitamin B6) 50 to 1,000 mg p.o. q.d.

—Methionine restricted, cysteine-supplemented diet.

—Avoid surgery if possible because of the risk of thromboembolic complications. If surgical intervention is necessary, anticoagulant therapy is indicated in conjunction with internist.

Follow-Up

Depends on the etiology, degree of subluxation or dislocation, and symptoms.

13.11 HYPOTONY SYNDROME

Definition

Decreased visual function and other ocular symptoms related to low IOP.

Symptoms

May have mild to severe pain. Vision may be reduced. Excessive tearing in patients after glaucoma filtering procedures. May be asymptomatic.

Signs

Critical. Low IOP, usually <6 mm Hg, but may occur with an IOP as high as 10 mm Hg.

Other. Corneal edema and folds, corneal decompensation, aqueous cell and flare, shallow or flat anterior chamber, retinal edema, hypotony maculopathy, chorioretinal folds, serous choroidal detachment, suprachoroidal hemorrhage, the appearance of optic disc swelling, and retinal vascular tortuosity.

Etiology

- Postsurgical: Wound leak, overfiltering bleb (more common with use of antimetabolites during surgery) or glaucoma drainage device, cyclodialysis cleft (disinsertion of the ciliary body from the sclera at the scleral spur), scleral perforation (e.g., from a superior rectus bridle suture or retrobulbar injection), iridocyclitis, retinal or choroidal detachment, and others.

- Posttraumatic: Same causes as postsurgical.

13

■ Pharmacologic: Usually from a carbonic anhydrase inhibitor in combination with a topical beta-blocker. Also associated with cidofovir.

■ Systemic (bilateral hypotony): Conditions that cause blood hypertonicity (e.g., dehydration, uremia, hyperglycemia), myotonic dystrophy, and others.

■ Vascular occlusive disease (e.g., ocular ischemic syndrome, giant cell arteritis, central retinal vein or artery occlusion): Usually mild hypotony.

■ Uveitis: Secondary to ciliary body shutdown.

Work-Up

1. History: Recent ocular surgery or trauma? Other systemic symptoms (nausea, vomiting, twitching, drowsiness, polyuria)? History of renal disease, diabetes, or myotonic dystrophy? Medications?

2. Complete ocular examination, including a slit-lamp evaluation of surgical or traumatic ocular wounds, IOP check, gonioscopy of the anterior chamber angle to rule out a cyclodialysis cleft, and indirect ophthalmoscopy to rule out a retinal or choroidal detachment.

3. Seidel test (with or without gentle pressure) to rule out a wound leak. See Appendix 5, *Seidel Test to Detect a Wound Leak*.

NOTE: A wound leak may drain under the conjunctiva, producing a filtering bleb. Seidel test will then be negative.

---

4. B-scan US when the fundus cannot be seen clinically. Consider US biomicroscopy for evaluation of the anterior chamber angle and to evaluate for cyclodialysis cleft.

5. Blood tests in bilateral cases: Glucose, blood urea nitrogen, and creatinine.

Treatment

Repair of the underlying disorder may be needed if symptoms are significant or progressive. Low IOP, even as low as 2 mm Hg, may not cause problems or symptoms and may be observed.

Wound Leak

1. Large wound leaks: Suture the wound closed.

2. Small wound leaks: Can be sutured closed or can be patched with a pressure dressing and an antibiotic ointment (e.g., erythromycin) for 1 night to allow the wound to close spontaneously. A carbonic anhydrase inhibitor and a nonselective topical beta-blocker (e.g., acetazolamide 500 mg sequel p.o. and a drop of timolol 0.5%) are usually given if patching is to be used to reduce aqueous flow through the wound.

NOTE: Occasionally, cyanoacrylate glue is applied to small wound leaks and covered with a bandage contact lens.

---

3. Wound leaks under a conjunctival flap: Repair required only if vision affected or for secondary ocular complication such as a flat anterior chamber. Consider cryotherapy or argon laser therapy after painting the conjunctiva with methylene blue or rose bengal, or autologous blood injection.

Cyclodialysis Cleft

Reattach the ciliary body to the sclera by chronic atropine therapy, diathermy, suturing, cryotherapy, laser photocoagulation, external plombage. See 3.7, *Iridodialysis/Cyclodialysis*.

Scleral Perforation

The site may be closed by suturing or cryotherapy.

Iridocyclitis

Topical steroid (e.g., prednisolone acetate 1% q1–6h) and a topical cycloplegic (e.g., scopolamine 0.25% t.i.d.). See 12.1, *Anterior Uveitis (Iritis/Iridocyclitis)*.

Retinal Detachment

Surgical repair. See 11.3, *Retinal Detachment*.

Choroidal Detachment

See 11.27, *Choroidal Effusion/Detachment*. Surgical drainage of the choroidal effusion along with reformation of the eye and anterior chamber is indicated for any of the following:

1. Retinal apposition ("kissing" choroidal detachments).

2. Lens–corneal touch (needs emergency attention).

3. A flat or persistently shallow anterior chamber accompanied by a failing filtering bleb or an inflamed eye.

4. Corneal decompensation.

Pharmacologic

Reduce or discontinue the IOP-reducing medications.

Systemic Disorder

Refer to an internist.

NOTE: In myotonic dystrophy, the hypotony is rarely severe enough to produce deleterious effects, and treatment of hypotony, from an ocular standpoint, is unnecessary.

Follow-Up

If vision is good, the anterior chamber is well formed, and there is no wound leak, retinal detachment, or kissing choroidal detachments, then the low IOP poses no immediate problem, and treatment and follow-up are not urgent. Fixed retinal folds in the macula may develop from long-standing hypotony.

13.12 BLIND, PAINFUL EYE

A patient with a non-seeing eye and unsalvageable vision can experience mild to severe ocular pain for a variety of reasons.

Causes of Pain

▪ Corneal decompensation: Fluorescein-staining defect on slit-lamp examination. Improvement of pain with topical anesthetic.

▪ Uveitis: Anterior chamber or vitreous white blood cells. If the cornea is opaque, the cells might not be seen.

▪ Glaucoma with elevated IOP.

▪ Hypotony: Ciliary body shutdown, retinal detachment, choroidal detachment, ciliary body detachment. See 13.11, *Hypotony Syndrome*.

Work-Up

1. History: Determine the etiology and duration of the blindness.

2. Ocular examination: Stain the cornea with fluorescein to detect an epithelial defect and measure the IOP. Tono-Pen measurements may be required if the corneal surface is irregular. If the cornea is clear, look for neovascularization of the iris and angle by gonioscopy, and inspect the anterior chamber for cells and flare. Attempt a dilated retinal examination to rule out an intraocular tumor or retinal detachment.

3. B-scan US of the posterior segment is required to rule out an intraocular tumor, retinal detachment, or choroidal or ciliary body detachment, when the fundus cannot be adequately visualized.

Treatment

1. Sterile corneal decompensation (if it appears infected, see 4.11, *Bacterial Keratitis*).

   —Antibiotic ointment (e.g., erythromycin), cycloplegia (e.g., atropine 1%), and a pressure patch for 24 to 48 hours.

   —Antibiotic or lubricating ointment q.d. to q.i.d. (after the patch is removed) for weeks to months (or even permanently).

   —Consider nightly patching.

   —Consider a tarsorrhaphy, amniotic membrane graft, or Gunderson conjunctival flap in refractory cases.

2. Uveitis.

   —Cycloplegia (e.g., atropine 1% t.i.d.).

   —Topical steroid (e.g., prednisolone acetate 1% q1–6h).

   —Treat uveitis if it is present. See 12.1, *Anterior Uveitis (Iritis/Iridocyclitis)*.

13

—Endophthalmitis should be ruled out if severe uveitis or a hypopyon is present.

3. Markedly increased IOP.

—Topical beta-blocker (e.g., timolol 0.5% b.i.d.) with or without an adrenergic agonist (e.g., brimonidine 0.2% b.i.d. to t.i.d.). Topical carbonic anhydrase inhibitors (e.g., dorzolamide 2% t.i.d.) are effective, but potential systemic side effects may not warrant their use for pain relief; miotics may increase ocular irritation.

—If the IOP remains markedly increased and is thought to be responsible for the pain, a cyclodestructive procedure [e.g., yttrium-aluminum garnet (YAG) or diode laser cyclophotocoagulation or cyclocryotherapy] may be attempted. The potential for sympathetic ophthalmia must be considered.

—If pain persists despite the previously described treatment, a retrobulbar alcohol block may be given. This is typically effective for approximately 3 to 6 months. Technique: 2 to 3 mL of lidocaine is administered in the retrobulbar region. The needle is then held in place while the syringe of lidocaine is replaced with a 1-mL syringe containing 95% to 100% alcohol (some physicians use 50% alcohol). The contents of the alcohol syringe are then injected into the retrobulbar space through the needle. The syringes are again switched, so a small amount of lidocaine can rinse out the remaining alcohol. The retrobulbar needle is then withdrawn. Patients are warned that transient eyelid droop or swelling, limitation of eye movement, or anesthesia may result. Retrobulbar chlorpromazine (25 to 50 mg, using 25 mg/mL) or phenol can also be used. See Appendix 10, *Technique for Retrobulbar/Subtenon/Subconjunctival Injections.*

4. Hypotony.

a. Resolve causes of hypotony (e.g., repair wound leak, treat uveitis or ciliochoroidal detachment). If retinal detachment is found, repair could resolve hypotony.

5. Cause of pain unknown.

a. Cycloplegic (e.g., atropine 1% t.i.d.).

b. Topical steroid (e.g., prednisolone acetate 1% q1–6h).

c. Retrobulbar injections of neurolytic agents can be considered. See Appendix 10, *Technique for Retrobulbar/Subtenon/Subconjunctival Injections.*

6. Enucleation or evisceration: Patients with ocular pain refractory to topical or retrobulbar injections should be considered for enucleation or evisceration of the eye. Evisceration should not be performed if intraocular malignancy is suspected. Enucleation does not relieve facial paresthesias.

7. All patients should wear protective eye wear (e.g., polycarbonate lenses) at all times to prevent injury to the contralateral eye.

Follow-Up

Depends on the degree of pain and the clinical abnormalities present. Once the pain resolves, patients are reexamined every 6 to 12 months. B-scan US should be performed periodically (typically every 5 years) to rule out an intraocular tumor when the posterior pole cannot be visualized.

13

13.13   PHAKOMATOSES

NEUROFIBROMATOSIS: TYPE 1 (VON RECKLINGHAUSEN SYNDROME) AND TYPE 2

Criteria for Diagnosis

See Table 13.13.1.

NOTE: Lisch nodules (light brown nodules on the iris surface) are sensitive and specific for neurofibromatosis 1 and precede the development of cutaneous neurofibromas. Occur in most by age 10. Unusual in neurofibromatosis 2.

TABLE 13.13.1 Characteristics of Neurofibromatosis 1 and 2	
Neurofibromatosis 1	**Neurofibromatosis 2**
At least two of the following:	Either A or B:
1. At least six café au lait spots	A. Bilateral acoustic nerve masses (by computed
• 5 mm prepubertal or	tomography or magnetic resonance imaging) or
• 15 mm postpubertal	B. Affected first-degree relative and
2. Neurofibromas	1. Unilateral acoustic nerve mass or
• One plexiform neurofibroma or	2. At least two of the following:
• At least two of any other type	• Neurofibroma
3. Intertriginous freckling	• Meningioma
4. Optic nerve glioma	• Glioma
5. At least two Lisch nodules (iris hamartomas)	• Schwannoma
6. Distinctive osseous dysplasia (sphenoid or tibial)	• Juvenile posterior subcapsular cataract
7. Affected first-degree relative	
Inheritance: Autosomal dominant	Autosomal dominant
Gene location: Chromosome 17	Chromosome 22
Frequency: 1:4,000	1:50,000

Signs

(See Figures 13.13.1 and 13.13.2.)

NF1 Ocular. Glaucoma (associated with plexiform neuromas of the ipsilateral upper eyelid), pulsating proptosis or "Orphan Annie Sign" secondary to absence of the greater wing of the sphenoid bone with a herniated encephalocele, optic nerve gliomas, prominent corneal nerves, combined hamartoma of the retina and RPE, diffuse uveal thickening, orbital Schwannoma, choroidal hamartomas (e.g., ovoid bodies).

NF1 Systemic. See Table 13.13.1. Intracranial astrocytoma (glioma), slightly decreased IQ, pheochromocytoma, vertebral dysplasias, short stature, scoliosis, cardiovascular abnormalities, pituitary adenoma, medullary carcinoma of the thyroid, neurofibrosarcomas.

NF2 Ocular. Presenile PSC cataract, optic nerve sheath meningioma, oculomotor paresis.

NF2 Systemic. See Table 13.13.1.

Inheritance

Autosomal dominant. NF1: Chromosome 17; NF2: Chromosome 22.

Work-Up

1. Family history. Complete general and ophthalmic examination of patient and family members.

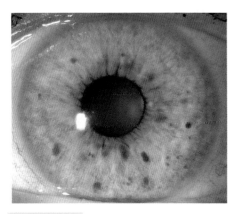

FIGURE 13.13.1. Lisch nodules.

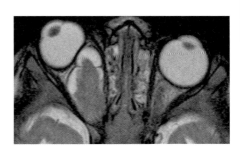

FIGURE 13.13.2. Optic nerve glioma.

13

2. MRI of the orbit and brain: Ophthalmic indications include orbital pain, proptosis, optic disc changes, decreased vision, visual field defect in NF1 or NF2. For NF2, a gadolinium-enhanced MRI of the brain and auditory canals should be performed for screening.

3. Others: Psychological testing, electroencephalography, and audiography.

Treatment/Follow-Up

Dependent upon the findings. Neonates with an eyelid plexiform neurofibroma should be seen more frequently because of a 50% risk of early glaucoma and risk of amblyopia.

STURGE–WEBER SYNDROME (ENCEPHALOFACIAL CAVERNOUS HEMANGIOMATOSIS)

Signs

(See Figure 13.13.3.)

Ocular. Diffuse choroidal hemangioma ("tomato catsup" fundus with uniform red background obscuring choroidal vasculature), unilateral glaucoma particularly with upper eyelid hemangioma, iris heterochromia, blood in the Schlemm canal (seen on gonioscopy), secondary serous retinal detachment, secondary RPE alterations (retinitis pigmentosa-like picture).

Systemic. Port-wine stain or nevus flammeus (congenital facial hemangioma in CN V_1 or V_2 distribution), subnormal intelligence or mental retardation, Jacksonian-type seizures, peripheral arteriovenous communications, facial hemihypertrophy ipsilateral to nevus flammeus, leptomeningeal angiomatosis, cerebral calcifications. *Klippel–Trenaunay–Weber syndrome* is an associated syndrome that involves limb hemihypertrophy, intracranial angiomas, varicosities, and cutaneous nevus flammeus.

Inheritance

Nonheritable.

Work-Up

Complete general and ophthalmic examinations with CT scan or MRI of the brain. Electroencephalography.

Treatment

1. Treat glaucoma if present. First-line drugs are aqueous suppressants. Latanoprost, pilocarpine, and epinephrine compounds are less effective because of high episcleral venous pressure. Surgery (goniotomy or trabeculectomy, or both) is often required. See 9.1, *Primary Open-Angle Glaucoma.*

2. Consider treating serous retinal detachments that threaten or involve the macula. Laser photocoagulation success rate is low. Low-dose radiotherapy often resolves the subretinal fluid. Photodynamic therapy is also successful for circumscribed tumors.

Follow-Up

Every 6 months or sooner for glaucoma screening and retinal examination.

TUBEROUS SCLEROSIS COMPLEX (BOURNEVILLE SYNDROME)

Signs

(See Figures 13.13.4 and 13.13.5.)

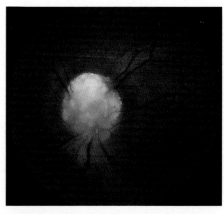

FIGURE 13.13.4. Retinal astrocytic hamartoma.

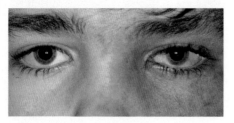

FIGURE 13.13.3. Nevus flammeus.

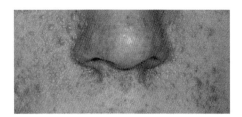

FIGURE 13.13.5. Adenoma sebaceum.

Ocular. Astrocytic hamartoma of the retina or optic disc (a white, semitransparent, or mulberry-appearing tumor in the superficial retina that may undergo calcification with age; no prominent feeder vessels, no associated retinal detachment; often multifocal and bilateral), punched-out chorioretinal depigmentation, iris abnormalities (e.g., atypical colobomas).

Systemic. Classic triad of adenoma sebaceum (yellow–red angiofibromas in a butterfly distribution on the upper cheeks), seizures (caused by CNS astrocytic hamartomas), and subnormal intelligence. Other findings include: subungual angiofibromas (yellow–red papules around and beneath the nails of the fingers or toes); shagreen patches; ash-leaf sign (depigmented macules on the skin); café au lait spots; renal angiomyolipoma; renal cell carcinoma; cardiac rhabdomyoma; spontaneous pneumothorax; cystic bone lesions; hamartomas of the liver, thyroid, pancreas, or testes.

Differential Diagnosis of Astrocytic Hamartoma

Retinoblastoma. See 8.1, *Leukocoria*.

Inheritance

Autosomal dominant with incomplete penetrance, though most cases occur as a sporadic mutation of the TSC1 gene on chromosome 9q34 or the TSC2 gene on chromosome 16p13.

Work-Up

1. Family history. Complete general physical and ophthalmic examinations of patient and family members in conjunction with an internist or pediatrician.

2. CBC and electrolytes. CT or MRI of the brain (calcified astrocytic hamartomas may be evident on CT). Electroencephalography, echocardiography, chest radiography, and abdominal CT scan.

Treatment/Follow-Up

Genetic counseling. Retinal astrocytomas usually require no treatment. Annual ophthalmic examinations.

VON HIPPEL–LINDAU SYNDROME (RETINOCEREBELLAR CAPILLARY HEMANGIOMATOSIS)

Signs

(See Figure 13.13.6.)

Critical. Retinal capillary hemangioma/hemangioblastoma (small, round, orange–red tumor with a prominent dilated feeding artery and draining vein), sometimes associated with subretinal exudates, subretinal fluid, and total retinal detachment. Bilateral in 50% of cases. Can produce macular traction and epiretinal membrane.

Systemic. CNS hemangioma (cerebellum and spinal cord most common, 25% of cases), renal cell carcinoma, renal cysts, pheochromocytoma, pancreatic cysts, epididymal cystadenoma.

Inheritance

Autosomal dominant. VHL gene on chromosome 3p25-p26.

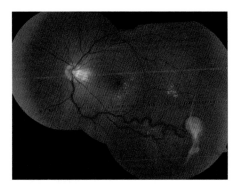

FIGURE 13.13.6. Retinal capillary hemangioma/hemangioblastoma.

13

Differential Diagnosis of Retinal Capillary Hemangioma

■ Coats disease: Aneurysmal dilation of blood vessels with prominent subretinal exudate and no identifiable tumor. See 8.1, *Leukocoria*.

■ Racemose hemangiomatosis: Large, dilated, tortuous vessels form arteriovenous communications void of intervening capillary beds without exudation or subretinal fluid.

■ Retinal cavernous hemangioma: Small vascular dilations around retinal vein without feeder vessels.

■ Retinal vasoproliferative tumor: Peripheral inferior retina usually in older patient. Feeder vessels can be slightly dilated and tortuous but not to the extent of capillary hemangioma.

■ Retinal macrovessel: Large, solitary, nontortuous vessel without arteriovenous connection that supplies or drains the macular area and crosses the horizontal raphe. More commonly veins than arteries.

■ Congenital retinal vascular tortuosity: Tortuous retinal vessels without racemose component.

■ Familial exudative vitreoretinopathy: Bilateral, temporal, peripheral exudation with retinal vascular abnormalities and traction. See 8.3, *Familial Exudative Vitreoretinopathy*.

Work-Up

Prompt referral to internist for systemic evaluation is indicated for all patients with retinal capillary hemangioma. Solitary tumors can occur without von Hippel–Lindau disease, but multiple or bilateral tumors are diagnostic of von Hippel–Lindau disease.

1. Family history. Complete general physical and ophthalmic examination of patient and family members.

2. CBC and electrolytes. Urine tests for levels of epinephrine and norepinephrine. MRI of the brain (visualizes the posterior fossa better than CT scan). Abdominal CT scan.

3. Intravenous fluorescein angiogram (IVFA) if treatment of the retinal capillary hemangioma is planned.

Treatment/Follow-Up

1. If retinal hemangioma is affecting or threatening vision, laser photocoagulation, cryotherapy, transpupillary thermotherapy, photodynamic therapy with verteporfin, or radiotherapy is indicated depending on size of tumor.

2. Genetic counseling. Systemic therapy, depending on findings. Follow-up every 3 to 6 months, depending on the extent of retinal involvement.

WYBURN–MASON SYNDROME (RACEMOSE HEMANGIOMATOSIS)

Signs

(See Figure 13.13.7.)

Ocular. Enormously dilated, tortuous retinal vessels with arteriovenous communications without communicating capillary beds and without mass or exudate. Rarely, proptosis from an orbital racemose hemangioma.

Systemic. Midbrain racemose hemangiomas, intracranial calcification, seizures, hemiparesis, mental changes, facial nevi, and ipsilateral pterygoid fossa, mandibular, and maxillary hemangiomas.

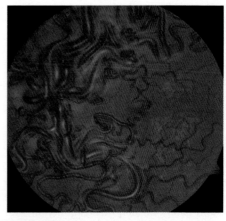

FIGURE 13.13.7. Racemose hemangioma.

Inheritence

Nonheritable.

Differential Diagnosis of Retinal Capillary Hemangioma

See von Hippel–Lindau syndrome above.

Work-Up

Complete general and ophthalmic examinations. MRI of the brain.

Treatment/Follow-Up

No treatment is indicated for retinal lesions. Complications include blindness and rarely intraocular hemorrhage, retinal vascular obstruction, and neovascular glaucoma. Warn of hemorrhage risk with ipsilateral dental and facial surgery. Annual follow-up.

ATAXIA-TELANGIECTASIA (LOUIS–BAR SYNDROME)

Signs

Ocular. Telangiectasias of the conjunctiva (delayed appearance, typically ages 3 to 5), oculomotor apraxia with supranuclear gaze palsies, nystagmus, and strabismus can be seen.

Systemic. Progressive cerebellar ataxia with gradual deterioration of motor function. Cutaneous telangiectases in a butterfly distribution. Recurrent sinopulmonary infections. Various immunologic abnormalities (e.g., IgA deficiency and T-cell dysfunction). High incidence of malignancy (mainly leukemia or lymphoma), mental retardation, seborrheic dermatitis, vitiligo, premature graying of the hair, testicular or ovarian atrophy, hypoplastic or atrophic thymus.

Inheritence

Autosomal recessive. ATM gene on chromosome 11q22.

Work-Up

1. Family history. Complete general and ophthalmic examinations of patient and family members.

2. CBC, urinalysis and urinary amino acids, immunoglobin panel. Chest radiography and MRI of the brain.

Treatment/Follow-Up

Genetic counseling. No specific ocular treatment. Annual follow-up.

13

14

Imaging Modalities in Ophthalmology

PLAIN FILMS

Description

Images of radiopaque tissues obtained by exposure of special photographic plates to ionizing radiation.

Uses in Ophthalmology

May be used to identify or exclude radiopaque intraorbital or intraocular foreign bodies. However, computed tomography (CT) is the study of choice to evaluate for foreign bodies, as CT has greater contrast sensitivity over radiography. Plain films remain a valid screening modality before magnetic resonance imaging (MRI) if an occult metallic foreign body is suspected. Plain films should not be used for the diagnosis of orbital fractures.

COMPUTED TOMOGRAPHY

Description

CT uses ionizing radiation and computer-assisted formatting to produce multiple cross-sectional planar images. Possible image planes include axial, direct coronal, reformatted coronal, and reformatted parasagittal images. Bone and soft-tissue windows should always be reviewed in both axial and coronal orientations (see Figures 14.2.1–14.2.3). Orbital studies use 3-mm or thinner slices. Radiopaque iodinated contrast allows more extensive evaluation of vascular structures and areas where there is a breakdown of the normal capillary endothelial barrier (as in inflammation).

Uses in Ophthalmology

1. Excellent for defining bone abnormalities such as fractures (orbital wall or optic canal), calcification, or bony involvement of a soft-tissue mass.

2. Locating suspected intraorbital or intraocular metallic foreign bodies. Glass, wood, and plastic are less radiopaque and therefore more difficult to isolate on CT.

3. Soft-tissue windows are good for determining some pathologic features, including orbital

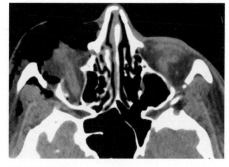

FIGURE 14.2.1. Axial soft-tissue window of inferior orbit shows abnormality, which is difficult to assess.

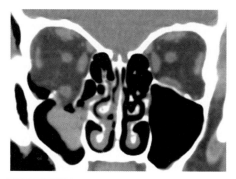

FIGURE 14.2.2. Coronal soft-tissue window shows a large blowout fracture of the orbital floor. This finding could have been missed on axial study, demonstrating the importance of reviewing both axial and coronal images.

cellulitis/abscess, noninfectious inflammation, and tumors. May be useful in determining posterior scleral rupture when clinical examination is inconclusive, but B-scan ultrasonography may be more sensitive.

4. Excellent for imaging paranasal sinus anatomy and disease.

5. Head CT helpful for locating parenchymal, subarachnoid, subdural, epidural, and retrobulbar hemorrhage in either acute or subacute setting.

6. Imaging modality of choice for thyroid-related orbitopathy. See 7.2.1, *Thyroid Eye Disease.*

7. Any loss of consciousness requires CT of the brain. CT of the brain does not provide

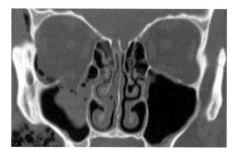

FIGURE 14.2.3. Coronal bone window shows the fracture again. In bone windows, the soft-tissue detail fades, but bone detail is enhanced, allowing for better examination of bony anatomy.

adequate detail of the orbital anatomy, and vice versa.

Guidelines for Ordering an Orbital Study

1. Always order a dedicated orbital study if ocular or orbital pathology is suspected. Always include views of paranasal sinuses and cavernous sinuses.

2. Order both axial and coronal views.

3. When evaluating traumatic optic neuropathy, request 1-mm cuts of the orbital apex and optic canal to rule out bony impingement of the optic nerve.

4. When attempting to localize ocular or orbital foreign bodies, order 1-mm cuts.

5. Contrast may be necessary for suspected infections or inflammatory conditions. Contrast is helpful in distinguishing orbital cellulitis from abscess. However, contrast is not mandatory to rule out orbital inflammation or postseptal involvement. Relative contraindications for contrast include renal failure, diabetes, congestive heart failure, myeloma, sickle cell disease, multiple severe allergies, and asthma. Check renal function in patients in whom renal insufficiency is suspected.

NOTE: The radiologist may recommend premedication with corticosteroids if contrast is required and a prior allergy is suspected. Follow the protocol recommended by your radiology department.

---

6. Obtain pregnancy test before obtaining CT scans in females of childbearing age if possible.

7. CT angiography (CTA) is helpful in diagnosing intracranial vascular pathology, including aneurysms. It is available on all multidetector CT scanners and in general is more sensitive than magnetic resonance angiography (MRA). However, it requires the use of intravenous iodinated contrast.

8. CT scans may be obtained in children with careful consideration of the risk of radiation

14

exposure versus benefits of performing the scan. Each CT scan exposes children to radiation with a cumulative risk over their lifetime. Radiation exposure from CT scans in children is of particular concern when serial imaging is required. In these cases, MRI is often a better choice for children, although sedation may be needed.

NOTE: Many radiology centers have pediatric protocols for CT scans that limit the amount of radiation exposure. If available, these should be considered when imaging children.

14.3 MAGNETIC RESONANCE IMAGING

Description

1. MRI uses a large magnetic field to excite protons of water molecules. The energy given off as the protons reequilibrate to their normal state is detected by specialized receivers (coils) and that information is reconstructed into a computer image.

2. Obtains multiplanar images without loss of resolution.

3. The basic principles of MRI are listed in Table 14.3.1. Figures 14.3.1 to 14.3.3 provide specific examples.

4. Contrast studies can be ordered using gadolinium, a well-tolerated non–iodine-based paramagnetic agent.

TABLE 14.3.1	Summary of MRI Sequences[a]			
	T1	**Fat Suppression**	**Gadolinium-DTPA[b]**	**T2**
Properties	Useful for intraorbital structures such as optic nerve, extraocular muscles, and orbital veins. The strong fat signal within the orbit gives poor resolution of lacrimal gland and may also mask intraocular structures.	T1-weighted images with bright intraconal fat signal suppressed in the orbit, allowing for better anatomic detail. Essential for all orbital MRIs.	A paramagnetic agent that distributes in the extracellular space and does not cross the intact blood–brain barrier. Gd-DTPA is best for T1, fat-suppressed images. The lacrimal gland and extraocular muscles "enhance" with Gd-DTPA. Essential for all orbital MRIs. Never order gadolinium without ordering fat suppression for orbital studies.	Suboptimal intraocular contrast. Demyelinating lesions (e.g., multiple sclerosis) are bright.
Interpretation	Fat is bright (high signal intensity). Vitreous and intracranial ventricles are dark.	Vitreous and fat are dark. Extraocular muscles are bright after Gd-DTPA is administered.	Most orbital masses are dark on T1 and become bright with gadolinium enhancement. Notable exceptions are listed in Table 14.3.2.	Fluid-containing structures such as vitreous and CSF are bright. Melanin is dark.

NOTE: Open MRI scanners cannot provide fat-suppressed images.
[a]Note: that high-flow areas create a dark area, "flow void," which is helpful in identifying arterial structures (e.g., carotid siphon within the cavernous sinus).
[b]Gd-DTPA is gadolinium-diethylenetriamine pentaacetic acid.

14

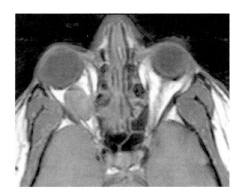

FIGURE 14.3.1. Axial T-1-weighted image without fat suppression or gadolinium. The vitreous is dark (hypointense) relative to the bright signal from fat. A well-circumscribed mass is clearly visible in the right orbit, also hypointense. Most orbital lesions are dark in T1 prior to gadolinium injection. The notable exceptions are listed in Table 14.3.2.

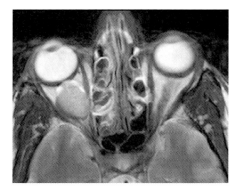

FIGURE 14.3.3. Axial T-2-weighted image. The vitreous is hyperintense (bright) relative to the orbital fat. The lesion is also bright but in some cases may be isointense with the surrounding fat.

Uses in Ophthalmology

1. Excellent for defining the extent of orbital/central nervous system masses. Signal-specific properties of certain pathology may be helpful in diagnosis (see Table 14.3.2).

2. Poor bone definition (e.g., fractures).

3. Excellent for diagnosing intracranial, cavernous sinus, and orbital apex lesions, many of which affect neuro-ophthalmic pathways.

4. For suspected neurogenic tumors (meningioma, glioma), gadolinium is essential in defining lesion extent.

5. All patients with clinical signs or symptomatic optic neuritis from suspected demyelinating disease should undergo brain MRI [fluid-attenuated inversion recovery (FLAIR) images are especially useful]. See Figure 14.3.4 and 10.14, *Optic Neuritis*.

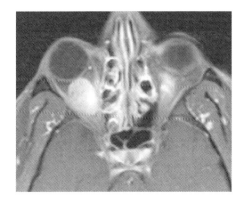

FIGURE 14.3.2. Axial T-1 image with fat suppression and gadolinium. Note how both the vitreous and fat are dark, but the extraocular muscles become bright. The orbital mass is now clearly visible. This technique should be performed in all orbital MRIs.

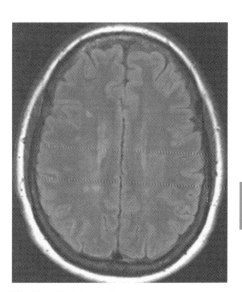

FIGURE 14.3.4. MRI with FLAIR sequence of demyelinating lesions in multiple sclerosis.

14

TABLE 14.3.2	Tissues/Lesions That Appear Bright (Hyperintense) Relative to Vitreous Before Gadolinium Injection
Tissues/Lesions	**Examples**
Fat	Lipoma, liposarcoma
Mucus/proteinaceous material	Dermoid cyst, mucocele, dacryocele, craniopharyngioma
Melanin	Melanoma
Subacute blood (3–14 days old)	Lymphangioma with blood cyst, hemorrhagic choroidal detachment
Certain fungal infections (iron scavengers)	Aspergillus

6. Fat suppression should always be used in conjunction with intravenous gadolinium to enhance the visualization of the underlying pathology (e.g., optic neuritis, fat-containing lesions).

7. Diffusion-weighted imaging can help differentiate the various phases of cerebral infarction (e.g., hyperacute, acute, subacute, and chronic).

Guidelines for Ordering the Study

1. For the vast majority of orbital studies, a head coil is indicated to provide bilateral orbital views extending to the optic chiasm.

2. Intravenous gadolinium is useful for augmenting ocular, orbital, and perineural masses. In patients who have kidney failure, nephrogenic systemic fibrosis is a rare complication of gadolinium that occurs weeks to months after administration. It is characterized by a thickening and hardening of the skin, especially over extremities and trunk. There is no known proven therapy. Evaluate renal function in patients in whom renal insufficiency is suspected.

3. Contraindications to MRI: Severe claustrophobia, marked obesity, cardiac pacemakers, some cardiac valves, suspected magnetic intraocular/intraorbital foreign bodies, spinal stimulators, vagal nerve stimulators, stapes implants, and specific breast and penile implants. Titanium plates and newer aneurysm clips are MRI safe as are gold weights placed in the eyelids. When in doubt, ask the radiologist to look up the specific device in an MRI safety catalog. Any patient with a poorly documented implanted device should NOT be scanned with MRI.

14.4   MAGNETIC RESONANCE ANGIOGRAPHY

14

Description

Special application of MRI technology in which signal from flowing blood is augmented while signal from stationary tissues is suppressed. MRA allows for three-dimensional rotational reconstruction.

Uses in Ophthalmology

1. Suspected carotid stenosis, occlusion, or dissection.

2. Suspected intracranial and orbital arterial aneurysms (e.g., pupil involving third cranial

nerve palsy), arteriovenous malformations, and acquired arteriovenous communications.

3. Suspected orbital or intracranial vascular mass. Note that MRA is best for imaging high-flow and large-caliber lesions. Lower-flow lesions (e.g., varix) are not well seen. MRA also has limited potential in visualizing cavernous sinus fistulas; color Doppler studies and conventional arteriography are more sensitive in making this diagnosis.

Guidelines for Ordering the Study

Cerebral arteriography remains the gold standard for diagnosis of vascular lesions but carries significant morbidity and mortality in certain populations. Currently, the limit of MRA is an aneurysm larger than 2 mm. However, the sensitivity is highly dependent on several factors: hardware, software, and the experience of the neuroradiologist. Despite these potential limitations, MRA remains a safe and sensitive screening test, especially when coupled with MRI for concomitant soft-tissue imaging. CTA in many situations can provide a suitable replacement for conventional angiography.

14.5　MAGNETIC RESONANCE VENOGRAPHY

Magnetic resonance venography is helpful in diagnosing venous thrombosis. MRI and magnetic resonance venography are an essential part of the workup of any patient presenting with bilateral optic disc swelling. See 10.15, *Papilledema*.

14.6　CEREBRAL ARTERIOGRAPHY

Description

This interventional examination entails intra-arterial injection of radiopaque contrast followed by rapid-sequence x-ray imaging of the region of interest to evaluate the transit of blood through the regional vasculature. Unlike MRA or CTA, catheter arteriography allows the option of simultaneous treatment of lesions by intravascular techniques. Arteriography is the gold standard for diagnosing intracranial aneurysms but is being replaced in many centers by CTA.

Uses in Ophthalmology

1. Suspected arteriovenous malformations, carotid cavernous fistulas, cavernous sinus fistula, and vascular masses (e.g., hemangioma, varix).

2. Evaluation of ocular ischemic syndrome or amaurosis fugax due to suspected atherosclerotic carotid, aortic arch, or ophthalmic artery occlusive disease. Usually carotid Doppler US, MRA, or CTA is adequate for diagnosis.

NOTE: Conventional arteriography is contraindicated in patients with suspected carotid artery dissection (catheter placement may propagate the dissection).

14

14.7 NUCLEAR MEDICINE

Description

Nuclear medicine imaging uses radioactive contrast (radionuclide) that emits gamma radiation, which is then gathered by a gamma ray detector. The classic types of radionuclide scanning known to ophthalmologists include bone scanning, liver–spleen scanning, and gallium scanning. Positron emission tomography (PET) is useful in determining metabolic activity within a lesion and may be coupled with CT for anatomic detail.

Uses in Ophthalmology

1. Scintigraphy (e.g., with technetium-99): Useful for assessing lacrimal drainage physiology in patients with contradictory or inconsistent irrigation testing.

2. Systemic gallium scan: Useful for detecting extraocular sarcoidosis and Sjogren syndrome.

3. Technetium 99m-tagged red blood cell study: Occasionally used to distinguish cavernous hemangioma/hemangiopericytoma from other solid masses in the orbit.

4. PET: The use of PET for the diagnosis and management of orbital disease is still an evolving technique. Limitations in this area include the high background metabolic activity of the adjacent brain which may mask orbital abnormalities, the size of the orbital pathology (current PET scanners have a resolution of about 7 mm), and the relatively indolent nature of most orbital lymphomas (decreasing the intensity of the signal on PET). PET is extremely useful in the diagnosis and surveillance of systemic pathologies, including lymphoma and metastases, and at present, this remains the primary role of PET in the management of orbital disease.

14.8 OPHTHALMIC ULTRASONOGRAPHY

A-SCAN

Description

(See Figure 14.8.1.)

A-scan, or amplitude-modulated ultrasound (US), uses ultrasonic waves (8 to 12 MHz) to generate linear distance versus amplitude of reflectivity curves of the evaluated ocular and orbital tissues. A-scans are one dimensional and used for measuring and characterizing the composition of tissues on the basis of the reflectivity curves. Not all A-scan instruments are standardized.

Uses in Ophthalmology

1. Primary use in ophthalmology is measurement of axial length of the globe. This information is critical for intraocular lens (IOL) power calculations for cataract surgery. Axial length information can also be used to identify certain congenital disorders such as microphthalmia, nanophthalmos, intraocular tumor size, intrinsic tumor vascularity, and congenital glaucoma.

2. Diagnostic identification of the echogenicity characteristics of masses in the globe or orbit with standardized A-scan probe.

3. Specialized A-mode ultrasonography can be used for corneal pachymetry (measurement of corneal thickness).

Guidelines for Ordering the Study

1. When used for IOL power calculations, make sure to check both eyes. The two eyes should be within 0.2 mm of each other.

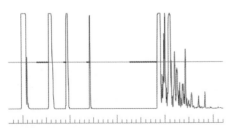

FIGURE 14.8.1.   Normal A-scan US.

14

2. Spikes along the baseline should be sharply rising at 90 degrees.

3. If needed, keratometry readings should be obtained prior to scan or 30 minutes after the scan for accurate results.

B-SCAN

Description

(See Figure 14.8.2.)

B-scan, or brightness-modulated US, gives real-time, two-dimensional (cross-sectional) images of the eye posterior to the iris to the posterior aspect of the globe. Both contact and water-bath techniques may be used, but the contact method does not visualize the anterior chamber well.

Uses in Ophthalmology

1. Define ocular anatomy in the presence of media opacities (e.g., mature cataract, hyphema, corneal opacity, vitreous hemorrhage, trauma) to evaluate retinal and/or choroidal pathology.

2. Diagnosis of scleral rupture posterior to the muscle insertions or when media opacities prevent direct visualization.

3. Identify intraocular foreign bodies especially if made of metal or glass (spherical objects have a specific echo shadow); wood or vegetable matter has variable echogenicity; can also give a more precise location if the foreign body is next to the scleral wall.

4. Evaluation of intraocular tumor/mass consistency, retinal detachment, choroidal detachment (serous vs. hemorrhagic), and optic disc abnormalities (e.g., optic disc drusen, coloboma).

Guidelines for Ordering the Study

1. If used in the setting of trauma to determine unknown scleral rupture, the probe is used over closed eyelids with immersion in copious amounts of sterile methylcellulose, such that no pressure is placed on the globe. The gain must be set higher to overcome the sound attenuation of the eyelids. Known ruptured globe is a relative contraindication to B-scan US.

2. When scleral integrity is not in question, B-scan US should be performed dynamically to help differentiate pathologic conditions, such as retinal detachment versus posterior vitreous detachment.

3. Dense intraocular calcifications (such as those occurring in many eyes with phthisis bulbi) result in poor-quality images.

4. Silicone oil and intraocular gas in the vitreous cause distortion of the scanned image, and therefore the study should be performed in an upright patient.

ULTRASONOGRAPHIC BIOMICROSCOPY

Description

(See Figure 14.8.3.)

Uses ultra–high-frequency (50 MHz) B-mode US of the anterior one-fifth of the globe to give cross sections at near-microscopic resolution. Uses a water-bath eyelid speculum with viscous liquid in the bowl of the speculum.

Uses in Ophthalmology

1. Excellent for defining corneoscleral or limbal pathologic conditions, anterior chamber angle, ciliary body, pathologic iris conditions (e.g., ciliary body masses/cysts, plateau iris, location of IOL), and small anterior foreign bodies.

2. Unexplained unilateral angle narrowing or closure.

3. Suspected cyclodialysis.

Guidelines for Ordering the Study

Known ruptured globe is a contraindication to the study.

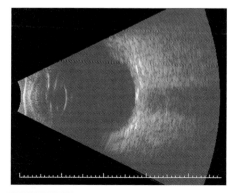

FIGURE 14.8.2. Normal B-scan US.

14

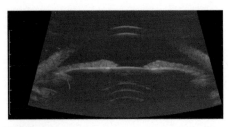

FIGURE 14.8.3. Normal anterior ultrasonographic biomicroscopy.

ORBITAL ULTRASONOGRAPHY/DOPPLER

Description

Uses B-mode US coupled with Doppler technology to visualize flow in the vessels in the orbit.

Uses in Ophthalmology

1. Superior ophthalmic vein pathology: High-flow cavernous sinus fistulas, superior ophthalmic vein thrombosis.

2. Orbital varix.

3. Arteriovenous malformations.

4. Vascular disease including central retinal artery occlusion, central retinal vein occlusion, ocular ischemic syndrome, and giant cell arteritis.

14.9 PHOTOGRAPHIC STUDIES

Description

Various methods of imaging the eyes or selected regions of the eye, using white light or various spectral wavelengths of light.

Types of Ophthalmic Photographic Imaging Studies

1. Documentary photography: Color pictures of face, external eye, anterior segment, and fundus (white light or red-free lighting) (see Figure 14.9.1).

2. Fundus autofluorescence (FAF): Imaging modality that takes advantage of the naturally and pathologically occurring fluorophores in the fundus. Provides sensitive information regarding the health of the retinal pigment epithelium and allows early detection and monitoring of a variety of conditions such as AMD, macular dystrophies, and medication toxicity. Addtionally, FAF is useful in the evaluation of certain ocular tumors, specifically, choroidal nevi and melanomas (see Figure 14.9.2).

3. Specular microscopy: Contact and noncontact photographic techniques used to image the corneal endothelium. The images can then be used to evaluate the quality and quantity of the endothelial cells.

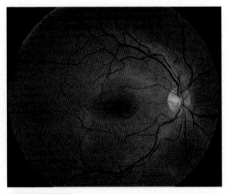

FIGURE 14.9.1. Normal fundus photograph.

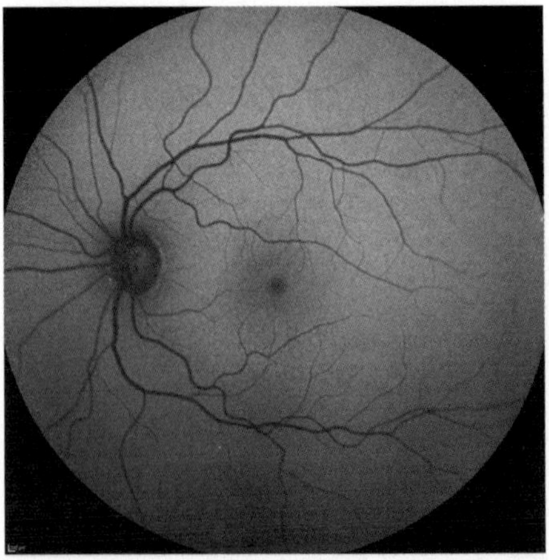

FIGURE 14.9.2. Normal fundus autofluorescence.

14

14.10 INTRAVENOUS FLUORESCEIN ANGIOGRAPHY

Description

(See Figure 14.10.1.)

Intravenous fluorescein angiography is a type of angiographic photography that does not rely on ionizing radiation or iodine-based contrast. After intravenous injection of fluorescein solution (usually in a hand or arm vein), rapid-sequence photography is performed by using a camera with spectral excitation and barrier filters. Fluorescein sodium absorbs blue light, with peak absorption and excitation occurring at wavelengths of 465 to 490 nm. Fluorescence then occurs at the yellow-green wavelengths of 520 to 530 nm. The fluorescein molecule is 80% protein-bound and does not pass through the tight junctions of a healthy blood–retinal barrier (pigment epithelium and retinal capillaries are impermeable, whereas Bruch membrane and choriocapillaris lack tight junctions and are freely permeable).

Phases of the Intravenous Fluorescein Angiography

1. Choroidal filling (background fluorescence): 8 to 15 seconds after injection. Choroid is normally completely filled within 5 seconds after dye appearance within it.

2. Arterial phase: Starts 1 to 2 seconds after choroidal filling.

3. Arteriovenous phase (laminar flow).

4. Venous phase: Arteriovenous transit time is the time from the first appearance of dye within the retinal arteries of the temporal arcade until the corresponding veins are completely filled; normal, <11 seconds.

5. Recirculation phase: 45 to 60 seconds after arterial phase.

6. Late phase: 10 to 30 minutes post-injection.

Foveal dark spot can result from xanthophyll pigment in the outer plexiform layer or tall retinal pigment epithelium (RPE) cells with increased melanin or lipofuscin. The foveal avascular zone is the central area which has no retinal capillaries (300 to 500 microns in diameter).

Describing an Abnormal Study

Hyperfluorescence

1. Leakage: Fluorescein penetrates the blood–retinal barrier and accumulates sub-, intra-, or preretinally. Hyperfluorescence increases in size and brightness as study progresses [e.g., choroidal or retinal neovascularization, central serous chorioretinopathy (CSCR), cystoid macular edema (CME)].

2. Staining: Fluorescence gradually increases in brightness but its borders remain fixed (e.g., scar or scleral show).

3. Pooling: Accumulation of fluorescein in fluid-filled space in retina or choroid. The margins of the space trapping fluorescein are distinct [e.g., pigment epithelial detachment (PED), CSCR].

4. Window or transmission defect. Focal area of hyperfluorescence without leakage usually due to RPE atrophy (e.g., geographic atrophy, RPE rip, laser scar).

5. Autofluorescence: Structures that naturally fluoresce can be captured on film prior to intravenous fluorescein injection (e.g., optic nerve drusen and lipofuscin).

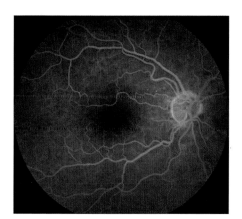

FIGURE 14.10.1. Normal intravenous fluorescein angiography.

14

Hypofluorescence

1. Blockage: Due to optical density such as blood, pigment, or fibrous tissue interposed between the camera and the choriocapillaris.

2. Vascular occlusion: Nonfilling vessel(s) causing relative or absolute hypofluorescence (e.g., central retinal artery occlusion). Applies to both capillaries and larger vessels.

Uses in Ophthalmology

1. Used to image retinal, choroidal, optic disc, iris vasculature, or a combination of these. It is used for diagnosis and therapeutic planning (e.g., retinal lasers).

2. Transit times between injection and appearance of dye in the choroid, retinal arteries, and veins also can be used to evaluate vascular flow. Arm to retina time is less accurate than intraretinal circulation.

3. Suspected retinal ischemia (capillary nonperfusion) and neovascularization from various conditions (e.g., diabetes).

4. Suspected choroidal neovascularization (CNV) from various diseases (e.g., age-related macular degeneration).

Guidelines for Ordering the Study

1. Side effects of intravenous fluorescein are nausea (10%), vomiting (2%), hives, pruritus, and vasovagal response. True anaphylaxis is rare. Death may occur in 1 out of 220,000 injections. Extravasation into extracellular space at the injection site can produce local necrosis. Treat with cool compresses. Excreted in urine in 24 to 36 hours. Urine will be bright yellow.

2. Because it is a photographic method, moderately clear media is required for visualization.

14.11 INDOCYANINE GREEN ANGIOGRAPHY

Description

Photographic method of ocular angiography similar to intravenous fluorescein angiography utilizing tricarbocyanine dye, an iodine-based dye. Indocyanine green (ICG) angiography differs in that fluorescence occurs in the infrared spectrum (835 nm), allowing for penetration through pigment, fluid, and blood. ICG provides better evaluation of the choroidal vasculature. ICG excitation occurs at 805 nm, with fluorescence at 835 nm. The ICG molecule is approximately 95% protein-bound.

Uses in Ophthalmology

1. Suspected occult CNV.

2. Suspected recurrent CNV after prior treatment.

3. Suspected CNV with retinal pigment epithelial detachment.

4. Suspected polypoidal choroidal vasculopathy. See 11.18, *Idiopathic Polypoidal Choroidal Vasculopathy (Posterior Uveal Bleeding Syndrome)*.

5. Other accepted uses: Identifying feeder vessels in retinal angiomatous proliferation lesions in age-related macular degeneration, chronic CSCR, certain inflammatory conditions, and occasionally helpful in diagnosing certain posterior-segment tumors).

Guidelines for Ordering the Study

1. Contraindicated in patients with iodine or shellfish allergies.

2. Most common side effect of ICG dye administration is a vasovagal response.

3. Excreted by hepatic parenchymal cells via bile.

14

14.12 OPTICAL COHERENCE TOMOGRAPHY

Description

(See Figure 14.12.1.)

Optical coherence tomography (OCT) provides noninvasive, noncontact two- or three-dimensional images by measuring optical reflections of light. In this manner, OCT is similar to US except that OCT is based on the reflection of light, not sound. The OCT scanner sends low-coherence light (820-nm wavelength) emitted by a superluminescent diode to the tissue to be examined and to a reference beam. The time delays of the light reflections from retinal structures are recorded by an interferometer. Using a reference mirror, these light reflections are then translated into an imaged object with a high resolution of up to 3 microns. The most highly reflective structures are the nerve fiber layer and the RPE. Highly reflective lesions include dense pigmentation, scar tissue, neovascularization, and hard exudates. Low-reflectivity in pathologic conditions include areas of edema.

Enhanced depth imaging OCT is a technique used to improve the detail of the choroid.

Uses in Ophthalmology

1. Retinal diseases including macular edema, macular atrophy, CSCR, age-related macular degeneration, CNV, CME, retinal detachment, PED, retinal tumors, drusen, and hard exudates.

2. Vitreoretinal interface abnormalities including macular holes, cysts, epiretinal membranes, and vitreoretinal strands or traction.

3. Suspected glaucoma, including quantification of the nerve fiber layer thickness and optic nerve cup characteristics.

4. Suspected optic neuritis, other optic neuropathies, and multiple sclerosis.

5. Anterior-segment pathology.

Guidelines for Ordering the Study

Requires patient's ability to fixate and relatively clear media.

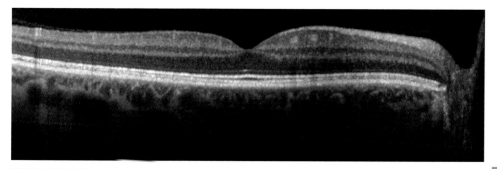

FIGURE 14.12.1. Normal optical coherence tomography.

14

14.13   CONFOCAL SCANNING LASER OPHTHALMOSCOPY

Description

Confocal scanning laser ophthalmoscopy is a noninvasive imaging technique to obtain high-resolution optical images and evaluate the topography of ocular structures. This confocal optical system provides a contour map of the desired structure in a process known as "optical sectioning." The system aims to detect reflected light from a very thin optical plane, the focal plane. A series of "focal planes" or images may be recorded and combined to create a three-dimensional image (e.g., Heidelberg retinal tomography).

Uses in Ophthalmology

1. Suspected optic nerve disease, including glaucoma and papilledema.

2. Suspected fundus elevations, including macular edema and choroidal nevi.

Guidelines for Ordering the Study

1. Requires patient's ability to fixate and relatively clear media.

2. Because the hallmark of the test is to provide comparative data, subsequent tests in the same patient need accurate alignment in the same focal plane to provide useful information.

14.14   CONFOCAL BIOMICROSCOPY

Description

The confocal microscope optically sections the cornea to noninvasively obtain structural and functional information of the different corneal layers.

Uses in Ophthalmology

The high level of detail available may be helpful in the detection of corneal microorganisms such as *Acanthamoeba* and fungi. It may also permit visualization of noninfectious changes seen in corneal dystrophies, iridocorneal endothelial syndrome, and epithelial downgrowth.

14.15   CORNEAL TOPOGRAPHY AND TOMOGRAPHY

14

Description

Standard keratometry measures the radius of corneal curvature and then converts the radius into dioptric corneal power. Computerized corneal topography is performed using various methods, including Placido disc analysis, scanning slit beam, and rasterstereography. These techniques project an image onto the cornea, most commonly a series of concentric rings, and analyze the reflection to determine corneal shape. They can provide information on anterior (and in some cases posterior) corneal curvature and regularity. Simulated keratometry readings can be generated and represented in graphical formats, such as a sagittal map.

Corneal tomography, the computerized reconstruction of multiple images of cornea, may help give detailed information about the anterior, posterior, and central cornea. These techniques include anterior-segment OCT, scanning slit, and rotating Scheimpflug photography–based systems. Scanning slit and rotating Scheimpflug imaging are particularly helpful in imaging posterior corneal elevation and anterior-segment anatomy. All tomographic systems also measure corneal thickness.

Uses in Ophthalmology

Detecting irregular astigmatism secondary to keratoconus, pellucid marginal degeneration, corneal surgery, corneal trauma, contact lens warpage, inherited corneal dystrophies, and corneal scars from inflammatory or infectious etiologies. It may be helpful in identifying the cause of decreased vision in patients with no known cause. It is useful for refractive surgical screening and imaging the post-keratorefractive cornea.

14.16   DACRYOCYSTOGRAPHY

Description

Dacryocystography utilizes special application of plain film or CT imaging to image the nasolacrimal drainage system after injection of radiopaque contrast into the system.

Uses in Ophthalmology

1. Suspected nasolacrimal drainage obstruction.

2. May be used for defining lacrimal drainage system anatomy when the cause of obstruction is maldevelopment, tumor, or even lacrimal stones with visualization of bony landmarks.

3. May be helpful in determining lacrimal pump function.

14

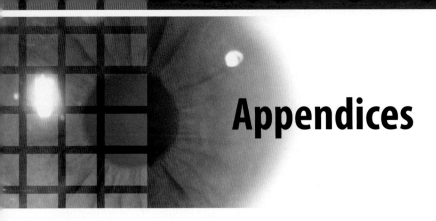

Appendices

DILATING DROPS

MYDRIATIC AND CYCLOPLEGIC AGENTS

	Approximate Maximal Effect	Approximate Duration of Action
Mydriatic agent		
Phenylephrine, 2.5%, 10%	20 min	3 h
Cycloplegic/mydriatic agents		
Tropicamide, 0.5%, 1%	20–30 min	3–6 h
Cyclopentolate, 0.5%, 1%, 2%	20–45 min	24 h
Homatropine, 2%, 5%	20–90 min	2–3 days
Scopolamine, 0.25%	20–45 min	4–7 days
Atropine, 0.5%, 1%, 2%	30–40 min	1–2 wk

The usual regimen for a dilated examination is:

- Adults: Phenylephrine, 2.5%, and tropicamide, 1%. Repeat these drops in 15 to 30 minutes if the eye is not dilated.

- Children: Phenylephrine, 2.5%, tropicamide, 1%, and cyclopentolate, 1% to 2%. Repeat these drops in 25 to 35 minutes if the eye is not dilated.

- Infants: Phenylephrine, 1%, and tropicamide, 0.2%. Homatropine, 2%, or cyclopentolate, 0.5% (usually reserved for infants older than 1 to 2 months of age) may also be used. The drops can be repeated in 35 to 45 minutes if the eye is not dilated.

NOTE:

1. Dilating drops are contraindicated in most types of angle-closure glaucoma and in eyes with severely narrow anterior-chamber angles.

2. Dilating drops tend to be less effective at the same concentration in darkly pigmented eyes.

APP

APPENDIX 2 — TETANUS PROPHYLAXIS

History of Tetanus Immunization (doses)	Clean Minor Wounds		All Other Wounds	
	Tetanus Toxoid	Immune Globulin	Tetanus Toxoid	Immune Globulin
Uncertain	Yes	No	Yes	Yes
0–1	Yes	No	Yes	Yes
2	Yes	No	Yes	No (a)
3 or more	No (b)	No	No (c)	No

Dose of tetanus toxoid is 0.5 mL intramuscularly.

(a) Unless wound is >24 hours old.

(b) Unless > 10 years since last dose.

(c) Unless >5 years since last dose.

APPENDIX 3 — COVER/UNCOVER AND ALTERNATE COVER TESTS

COVER/UNCOVER TEST

The primary purpose is to detect a tropia (a deviation when both eyes are open) and/or a phoria (a latent deviation that manifests when binocular fusion is disrupted).

Requirements

Full range of ocular motility, vision adequate to see the target of fixation, foveal fixation in each eye, and patient cooperation. This test should be performed before the alternate cover test (see below).

Method

1. Ask the patient to fixate on a non-accommodative target at distance (e.g., a letter on the vision chart).

2. Cover one of the patient's eyes while observing the uncovered eye. A refixation movement of the uncovered eye indicates the presence of a manifest deviation (tropia). Prisms may be used to quantify this. In the absence of a tropia, deviation of the covered eye that refixates when the cover is removed indicates a latent deviation (phoria).

3. Repeat the procedure, covering the opposite eye.

4. If there is no movement of either eye, the eyes are aligned with both eyes open (no tropia).

5. Ask the patient to fixate on an accommodative target at near. Both eyes are tested at near in the manner described previously.

NOTE: An esodeviation is detected by a refixation movement temporally (the eye being observed turns away from the nose). An exodeviation is detected by a refixation movement nasally (the eye being observed turns toward the nose). A hyperdeviation is detected by a refixation movement inferiorly.

APP

ALTERNATE COVER TEST

When it has been determined by the cover/ uncover test if there is a tropia or phoria, the alternate cover test may be use to dissociate the two eyes and further quantify the total deviation. The alternate cover test does not distinguish manifest from latent deviations.

Requirements

Same as for the cover/uncover test above.

Method

1. Ask the patient to fixate on a non-accommodative target at distance. To make certain that he or she is fixing on the target, ask that the letters be read or the picture described.

2. Repeatedly cover one eye and then quickly move the cover to the other eye. The eye being uncovered may be noted to swing into position to refixate on the target, indicating the presence of a deviation. Then repeat the test at near.

ALTERNATE COVER TEST WITH PRISM

Measures the size of the total deviation, regardless of whether a phoria or tropia is present.

Method

1. To measure a deviation, prisms are placed in front of one eye with the prism base placed in the direction of eye movement. While continuing to alternately cover, as described above, increase the prism strength until eye movement ceases. The strength of the weakest prism that eliminates eye movement during the alternate cover is the amount of the deviation.

2. Measurements may be done for any direction of gaze by turning the patient's head away from the target while asking him or her to maintain fixation on it (e.g., right gaze is measured by turning the patient's head toward his or her left shoulder and asking the patient to look at the target).

3. In general, measurements are taken in the straight-ahead position (both at distance and near), in right gaze, left gaze, downgaze (the head is tilted up while the patient focuses on the target), upgaze (the head is tilted down while the patient focuses on the target), and with the patient's head tilted toward either shoulder. Measurements are taken both with and without glasses in the straight-ahead position.

APPENDIX 4 — AMSLER GRID

Used to test macular function or to detect a central or paracentral scotoma.

1. Have the patient wear his or her glasses and occlude the left eye while an Amsler grid is held approximately 12 inches in front of the right eye (Figure A.4.1).

2. The patient is asked what is in the center of the page. Failure to see the central dot may indicate a central scotoma.

3. Have the patient fixate on the central dot (or the center of the page if he or she cannot see the dot). Ask if all four corners of the diagram are visible and if any of the boxes are missing.

4. Again, while staring at the central dot, ask the patient if all of the lines are straight and continuous or if some are distorted and broken.

5. The patient is asked to outline any missing or distorted areas on the grid with a pencil.

6. Repeat the procedure, covering the right eye and testing the left.

NOTE:

1. It is very important to monitor the patient's eye for movement away from the central dot.

2. A red Amsler grid may define more subtle defects.

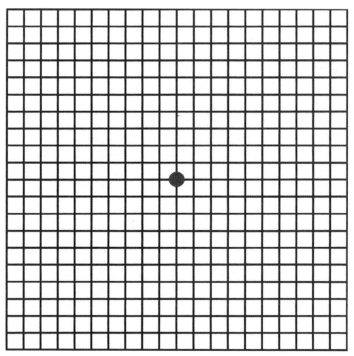

FIGURE A.4.1. Amsler grid.

SEIDEL TEST TO DETECT A WOUND LEAK

Concentrated fluorescein dye (from a moistened fluorescein strip) is applied directly over the potential site of perforation while observing the site with the slit lamp (Figure A.5.1). If a perforation and leak exist, the fluorescein dye is diluted by the aqueous and appears as a green (dilute) stream within the dark orange (concentrated) dye. The stream of aqueous is best seen with the cobalt blue light of the slit lamp.

FORCED-DUCTION TEST AND ACTIVE FORCE GENERATION TEST

Forced-Duction Test (Figure A.6.1)

This test distinguishes restrictive causes of decreased ocular motility from other motility disorders. One technique is the following:

1. Place a drop of topical anesthetic (e.g., proparacaine) into the eye.

2. Apply viscous lidocaine to further anesthetize the eye.

APP

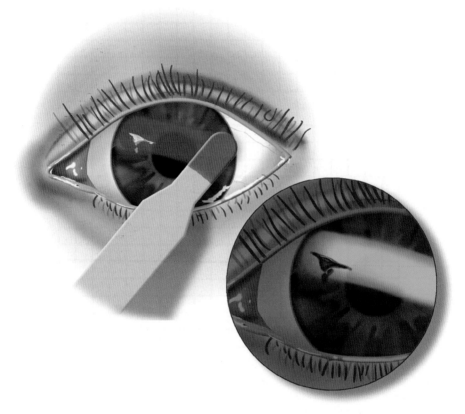

FIGURE A.5.1.   Seidel test.

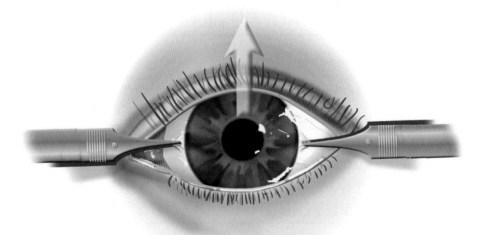

FIGURE A.6.1.   Forced-duction test.

3. Use toothed forceps (e.g., Graefe fixation forceps) to firmly grasp Tenon's close to the limbus at both locations perpendicular to the desired direction of movement. Doing so helps prevent corneal abrasions should the forceps slip. Rotate the eye in the "paretic" direction. If there is resistance to passive rotation of the eye, a restrictive disorder is diagnosed. This test does not require the patient to be conscious.

Active Force Generation Test

The patient is asked to look in the "paretic" direction while a sterile cotton swab is held just beneath the limbus on that same side. The amount of force generated by the "paretic" muscle is compared with that generated in the normal contralateral eye. The test can only be used in a cooperative, alert patient.

APPENDIX 7

TECHNIQUE FOR DIAGNOSTIC PROBING AND IRRIGATION OF THE LACRIMAL SYSTEM

1. Anesthetize the eye with a drop of topical anesthetic (e.g., proparacaine) and hold a cotton-tipped applicator soaked in the topical anesthetic on the involved punctum for several minutes.

2. Dilate the punctum with a punctum dilator (Figure A.7.1).

3. Gently insert a #00 Bowman probe into the punctum 2 mm vertically, and then 8 mm horizontally, toward the nose. Avoid using smaller probes, as they can create a false passage. Pull the involved eyelid laterally while slowly moving the probe horizontally to facilitate the procedure and to avoid creating a false passageway.

4. In the presence of an eyelid laceration, a torn canaliculus may be diagnosed by the appearance of the probe in the site of the eyelid laceration. See 3.8, *Eyelid Laceration*.

5. Irrigation of the lacrimal system is performed after removing the probe and inserting an irrigation cannula in the same manner in which the probe was inserted. Warn the patient before irrigation to expect a gag reflex. Two to 3 mL of saline is gently pushed into the system. Leakage through a torn eyelid also diagnoses a severed canaliculus. Resistance to injection of the saline, ballooning of the lacrimal sac, or leakage of the saline out of either punctum may be the result of a lacrimal system obstruction. If soft-tissue edema occurs during irrigation, stop immediately—a false passage may have been created. A patent lacrimal system usually drains into the throat quite readily, and the arrival of saline may be noted by the patient. Stop irrigating as soon as the patient tastes the fluid.

NOTE: If only evaluating the patency of the lacrimal system, and not ruling out a laceration, the system can be irrigated immediately after punctum dilation.

APPENDIX 8

CORNEAL CULTURE PROCEDURE

Indications

Small (<1 mm) infiltrates may be treated empirically with intensive commercially available broad-spectrum antibiotics without prior scraping. We routinely culture infiltrates larger than 1 to 2 mm, in the visual axis, unresponsive to initial treatment, or if we suspect an unusual organism based on history or examination. See 4.11, *Bacterial Keratitis*.

APP

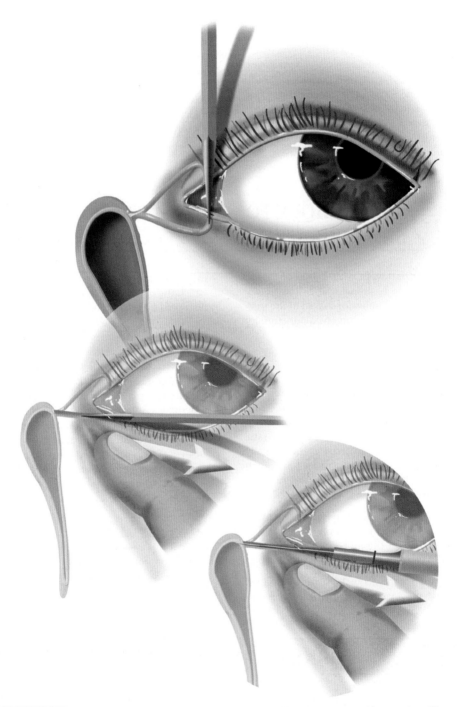

APP

FIGURE A.7.1.   Probing and irrigation: After anesthetizing the eye, dilate the punctum with a punctum dilator. Insert the dilator 2 mm vertically. Pull the eyelid laterally. Rotate the dilator 90 degrees and continue to advance it horizontally. Using a similar insertion technique, advance the irrigation cannula.

Equipment

Slit lamp; sterile Kimura spatula, knife blade, or moistened calcium alginate swab (e.g., with sterile saline, or thioglycolate or trypticase soy broth); culture media; microscopy slides; alcohol lamp.

Procedure

1. Anesthetize the cornea with topical drops. Proparacaine is best because it appears to be less bactericidal than others.

2. At the slit lamp, scrape the ulcer base (unless significant corneal thinning has occurred) and the leading edge of the infiltrate firmly with the spatula, blade, or swab. Place the specimens on the slides first, then the culture media. Sterilize the spatula over the flame of the alcohol lamp between each separate culture or slide. Be certain that the spatula tip temperature has returned to normal before touching the cornea again.

Media

Routine:

1. Blood agar (most bacteria).

2. Sabouraud dextrose agar without cyclo-heximide; place at room temperature (fungi).

3. Thioglycolate broth (aerobic and anaerobic bacteria).

4. Chocolate agar; place into a CO_2 jar (Haemophilus species, *Neisseria gonorrhoeae*).

Optional:

1. Löwenstein–Jensen medium (mycobacteria, Nocardia species) should be included in patients with a history of LASIK or an atypical ulcer appearance.

2. Nonnutrient agar with *Escherichia coli* overlay if available (Acanthamoeba).

Slides

Routine:

1. Gram stain (bacteria, fungi).

2. Calcofluor white; a fluorescent microscope is needed (Acanthamoeba, fungi).

Optional:

1. Giemsa stain (bacteria, fungi, Acanthamoeba).

2. Acid-fast stain (mycobacteria, Nocardia species).

3. Gomori methenamine silver stain, periodic acid–Schiff (PAS) stain (Acanthamoeba, fungi).

4. KOH wet mount (fungi, Nocardia species, Acanthamoeba).

5. Extra slide to send to pathology at a local institution.

NOTE: When a fungal infection is suspected, deep scrapings into the base of the ulcer are essential. Sometimes a corneal biopsy is necessary to obtain diagnostic information for fungal, atypical mycobacterial, and Acanthamoeba infections.

APPENDIX 9

FORTIFIED TOPICAL ANTIBIOTICS/ ANTIFUNGALS

Fortified Bacitracin (10,000 U/mL)

Add enough sterile water (without preservative) to 50,000 U bacitracin dry powder to form 5 mL of solution. This provides a concentration of 10,000 U/mL. Refrigerate. Expires after 7 days.

Fortified Cefazolin (50 mg/mL)

Add enough sterile water (without preservative) to 500 mg of cefazolin dry powder to form 10 mL of solution. This provides a strength of 50 mg/mL. Refrigerate. Expires after 7 days.

Fortified Ceftazidime (50 mg/mL)

Add 10ml of sterile water to 1 g of ceftazidime. Draw up 7.5 mL of this solution and add it to a sterile dropper bottle. Then add 7.5 mL of sterile water to the dropper bottle to produce a concentration of 50 mg/mL. Refrigerate. Expires after 7 days.

Fortified Tobramycin (or Gentamicin) (15 mg/mL)

With a syringe, inject 2 mL of tobramycin, 40 mg/mL, directly into a 5-mL bottle of tobramycin, 0.3%, ophthalmic solution. This gives a 7-mL solution of fortified tobramycin (approximately 15 mg/mL). Refrigerate. Expires after 14 days.

Fortified Vancomycin (25 mg/mL)

Add enough sterile water (without preservative) to 500 mg of vancomycin dry powder to form 10 mL of solution. This provides a strength of 50 mg/mL. To achieve a 25 mg/mL concentration, take 5 mL of 50-mg/mL solution and add 5 mL sterile water. Refrigerate. Expires after 7 days.

Fortified Voriconazole (0.5 mg/mL)

Dilute 1 mL of IV voriconazole (10 mg/mL) with 19 mL of sterile water. Filter the solution prior to topical administration.

APPENDIX 10

TECHNIQUE FOR RETROBULBAR/ SUBTENON/SUBCONJUNCTIVAL INJECTIONS

Retrobulbar Injection

1. Clean the skin of the lower lid and upper cheek around the area of the inferior orbital rim with an alcohol swab.

2. With the patient in primary gaze, use a 1.25-inch 25- or 27-gauge needle (preferably a short-beveled blunt retrobulbar needle) to penetrate the skin just superior to the inferior orbital rim in line with the lateral limbus.

3. Advance the needle parallel to the orbital floor. After passing parallel to the equator of the globe, redirect the needle superonasally into the muscle cone.

4. Lateral motions of the needle are made to ensure that the needle has not penetrated the sclera (at which point, lateral motion would be inhibited).

5. Pull back on the syringe to ensure no vascular structures have been penetrated. If no aspiration occurs, slowly inject the contents of syringe. In a successful injection, the globe may move anteriorly due to the retrobulbar pressure.

6. Withdraw the needle along the same contour as insertion. Perform orbital compression for at least 2 minutes.

Subtenon Injection

1. Apply topical anesthesia to the area to be injected (e.g., topical proparacaine or a cotton-tipped applicator soaked in proparacaine, or both, held on the area for 1 to 2 minutes). Place a drop of topical 5% povidone-iodine on the surface of the eye. If subtenon steroids are to be injected, 0.1 mL of lidocaine may be injected in the same manner as described next, several minutes before the steroids. The inferotemporal quadrant is usually the easiest location for injection.

2. With the aperture of a 25-gauge, 5/8-inch needle facing the sclera, the bulbar conjunctiva is penetrated 2 to 3 mm from the fornix, avoiding conjunctival blood vessels.

3. As the needle is inserted, lateral motions of the needle are made to ensure that the needle has not penetrated the sclera (at which point, lateral motion would be inhibited).

4. The curvature of the eyeball is followed, attempting to place the aperture of the needle near the posterior sclera.

5. When the needle has been pushed in to the hilt, the stopper of the syringe is withdrawn to ensure the needle is not intravascular.
6. The contents of the syringe are injected, and the needle is removed.

Subconjunctival Injection

1. Apply topical anesthesia and antiseptic as above.
2. Forceps are used to tent the conjunctiva, allowing the tip of a 25-gauge, 5/8-inch needle to penetrate the subconjunctival space. The needle is placed several millimeters below the limbus at the 4- or 8-o'clock position, with the aperture facing the sclera and the needle pointed inferiorly toward the fornix.
3. When the entire tip of the needle is beneath the conjunctiva, the stopper of the syringe is withdrawn to ensure the needle is not intravascular.
4. The contents of the syringe are injected, and the needle is removed.

NOTE: An eyelid speculum may be helpful in keeping the eyelids open during subtenon and subconjunctival injections.

APPENDIX 11 INTRAVITREAL TAP AND INJECT

1. Anesthetize the eye with a topical anesthetic (e.g., proparacaine) and place an eyelid speculum.Place a drop of topical 5% povidone-iodine on the surface of the eye.
2. Consider further ocular anesthesia with viscous lidocaine, a cocaine-soaked cotton-tip applicator directly on the anticipated site of needle insertion, subconjunctival, subtenon or retrobulbar lidocaine.
3. The site of needle insertion should be in the inferotemporal quadrant, 3.5 mm from the limbus in a pseudophakic eye or 4 mm in a phakic eye (Figure A.11.1).
4. Penetrate the eye with a 27-gauge needle on a 3 mL syringe. Aspirate about 0.2 mL of vitreous.

NOTE: Always aim the needle toward the optic nerve (Figure A.11.2).

5. Through the same insertion site, inject 0.2 mL of intravitreal antibiotics. See Appendix 12, *Intravitreal Antibiotics* for preparation instructions.

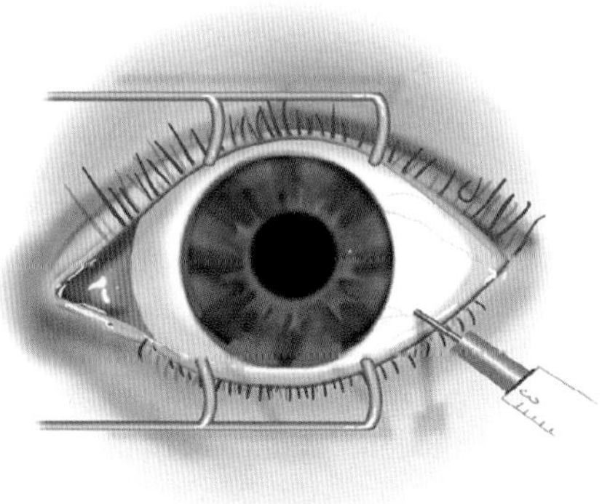

FIGURE A.11.1. Tap and inject: Anterior view of inferotemporal needle insertion.

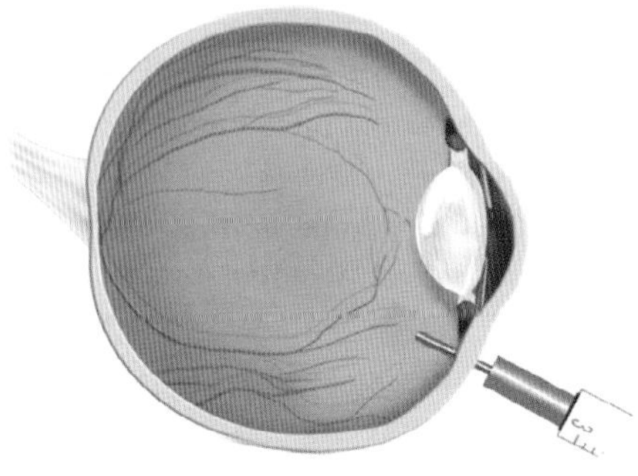

FIGURE A.11.2. Tap and inject: Horizontal view, with needle in the mid-vitreous pointing toward the optic nerve.

APPENDIX 12 — INTRAVITREAL ANTIBIOTICS

Intravitreal Cefazolin (2.25 mg/0.1 mL)

Reconstitute 500-mg vial of cefazolin with 2 mL of sterile water. Draw 1 mL of the solution into a Tb syringe and inject into an empty 30-mL vial. Add 9 mL of sterile water. Mix. Withdraw 0.2 mL of solution from the 30-mL vial into a Tb syringe. Remove the Tb syringe needle and replace with a 25-gauge needle. Expel 0.1 mL to leave 0.1 mL of 2.25 mg/0.1 mL cefazolin solution.

Intravitreal Vancomycin (1 mg/0.1 mL)

Reconstitute a 500-mg vial of vancomycin with 10 mL of sterile water. Withdraw 1 mL of the solution and inject into a sterile 10-mL vial. Add 4 mL of sterile water to the 10-mL vial. Mix. Withdraw 0.2 mL of vancomycin solution with a Tb syringe. Remove the Tb syringe needle and replace with a 25-gauge needle. Expel 0.1 mL to leave 0.1 mL of 1 mg/0.1 mL vancomycin solution.

Intravitreal Amikacin (400 mcg/0.1 mL)

Withdraw 0.8 mL (40 mg) of amikacin from a 100 mg/2 mL amikacin vial. Inject into a sterile 10 mL vial. Add 9.2 mL of nonpreserved sodium chloride and mix. Withdraw 0.3 mL into sterile Tb syringe and replace needle with a 25-gauge needle. Expel 0.2 mL to leave 0.1 mL of 400 mcg/0.1 mL amikacin solution.

Intravitreal Ceftazidime (2 mg/0.1 mL)

Add 9.4 mL of sterile water to 1 g of ceftazidime injection (in a vial). After dissolving, vent the vial. From the ceftazidime vial, transfer 2 mL to a 10 mL sterile vial. To this sterile vial, add 8 mL of sodium chloride 0.9% nonpreserved. Withdraw 0.3 mL of the solution into a Tb syringe. Change the needle to a 25 gauge and expel to 0.1 mL.

APPENDIX 13 — ANTERIOR CHAMBER PARACENTESIS

1. Place a drop of topical anesthetic (e.g., proparacaine) on the surface of the eye.

2. Retract the eyelid with an eyelid speculum.

3. Place a drop of topical 5% povidone-iodine on the surface of the eye.

4. Use an operating microscope or slit lamp (a microscope is easier).

5. In an eye with normal or elevated intraocular pressure, fixation forceps are not needed.

6. In eyes with intraocular pressure <8 mm Hg, fixation forceps may be necessary. Anesthetize the base of the lateral rectus muscle by holding a cotton-tipped applicator dipped in the topical anesthetic against the muscle for 1 minute. Grasp the base of the lateral rectus muscle with fixation forceps at the anesthetized site.

NOTE: To best provide countertraction and minimize globe rotation, the eye is fixated at the same side of needle insertion.

7. Use a 30-gauge short needle on a syringe and remove the plunger.

8. Enter the eye at an area with a sufficiently formed anterior chamber. Keep the bevel of the needle pointing anteriorly (toward the epithelium) and away from the lens. Keep the tip of the needle over the iris (not the lens) when entering the anterior chamber (Figure A.13.1).

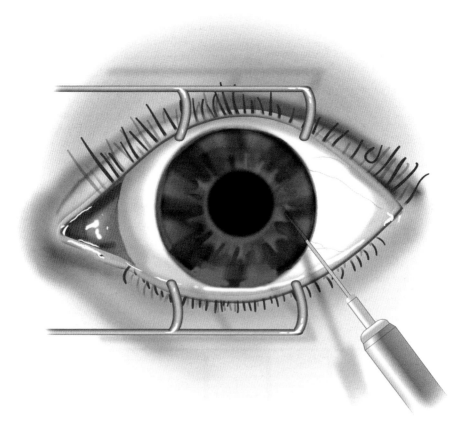

FIGURE A.13.1. Anterior chamber paracentesis.

NOTE: Make sure the plane of the needle is parallel to the plane of the iris.

NOTE: In some instances (e.g., when an aqueous specimen is necessary), it may be necessary to withdraw aqueous. This greatly increases the risk of complication and is to be avoided if possible.

9. Leave the tip of the needle in the anterior chamber for about 2 to 3 seconds. Aqueous will passively egress into the plunger-less syringe.

10. Withdraw the needle and place a drop of antibiotic on the eye (e.g., gatifloxacin or moxifloxacin) and consider antibiotics q.i.d. for 4 to 7 days.

APPENDIX 14 — ANGLE CLASSIFICATION

Proper evaluation of the configuration of the anterior chamber requires the use of at least three descriptors: the point at which the peripheral iris is adherent to the cornea or uvea, the depth of the anterior chamber, and the curvature of the peripheral iris. The Spaeth grading system of the anterior chamber angle takes into account all three of these attributes.

Spaeth Grading System (Figure A.14.1)

Iris Insertion

A = Anterior to Schwalbe line (SL)

B = Between SL and scleral spur

C = Scleral spur visible (common in blacks and Asians)

D = Deep: ciliary body visible (common in whites)

E = Extremely deep: >1 mm of ciliary body is visible

Indentation gonioscopy may be necessary to differentiate false opposition of the iris against structures in the iridocorneal angle from the true iris insertion. First, make note of the most posterior portion of the inner wall of the eye that can be seen without indenta-tion. The iris is then displaced posteriorly by indenting the cornea. This allows determina-tion of the true iris insertion. When the true iris insertion is different from the preindenta-tion appearance, the preindentation appear-ance is placed in parentheses. For example, a (B)D means that without indentation it is not possible to see any of the scleral spur or ciliary body, but with indentation the ciliary body can be seen.

Angle of Anterior Chamber

The angular width that is measured as the angle between a line parallel to the corneal endothelium at Schwalbe line and a line par-allel to the anterior surface of the iris.

Curvature of Iris

b = bowing anteriorly

p = plateau configuration

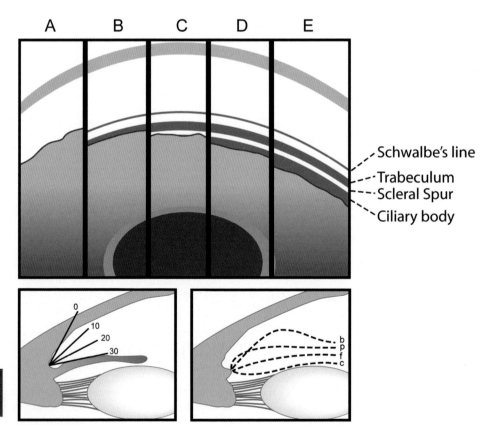

FIGURE A.14.1. Spaeth angle classification.

APP

f = flat

c = concave posterior bowing

Pigmentation of Posterior Trabecular Meshwork (PTM)

Viewing at 12 o'clock in the angle with mirror at 6 o'clock position, pigmentation graded on a scale of 0 (no PTM pigment seen) to 4 + (intense PTM pigment).

General Guidelines

1. Occludable angles would include the following:

   —Any angle narrower than 10 degrees

   —Any *p* angle configuration

2. Potentially occludable angles include

   —Any angle narrower than 20 degrees

   —Any B insertion

3. Abnormal iris insertions include:

   —Any A insertion

   —Any B insertion

   —C attachment in certain populations

4. Iris bow >1+ usually indicates pupillary block.

5. Pigmentation >2+ is usually pathologic.

Examples of Spaeth Grading System

1. C15b 2+ ptm = Open but narrow occludable angle

2. A40f = closed angle

3. (B)D30p 0ptm = open, atypical narrow angle, occludable with dilation

4. D40c 4+ ptm = open angle characteristic of patients with myopia or iris pigment dispersion syndrome.

Shaffer Classification (Figure A.14.2)

Grade 0: The angle is closed.

Grade 1: Extremely narrow angle (10 degrees). Only Schwalbe line, and perhaps also the top of the trabecula, can be visualized. Closure is probable.

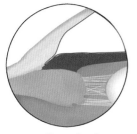

Grade 0

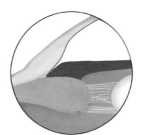

Grade 1

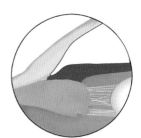

Grade 2

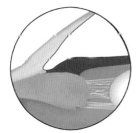

Grade 3

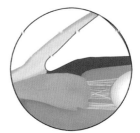

Grade 4

FIGURE A.14.2. Shaffer angle classification.

APP

Grade 2: Moderately narrow angle (20 degrees). Only the trabecular meshwork can be seen. Closure is possible.

Grade 3: Moderately open angle (20 to 35 degrees). The scleral spur can be seen. Closure is not possible.

Grade 4: Angle wide open (35 to 45 degrees). The ciliary body can be visualized with ease. Closure is not possible.

APPENDIX 15 — YAG LASER PERIPHERAL IRIDOTOMY

Also see 9.4, *Acute Angle-Closure Glaucoma.*

1. Perform pre-laser peripheral iridotomy (LPI) gonioscopy to assess baseline angle.

2. Inform the patient that they may experience ghost imaging after LPI due to the newly created iris defect. In effort to minimize this risk, note the position of the upper eyelid with respect to the superior iris. If the upper eyelid covers the superior iris, create the LPI through the superior iris. If the upper eyelid only partially covers the superior iris, there is increased risk of post-LPI ghost image due to the tear film meniscus. In such cases, consider creating the LPI at either 3- or 9-o'clock where there is no tear film meniscus.

3. Pretreat the eye with one drop each of apraclonidine 1% and pilocarpine (1% for lightly pigmented irides, 2% for darkly pigmented). As an alternative to pilocarpine, some ophthalmologists prefer to shine a bright light into the fellow eye immediately before engaging the laser. This light allows for physiologic constriction of the operative pupil.

4. Laser settings:

    —Power: 4 to 7 mJ

    —Spot Size: 10 to 70 um

    —Shots/pulse: 3

NOTE: Darker irides usually require more total power.

---

5. Anesthetize the eye (e.g., proparacaine).

6. Place an Abraham YAG iridotomy contact lens cushioned with 2.5% hydroxypropyl-methyl cellulose, positioning the magnification button above the anticipated site of iris penetration.

NOTE: Keep the lens perpendicular to the YAG beam to ensure good focus and laser concentration.

---

7. Focus the YAG beam on the predetermined iris location (see #2, above). Focus within an iris crypt if possible (Figure A.15.1).

8. Engage the laser. There will be a gush of posterior iris pigment when the iris

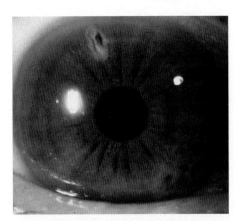

FIGURE A.15.1. Laser peripheral iridotomy.

is completely penetrated. If not penetrated, advance the YAG beam to refocus on the newly created crater. Reengage the laser until the iris is completely penetrated.

9. Administer one drop of prednisolone 1% and apraclonidine 1%.

10. Check post-LPI intraocular pressure and gonioscopy.

11. Treat inflammation with prednisolone 1% q.i.d. for 4 to 7 days. If the LPI required a significant amount of power (e.g., more than six triple shots), taper the steroids before discontinuation.

YAG CAPSULOTOMY

Typically performed for symptomatic posterior capsule opacity in pseudophakic patients (Figure A.16.1).

1. Assess the pupillary aperture prior to dilation.

2. Dilate the pupil.

3. Laser settings:

   —Power: 1 to 3 mJ

   —Shots/pulse: 1

   —Mode: fm

   —Focus: 0 to 1

NOTE: In an effort to minimize total energy, start with a lower power and titrate up as needed.
To prevent pitting the intraocular lens, displace or focus the laser beam posteriorly.

4. Anesthetize the eye (e.g., proparacaine).

5. Consider placing a YAG capsulotomy contact lens cushioned with 2.5% hydroxypropylmethyl cellulose. Some prefer to not use a contact lens.

6. Focus on the posterior lens capsule and engage the laser. A common technique is a cruciate capsulotomy.

NOTE: The capsulotomy only needs to be as big as the undilated pupil.

7. Upon completion, treat the eye with one drop each of prednisolone 1% and apraclonidine 1%.

8. Optional: treat postcapsulotomy inflammation with prednisolone 1% q.i.d. for 4 to 7 days. Inflammation after capsulotomy is usually minimal.

9. Check the intraocular pressure in 20 to 40 minutes, and in 1 week.

NOTE: Lens pitting and a rise in intraocular pressure (usually temporary) are the most common complications.

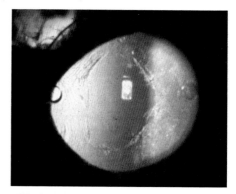

FIGURE A.16.1. YAG capsulotomy.

Ophthalmic Acronyms and Abbreviations

A

ABK	Aphakic bullous keratopathy
ABMD	Anterior basement membrane dystrophy
AC	Anterior chamber
AC/A	Accommodative convergence/accommodation angle
ACIOL	Anterior chamber intraocular lens
AFB	Acid fast bacillus
AFGE	Air-fluid gas exchange
AFX	Air-fluid exchange
AGIS	Advanced Glaucoma Intervention Study
AION	Arteritic ischemic optic neuropathy
AK	Astigmatic keratotomy
ALT	Argon laser trabeculoplasty
AMD or ARMD	Age-related macular degeneration
AMPPE	Acute multifocal placoid pigment epitheliopathy
APD or RAPD	(Relative) afferent pupillary defect
ARC	Abnormal retinal correspondence
ARMD or AMD	Age-related macular degeneration
ARN	Acute retinal necrosis
ASC	Anterior subcapsular cataract
AV	Arteriovenous
AZOOR	Acute zonal occult outer retinopathy

B

BARN	Bilateral acute retinal necrosis
BCVA	Best corrected visual acuity
BDR	Background diabetic retinopathy
BRAO	Branch retinal artery occlusion
BRVO or BVO	Branch retinal vein occlusion
BSS	Balanced salt solution
Bx	Biopsy

C

C_3F_8	Perfluoropropane
CACG	Chronic angle-closure glaucoma
CAI	Carbonic anhydrase inhibitor
CB	Ciliary body
CBC	Complete blood count
CCF	Carotid-cavernous (sinus) fistula
CCT	Central corneal thickness
C/D	Cup/disc ratio
CE	Cataract extraction
C/F	Cell/flare
CF	Count fingers
CHED	Congenital hereditary endothelial dystrophy
CHRPE	Congenital hypertrophy of the retinal pigment epithelium
CIN	Conjunctival intraepithelial neoplasia
CL	Contact lens
CLW	Contact lens wearer
CME	Cystoid macular edema
CMV	Cytomegalovirus
CN	Cranial nerve
CNV or CNVM	Choroidal neovascular membrane
COAG	Chronic open-angle glaucoma
CPA	Cerebellopontine angle
CPEO	Chronic progressive external ophthalmoplegia

CRA	Chorioretinal atrophy
CRAO	Central retinal artery occlusion
CRVO or CVO	Central retinal vein occlusion
CSCR or CSR	Central serous (chorio)retinopathy
CSM	Central, steady and maintained fixation
CSME	Clinically significant macular edema
CSNB	Congenital stationary night blindness
CVOS	Central Vein Occlusion Study
CWS	Cotton–wool spot

D

DCR	Dacryocystorhinostomy
DDT	Dye disappearance test
DD	Disc diameter(s)
DFE	Dilated fundus examination
DLK	Diffuse lamellar keratitis
DM	Diabetes mellitus
D/Q	Deep and quiet
DR	Diabetic retinopathy
DRS	Diabetic Retinopathy Study
DS(A)EK	Descemet stripping (automated) endothelial keratoplasty
DUSN	Diffuse unilateral subacute neuroretinitis
DVD	Dissociated vertical deviation

E

E	Esophoria
ECCE	Extracapsular cataract extraction
EDTA	Ethylene diamine-tetra-acetate
EKC	Epidemic keratoconjunctivitis
EL	Endolaser
EOG	Electrooculogram
EOM	Extraocular muscles or motility
ERG	Electroretinogram
ERM	Epiretinal membrane
ESR	Erythrocyte sedimentation rate
ET	Esotropia
ETDRS	Early Treatment Diabetic Retinopathy Study
EUA	Examination under anesthesia

F

FA	Fluorescein angiogram
FAZ	Foveal avascular zone
FB	Foreign body
FBS	Fasting blood sugar or foreign body sensation
FEVR	Familial exudative vitreal retinopathy
FNA	Fine needle aspiration
FTFC	Full to finger counting
FTN	Finger tension normal

G

GA	Geographic atrophy
GC	Gonococcus
GCA	Giant cell arteritis
GLT	Glaucoma Laser Trial
GPC	Giant papillary conjunctivitis

H

H	Hemorrhage
HA	Headache
HM	Hand motion
HSV	Herpes simplex virus
HT	Hypertropia
HVF	Humphrey visual field
HZV	Herpes zoster virus

I

ICCE	Intracapsular cataract extraction
ICE	Iridocorneal endothelial syndrome
ICG	Indocyanine green
IK	Interstitial keratitis
ILM	Internal limiting membrane
INO	Internuclear ophthalmoplegia
IO	Inferior oblique muscle
IOFB	Intraocular foreign body
IOL	Intraocular lens
IOOA	Inferior oblique overaction
IOP	Intraocular pressure
IR	Inferior rectus muscle
IRMA	Intraretinal microvascular abnormalities
IVFA	Intravenous fluorescein angiography

ABB

J

JOAG	Juvenile-onset open-angle glaucoma
JRA	Juvenile rheumatoid arthritis
JXG	Juvenile xanthogranuloma

K

K	Keratometry or cornea
KP	Keratic precipitates

L

LASER	Light amplification by stimulated emission of radiation
LASIK	Laser in situ keratomileusis
LASEK	Laser subepithelial keratomileusis
LL	Lower lid
LF	Levator function
LP	Light perception
LPI	Laser peripheral iridotomy
LR	Lateral rectus muscle
LTG	Low-tension glaucoma

M

MA	Microaneurysm
MCE	Microcystic corneal edema
ME	Macular edema
MEWDS	Multifocal evanescent white dot syndrome
MG	Myasthenia gravis
MGD	Meibomian gland dysfunction
MM	Malignant Melanoma
MMC	Mitomycin C
MP	Membrane peel
MPS	Macular Photocoagulation Study
MR	Medial rectus muscle
MRD	Margin to reflex distance
MS	Multiple sclerosis
MVR	Microvitreoretinal (blade)

N

Nd-YAG	Neodymium-doped yttrium-aluminum-garnet laser
NI	No improvement
NLDO	Nasolacrimal duct obstruction
NLP	No light perception
NPA	Near point of accommodation
NPC	Near point of convergence
NPDR	Nonproliferative diabetic retinopathy
NRC	Normal retinal correspondence
NS	Nuclear sclerosis
NTG	Normal tension glaucoma
NV(A, D, E, or I)	Neovascularization (angle, disc, elsewhere, or iris)
NVG	Neovascular glaucoma

O

OCP	Ocular cicatricial pemphigoid
OCT	Optical coherence tomography
OD	Oculus dexter, or right eye
OHT	Ocular hypertension
OKN	Optokinetic nystagmus
ON	Optic nerve
OS	Oculus sinister, or left eye
OU	Oculus uterque, or both eyes

P

P	Pupils
PAM	Primary acquired melanosis or potential acuity meter
PAS	Peripheral anterior synechiae
PBK	Pseudophakic bullous keratopathy
PC	Posterior chamber
PCIOL	Posterior chamber intraocular lens
PCO	Posterior capsular opacity
PD	Prism diopters or pupillary distance
PDT	Photodynamic therapy
PE	Phacoemulsification or physical examination
PED	Pigment epithelial detachment
PERRL(A)	Pupils equal, round, and reactive to light (and accommodation)
PF	Palpebral fissure

ABB

PH	Pinhole
PI	Peripheral iridectomy/ iridotomy
PK	Penetrating keratoplasty
PLE	Pen light examination
PMMA	Polymethylmethacrylate
POAG	Primary open-angle glaucoma
POHS	Presumed ocular histoplasmosis syndrome
PORT	Punctate outer retinal toxoplasmosis
PPL	Pars plana lensectomy
PPV	Pars plana vitrectomy
PRP	Panretinal photocoagulation
PRK	Photorefractive keratectomy
PSC	Posterior subcapsular cataract
PTK	Phototherapeutic keratectomy
PVD	Posterior vitreous detachment
PVR	Proliferative vitreoretinopathy
PXE	Pseudoxanthoma elasticum
PXF	Pseudoexfoliation

R

RA	Rheumatoid arthritis
RAPD or APD	Relative afferent pupillary defect
Rb	Retinoblastoma
(R)RD	(Rhegmatogenous) retinal detachment
RGP	Rigid gas permeable (contact lens)
RK	Radial keratotomy
ROP	Retinopathy of prematurity
RP	Retinitis pigmentosa
RPE	Retinal pigment epithelium

S

SAP	Spontaneous arterial pulsation
SB(P)	Scleral buckle (procedure)
SCH	Subconjunctival hemorrhage
SF$_6$	Sulfur hexafluoride

SLE	Slit-lamp examination or systemic lupus erythematosus
SLT	Selective laser trabeculoplasty
SO	Superior oblique muscle or sympathetic ophthalmia or silicone oil
SPK	Superficial punctate keratopathy or keratitis
SR	Superior rectus muscle
SRF	Subretinal fluid
SS	Scleral spur
SVP	Spontaneous venous pulsation

T

$T_{(a, p, t)}$	Tension or tonometry (applanation, palpation or pen, Tonopen)
TBUT	Tear break-up time
TM	Trabecular meshwork
TRD	Tractional retinal detachment
TTT	Transpupillary thermotherapy

U

UGH	Uveitis–glaucoma–hyphema syndrome

V

VA(cc or sc)	Visual acuity (with correction or without correction)
VER	Visually evoked response
VF	Visual field(s)
VH	Vitreous hemorrhage
VKH	Vogt–Koyanagi–Harada syndrome

X

X	Exophoria
XT	Exotropia

Y

YAG	Yttrium aluminum garnet

ABB

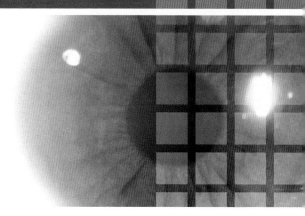

Index

Page numbers followed by *f* refer to figures; page numbers followed by *t* refer to tables.